# HANDBOOK OF STATISTICS
# IN
# CLINICAL ONCOLOGY
## THIRD EDITION

# HANDBOOK OF STATISTICS IN CLINICAL ONCOLOGY

## THIRD EDITION

Edited by

## John Crowley, PhD

*CEO, Cancer Research And Biostatistics (CRAB)*
*Seattle, Washington, USA*

## Antje Hoering, PhD

*Senior Biostatistician, Cancer Research And Biostatistics (CRAB)*
*Affiliate Assistant Professor, Department of Biostatistics, University of Washington*
*Affiliate Investigator, Fred Hutchinson Cancer Research Center*
*Seattle, Washington, USA*

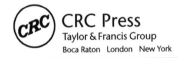

CRC Press
Taylor & Francis Group
Boca Raton  London  New York

CRC Press is an imprint of the
Taylor & Francis Group, an **informa** business

A CHAPMAN & HALL BOOK

CRC Press
Taylor & Francis Group
6000 Broken Sound Parkway NW, Suite 300
Boca Raton, FL 33487-2742

First issued in paperback 2017

© 2012 by Taylor & Francis Group, LLC
CRC Press is an imprint of Taylor & Francis Group, an Informa business

No claim to original U.S. Government works

ISBN 13: 978-1-138-19949-1 (pbk)
ISBN 13: 978-1-4398-6200-1 (hbk)

Version Date: 20120215

### Library of Congress Cataloging-in-Publication Data

Handbook of statistics in clinical oncology / editors, John Crowley, Antje Hoering. -- 3rd ed.
    p. ; cm.
    Rev. ed. of: Handbook of statistics in clinical oncology / [edited by] John Crowley, Donna Pauler Ankerst. 2006.
    Includes bibliographical references and index.
    ISBN 978-1-4398-6200-1 (hardcover : alk. paper)
    I. Crowley, John, 1946- II. Hoering, Antje.
    [DNLM: 1. Neoplasms--therapy. 2. Research Design. 3. Clinical Trials as Topic. 4. Computational Biology. 5. Data Interpretation, Statistical. 6. Translational Medical Research. QZ 20.5]

616.99'400727--dc23

2012001496

**Visit the Taylor & Francis Web site at**
**http://www.taylorandfrancis.com**

**and the CRC Press Web site at**
**http://www.crcpress.com**

*To my wife, Catherine Abram Crowley, my
patient partner of over 40 years.*

**John Crowley**

*In memory of my father, Heinz Ferdinand Felix Höring,
who died much too young of colon cancer; and to my
husband, Peter Tadych, for his love and support.*

**Antje Hoering**

# Contents

## PART I Phase I Trials

## PART II Phase II Trials

## PART III   Phase III Trials

## PART IV   *Exploratory and High-Dimensional Data Analyses*

# Preface

This third edition expands on the first and second editions as a compilation of statistical topics relevant to cancer research in general, and to oncology clinical trials and translational research in particular. Since the last edition, published in 2006, many new challenges have arisen in this area. New cancer therapies are often based on cytostatic or targeted agents, which pose new challenges in the design and analysis of all phases of oncology clinical trials. New chapters specifically addressing trial design issues pertaining to targeted agents have been added. The literature on adaptive trial designs and early stopping has been exploding, and new chapters on these topics have been added. Inclusion of high-dimensional data and imaging techniques have become common practice in oncology clinical trials, and statistical methods on how to analyze such data have been refined in this area. Many tools have become available to help statisticians design clinical trials, and a chapter has been added to review these tools and to provide a reference on where to find them. In addition, previous sections of the second edition have been revised to reflect the current state of the art. As in the first two editions, the intended audience is primarily statisticians and other researchers involved in designing and analyzing cancer clinical trials. Experts in the field have contributed individual chapters making this an invaluable reference.

This third edition is divided into four parts:

1. **Phase I Trials.** Updated recommendations regarding the standard $3 + 3$ and continual reassessment approaches along with new chapters on phase 0 trials and on phase I trial design for targeted agents are provided.
2. **Phase II Trials.** Current experience in single-arm and randomized phase II trial designs has been updated. New chapters added to this part include phase II designs with multiple strata and phase II/III designs.
3. **Phase III Trials.** Many new chapters have been added to this part, including interim analyses and early stopping considerations, phase III trial designs for targeted agents and for testing the ability of markers, adaptive trial designs, cure-rate survival models, statistical methods of imaging, as well as a thorough review of software for the design and analysis of clinical trials.
4. **Exploratory and High-Dimensional Data Analyses.** All chapters in this part have been thoroughly updated since the last edition. New chapters have been added to address methods for analyzing SNP data and for developing a score based on gene expression data. In addition, chapters on risk calculators and forensic bioinformatics have been added to this part.

# Editors

**John J. Crowley**, PhD, is president and CEO of Cancer Research And Biostatistics (CRAB), Seattle, Washington; director of the SWOG Statistical Center; and a faculty member at the Fred Hutchinson Cancer Research Center. The author or coauthor of more than 350 refereed articles, book chapters, and other publications, Dr. Crowley is a fellow of the American Statistical Association and the American Association for the Advancement of Science and a member of the International Biometrics Society, the American Society for Clinical Oncology, and the International Association for the Study of Lung Cancer. He received his BA (1968) from Pomona College, Claremont, California, and his MS (1970) and PhD (1973) in biomathematics from the University of Washington, Seattle.

**Antje Hoering**, PhD, is a senior biostatistician at Cancer Research And Biostatistics (CRAB), Seattle, Washington. She is also an affiliate faculty member in the Department of Biostatistics at the University of Washington and an affiliate investigator at the Fred Hutchinson Cancer Research Center. Dr. Hoering is the lead statistician of the SWOG Myeloma Committee, the SWOG Early Therapeutics Subcommittee, and the Stand Up To Cancer, Pancreatic Dream Team. She is the coordinating statistician for the Myeloma Institute for Research and Therapy, the International Myeloma Foundation, and the Pancreatic Cancer Research Team. She serves as a consultant on a variety of industry-sponsored studies and has been the biostatistics representative on two Type B meetings with the FDA. She is a member of the American Statistical Association, the International Biometrics Society, and the International Myeloma Society. She received her BS (1985) from the University of Tubingen, Germany, her MS (1988) in physics from Oregon State University, Corvallis, and her PhD (1991) in physics from the Max Planck Institute for Theoretical Nuclear Physics, Heidelberg, Germany. She transitioned into biostatistics with a three-year NRSA postdoctoral fellowship with the Department of Biostatistics at the University of Washington and the Fred Hutchinson Cancer Research Center.

# Contributors

**Garnet L. Anderson**
Division of Public Health Sciences
Fred Hutchinson Cancer Research
   Center
and
Department of Biostatistics
University of Washington
Seattle, Washington

**Donna Pauler Ankerst**
Department of Mathematics
Technical University of Munich
Munich, Germany

**Keith A. Baggerly**
Bioinformatics and Computational
   Biology
MD Anderson Cancer Center
The University of Texas
Houston, Texas

**Bart Barlogie**
Myeloma Institute for Research and
   Therapy
University of Arkansas for Medical
   Sciences
Little Rock, Arkansas

**William E. Barlow**
Cancer Research And Biostatistics
and
Department of Biostatistics
University of Washington
and
Fred Hutchinson Cancer Research
   Center
Seattle, Washington

**Harald Binder**
Institute of Medical Biostatistics,
   Epidemiology, and Informatics
University Medical Center Mainz
and
University of Mainz
Mainz, Germany

**Nan Chen**
Department of Biostatistics
MD Anderson Cancer Center
The University of Texas
Houston, Texas

**Mark R. Conaway**
Division of Translational Research and
   Applied Statistics
University of Virginia Health System
Charlottesville, Virginia

**Kevin R. Coombes**
Bioinformatics and Computational
   Biology
MD Anderson Cancer Center
The University of Texas
Houston, Texas

**John J. Crowley**
Cancer Research And Biostatistics
and
Fred Hutchinson Cancer Research
   Center
Seattle, Washington

**Bryan Goldman**
Southwest Oncology Group Statistical
   Center
Fred Hutchinson Cancer Research
   Center
Seattle, Washington

**Stephanie Green**
Biostatistics
Pfizer, Inc
Groton, Connecticut


**Alexander Hapfelmeier**
Institute for Medical Statistics and
    Epidemiology
Technische Universität München
Munich, Germany


**Brian P. Hobbs**
Department of Biostatistics
MD Anderson Cancer Center
The University of Texas
Houston, Texas


**Antje Hoering**
Cancer Research And Biostatistics and
    Department of Biostatistics
University of Washington
and
Fred Hutchinson Cancer Research
    Center
Seattle, Washington


**Norbert Holländer**
Novartis Oncology
Biometrics and Data Management
Novartis Pharma AG
Basel, Switzerland


**Sally Hunsberger**
National Cancer Institute
Biostatistics Research Branch
Rockville, Maryland


**Alexia Iasonos**
Memorial Sloan-Kettering Cancer
    Research Center
New York, New York

**Charles Kooperberg**
Public Health Sciences Division
Fred Hutchinson Cancer Research
    Center
and
Department of Biostatistics
University of Washington
Seattle, Washington


**Kenneth J. Kopecky**
Southwest Oncology Group Statistical
    Center
and
Fred Hutchinson Cancer Research Center
and
Department of Biostatistics
University of Washington
Seattle, Washington


**Brenda F. Kurland**
Clinical Research Division
Fred Hutchinson Cancer Research
    Center
Seattle, Washington


**Michael LeBlanc**
Southwest Oncology Group Statistical
    Center
and
Fred Hutchinson Cancer Research Center
and
Department of Biostatistics
University of Washington
Seattle, Washington


**J. Jack Lee**
Department of Biostatistics
MD Anderson Cancer Center
The University of Texas
Houston, Texas


**Yuanyuan Liang**
Department of Epidemiology and
    Biostatistics
University of Texas Health Science
    Center at San Antonio
San Antonio, Texas

**P.Y. Liu (Retired)**
Fred Hutchinson Cancer Research
    Center
Seattle, Washington

**Simon Lunagomez**
Department of Statistics
Harvard University
Cambridge, Massachusetts

**Sumithra J. Mandrekar**
Division of Biomedical Statistics and
    Informatics
Department of Health Sciences
    Research
Mayo Clinic
Rochester, Minnesota

**David A. Mankoff**
Department of Radiology
University of Washington
and
Seattle Cancer Care Alliance
Seattle, Washington

**Shigeyuki Matsui**
Department of Data Science
The Institute of Statistical Mathematics
Tokyo, Japan

**Carol M. Moinpour**
Southwest Oncology Group Statistical
    Center
and
Public Health Sciences Division
Fred Hutchinson Cancer Research
    Center
Seattle, Washington

**James Moon**
Southwest Oncology Group Statistical
    Center
and
Fred Hutchinson Cancer Research Center
Seattle, Washington

**Peter Müller**
Department of Mathematics
The University of Texas at Austin
Austin, Texas

**Hisashi Noma**
Department of Biostatistics
School of Public Health
Kyoto University
Kyoto, Japan

**John O'Quigley**
Laboratoire de Statistique Théorique et
    Appliquée
Université Paris VI
Paris, France

**Megan Othus**
Southwest Oncology Group Statistical
    Center
Fred Hutchinson Cancer Research Center
Seattle, Washington

**Gina R. Petroni**
Division of Translational Research and
    Applied Statistics
University of Virginia Health System
Charlottesville, Virginia

**Pingping Qu**
Cancer Research And Biostatistics
Seattle, Washington

**Scott D. Ramsey**
Public Health Sciences Division
Fred Hutchinson Cancer Research
    Center
Seattle, Washington

**Cathryn Rankin**
Southwest Oncology Group Statistical
    Center
and
Fred Hutchinson Cancer Research Center
Seattle, Washington

**Mary W. Redman**
Southwest Oncology Group Statistical
    Center
and
Fred Hutchinson Cancer Research Center
Seattle, Washington


**Dean A. Regier**
Canadian Centre for Applied Research
    in Cancer Control
BC Cancer Agency
Vancouver, British Columbia, Canada


**Robert Rosenberg**
Department of Radiology
University of New Mexico Health
    Sciences Center
Albuquerque, New Mexico


**Gary L. Rosner**
Division of Biostatistics &
    Bioinformatics
Sidney Kimmel Comprehensive Cancer
    Center
and
Department of Biostatistics
Johns Hopkins University
Baltimore, Maryland


**Larry Rubinstein**
Biometric Research Branch
National Cancer Institute
Bethesda, Maryland


**Daniel J. Sargent**
Division of Biomedical Statistics and
    Informatics
Department of Health Sciences
    Research
Mayo Clinic
Rochester, Minnesota


**Willi Sauerbrei**
Institute of Medical Biometry and
    Medical Informatics
University Medical Center Freiburg
Freiburg, Germany


**Martin Schumacher**
Institute of Medical Biometry and
    Medical Informatics
University Medical Center Freiburg
Freiburg, Germany


**Guido Schwarzer**
Institute of Medical Biometry and
    Medical Informatics
University Medical Center Freiburg
Freiburg, Germany


**John D. Shaughnessy Jr.**
Myeloma Institute for Research and
    Therapy
University of Arkansas for Medical
    Sciences
Little Rock, Arkansas


**Barry E. Storer**
Clinical Research Division
Fred Hutchinson Cancer Research
    Center
and
Department of Biostatistics
University of Washington
Seattle, Washington


**Catherine M. Tangen**
Southwest Oncology Group Statistical
    Center
and
Fred Hutchinson Cancer Research Center
Seattle, Washington

**Patrick A. Thompson**
Texas Children's Cancer Center
Baylor College of Medicine
Houston, Texas

**Andrea B. Troxel**
Department of Biostatistics and
    Epidemiology
Perelman School of Medicine
University of Pennsylvania
Philadelphia, Pennsylvania

**Kurt Ulm**
Institute for Medical Statistics and
    Epidemiology
Technische Universität München
Munich, Germany

**Ronghui Xu**
Department of Mathematics
and
School of Medicine
University of California, San Diego
San Diego, California


**Waheed Babatunde Yahya**
Department of Statistics
University of Ilorin
Ilorin, Nigeria

# Part I

## Phase I Trials

# 1 Choosing a Phase I Design

*Barry E. Storer*

## CONTENTS

## 1.1 INTRODUCTION AND BACKGROUND

Although the term phase I is sometimes applied generically to almost any "early" trial, in cancer drug development, it usually refers specifically to a dose finding trial whose major endpoint is toxicity. The goal is to find the highest dose of a potential therapeutic agent that has acceptable toxicity; this dose is referred to as the MTD ("maximum tolerable dose"), and is presumably the dose that will be used in subsequent phase II trials evaluating efficacy. Occasionally, one may encounter trials that are intermediate between phase I and phase II and are referred to as phase IB trials. This is a more heterogeneous group, but typically includes trials that are

3

evaluating some measure of biologic efficacy over a range of doses that have been found to have acceptable toxicity in a phase I trial. In that context, the trial determining the MTD may be referred to as a phase IA trial. This chapter will focus exclusively on phase I trials with a toxicity endpoint.

What constitutes acceptable toxicity of course depends on the potential therapeutic benefit of the drug. There is an implicit assumption with most anticancer agents that there is a positive correlation between toxicity and efficacy, but most drugs that will be evaluated in phase I trials will prove ineffective at any dose. The problem of defining an acceptably toxic dose is complicated by the fact that patient response is heterogeneous: at a given dose, some patients may experience little or no toxicity, while others may have severe or even fatal toxicity. Since the response of the patient will be unknown before the drug is given, acceptable toxicity is typically defined with respect to the frequency of toxicity in the population as a whole. For example, given a toxicity grading scheme ranging from 0 to 5 (none, mild, moderate, severe, life-threatening, fatal), one might define the MTD as the dose where, on average, one out of three patients would be expected to experience a grade 3 or worse toxicity. In that case, grade 3 or worse toxicity in an individual patient would be referred to as "dose limiting toxicity" (DLT). The definition of DLT may vary from one trial to another depending on what toxicities are expected and how manageable they are.

When defined in terms of the presence or absence of DLT, the MTD can be represented as a quantile of a dose–response curve. By notation, if $Y$ is a random variable whose possible values are 1 and 0, respectively, depending on whether a patient does or does not experience DLT, and for dose $d$ we have $\psi(d) = \Pr(Y = 1|d)$, then the MTD is defined by $\psi(d_{MTD}) = \theta$, where $\theta$ is the desired probability of toxicity. Alternately, one could define $Y$ to be the random variable representing the threshold dose at which a patient would experience DLT. The distribution of $Y$ is referred to as a tolerance distribution and the dose–response curve is the cumulative distribution function for $Y$, so that the MTD would be defined by $\Pr(Y \leq d_{MTD}) = \theta$. For a given sample size, the most effective way of estimating this quantile would be from a sample of threshold doses. Such data are nearly impossible to gather, however, as it is impractical to give each patient more than a small number of discrete doses. Further, the data obtained from sequential administration of different doses to the same patient would almost surely be biased, as one could not practicably distinguish the cumulative effects of the different doses from the acute effects of the current dose level. For this reason, almost all phase I trials involve the administration of only a single dose level to each patient and the observation of the frequency of occurrence of DLT in all patients treated at the same dose level.

There are two significant constraints on the design of a phase I trial. The first is the ethical requirement to approach the MTD from below, so that one must start at a dose level believed almost certainly to be below the MTD and gradually escalate upward. The second is the fact that the number of patients typically available for a phase I trial is relatively small, say 15–30, and is not driven traditionally by rigorous statistical considerations requiring a specified degree of precision in the estimate of MTD. The pressure to use only small numbers of patients is large—literally dozens of drugs per year may come forward for evaluation, and each combination with other drugs, each schedule, and each route of administration requires a separate trial. Furthermore, the number of patients for whom it is considered ethically justified to participate in a trial with little evidence of efficacy is limited. The latter limitation also has implications for the relevance of the MTD in subsequent phase II trials of efficacy. Since the patient populations are different, it is not clear that the MTD estimated in one population will yield the same result when implemented in another.

## 1.2 DESIGNS FOR PHASE I TRIALS

As a consequence of the previous considerations, the traditional phase I trial design utilizes a set of fixed dose levels that have been specified in advance, that is $d \in \{d_1, d_2,..., d_K\}$. The choice of the initial dose level $d_1$, and the dose spacing, are discussed in more detail hereafter. Beginning at the first dose level, small numbers of patients are entered, typically 3–6, and the decision to escalate or not depends on a prespecified algorithm related to the occurrence of DLT. When a dose level is reached with unacceptable toxicity, then the trial is stopped.

### 1.2.1 INITIAL DOSE LEVEL AND DOSE SPACING

The initial dose level is generally derived either from animal experiments, if the agent in question is completely novel, or by conservative consideration of previous human experience, if the agent in question has been used before but with a different schedule, route of administration, or with other concomitant drugs. A common starting point based on the former is from 1/10 to 1/3 of the mouse $LD_{10}$, the dose that kills 10% of mice, adjusted for the size of the animal on a per kilogram basis or by some other method.

Subsequent dose levels are determined by increasing the preceding dose level by decreasing multiples, a typical sequence being $\{d_1, d_2 = 2d_1, d_3 = 1.67d_2, d_4 = 1.4d_3,..., d_k = 1.33d_{k-1}\}$. Such sequences are often referred to as "modified Fibonacci," although in a true Fibonacci sequence the increments would be approximately 2, 1.5, 1.67, 1.60, 1.63, and then 1.62 thereafter, converging on the golden ratio. Note that after the first few increments, the dose levels are equally spaced on a log scale. With some agents, particularly biological agents, the dose levels may be determined by log spacing, that is, $\{d_1, d_2 = 10d_1,..., d_k = 10d_{k-1}\}$, or approximate half-log spacing, that is, $\{d_1, d_2 = 3d_1, d_3 = 10d_1,..., d_k = 10d_{k-2}\}$.

### 1.2.2 TRADITIONAL ESCALATION ALGORITHMS

A wide variety of dose escalation rules may be used. For purposes of illustration, we describe the following, which is often referred to as the traditional "3+3" design. Beginning at $k = 1$,

[A] Evaluate three patients at $d_k$:
    [A1]  If zero of three patients have DLT, then increase dose to $d_{k+1}$ and go to [A].
    [A2]  If one of three patients has DLT, then go to [B].
    [A3]  If ≥ two of three patients have DLT, then go to [C].

[B]  Evaluate an additional three patients at $d_k$:
    [B1]  If one of six patients has DLT, then increase dose to $d_{k+1}$ and go to [A].
    [B2]  If $\geq$ two of six patients have DLT, then go to [C].
[C]  Discontinue dose escalation.

If the trial is stopped, then the dose level below that at which excessive DLT was observed is the MTD. Some protocols may specify that if only three patients were evaluated at that dose level, then an additional three should be entered, for a total of six, and that process should proceed downward, if necessary, so that the MTD becomes the highest dose level where no more than one toxicity is observed in six patients. The actual $\theta$ that is desired is generally not defined when such algorithms are used, but implicitly $0.17 \leq \theta \leq 0.33$, so we could take $\theta \approx 0.25$.

Another example of a dose escalation algorithm, referred to as the "best-of-5" design, is described here. Again, the value of $\theta$ is not explicitly defined, but one could take $\theta \approx 0.40$. Beginning at $k=1$,

[A]  Evaluate three patients at $d_k$:
    [A1]  If zero of three patients have DLT, then increase dose to $d_{k+1}$ and go to [A].
    [A2]  If one or two of three patients have DLT, then go to [B].
    [A3]  If three of three patients have DLT, then go to [D].
[B]  Evaluate an additional patient at $d_k$:
    [B1]  If one of four patients has DLT, then increase dose to $d_{k+1}$ and go to [A].
    [B2]  If two of four patients have DLT, then go to [C].
    [B3]  If three of four patients have DLT, then go to [D].
[C]  Evaluate an additional patient at $d_k$:
    [C1]  If two of five patients have DLT, then increase dose to $d_{k+1}$ and go to [A].
    [C2]  If three of five patients have DLT, then go to [D].
[D]  Discontinue dose escalation.

Although traditional designs reflect an empirical common sense approach to the problem of estimating the MTD under the noted constraints, only brief reflection is needed to see that the determination of MTD will have a rather tenuous statistical basis. Consider the outcome of a trial employing the "3+3" design where the frequency of DLT for dose levels $d_1$, $d_2$, and $d_3$ is zero of three, one of six, and two of six, respectively. Ignoring the sequential nature of the escalation procedure, the pointwise 80% confidence intervals for the rate of DLT at the three dose levels are, respectively, 0–0.54, 0.02–0.51, and 0.09–0.67. Although the middle dose would be taken as the estimated MTD, there is not even reasonably precise evidence that the toxicity rate for *any* of the three doses is either above or below the implied $\theta$ of approximately 0.25.

Crude comparisons among traditional dose escalation algorithms can be made by examining the level-wise operating characteristics of the design, that is, the probability of escalating to the next dose level given an assumption regarding the underlying probability of DLT at the current dose level. Usually this calculation is a function of simple binomial success probabilities. For example, in the "3+3" algorithm described earlier, the probability of escalation is $\text{Bin}(0, 3; \psi(d)) + \text{Bin}(1, 3; \psi(d))$

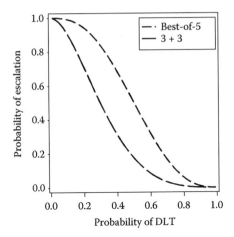

**FIGURE 1.1** Level-wise operating characteristics of two traditional dose escalation algorithms. The probability of escalating to the next higher dose level is plotted as a function of the true probability of DLT at the current dose.

Bin(1, 3;$\psi(d)$), where Bin($r$, $n$;$\psi(d)$) is the binomial probability of $r$ successes (toxicities) out of $n$ trials (patients) with underlying success probability at the current dose level $\psi(d)$. The probability of escalation can then be plotted over a range of $\psi(d)$, as is done in Figure 1.1 for the two algorithms described previously. Although it is obvious from such a display that one algorithm is considerably more aggressive than another, the level-wise operating characteristics do not provide much useful insight into whether or not a particular design will tend to select an MTD that is close to the target. More useful approaches to choosing among traditional designs and the other designs described hereafter are discussed in Section 1.3.

### 1.2.3 BAYESIAN APPROACH: THE CONTINUAL REASSESSMENT METHOD

The small sample size and low information content in the data derived from traditional methods have suggested to some the usefulness of Bayesian methods to estimate the MTD. In principle, this approach allows one to combine any prior information available regarding the value of the MTD with subsequent data collected in the phase I trial to obtain an updated estimate reflecting both.

The most clearly developed Bayesian approach to phase I design is the continual reassessment method (CRM) proposed by O'Quigley and colleagues (O'Quigley et al. 1990, O'Quigley and Chevret 1991). From among a small set of possible dose levels, say $\{d_1, \ldots, d_6\}$, experimentation begins at the dose level which the investigators believe, based on all available information, is the most likely to have an associated probability of DLT equal to the desired $\theta$. It is assumed that there is a simple family of monotone dose–response functions $\psi$ such that for any dose $d$ and probability of toxicity $p$ there exists a unique $a$ where $\psi(d, a)=p$, in particular $\psi(d_{MTD}, a_0)=\theta$. An example of such a function is $\psi(d, a)=[(\tanh d+1)/2]^a$. Note that $\psi$ is not assumed to be necessarily a dose–response function relating a characteristic of the dose levels to the probability of toxicity. That is, $d$ does not need to correspond literally to the dose of a drug. In fact, the treatments at each of the dose levels may be completely unrelated, as long as the probability of toxicity increases from each dose level to the next; in this case $d$ could be just the index of the dose levels. The uniqueness constraint implies in general the use of one-parameter models, and explicitly eliminates popular two-parameter dose–response models like the logistic. In practice, the latter have a tendency to become "stuck" and oscillate between dose levels when any data configuration leads to a large estimate for the slope parameter.

A prior distribution $g(a)$ is assumed for the parameter $a$ such that for the initial dose level, for example, $d_3$, either $\int_0^\infty \psi(d_3,a)g(a)da = \theta$ or, alternatively, $\psi(d_3, \mu_a) = \theta$, where $\mu_a = \int_0^\infty ag(a)da$. The particular prior used should also reflect the degree of uncertainly present regarding the probability of toxicity at the starting dose level; in general this will be quite vague.

After each patient is treated and the presence or absence of toxicity observed, the current distribution $g(a)$ is updated along with the estimated probabilities of toxicity at each dose level, calculated by either of the previous methods (O'Quigley et al. 1990). The next patient is then treated at the dose level minimizing some measure of the distance between the current estimate of the probability of toxicity and $\theta$. After a fixed number $n$ of patients has been entered sequentially in this fashion, the dose level selected as the MTD is the one which would be chosen for a hypothetical $n+1$ th patient.

An advantage of the CRM design is that it makes full use of all the data at hand in order to choose the next dose level. Even if the dose–response model used in updating is misspecified, CRM will tend eventually to select the dose level which has a probability of toxicity closest to $\theta$ (Shen and O'Quigley 1996), although its practical performance should be evaluated in the small sample setting typical of phase I trials. A further advantage is that, unlike traditional algorithms, the design is easily adapted to different values of $\theta$.

In spite of these advantages, some practitioners object philosophically to the Bayesian approach, and it is clear in the phase I setting that the choice of prior can have a measurable effect on the estimate of MTD (Gatsonis and Greenhouse 1992). On the other hand, the basic framework of CRM can easily be adapted to a non-Bayesian setting and can conform in practice more closely to traditional methods (O'Quigley and Shen 1996). For example, there is nothing in the approach that prohibits one from starting at the same low initial dose as would be common in traditional trials, or from updating after groups of three patients rather than single patients. In fact, the Bayesian prior can be abandoned entirely and the updating after each patient can be fully likelihood based. Without a prior, however, the dose–response model cannot be fit to the data until there is some heterogeneity in outcome, that is, at least one patient with DLT and one patient without DLT. Thus, some simple rules are needed to guide the dose escalation until heterogeneity is achieved. A number of other modifications to the CRM design have been proposed that address practical issues of implementation. These include limiting the rate of dose escalation (Goodman et al. 1995), stopping rules based on the width of the posterior probability interval (Heyd and Carlin 1999), and interpolation between doses (Piantadosi and Liu 1996).

## 1.2.4 STORER'S TWO-STAGE DESIGN

Storer (1989, 1993) has explored a combination of more traditional methods implemented in such a way as to minimize the numbers of patients treated at low dose levels and to focus sampling around the MTD; these methods also utilize an explicit dose–response framework to estimate the MTD.

The design has two stages and uses a combination of simple dose–escalation algorithms. The first stage assigns single patients at each dose level, and escalates upward until a patient has DLT, or downward until a patient does not have DLT. Algorithmically, beginning at $k = 1$,

[A] Evaluate one patient at $d_k$:
   [A1] If no patient has had DLT, then increase dose to $d_{k+1}$ and go to [A].
   [A2] If all patients have had DLT, then decrease dose to $d_{k-1}$ and go to [A].
   [A3] If at least one patient has had DLT and at least one patient has not had DLT, then if the current patient has not had DLT, go to [B], otherwise decrease the dose to $d_{k-1}$ and go to [B].

Note that the first stage meets the requirement for heterogeneity in response needed to start off a likelihood-based CRM design, and could be used for that purpose. The second stage incorporates a fixed number of cohorts of patients. If $\theta = 1/3$, then it is natural to use cohorts of size three, as follows:

[B] Evaluate three patients at $d_k$:
   [B1] If zero of three patients have DLT, then increase dose to $d_{k+1}$ and go to [B].
   [B2] If one of three patients has DLT, then go to [B].
   [B3] If $\geq$ two of three patients have DLT, then decrease dose to $d_{k-1}$ and go to [B].

After completion of the second stage a dose–response model is fit to the data and the MTD estimated by maximum likelihood or other method. For example, one could use a logistic model where $\mathrm{logit}[\psi(d)] = \alpha + \beta \log(d)$, whence the estimated MTD is determined from $\log(\hat{d}_{MTD}) = (\mathrm{logit}(\theta) - \hat{\alpha})/\hat{\beta}$. A two-parameter model is used here in order to make fullest use of the final sample of data; however, as noted earlier, two-parameter models have undesirable properties for purposes of dose escalation. In order to obtain a meaningful estimate of the MTD, one must have $0 < \hat{\beta} < \infty$. If this is not the case, then one needs either to add additional cohorts of patients or substitute a more empirical estimate, such as the last dose level or hypothetical next dose level.

As noted, the algorithm described previously is designed with a target $\theta = 1/3$ in mind. Although other quantiles could be estimated from the same estimated dose–response curve, a target $\theta$ different from 1/3 would probably lead one to use a modified second stage algorithm.

Extensive simulation experiments using this trial design in comparison to more traditional designs demonstrated the possibility of reducing the variability of point estimates of the MTD, and reducing the proportion of patients treated at very low dose levels, without markedly increasing the proportion of patients treated at dose levels where the probability of DLT is excessive. Storer (1993) also evaluated different methods of providing confidence intervals for the MTD, and found that standard likelihood-based methods that ignore the sequential sampling scheme are often markedly anticonservative; these methods included the delta method, a method based on Fieller's theorem, and a likelihood ratio method. More accurate confidence sets can be constructed by simulating the distribution of any of those test statistics at trial values of the MTD; however, the resulting confidence intervals are often extremely wide. Furthermore, the methodology is purely frequentist, and may be unable to account for minor variations in the implementation of the design when a trial is conducted.

With some practical modifications, the two-stage design described earlier has been implemented in a real phase I trial (Berlin et al. 1998). The major modifications included: (a) a provision to add additional cohorts of three patients, if necessary, until the estimate of $\beta$ in the fitted logistic model becomes positive and finite; (b) a provision that if the estimated MTD is higher than the highest dose level at which patients have actually been treated, the latter will be used as the MTD; and (c) a provision to add additional intermediate dose levels if, in the judgment of the protocol chair, the nature or frequency of toxicity at a dose level precludes further patient accrual at that dose level.

## 1.2.5 OTHER APPROACHES

### 1.2.5.1 Accelerated Titration

If the starting dose level has been chosen too conservatively, then the $3+3$ design may use large numbers of patients before reaching a dose level where the probability of toxicity is nonnegligible. Although one cannot know in advance that the starting dose level is far below the MTD, a feature of the CRM and two-stage designs described previously is that they have the potential to escalate the dose level using smaller numbers of patients than a traditional $3+3$ design. Naturally, there is a trade-off with the potential to escalate above the MTD, but the ability to escalate quickly could be an attractive feature of the design if the toxicity profile of the drug is reasonably well understood and the dose limiting toxicities are thought to be manageable even at doses above the MTD.

An example of a design that is more similar to the $3+3$ design but also permits more rapid dose escalation is the "accelerated titration" design proposed by Simon et al. (1997). This design permits dose escalation using single patient cohorts, but then reverts to the traditional $3+3$ design at a dose level where a patient experiences DLT or a second patient experiences grade 2 toxicity (or other specified level of toxicity less than a DLT). The original description of this design also allowed for intra-patient dose escalation and a final model fitting procedure using all patients at all dose levels, although this component is generally not implemented in actual trials using this design framework.

### 1.2.5.2  Another Bayesian Approach (EWOC)

Another Bayesian approach to phase I design has been described by Babb et al. (1996) and Tighiouart et al. (2005). The approach is referred to as EWOC (escalation with overdose control). The general framework is similar to that of CRM, and the MTD has the usual definition in terms of the probability of DLT; however, in contrast to CRM the MTD is related explicitly to an underlying continuous tolerance distribution. The dose for each patient is selected such that, based on all available information, the posterior probability that the dose exceeds the MTD is equal to $\alpha$. The feasibility bound $\alpha$ controls the aggressiveness of the escalation; a typical value would be $\alpha \approx 0.25$. In the usual case that there are a few fixed dose levels available for testing, additional tolerance parameters are used to select one that is closest to the optimal exact dose. Note that, unlike CRM, the dose chosen during dose escalation is not necessarily the one estimated to be closest to the MTD. After a predetermined number of patients have been evaluated, the final estimate of MTD is determined by minimizing the posterior expected loss with respect to some loss function.

### 1.2.5.3  Late Toxicity

In the majority of phase I settings dose escalation is based on the evaluation of DLT within a relatively limited period of observation, typically no more than 4–6 weeks. This is acceptable in the usual case that the toxicities of interest are expected to occur acutely; however, there may be other settings where toxicities may not be manifest immediately but may occur after chronic dosing over an extended period of time, or are simply delayed in appearance. Any of the designs mentioned earlier can be implemented in such a setting, but obviously will extend the duration of the trial if cohorts of patients must be observed for an extended period of time before dose escalation is permitted.

Relatively little attention has been paid to this design situation, the most notable exception being the TITE (time to event)—CRM design (Cheung and Chappell 1996; Braun 2006). This is a weighted version of CRM, with the weights related in some way to the amount of time that patients have been observed relative to the maximum period of time where the occurrence of DLT is of interest. For example, if $T$ is the maximum time (e.g., 6 months), and $u_i$ is the amount of time the $i$th patient has been observed, then a very simple weighting scheme might take $w_i = u_i/T$ for patients that have not experienced DLT, and $w_i = 1$ for patients that have. The Bayesian updating is performed in the usual manner, but patients who have not experienced DLT do not contribute fully until they have been observed until $T$. More complex versions of the weighting can also be devised, for example, by making some assumptions about the distribution of the time to DLT during the interval up to $T$. As with the basic CRM design, similar weighting schemes could also be applied to likelihood-based updating.

### 1.2.5.4  MTD Defined by a Continuous Parameter

Although not common in practice, it is useful to consider the case where the major outcome defining toxicity is a continuous measurement, for example, the nadir WBC. This may or may not involve a fundamentally different definition of the MTD in terms of the occurrence of DLT. For example, suppose that DLT is determined by the outcome $Y < c$, where $c$ is a constant, and we have $Y \sim \text{Normal}(\alpha + \beta d, \sigma^2)$. Then $d_{MTD} = (c - \alpha - \Phi^{-1}(\theta)\sigma)/\beta$ has the traditional definition that the probability of DLT is $\theta$. The use of such a model in studies with small sample size makes some distributional assumption imperative. Some sequential design strategies in this context have been described by Eichhorn and Zacks (1973).

Alternatively, the MTD might be defined in terms of the mean response, that is, the dose where $E(Y) = c$. For the same simple linear model, we then have that $d_{MTD} = (c - \alpha)/\beta$. An example of a two-stage design using a regression model for WBC is given in Mick and Ratain (1993). Fewer distributional assumptions are needed to estimate $d_{MTD}$, and stochastic approximation techniques might be applied in the design of trials with such an endpoint (Anbar 1984). Nevertheless, the use of a mean response to define MTD is not generalizable across drugs with different or multiple toxicities, and consequently has received little attention in practice.

## 1.3   CHOOSING A PHASE I DESIGN

As noted previously, only limited information regarding the suitability of a phase I design can be gained from the level-wise operating characteristics shown in Figure 1.1. Furthermore, for designs like CRM, which depend on data from prior dose levels to determine the next dose level, it is not even possible to specify a level-wise operating characteristic.

Useful evaluations of phase I designs must involve the entire dose–response curve, which of course is unknown. Many simple designs for which the level-wise operating characteristics can be specified can be formulated as discrete Markov chains (Storer 1989). The states in the chain refer to treatment of a patient or group of patients at a dose level, with an absorbing state corresponding to the stopping of the trial. For various assumptions about the true dose–response curve, one can then calculate exactly many quantities of interest, such as the number of patients treated at each dose level, from the appropriate quantities determined from successive powers of the transition probability matrix **P**. Such calculations are fairly tedious, however, and do not accommodate designs with nonstationary transition probabilities, such as CRM. Nor do they allow one to evaluate any quantity derived from all of the data, such as the MTD estimated after following Storer's two-stage design.

For these reasons, simulations studies are the only practical tool for evaluating phase I designs. As with exact computations, one needs to specify a range of possible dose–response scenarios, and then simulate the outcome of a large number of trials under each scenario. Here we give an example of such a study, in order to illustrate the kinds of information that can be used in the evaluation and some of the considerations involved in the design of the study. This study has also been presented in Storer (2001). Other examples of simulation studies comparing phase I designs are Korn et al. (1994) and Ahn (1998).

### 1.3.1   SPECIFYING THE DOSE–RESPONSE CURVE

We follow the modified Fibonacci spacing described in Section 1.2. For example, in arbitrary units, $\{d_1 = 100.0, d_2 = 200.0, d_3 = 333.3, d_4 = 500.0, d_5 = 700.0, d_6 = 933.3,$

$d_7 = 1244.4,...\}$. We also define hypothetical dose levels below $d_1$ that successively halve the dose above, that is, $\{d_0 = 50.0, d_{-1} = 25.0,...\}$. The starting dose is always $d_1$, and we assume that the true MTD is four dose levels higher, at $d_5$, with $\theta = 1/3$. In order to define a range of dose–response scenarios, we vary the probability of toxicity at $d_1$ from 0.01 to 0.20 in increments of 0.01, and graph our results as a function of that probability. The true dose–response curve is determined by assuming that a logistic model holds on the log scale. In the usual formulation one would have $\text{logit}[\psi(d)] = \alpha + \beta \log(d)$. In the present setup, we specify $d_1$, $\psi(d_1)$, and that $\psi(d_5) = 1/3$, whence $\beta = \text{logit}(1/3) - \text{logit}[\psi(d_1)]/\Delta$, where $\Delta = \log(d_5) - \log(d_1)$, and $\alpha = \text{logit}[\psi(d_1)] - \beta \log(d_1)$.

Varying the probability of DLT at $d_1$ while holding the probability at $d_5$ fixed at $\theta$ results in a sequence of dose–response curves ranging from relatively steep to relatively flat. An even greater range could be encompassed by also varying the number of dose levels between the starting dose and the true MTD, which of course need not be exactly at one of the predetermined dose levels. The point is to study the sensitivity of the designs to features of the underlying dose–response curve, which obviously is unknown.

### 1.3.2 SPECIFYING THE DESIGNS

This simulation will evaluate the two traditional designs described earlier, Storer's two-stage design, and a non-Bayesian CRM design. It is important to make the simulation as realistic as possible in terms of how an actual clinical protocol would be implemented, or at least to recognize what differences might exist. For example, the simulation does not place a practical limit on the highest dose level, although it is rare for any design to escalate beyond $d_{10}$.

An actual protocol might have an upper limit on the number of dose levels, with a provision for how to define the MTD if that limit is reached. Similarly, the simulation always evaluates a full cohort of patients, whereas in practice, where patients are more likely entered sequentially than simultaneously, a $3 + 3$ design might, for example, forego the last patient in a cohort of three if the first two patients had experienced DLT. Specifics of the designs used in the simulation study are given hereafter.

#### 1.3.2.1 Traditional 3 + 3 Design

This design is implemented as described in Section 1.2. In the event that excessive toxicity occurs at $d_1$, the MTD is taken to be $d_0$. Although this is an unlikely occurrence in practice, a clinical protocol should specify any provision to decrease dose if the stopping criteria are met at the first dose level.

#### 1.3.2.2 Traditional Best-of-5 Design

This design is implemented as described in Section 1.2, with the same rules applied to stopping at $d_1$.

#### 1.3.2.3 Storer's Two-Stage Design

This design is implemented as described in Section 1.2, using a second stage sample size of 24 patients. A standard logistic model is fit to the data. If it is not the case that

$0 < \hat{\beta} < \infty$, then the geometric mean of the last dose level used and the dose level that would have been assigned to the next cohort is used as the MTD. In either case, if that dose is higher than the highest dose at which patients have actually been treated, then the latter is taken as the MTD.

#### 1.3.2.4 Non-Bayesian CRM Design

We start the design using the first stage of the two-stage design as described earlier. Once heterogeneity has been achieved, 24 patients are entered in cohorts of three. The first cohort is entered at the same dose level as for the second stage of the two-stage design; after that, successive cohorts are entered using likelihood based updating of the dose–response curve. For this purpose we use a single parameter logistic model—a two parameter model with $\beta$ fixed at 0.75. This value does have to be tuned to the actual dose scale, but is not particularly sensitive to the precise value. That is, similar results would be obtained with $\beta$ in the range 0.5–1.0. For reference, on the natural log scale the distance $\log(d_{MTD}) - \log(d_1) \approx 2$, and the true value of $\beta$ in the simulation ranges from 2.01 to 0.37 as $\psi(d_1)$ ranges from 0.01 to 0.20. After each updating, the next cohort is treated at the dose level with estimated probability of DLT closest in absolute value to $\theta$; however, the next level cannot be more than one dose level higher than the current highest level at which any patients have been treated. The level that would be chosen for a hypothetical additional cohort is the MTD; however, if this dose is above the highest dose at which patients have been treated, the latter is taken as the MTD.

### 1.3.3 SIMULATION AND RESULTS

The simulation is performed by generating 5000 sequences of patients and applying each of the designs to each sequence for each of the dose–response curves being evaluated. The sequence of "patients" is really a sequence of pseudo-random numbers generated to be uniform $(0,1)$. Each patient's number is compared to the hypothetical true probability of DLT at the dose level the patient is entered at for the dose–response curve being evaluated. If the number is less than that probability, then the patient is taken to have experienced DLT.

Figure 1.2 displays results of the aforementioned simulation study which relate to the estimate $\hat{d}_{MTD}$. Since the dose scale is arbitrary, the results are presented in terms of $\psi(\hat{d}_{MTD})$. Panel (a) displays the mean probability of DLT at the estimated MTD. The horizontal line at 1/3 is a point of reference for the target $\theta$. Although none of the designs is unbiased, all except the conservative 3+3 design perform fairly well across the range of dose–response curves. The precision of the estimates, taken as the root MSE of the probabilities $\psi(\hat{d}_{MTD})$, is shown in panel (b). In this regard the CRM and two-stage designs perform better than the best-of-5 design over most settings of the dose–response curve. One should also note that, in absolute terms, the precision of the estimates is not high even for the best designs.

In addition to the average properties of the estimates, it is also relevant to look at the extremes. Panels (c) and (d) present the fraction of trials where $\psi(\hat{d}_{MTD}) < 0.20$ or $\psi(\hat{d}_{MTD}) > 0.50$, respectively. The seesaw pattern observed for all but the two-stage design is caused by changes in the underlying dose–response curve, as the

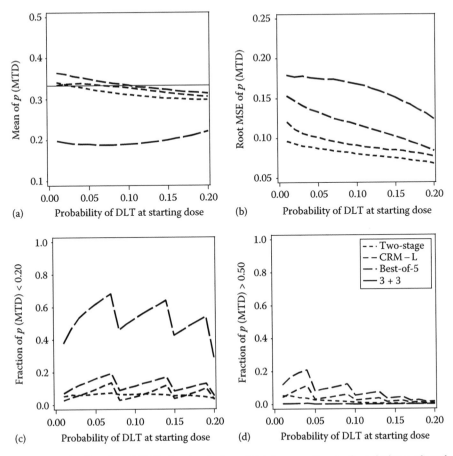

**FIGURE 1.2**   Results of 5000 simulated phase I trials according to four designs, plotted as a function of the probability of DLT at the starting dose level. The true MTD is fixed at four dose levels above the starting dose, with $\theta = 1/3$. Results are expressed in terms of $p_{MTD} = \psi(\hat{d}_{MTD})$.

probability of DLT at particular dose levels moves over or under the limit under consideration. Since the three designs select discrete dose levels as $\hat{d}_{MTD}$, this will result in a corresponding decrease in the fraction of estimates beyond the limit. The cutoff of 0.20 is the level at which the odds of DLT are half that of $\theta$. Although this may not be an important consideration, to the extent that the target $\theta$ defines a dose with some efficacy in addition to toxicity, the fraction of trials below this arbitrary limit may represent cases in which the dose selected for subsequent evaluation in efficacy trials is "too low." Because of their common first stage design that uses single patients at the initial dose levels, the two-stage and CRM designs do best in this regard. Conversely, the cutoff used in panel (d) is the level at which the odds of toxicity are twice that of $\theta$. Although the occurrence of DLT in and of itself is not necessarily undesirable, as the probability of DLT increases there is likely a corresponding increase in the probability of very severe or even fatal toxicity. Hence, the

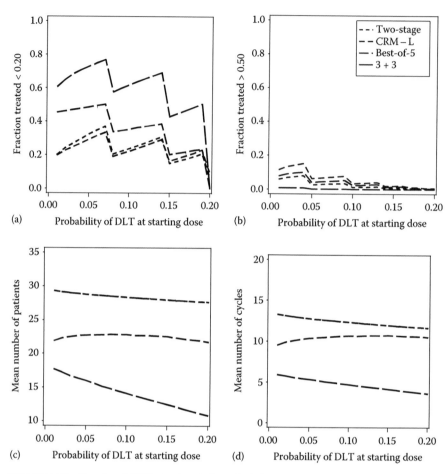

**FIGURE 1.3** Results of 5000 simulated phase I trials according to four designs, plotted as a function of the probability of DLT at the starting dose level. The true MTD is fixed at four dose levels above the starting dose, with $\theta = 1/3$.

trials where the probability of DLT is above this arbitrary level may represent cases in which the dose selected as the MTD is "too high." In this case there are not large differences among the designs, and in particular we find that the two designs that perform the best in panel (c) do not carry an unduly large penalty. One could easily evaluate other limits if desired.

Some results related to the outcome of the trials themselves are presented in Figure 1.3. Panels (a) and (b) present the overall fraction of patients that are treated below and above, respectively, the same limits as for the estimates in Figure 1.2. The two-stage and CRM designs perform best at avoiding treating patients at the lower dose levels; the two-stage design is somewhat better than the CRM design at avoiding treating patients at higher dose levels, although of course it does not do as well as the very conservative 3+3 design.

Sample size considerations are evaluated in panels (c) and (d). Panel (c) shows the mean number of patients treated. Because they share a common first stage and use the same fixed number of patients in the second stage, the two-stage and CRM designs yield identical results. The $3+3$ design uses the smallest number of patients, but this is because it tends to stop well below the target. On average, the best-of-5 design uses six to eight fewer patients than the two-stage or CRM design. Panel (d) displays the mean number of "cycles" of treatment that are needed to complete the trial, where a cycle is the period of time over which a patient or group of patients needs to be treated and evaluated before a decision can be made as to the dose level for the next patient or group. For example, the second stage in the two-stage or CRM designs always uses eight cycles; each dose level in the $3+3$ design uses one or two cycles, etc. This is a consideration only for situations where the time needed to complete a phase I trial is not limited by the rate of patient accrual but by the time needed to treat and evaluate each group of patients. In this case the results are qualitatively similar to that of panel (e).

## 1.4   SUMMARY AND CONCLUSION

Based only on the previous results, one would likely eliminate the $3+3$ design from consideration. The best-of-5 design would probably also be eliminated as well, owing to the lower precision and greater likelihood that the MTD will be well below the target. On the other hand, the best-of-5 design uses fewer patients. If small patient numbers are a priority, it would be reasonable to consider an additional simulation in which the second stage sample size for the two-stage and CRM designs is reduced to, say, 18 patients. This would put the average sample size for those designs closer to that of the best-of-5, and one could see whether they continued to maintain an advantage in the other aspects. Between the two-stage and CRM designs, there is perhaps a slight advantage to the former in terms of greater precision and a smaller chance that the estimate will be too far above the target; however, the difference is likely not important in practical terms and might vary under other dose–response conditions. The advantage of the two-stage design may seem surprising, given that the next dose level is selected only on the basis of the outcome at the current dose level, and ignores the information that CRM uses from all prior patients. However, the two-stage design also incorporates a final estimation procedure for the MTD that utilizes all the data, and uses a richer family of dose–response models. This issue is examined in Storer (2001).

A desirable feature of the results shown is that both the relative and absolute properties of the designs do not differ much over the range of dose–response curves. Additional simulations could be carried out which would vary also the distance between the starting dose and the true MTD, or place the true MTD between dose levels instead of exactly at a dose level.

To illustrate further some of the features of phase I designs, and the necessity of studying each situation on a case by case basis, we repeated the simulation study using a target $\theta = 0.20$. Exactly the same dose–response settings are used, so that the results for the two traditional designs are identical to those shown previously. The two-stage design is modified to use five cohorts of five patients, but follows

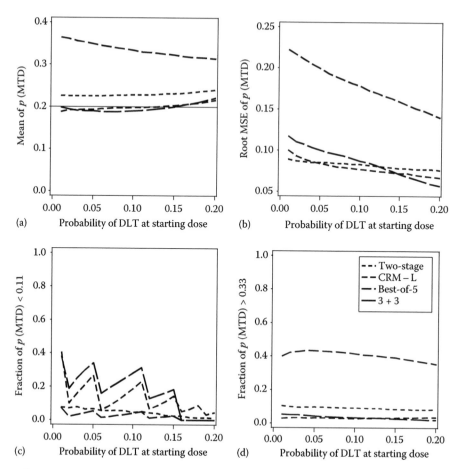

**FIGURE 1.4** Results of 5000 simulated phase I trials according to four designs, plotted as a function of the probability of DLT at the starting dose level. The dose–response curves are identical to those used for Figure 1.2, but with $\theta = 0.20$. Results are expressed in terms of $p_{MTD} = \psi(\hat{d}_{MTD})$.

essentially the same rule for selecting the next level described earlier with "3" replaced by "5". Additionally, the final fitted model estimates the MTD associated with the new target; and of course the CRM design selects the next dose level based on the new target.

The results for this simulation are presented in Figures 1.4 and 1.5. In this case the best-of-5 design is clearly eliminated as too aggressive. However, and perhaps surprisingly, the 3+3 design performs nearly as well, or better, than the supposedly more sophisticated two-stage and CRM designs. There is a slight disadvantage in terms of precision, but given that the mean sample size with the 3+3 design is nearly half that of the other two, this may be a reasonable trade-off. Of course, it could also be the case in this setting that using a smaller second stage sample size would not adversely affect the two-stage and CRM designs.

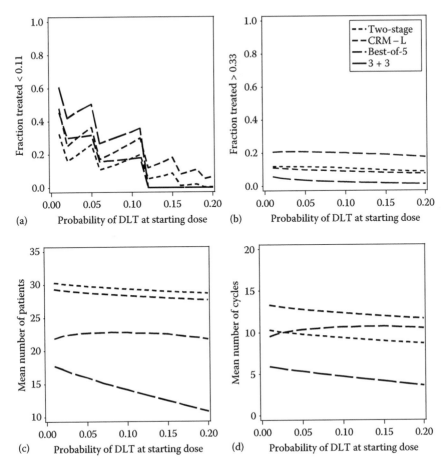

**FIGURE 1.5**  Results of 5000 simulated phase I trials according to four designs, plotted as a function of the probability of DLT at the starting dose level. The dose–response curves are identical to those used for Figure 1.3, but with $\theta = 0.20$.

Finally, we reiterate the point that the purpose of this simulation was to demonstrate some of the properties of phase I designs and of the process of simulation itself, not to advocate any particular design. Depending on the particulars of the trial at hand, any one of the four designs might be a reasonable choice. An important point to bear in mind is that traditional designs must be matched to the desired target quantile, and will perform poorly for other quantiles. CRM designs are particularly flexible in this regard; the two-stage design can be modified to a lesser extent.

## REFERENCES

Ahn, C. 1998. An evaluation of phase I cancer clinical trial designs. *Statistics in Medicine* 17: 1537–1549.

Anbar, D. 1984. Stochastic approximation methods and their use in bioassay and phase I clinical trials. *Communications in Statistics—Theory and Methods* 13: 2451–2467.

Babb, J., Rogatko, A., and Zacks, S. 1996. Cancer phase I clinical trials: Efficient dose escalation with overdose control. *Statistics in Medicine* 17: 1103–1120.

Berlin, J., Stewart, J.A., Storer, B., Tutsch, K.D., Arzoomanian, R.Z., Alberti, D., Feierabend, C., Simon, K., and Wilding, G. 1998. Phase I clinical and pharmacokinetic trial of penclomedine utilizing a novel, two-stage trial design. *Journal of Clinical Oncology* 16: 1142–1149.

Braun, T.M. 2006. Generalizing the TITE-CRM to adapt for early- and late-onset toxicities. *Statistics in Medicine* 25: 2071–2083.

Cheung, Y.K. and Chappell, R. 2000. Sequential designs for phase I clinical trials with late-onset toxicities. *Biometrics* 56: 1177–1182.

Eichhorn, B.H. and Zacks, S. 1973. Sequential search of an optimal dosage. *Journal of the American Statistical Association* 68: 594–598.

Gatsonis, C. and Greenhouse, J.B. 1992. Bayesian methods for phase I clinical trials. *Statistics in Medicine* 11: 1377–1389.

Goodman, S.N., Zahurak, M.L., and Piantadosi, S. 1995. Some practical improvements in the continual reassessment method for phase I studies. *Statistics in Medicine* 14: 1149–1161.

Heyd, J.M. and Carlin, B.P. 1999. Adaptive design improvements in the continual reassessment method for phase I studies. *Statistics in Medicine* 18: 1307–1321.

Korn, E.L., Midthure, D., Chen, T.T., Rubinstein, L.V., Christian, M.C., and Simon, R. 1994. A comparison of two phase I trial designs. *Statistics in Medicine* 13: 1799–1806.

Mick, R. and Ratain, M.J. 1993. Model-guided determination of maximum tolerated dose in phase I clinical trials: Evidence for increased precision. *Journal of the National Cancer Institute* 85: 217–223.

O'Quigley, J. and Chevret, S. 1991. Methods for dose finding studies in cancer clinical trials: A review and results of a Monte Carlo study. *Statistics in Medicine* 10: 1647–1664.

O'Quigley, J., Pepe, M., and Fisher, L. 1990. Continual reassessment method: A practical design for phase I clinical studies in cancer. *Biometrics* 46: 33–48.

O'Quigley, J. and Shen, L.Z. 1996. Continual reassessment method: A likelihood approach. *Biometrics* 52: 673–684.

Piantadosi, S. and Liu, G. 1996. Improved designs for dose escalation studies using pharmacokinetic measurements. *Statistics in Medicine* 15: 1142–1149.

Shen, L.Z. and O'Quigley, J. 1996. Consistency of continual reassessment method under model misspecification. *Biometrika* 83: 395–405.

Simon, R., Freidlin, B., Rubinstein, L., Arbuck, S.G., Collins, J., and Christian, M.C. 1997. Accelerated titration designs for phase I clinical trials in oncology. *Journal of the National Cancer Institute* 89: 1138–1147.

Storer, B. 1989. Design and analysis of phase I clinical trials. *Biometrics* 45: 925–937.

Storer, B. 1993. Small-sample confidence sets for the MTD in a phase I clinical trial. *Biometrics* 49: 1117–1125.

Storer, B. 2001. An evaluation of phase I designs for continuous dose response. *Statistics in Medicine* 20: 2399–2408.

Tighiouart, M., Rogatko, A., and Babb, J.S. 2005. Flexible Bayesian methods for cancer phase I clinical trials: Dose escalation with overdose control. *Statistics in Medicine* 24: 2183–2196.

# 2 Dose-Finding Designs Based on the Continual Reassessment Method

*John O'Quigley and Alexia Iasonos*

## CONTENTS

## 2.1 OVERVIEW

This review describes the basic ideas behind the continual reassessment method (CRM), as it is used in Phase I and Phase I/II dose finding. We recall some important technical considerations, some key properties of the method, and the possibility for substantial generalization, specifically, the use of graded information on toxicities, the incorporation of a stopping rule leading to potential reductions in sample size, the incorporation of information on patient heterogeneity, the incorporation of pharmacokinetics, and the possibility of modeling in the presence of drug combinations. In its most classical setting the CRM is used to identify the maximum tolerated dose (MTD) where only information on toxicities is used. For Phase I/II designs, in which information on efficacy can be obtained within a comparable time frame as that on toxicity, we can use the CRM structure, together with the sequential probability ratio test, to construct very effective designs to locate the dose producing the greatest rate of success. We consider more involved CRM designs, for example, designs that account for low-grade toxicities, pharmacokinetic endpoints, patient heterogeneity, partial ordering in drug combinations and model averaging techniques. The theory that backs up this extra complexity comes under the umbrella of Bayesian model choice.

## 2.2 GOALS AND OPERATING CHARACTERISTICS

We describe here the clinical goals for these studies and the method's operating characteristics. Essentially, the clinical goals correspond to the basic properties we would wish a suitable method to possess. The operating characteristics describe what we actually have, that is, how the method will behave in practice.

### 2.2.1 CLINICAL GOALS

Storer (1989) made explicit the goal of a Phase I dose finding study in chronic illness such as cancer, as being the identification of some dose corresponding to an acceptable rate of undesirable side effects, usually called toxicities. This would be the context for cytotoxic drugs in which we might view toxicity as a surrogate for longer-term efficacy. For Phase I/II studies we observe in a similar time frame both toxicity and some measure of effect. For these studies the goal is usually to maximize the overall success rate. O'Quigley et al. (1990) argued that, for a Phase I study, in addition to the goal of targeting some percentile, an acceptable design should aim to incorporate the following restrictions:

1. We should minimize the number of under-treated patients, that is, patients treated at unacceptably low dose levels.
2. We should minimize the number of patients treated at unacceptably high dose levels.
3. We should minimize the number of patients needed to complete the study (efficiency).

4. The method should respond quickly to inevitable errors in initial guesses, rapidly escalating in the absence of indication of drug activity (toxicity) and rapidly de-escalating in the presence of unacceptably high levels of observed toxicity.

Before describing just how the CRM meets the aforementioned requirements we will first look at the requirements themselves in the context of Phase I cancer dose finding studies.

Most Phase I cancer clinical trials are carried out on patients for whom all currently available therapies have failed. There will always be hope in the therapeutic potential of the new experimental treatment but such hope will often be tempered by the almost inevitable life-threatening toxicity accompanying the treatment. Given that candidates for these trials have no other options concerning treatment, their inclusion appears contingent upon maintaining some acceptable degree of control over the toxic side effects as well as trying to maximize treatment efficacy, which in the absence of information on efficacy itself translates as dose. Too high a dose, while offering in general better hope for treatment effect, will be accompanied by too high a probability of encountering unacceptable toxicity. Too low a dose, while avoiding this risk, may offer too little chance of seeing any benefit at all.

Given this context, the first two of the earlier numbered requirements appear immediate. The third requirement, a concern for all types of clinical studies, becomes of paramount importance here where very small sample sizes are inevitable. This is because of the understandable desire to proceed quickly with a potentially promising treatment to the Phase II stage. At the Phase II stage the probability of observing treatment efficacy is almost certainly higher than that for the Phase I population of patients. We have to do the very best we can with the relatively few patients available and the statistician involved in such studies should also provide some idea as to the error of our estimates, translating the uncertainty of our final recommendations based on such small samples. The fourth requirement is not an independent requirement and can be viewed as a partial reexpression of requirements 1 and 2, taking timeliness also into account.

Taken together, the requirements point toward a method where we converge quickly to the correct level, the correct level being defined as the one having a probability of toxicity as close as possible to some prespecified value $\theta$. The value is chosen by the investigator such that he or she considers probabilities of toxicity higher than $\theta$ (to be unacceptably high), while those lower than $\theta$ unacceptably low in that they indicate, indirectly, the likelihood of too weak an antitumor effect.

Figure 2.1 illustrates the comparative behavior of CRM with a fixed sample up and down design (Storer 1989) in which level 7 is the correct level. How does CRM work? The essential idea is similar to that of stochastic approximation, the main differences being the use of a nonlinear under-parameterized model, belonging to a particular class of models, and a small number of discrete dose levels rather than a continuum. Patients enter sequentially. The working dose–toxicity curve, taken from the CRM class (described hereafter), is refitted after observing each patient's outcome. The curve is then inverted to identify which of the available levels has an

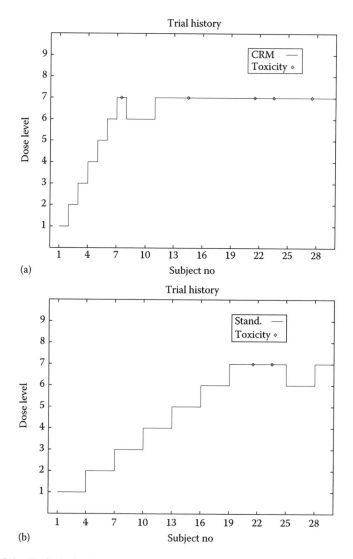

**FIGURE 2.1** Typical trial histories; CRM (a), standard design (b).

associated estimated probability as close as we can get to the targeted acceptable toxicity level. The next patient is then treated at this level. The cycle is continued until a fixed number of subjects have been treated or until we apply some stopping rule (see Section 2.4.1). Typical behavior is that shown in Figure 2.1.

## 2.2.2 Operating Characteristics

A large sample study (Shen and O'Quigley 1996) showed that, under certain conditions, the level to which a CRM design converges will indeed be the level with respective estimated toxicity probability closest to the target. As pointed out by Storer

(1998) large sample properties themselves will not be wholly convincing since, in practice, we are inevitably faced with small to moderate sample sizes. Nonetheless, if any scheme fails to meet such basic statistical criteria as large sample convergence, we need to investigate with great care its finite sample properties. The tool to use here is mostly that of simulation although for the standard up and down schemes, the theory of Markov chains enables us to carry out exact probabilistic calculations (Storer 1993, Reiner et al. 1998).

Whether Bayesian or likelihood based, once the scheme is under way, then it is readily shown that a nontoxicity always points in the direction of higher levels and a toxicity in the direction of lower levels, the absolute value of the change diminishing with the number of included patients. For the case of non-monotone likelihood it is impossible to be at some level, observe a toxicity and then for the model to recommend a higher level as claimed by some authors, unless pushed in such a direction by a strong prior. Furthermore, when targeting lower percentiles such as 0.2, it can be calculated, and follows our intuition, that a toxicity, occurring with a frequency, a factor of 4 less than that for the nontoxicities, will have a much greater impact on the likelihood or posterior density. This translates directly into an operating characteristic whereby model-based escalation is relatively cautious and de-escalation more rapid, particularly early on where little information is available. In the model and examples of O'Quigley et al. (1990) dose levels could never be skipped when escalating. However, if the first patient, treated at level 3, suffered a toxic side effect, the method skipped when de-escalating, recommending level 1 for the subsequent two entered patients before, assuming no further toxicities were seen, escalating to level 2.

Simulations in O'Quigley et al. (1990), O'Quigley and Chevret (1991, 1993), Goodman et al. (1995), Korn et al. (1994), and O'Quigley (2006) show the operating characteristics of CRM to be good, in terms of accuracy of final recommendation while simultaneously minimizing the numbers of overtreated and undertreated patients. As long as strong priors are not used in the Bayesian framework, and the model requirements are not violated, the method behaves very well (Cheung and Chappell 2002).

### 2.2.3 SAFETY

Safety is a concern for all clinical trials. Concern for safety in Phase I trials has been expressed because these are the first inhuman trials and the dose–toxicity profile obtained from preclinical studies may no longer be valid in the clinical context. Some investigators have expressed a worry that CRM may tend to treat the early included patients in a study at high dose levels. This can be seen to not be the case but the concern alone convinced many investigators that without some modification CRM was not "safe" to use routinely. Safety is in fact a statistical property of any method. When faced with some potential realities or classes of realities, we can ask ourselves questions such as: what is the probability of toxicity for a randomly chosen patient that has been included in the study or, say, what is the probability of toxicity for those patients entered into the study at the very beginning.

Once we know the realities or classes of realities we are facing, the operating rules of the method—obvious and transparent for up and down schemes and less transparent for model based schemes such as CRM—then, in principle, we can calculate the probability of toxicity for a randomly chosen patient or for those patients entered into the study at the very beginning. Theoretical work as well as extensive simulations (O'Quigley et al. 1990, O'Quigley and Chevret 1991, O'Quigley and Shen 1996, Ahn 1998, Reiner et al. 1998, O'Quigley 1999) indicates CRM to be a safer design than any of the commonly used up and down schemes, in that, for targets of less than ($\theta = 0.30$, the probability that a randomly chosen patient suffers a toxicity is lower. In practice, these calculations are involved and we may simply prefer to estimate them to any desired degree of accuracy via simulation.

Were the definition of safety to be widened to include the concept of treating patients at unacceptably low levels where the probability of toxicity is deemed too close to zero, then CRM does very much better than the standard designs. This finding is logical given that the purpose of CRM is to concentrate as much experimentation as possible around the prespecified target. In addition, it ought be emphasized that we can adjust the CRM to make it as safe as we require by changing the target level. For instance, were we to decrease the target from 0.20 to 0.10, the observed number of toxicities will, on average, be reduced and, in many cases, halved. This is an important point since it highlights the main advantages of the CRM over the standard designs in terms of flexibility and the ability to be adapted to potentially different situations. An alternative way to enhance conservatism is, rather than choose the closest available dose to the target, systematically take the dose immediately lower than the target or change the distance measure used to select the next level to recommend. This idea has been studied by Babb et al. (1998) who introduced criteria that control overdosing. The issue of safety has been further addressed by modified CRM designs that start at the lowest dose level, and do not allow skipping levels. Simulation studies have shown that the impact of such modifications on the reliability of final estimation is negligible (Garrett-Mayer 2006, Iasonos et al. 2008). In addition, in the Bayesian setting, we are at liberty to assign heavier priors to lower dose levels if those levels should be preferred.

## 2.3   TECHNICAL ASPECTS

The aim of CRM is to locate the most appropriate dose, the so-called target dose, the precise definition of which is provided as follows. This dose is taken from some given range of available doses. Dose spacing for single drug combinations is often addressed via a modified Fibonacci design, preclinical or earlier clinical studies. For the purposes of CRM we do not generally address the issue of dose spacing and we assume that we have available $K$ preselected fixed doses; $d_1, ..., d_k$. The need to add doses may arise in practice when the toxicity frequency is deemed too low at one level but the next highest level is considered too toxic. CRM can help with this affirmation but as far as extrapolation or interpolation of dose is concerned, the relevant insights will come from pharmacokinetics. These doses are not necessarily ordered directly in terms of the $d_i$ themselves, in particular, since each $d_i$ may be a vector, being a combination of different treatments, but rather in terms of the probability $R(d_i)$ of encountering toxicity at each dose $d_i$. We take monotonicity to mean that the dose levels, equally well identified by their integer subscripts $i$ ($i = 1, ..., k$), are ordered whereby the probability of toxicity at level $i$ is greater than that at level $i'$ (whenever $i > i'$). The monotonicity requirement or the assumption that we can so order our available dose levels in terms of toxicity is thus important. Currently all the dose information required to run a CRM trial is contained in the dose levels. Without wishing to preclude the possibility of exploiting information contained in the doses $d_i$ and not in the dose levels $i$, at present we lose no information when we replace $d_i$ by $i$.

The actual amount of drug therefore, so many mg/m$^2$ say, is typically not used. For a single agent trial it is in principle possible to work with the actual dose (see Piantadosi et al. 1998). This requires care, in particular, if working with Bayesian priors, and, generally, we advise working with conceptual dose levels. For multidrug or treatment combination studies there is no obvious univariate measure. We work instead with some conceptual dose, increasing when one of the constituent ingredients increases, and under our monotonicity assumption, translating itself as an increase in the probability of a toxic reaction. Choosing the dose levels amounts to selecting levels (treatment combinations) such that the lowest level hopefully has an associated toxic probability less than the target and the highest level possibly close or higher than the target.

The most appropriate dose, the "target" dose, is that dose having an associated probability of toxicity as close as we can get to the target "acceptable" toxicity $\theta$. Values for the target toxicity level, $\theta$, might typically be 0.2, 0.25, 0.3, 0.35, although there are studies in which this can be as high as 0.4 (Moller 1995). The value depends on the context and the nature of the toxic side effects.

The dose for the $j$th entered patient $X_j$ can be viewed as random taking values $x_j$, most often discrete in which case $x_j \in \{d_1, \ldots, d_k\}$ but possibly continuous where $X_j = x$; $x \in \mathcal{R}^+$. In light of the remarks of the previous two paragraphs we can, if desired, entirely suppress the notion of dose and retain only information pertaining to dose level. This is all we need and we may prefer to write $x_j \in \{1, \ldots, k\}$. Let $Y_j$ be a binary random variable $(0,1)$ where 1 denotes severe toxic response for the $j$th entered patient $(j = 1, \ldots, n)$. We model $R(x_j)$, the true probability of toxic response at $X_j = x_j$; $x_j \in \{d_1, \ldots, d_k\}$ or $x_j \in \{1, \ldots, k\}$ via

$$R(x_j) = \Pr(Y_j = 1 | X_j = x_j) = E(Y_j | x_j) = \psi(x_j, a)$$

for some one-parameter model $\psi(x_j, a)$.

For the most common case of a single homogeneous group of patients we are obliged to work with an under-parameterized model, notably a one-parameter model. Although a two-parameter model may appear more flexible, the sequential nature of CRM together with its aim to put the included patients at a single correct level means that we will not obtain information needed to fit two parameters. We are close to something like non-identifiability. A likelihood procedure will be unstable and may even break down, whereas a two-parameter fully Bayesian approach (O'Quigley et al. 1990, Gatsonis and Greenhouse 1992, Whitehead and Williamson 1998) may work initially, by virtue of the cohesion and structure created by the prior, but may become less stable as the sample size increases (Shu and O'Quigley 2008). The goal of CRM in not to fit an overall model to the full range of data, but is rather to identify some target percentile from the dose–toxicity curve.

### 2.3.1 MODEL REQUIREMENTS

The restrictions on $\psi(x,a)$ were described by O'Quigley et al. (1990). For given fixed $x$ we require that $\psi(x,a)$ be strictly monotonic in $a$. For fixed $a$ we require that $\psi(x,a)$ be monotonic increasing in $x$ or, in the usual case of discrete dose levels $d_i$, $i=1,\ldots,k$, that $\psi(d_i,a) > \psi(d_m,a)$ whenever $i > m$. The true probability of toxicity at whatever treatment combination has been coded by $x$, is given by $R(x)$ and we require that, for the specific doses under study $(d_1,\ldots,d_k)$ there exists values of $a$, say $a_1,\ldots,a_k$ such that $\psi(d_i,a_i) = R(d_i),(i=1,\ldots,k)$. In other words, our one-parameter model has to be rich enough to model the true probability of toxicity at any given level. We call this a working model since we do not anticipate a single value of $a$ to work precisely at every level, that is, we do not anticipate $a_1 = a_2 = \cdots = a_k = a$. Many choices are possible. We have obtained excellent results with the simple choice:

$$\psi(d_i, a) = \alpha_i^a, \quad (i=1,\ldots,k) \tag{2.1}$$

where $0 < \alpha_1 < \cdots \alpha_k < 1$ and $0 < a < \infty$. For the six levels studied in the simulations by O'Quigley et al. (1990) the working model had $\alpha_1 = 0.05$, $\alpha_2 = 0.10$, $\alpha_3 = 0.20$, $\alpha_4 = 0.30$, $\alpha_5 = 0.50$, and $\alpha_6 = 0.70$. In that paper this was expressed a little differently in terms of conceptual dose $d_i$ where $d_1 = -1.47$, $d_2 = -1.10$, $d_3 = -0.69$, $d_4 = -0.42$, $d_5 = 0.0$, and $d_6 = 0.42$ obtained from a model in which

$$\alpha_i = \frac{(\tanh d_i + 1)}{2} \quad i=1,\ldots,k \tag{2.2}$$

The preceding "tanh" model was first introduced in this context by O'Quigley et al. (1990), the idea being that $\tanh(x)$ increases monotonically from 0 to 1 as $x$ increases from $-\infty$ to $\infty$. This extra generality is not usually needed since attention is focused on the few fixed $d_i$. Note that, at least as far as maximum likelihood estimation is concerned (see Section 2.3.2), working with model (1) is equivalent to working with a model in which $\alpha_i$, $i=1,\ldots,k$ is replaced by $\alpha_i^*(i=1,\ldots,k)$ where $\alpha_i^* = \alpha_i^m$ for any real $m > 0$. Thus, we cannot really attach any concrete meaning to the $\alpha_i$. The spacing, however, between adjacent $\alpha_i$ will impact operating characteristics. Working with real doses corresponds to using some fixed dose spacing, although not necessarily one with nice properties. The spacings chosen here have proved satisfactory in terms of performance across a broad range of situations. An investigation into how to choose the $\alpha_i$ with the specific aim of improving certain aspects of performance has been carried out by Lee and Cheung (2009).

Some obvious choices for a model can fail the previous conditions leading to potentially poor operating characteristics. The one-parameter logistic model, $\psi(x,a) = w/(1+w)$, in which $b$ is fixed and where $w = \exp(b+ax)$ can be seen to fail the previous requirements (Shen and O'Quigley 1996). On the other hand the less intuitive model obtained by $w$ so that $w = \exp(a+bx)$, $b \neq 0$, belongs to the CRM class.

### 2.3.2  MAXIMUM LIKELIHOOD ESTIMATION

Once a model has been chosen and we have data in the form of the set $\Omega_{j-1} = \{y_1, x_1, \ldots, y_{j-1}, x_{j-1}\}$, the outcomes of the first $j-1$ patients we obtain estimates $\hat{R}(d_i)$, $(i=1,\ldots,k)$ of the true unknown probabilities $R(d_i)$, $(i=1,\ldots,k)$ at the $k$ dose levels (see the following). The target dose level is that level having associated with it a probability of toxicity as close as we can get to $\theta$. The dose or dose level $x_j$ assigned to the $j$th included patient is such that

$$|\hat{R}(x_j) - \theta| < |\hat{R}(d_i) - \theta|, \quad (i=1,\ldots,k; x_j \neq d_i)$$

Thus, $x_j$ is the closest level to the target level in the previous precise sense. Other choices of closeness could be made, incorporating cost or other considerations. We could also weight the distance, for example, multiply $|\hat{R}(x_j) - \theta|$ by some constant greater than 1 when $\hat{R}(x_j) > \theta$. This would favor conservatism, such a design tending to experiment more often below the target than a design without weights. Similar ideas have been pursued by Babb et al. (1998).

The estimates $\hat{R}(x_j)$ are obtained from the one-parameter working model. Two questions dealt with in this section arise: (1) How do we estimate $R(x_j)$ on the basis of $\Omega_{j-1}$? and (2) how do we obtain the initial data, in particular since the first entered patient or group of patients must be treated in the absence of any data-based estimates of $R(x_1)$? Even though our model is under-parameterized, leading us into the area of mis-specified models, it turns out that standard procedures of estimation work. Some care is needed to show this and we look at this in Section 2.4. The procedures themselves are described later. Obtaining the initial data is partially described in these same sections as well as being the subject of its own Section 2.4.2.

In order to decide, on the basis of available information and previous observations, the appropriate level at which to treat a patient, we need some estimate of the probability of toxic response at dose level $d_i$, $(i=1,\ldots,k)$. We would currently recommend use of the maximum likelihood estimator (O'Quigley and Shen 1996) described in Section 2.3.1. The Bayesian estimator, developed in the original paper by O'Quigley et al. (1990) will perform very similarly unless priors are strong. The use of strong priors in the context of an under-parameterized and mis-specified model may require deeper study. Bayesian ideas can nonetheless be very useful in addressing more complex questions such as patient heterogeneity and drug combinations. We return to this in the Section 2.8. After the inclusion of the first $j$ patients, the log-likelihood can be written as

$$\mathcal{L}_j(a) = \sum_{\ell=1}^{j} y_\ell \log \psi(x_\ell, a) + \sum_{\ell=1}^{j} (1 - y_\ell) \log(1 - \psi(x_\ell, a)) \tag{2.3}$$

and is maximized at $a = \hat{a}_j$. Maximization of $\mathcal{L}_j(a)$ can easily be achieved with a Newton–Raphson algorithm. Once we have calculated $\hat{a}_j$, we can next obtain an estimate of the probability of toxicity at each dose level $d_i$ via

$$\hat{R}(d_i) = \psi(d_i, \hat{a}_j), \quad (i=1,\ldots,k)$$

On the basis of this formula the dose to be given to the $(j+1)$th patient, $x_{j+1}$ is determined as already mentioned.

A requirement to be able to maximize the log-likelihood on the interior of the parameter space is that we have heterogeneity among the responses, that is, at least one toxic and one nontoxic response (Silvapulle 1981). Otherwise the likelihood is maximized on the boundary of the parameter space and our estimates of $R(d_i)$, $(i=1,\ldots,k)$ are trivially either zero, one, or, depending on the model we are working with, may not even be defined. Thus, the experiment is considered as not being fully underway until we have some heterogeneity in the responses. These could arise in a variety of different ways: the use of the standard up and down approach, the use of an initial Bayesian CRM as outlined in *two-stage designs*, or the use of a design believed to be more appropriate by the investigator. Once we have achieved heterogeneity, the model kicks in and we continue as prescribed earlier (estimation–allocation). Achieving the necessary heterogeneity to carry out the previous prescription is largely arbitrary.

## 2.4 IMPLEMENTATION

### 2.4.1 Fixed Sample or Stopping Rules

CRM can be implemented on the basis of a fixed sample or by making use of a stopping rule. If a fixed sample $n$ is used, then the recommended dose level is the level that would be recommended to patient $n+1$. However, given the convergence properties of CRM, it may occur in practice that we appear to have settled on a level before having included the full sample size $n$ of anticipated patients. In such a case we may wish to bring the study to an early close, thereby enabling the Phase II study to be undertaken more quickly. One possible approach suggested by O'Quigley et al. (1990) would be to use the estimated confidence interval for the probability of toxicity, $\psi(x_{j+1}, \hat{a}_j)$, at the currently recommended level and when this interval falls within some prespecified range; then we stop the study.

We can calculate an approximate $100(1 - \alpha)\%$ confidence interval for $\psi(x_{j+1}, \hat{a}_j)$ as $(\psi_j^-, \psi_j^+)$ where

$$\psi_j^- = \psi\{x_{j+1}, (\hat{a}_j + z_{1-\alpha/2} v\,(\hat{a}_j)^{1/2})\}, \psi_j^+ = \psi\{x_{j+1}, (\hat{a}_j - z_{1-\alpha/2} v(\hat{a}_j)^{1/2})\}$$

where

$z_\alpha$ is the $\alpha$th percentile of a standard normal distribution

$v(\hat{a}_j)$ is an estimate of the variance of $\hat{a}_j$

For the model of Equation 2.1 this turns out to be particularly simple and we can write

$$v^{-1}(\hat{a}_j) = \frac{\sum_{\ell \leq j, y_\ell = 0} \psi(x_\ell, \hat{a}_j)(\log \alpha_\ell)^2}{(1 - \psi(x_\ell, \hat{a}_j))^2}$$

Although based on a mis-specified model these intervals turn out to be quite accurate, even for sample sizes as small as 12 and thus helpful in practice (Natarajan and O'Quigley 2003). Another approach would be to stop after some fixed number of subjects have been treated at the same level. Such designs were used by Goodman et al. (1995) and Korn et al. (1994) and have the advantage of great simplicity. These modifications have been evaluated through simulations and they appear to work well in terms of MTD estimation (Goodman et al. 1995, Iasonos et al. 2008) if the sample size is no less than 20, but their theoretical properties remain to be studied.

One stopping rule that has been studied in detail (O'Quigley and Reiner 1998) is based on the convergence of CRM so that, as we appear to settle at some level, the accumulating information can enable us to quantify this notion. Specifically, given the data of $j$ patients, $\Omega_j$, we would like to be able to say something about the levels at which the remaining patients, $j+1$ to $n$, are likely to be treated. The quantity we are interested in is

$$\mathcal{P}_{j,n} = \Pr\left\{x_{j+1} = x_{j+2} = \cdots = x_{n+1} \middle| \Omega_j\right\}$$

In other words, $\mathcal{P}_j n$ is the probability that $x_{j+1}$ is the dose recommended to all remaining patients in the trial as well as being the final recommended dose. Thus, to find $\mathcal{P}_j n$ one needs to determine all the possible outcomes of the trial based on the results known for the first $j$ patients. Details regarding estimating $\mathcal{P}_j n$ are given in O'Quigley and Reiner (1998). The rule, based on precise probabilistic calculation, is quite involved. A much simpler rule was constructed based on the idea of having settled at some level in O'Quigley (2002) where the operating characteristics were more closely evaluated. In addition, Zohar and Chevret (2001) compared various Bayesian stopping rules and confirmed the requirement of including at least 20 patients to reach an accurate estimate of MTD when testing 5–6 dose levels.

### 2.4.2   TWO-STAGE DESIGNS

It may be felt that we know so little before undertaking a given study that it is worthwhile splitting the design into two stages, an initial exploratory escalation followed by a more refined homing in on the target. Such an idea was first proposed by Storer (1989) in the context of the more classical up and down schemes. His idea was to enable more rapid escalation in the early part of the trial where we may be quite far from a level at which treatment activity could be anticipated. Moller (1995) was the first to use this idea in the context of CRM designs. Her idea was to allow the first stage to be based on some variant of the usual up and down procedures. In the context of sequential likelihood estimation, the necessity of an initial stage was pointed out by O'Quigley and Shen (1996) since the likelihood equation fails to have a solution on the interior of the parameter space unless some heterogeneity in the responses has been observed. Their suggestion was to work with any initial scheme, Bayesian CRM or up and down, and, for any reasonable scheme, the operating characteristics appear relatively insensitive to this choice.

However, we believe there is something very natural and desirable in two-stage designs and that currently they could be taken as the designs of choice. The reason is the following: Early behavior of the method, in the absence of heterogeneity, appears to be rather arbitrary. A decision to escalate after inclusion of three patients tolerating some level, or after a single patient tolerating a level or according to some Bayesian prior corresponds to the simple desire to try a higher dose. This follows some kind of evidence of a low rate of toxicity at the current level. Rather than lead the clinician into thinking that something subtle and carefully analytic is taking place, our belief is that it is preferable that he or she be involved in the design of the initial phase. Operating characteristics that do not depend on data ought to be driven by clinical rather than statistical concerns. More importantly, the initial phase of the design, in which no toxicity has yet been observed, can be made much more efficient, from both the statistical and ethical angles, by allowing information on toxicity grade to determine the rapidity of escalation.

The simplest example of a two-stage design would be to include an initial escalation stage which exactly replicates the old standard design: starting at the lowest level, three patients are treated and only if all three tolerate the dose do we escalate to a higher level. As soon as the first dose limiting toxicity (DLT) is encountered, we close the first stage and open the second stage based on CRM modeling and using all the available data. Such a scheme could be varied in many ways, for example, including only a single patient at the lowest, then two patients at the second lowest and then as before. Another simple design, using information on toxicity severity (Table 2.1), enables rapid escalation through the lower levels. Assume there were many dose levels and the first included patient was treated at a low level. As long as we observe very low–grade toxicities then we escalate quickly, including only a single patient at each level. As soon as we encounter more serious toxicities then escalation is slowed down. Ultimately, we encounter dose limiting toxicities at which time the second stage, based on fitting a CRM model, comes fully into play. This is done by integrating this information and that obtained on all the earlier non-dose-limiting toxicities to estimate the most appropriate dose level.

It was decided to use information on low-grade toxicities in the first stage of a two-stage design in order to allow rapid initial escalation since it is possible that we could be far below the target level. Specifically, we define a grade severity variable $S(i)$ to be the average toxicity severity observed at dose level $i$, in this case the sum of the severities at that level divided by the number of patients treated at that level.

The rule is to escalate providing $S(i)$ is less than two. Furthermore, once we have included three patients at some level then escalation to higher levels only occurs if each cohort of three patients does not experience DLT. This scheme means that, in

---

**TABLE 2.1**

**Toxicity "Grades" (Severities) for Trial**

| Severity | Degree of Toxicity |
| --- | --- |
| 0 | No toxicity |
| 1 | Mild toxicity (non-dose limiting) |
| 2 | Moderate toxicity (non-dose limiting) |
| 3 | Severe toxicity (non-dose limiting) |
| 4 | DLT |

practice, if we see toxicities of severities coded 0 or 1, then we escalate. The first severity, coded 2, necessitates a further inclusion at this same level and, anything other than a 0 severity for this inclusion, would require yet a further inclusion and a non-dose-limiting toxicity before being able to escalate. This design also has the advantage that, should we be slowed down by a severe (severity 3), albeit non-dose-limiting toxicity, we retain the capability of picking up speed (in escalation) should subsequent toxicities be of low degree (0 or 1). This can be helpful in avoiding being handicapped by an outlier or an unanticipated and possibly not drug related toxicity. Once DLT is encountered, this phase of the study (the initial escalation scheme) comes to a close and we proceed on the basis of CRM recommendation. Although the initial phase is closed, the information on both dose limiting and non-dose-limiting toxicities thereby obtained is used in the second stage.

### 2.4.3 GROUPED DESIGNS

O'Quigley et al. (1990) describe the situation of delayed response in which new patients become available to be included in the study while we are still awaiting the toxicity results on already entered patients. The suggestion was, in the absence of information on such recently included patients, that the logical course to take was to treat at the most recent recommended level. This is the level indicated by all the currently available information. The likelihood for this situation was written down by O'Quigley et al. (1990) and, apart from a constant term not involving the unknown parameter, is just the likelihood we obtain had the subjects been included one by one. There is therefore, operationally, no additional work required to deal with such situations.

The question does arise, however, as to the performance of CRM in such cases. The delayed response can lead to grouping or we can simply decide upon the grouping by design. Three papers (Goodman et al. 1995, O'Quigley and Shen 1996, Iasonos et al. 2008) have studied the effects of grouping. The more thorough study was that of Goodman et al. in which cohorts of sizes 1, 2, and 3 were evaluated. Broadly speaking the cohort size had little impact upon operating characteristics and the accuracy of final recommendation. O'Quigley and Shen (1996) indicated that for groups of three, and relatively few patients (16), when the correct level was the highest available level and we started out at the lowest or a low level, we might anticipate some marked drop in performance when contrasted with, say, one-by-one inclusion, but the differences disappeared for samples of size 25. One-by-one inclusion tends to maximize efficiency but, should stability throughout the study be an issue, then this extra stability can be obtained through grouping. The cost of this extra stability in terms of efficiency loss appears to be generally small. The findings of Goodman et al. (1995), O'Quigley and Shen (1996), O'Quigley (1999), and Iasonos et al. (2008) show that grouping would not lead to any noticeable efficiency losses, a finding which contradicts the fears expressed by some workers in the field.

### 2.4.4 ILLUSTRATION

This brief illustration is recalled from O'Quigley and Shen (1996). The study concerned 16 patients and there was no stopping rule in effect. Their toxic responses were simulated from the known dose–toxicity curve. There were six levels in the study, maximum likelihood was used, and the first entered patients were treated at the lowest level. The design was two stage. The true toxic probabilities were $R(d_1)=0.03$, $R(d_2)=0.22$, $R(d_3)=0.45$, $R(d_4)=0.6$, $R(d_5)=0.8$, and $R(d_6)=0.95$. The working model was that given by Equation 2.1 where $\alpha_1=0.04$, $\alpha_2=0.07$, $\alpha_3=0.20$, $\alpha_4=0.35$, $\alpha_5=0.55$, and $\alpha_6=0.70$. The targeted toxicity was given by $\theta=0.2$ indicating that the best level for the MTD is given by level 2 where the true probability of toxicity is 0.22. A grouped design was used until heterogeneity in toxic responses was observed, patients being included, as for the classical schemes, in groups of three. The first three patients experienced no toxicity at level 1. Escalation then took place to level 2 and the next three patients treated at this level did not experience any toxicity either. Subsequently two out of the three patients treated at level 3 experienced toxicity. Given this heterogeneity in the responses the maximum likelihood estimator for $a$ now exists and, following a few iterations, could be seen to be equal to 0.715. We then have that $\hat{R}(d_1)=0.101$, $\hat{R}(d_2)=0.149$, $\hat{R}(d_3)=0.316$, $\hat{R}(d_4)=0.472$, $\hat{R}(d_5)=0.652$, and $\hat{R}(d_6)=0.775$. Table 2.2 shows the visited dose levels, the toxicity outcomes, the estimated parameter $\hat{a}$, and the estimated probabilities of toxicity at each of the six dose level for each inclusion. Note that the modeling stage begins after observing the outcome from the ninth patient. The 10th entered patient is then treated at level 2 for which $\hat{R}(d_2)=0.149$ since, from the

**TABLE 2.2**

**Sequential Trial for 16 Patients. The 3+3**
**Design Is Followed for the First Nine**
**Patients. CRM Estimation Starts after**
**Observing the Ninth Patient**

| j | xj | yj | âj | R̂(dj) |
|---|----|----|------|-------|
| 1 | 1 | 0 | | |
| 2 | 1 | 0 | | |
| 3 | 1 | 0 | | |
| 4 | 2 | 0 | | |
| 5 | 2 | 0 | | |
| 6 | 2 | 0 | | |
| 7 | 3 | 0 | | |
| 8 | 3 | 1 | | |
| 9 | 3 | 1 | 0.7151 | 0.10, 0.15, 0.32, 0.47, 0.65, 0.77 |
| 10 | 2 | 0 | 0.7592 | 0.09, 0.13, 0.29, 0.45, 0.64, 0.76 |
| 11 | 2 | 1 | 0.5711 | 0.16, 0.22, 0.40, 0.55, 0.71, 0.82 |
| 12 | 2 | 0 | 0.6066 | 0.14, 0.20, 0.38, 0.53, 0.70, 0.81 |
| 13 | 2 | 0 | 0.6391 | 0.13, 0.18, 0.36, 0.51, 0.68, 0.80 |
| 14 | 2 | 0 | 0.6691 | 0.12, 0.17, 0.34, 0.50, 0.67, 0.79 |
| 15 | 2 | 1 | 0.5563 | 0.17, 0.23, 0.41, 0.56, 0.72, 0.82 |
| 16 | 2 | 0 | 0.582 | 0.15, 0.21, 0.39, 0.54, 0.71, 0.81 |

available estimates, this is the closest to the target $\theta = 0.2$. The 10th included patient does not suffer toxic effects and the new maximum likelihood estimator becomes 0.759. Level 2 remains the level with an estimated probability of toxicity closest to the target. This same level is in fact recommended to the remaining patients so that after 16 inclusions the recommended MTD is level 2. The estimated probability of toxicity at this level is 0.212 and a 90% confidence interval for this probability is estimated as (0.07, 0.39).

## 2.5  STATISTICAL PROPERTIES

Recall that CRM is a class of methods rather than a single method, the members of the class depending on arbitrary quantities chosen by the investigator such as the form of the model, the spacing between the doses, the starting dose, whether single or grouped inclusions, the initial dose escalation scheme in two-stage designs, or the prior density chosen for Bayesian formulations. The statistical properties described in this section apply broadly to all members of the class, the members nonetheless maintaining some of their own particularities.

### 2.5.1  CONVERGENCE

Convergence arguments obtain from considerations of the likelihood. The same arguments apply to Bayesian estimation as long as the prior is other than degenerate. Usual likelihood arguments based on large sample theory break down since our models are mis-specified. The maximum likelihood estimate, $\hat{R}(d_i) = \psi(d_i, \hat{a}_j)$, exists as soon as we have some heterogeneity in the responses (Silvapulle 1981). We need to assume that the dose toxicity function, $\psi(x,a)$, satisfies the conditions described in Shen and O'Quigley (1996); in particular the condition that, for $i = 1,\ldots,k$, there exists a unique $a_i$ such that $\psi(d_i, a_i) = R(d_i)$. Note that the $a_i$s depend on the actual probabilities of toxicity and are therefore unknown. We also require the following:

1. For each $0 < t < 1$ and each $x$, the function

$$s(t,x,a) := t\frac{\psi'}{\psi}(x,a) + (1-t)\frac{-\psi'}{1-\psi}(x,a)$$

   is continuous and is strictly monotone in $a$.
2. The parameter $a$ belongs to a finite interval $[A,B]$.

The first condition is standard for estimating equations to have unique solutions. The second imposes no real practical restriction. We will also require the true unknown dose toxicity function, $R(x)$, to satisfy the following conditions:

1. The probabilities of toxicity at $d_1,\ldots,d_k$ satisfy $0 < R(d_1) < ,\ldots, R(d_k) < 1$.
2. The target dose level is $x_0 \in \{d_1,\ldots,d_k\}$ where $|\hat{R}(x_0) - \theta| < |\hat{R}(d_i) - \theta|$, $(i = 1,\ldots, k; x_0 \neq d_i)$.

3. Before writing down the third condition, note that, since our model is misspecified, it will generally not be true that $\psi(d_i, a_0) \equiv R(d_i)$ for $i = 1, \ldots, k$. We will nonetheless require that the working model be not "too distant" from the true underlying dose toxicity curve and this can be made precise with the help of the set

$$S(a_0) = \{a : |\, \psi(x_0, a) - \theta\,| < |\, \psi(x_i, a) - \theta\,|, \text{ for all } d_i \neq x_0\} \tag{2.4}$$

The condition we require is that for $i = 1, \ldots, k$, $a_i \in S(a_0)$.

At the target level $x_0$ we have $R(x_0) = \theta_0$ and $a_0$ is defined as the value of $a$ so that $\psi(x_0, a_0) = R(x_0)$. Under these conditions, Shen and O'Quigley (1996) showed that the estimator $\hat{a}_n$ converges to $a_n$ and that the asymptotic distribution of $\sqrt{n}(\hat{a}_n - a_0)$ is $N(0, \sigma^2)$, with $\sigma^2 = \{\psi'(x_0, a_0)\}^{-2}\theta_0(1 - \theta_0)$.

### 2.5.2 EFFICIENCY

We can use $\hat{\theta}_n = \psi(x_{n+1}, \hat{a}_n)$ to estimate the probability of toxicity at the recommended level $x_{n+1}$, where $\hat{a}_n$ is the maximum likelihood estimate (O'Quigley 1992). An application of the $\delta$-method shows that the asymptotic distribution of $\sqrt{n}\{\hat{\theta}_n - R(x_0)\}$ is $N\{0, \theta_0(1 - \theta_0)\}$. The estimate then provided by CRM is fully efficient. This is what our intuition would suggest given the convergence properties of CRM and the variance of a binomial variate. What actually takes place in finite samples needs to be investigated on a case-by-case basis. Nonetheless the relatively broad range of cases studied by O'Quigley (1992) show a mean squared error for the estimated probability of toxicity at the recommended level under CRM to correspond well with the theoretical variance for samples of size $n$, were all subjects to be experimented at the correct level. Some of the cases studied showed evidence of superefficiency, translating nonnegligible bias that happens to be in the right direction while a few others indicated efficiency losses large enough to suggest the potential for improvement.

Large sample results are helpful in as much as they provide some assurance as to the basic statistical soundness of the approach. For instance, some suggested approaches using richer parametric models turn out to be not only inefficient but also inconsistent. However, in practice, we are typically interested in behavior at small sample sizes. For some arbitrarily chosen true dose–toxicity relations, authors have studied the relative behavior of competing schemes, case by case, in terms of percentage of final recommendation, in-trial allocation, probability of toxicity, average number of subjects included etc. The operating characteristics are to some extent dependent upon the true dose–toxicity relation (Gooley et al. 1994). The choice then of such relations and their influence on the evaluation of the performance of the method under study raises questions of generalizability.

Nonetheless, it can be seen (O'Quigley et al. 2002) that there does exist an optimal scheme making the fullest use of all the information in the experiment. The scheme is optimal in that the mean squared error of estimate of the probability of toxicity at the recommended dose is less than or equal to all other asymptotically unbiased estimates. Of course, Bayesian schemes could outperform the optimal design by including accurate information. It is also helpful to think in terms of the complementary idea, suboptimality, since we will see that suboptimality can be seen to be equivalent to the concept of incomplete information.

Most experiments have incomplete information in that it is not usually possible to replicate experiments for each subject at each level. Were it possible to experiment each subject independently at each level then such a scheme would in fact be equivalent to the nonparametric optimal method. In a real experiment each patient provides partial or incomplete information. The monotonicity of toxicity assumption implies that if a subject had a toxic reaction at level $d_k (k \leq 6)$, then he or she would necessarily have had a toxic reaction at $d_\ell (k \leq \ell \leq 6)$. As for his or her response at levels below $d_k$, we have no information on this. The information is partial or incomplete. For instance, a subject experiencing a toxicity at $d_5$ provides the information shown in Table 2.3 where a "*" indicates missing or incomplete information. On the other hand, should the subject tolerate the treatment at level $d_k (1 \leq k \leq 6)$ then he or she would necessarily tolerate the treatment at all levels $d_\ell (1 \leq \ell \leq k)$. Thus, if a subject had been included at $d_3$ without a toxic response, the experiment would provide the tabulated information as in Table 2.4. The preceding considerations help us understand in a precise way why we describe our data as being incomplete. If all the information were available, for each patient, we would know the response at every dose level. In other words, the highest tolerated dose level would be known. For instance, instead of the previous two tables, we could imagine a table for a subject for whom DLT appears from dose level 3. The complete information would be as shown in Table 2.5.

Of course in a real trial, such information is not available. However, in the framework of simulations or probabilistic calculation, complete information can be obtained. As an illustration we take the dose–toxicity relation from O'Quigley et al. (2002). We carried out 5000 simulations of the two procedures. Table 2.6 gives the recommendation distribution when the target is 0.2. We denote by $q_k(16)$ the proportion of times that the optimal method recommends level $k$ based on 16 patients and $p_k(16)$ the analogous quantity for a CRM design.

**TABLE 2.3**

**Incomplete Information for a Subject with a Toxicity**

| Dose | d1 | d2 | d3 | d4 | d5 | d6 |
|------|-----|-----|-----|-----|-----|-----|
| $Y_k$ | * | * | * | * | 1 | 1 |

**TABLE 2.4**

**Incomplete Information for a Subject without a Toxicity**

| Dose | d1 | d2 | d3 | d4 | d5 | d6 |
|------|-----|-----|-----|-----|-----|-----|
| $Y_k$ | 0 | 0 | 0 | * | * | * |

**TABLE 2.5**

**Complete Information for a Given Patient**

| Dose | d1 | d2 | d3 | d4 | d5 | d6 |
|------|----|----|----|----|----|----|
| $Y_k$ | 0 | 0 | 1 | 1 | 1 | 1 |

**TABLE 2.6**

**Compared Frequency of Final Recommendations of the Optimal Method and the CRM for Simulated Examples Based on the Probabilities Given on Line 2**

| dk | 1 | 2 | 3 | 4 | 5 | 6 |
|------|------|------|------|------|------|------|
| $R_k$ | 0.05 | 0.11 | 0.22 | 0.35 | 0.45 | 0.60 |
| $p_k(16)$ | 0.05 | 0.26 | 0.42 | 0.21 | 0.06 | 0.0 |
| $q_k(16)$ | 0.04 | 0.27 | 0.48 | 0.17 | 0.04 | 0.0 |

Only 16 patients were available for study and we might imagine that, for such a small sample, we could hope for large gains were we to work with the correct model instead of an under-parameterized working model. However, there appears to be very little room for improvement over the CRM model used since the optimal method only performs slightly better. The improvement would be worth having nonetheless, but we would need quite good evidence that any model that we use is justified. For larger sample sizes the difference between the CRM and the optimal method quickly diminishes to the point at which they can be neglected.

## 2.6 MORE COMPLEX CRM DESIGNS

The different up and down designs amount to a collection of ad hoc rules for making decisions when faced with accumulating observations. The CRM leans on a model which, although not providing a broad summary of the true underlying probabilistic phenomenon, in view of its being under-parameterized, does nonetheless provide structure enabling better control in an experimental situation. In principle at least, a model enables us to go further and accommodate greater complexity. Care is needed, but it has been shown that within the CRM framework we can capture some of the more complex aspects of dose-finding studies, that are necessarily ignored by the rule-based designs. The following sections consider some examples.

### 2.6.1 PHARMACOKINETIC STUDIES

Statistical modeling of Phase I dose finding studies, such as the modeling that takes place with the CRM, has been introduced in the last two decades. Much more fully studied in the Phase I context are pharmacokinetics and pharmacodynamics (see Chapter 3). Roughly speaking, pharmacokinetics deals with the study of concentration and elimination characteristics of given compounds in specified organ systems, most often blood plasma, whereas pharmacodynamics focuses on how the compounds affect the body. This is a vast subject referred to as PK/PD modeling. Clearly such information will have a bearing on whether or not a given patient is likely to encounter DLT or, in retrospect, why some patients and not others were able to tolerate some given dose. There are many parameters of interest to the pharmacologist, for example, the area under the concentration time curve, the rate of clearance of the drug, and the peak concentration.

For our purposes, a particular practical difficulty arises in the Phase I context, in which any such information only becomes available once the dose has been administered. Most often then the information will be of most use in terms of retrospectively explaining the toxicities. However, it is possible to have pharmacodynamic information and other patient characteristics relating to the patient's ability to synthesize the drugs, available before selecting the level at which the patient should be treated.

The strength of CRM is to locate with relatively few patients the target dose level. The remaining patients are then treated at this same level. A recommendation is made for this level. Further studies, following the Phase I clinical study, can now be made and this is where we see the main advantage of pharmacokinetics. Most patients will have been studied at the recommended level and a smaller amount at adjacent levels. At any of these levels we will have responses and a great deal of pharmacokinetic information. The usual models, in particular the logistic model, can be used to see if this information helps explain the toxicities. If so we may be encouraged to carry out further studies at higher or lower levels for certain patient profiles, indicated by the retrospective analysis to have probabilities of toxicity much lower or much higher than suggested by the average estimate. This can be viewed as the fine tuning and may itself give rise to new more highly focused Phase I studies. At this point, we do not see the utility of a model in which all the different factors are included as regressors. These further analyses are necessarily very delicate, requiring great statistical and/or pharmacological skill, and a mechanistic approach based on a global umbrella model is probably unrealistic. In principle we can write down any model, say one including all the relevant factors believed to influence the probability of encountering toxicity. We can then proceed to estimate the parameters. However, we must remain realistic in terms of what can be achieved given the maximum obtainable sample size. Some pioneering work has been carried out here by Piantadosi and Liu (1996), indicating the potential for improved precision by the incorporation of pharmacokinetic information.

Recently, O'Quigley et al. (2010) introduced a dose-finding algorithm to be used to identify a level of dose that corresponds to some given targeted response, where the response is a continuously measured quantity, typically some pharmacokinetic parameter. Consider the case where an agreed level of response has been determined from earlier studies on some population and the purpose of the current trial is to obtain the same, or a comparable, level of response in a new population. This relates to bridging studies. The example came from studies on drugs for HIV that have already been evaluated in adults and where the new studies are to be carried out in children. These drugs have the ability to produce some given mean pharmacokinetic response in the adult population, and the goal is to calibrate the dose in order to obtain a comparable response in the childhood population. In practice, it may turn out that the dose producing some desired mean response is also associated with an unacceptable rate of toxicity. In this case, we may need to reevaluate the target response and this is readily achieved. In simulations, the algorithm can be seen to work very well. In the most challenging situations for the method, those where the targeted response corresponds to a region of the dose–response curve that is relatively flat, the algorithm can still perform satisfactorily. This is a large field awaiting further exploration.

## 2.6.2    GRADED TOXICITIES

Although we refer to dose limiting toxicities as a binary (0,1) variable, most studies record information on the degree of toxicity, from 0, complete absence of side effects, to 4, life threatening toxicity. The natural reaction for a statistician is to consider that the response variable, toxicity, has been simplified when going from 5 levels to 2 and that it may help to employ models accommodating multilevel responses. The issue is not that of modeling a response (toxicity) at 5 levels but of controlling DLT, mostly grade 4 but possibly also certain kinds of grade 3. Lower grades are helpful in that their occurrence indicates that we are approaching a zone in which the probability of encountering a DLT is becoming large enough to be of concern. This idea is used implicitly in the two-stage designs described in Section 2.4. If we are to proceed more formally and hopefully extract yet more information from the observations, then we need models relating the occurrence of dose limiting toxicities to the occurrence of lower-grade toxicities. In the unrealistic situation in which we can accurately model the ratio of the probabilities of the different types of toxicity, we can make small gains in efficiency since the more frequently observed lower-grade toxicities carry some information on the potential occurrence of dose limiting toxicities. Such a situation would also allow gains in safety since it would allow the method to concentrate the experimentation at the MTD even faster and result in a smaller variance in the estimation of the parameter of interest. At the opposite end of the model/hypothesis spectrum we might decide we know nothing about the relative rates of occurrence of the different toxicity types and simply allow the accumulating observations to provide the necessary estimates. In this case it turns out that we neither lose nor gain efficiency, and the method behaves identically to one in which the only information we obtain is whether or not the toxicity is dose limiting. These two situations suggest there may be a middle road, using a Bayesian prescription, in which very careful modeling can lead to efficiency improvements, if only moderate, without making strong assumptions.

To make this more precise let us consider the case of three toxicity levels, the highest being dose limiting, the middle level indicating moderate toxicities, and the lowest level indicating no toxicities at all. Let $Y_j$ denote the toxic response for patient $j$ who is treated at level $x_j$, and let $Y_j$ take three values 1, 2, 3. The goal of the trial is still to identify a level of dose whose probability of DLT is closest to a given percentile of the dose–toxicity curve. A working model for the CRM could be

$$\Pr(Y_j = 3) = \psi_1(x_j, a)$$

$$\Pr(Y_j = 2 \text{ or } Y_j = 3) = \psi_2(x_j, a, b)$$

$$\Pr(Y_j = 1) = 1 - \psi_2(x_j, a, b)$$

The contributions to the likelihood are $1 - \psi_2(x_j, a, b)$ when $Y_j = 1$, $\psi_1(x_j, a)$ when $Y_j = 3$ and $\psi_2(x_j, a, b) - \psi_1(x_j, a)$ when $Y_j = 2$. To begin with, we make the (generally unrealistic) assumption that the parameter $b$ is known precisely. The model need not be correctly specified although $b$ should maintain interpretation outside the model, for instance some simple function of the ratio of dose-limiting toxicities $\Pr(Y=3)$ to moderate toxicities $\Pr(Y=2)$. The known value might have been obtained from other data although, mostly, the use of a known value is for theoretical purposes, providing us with some kind of a bound when compared with the more realistic situation in which $b$ is not known precisely. Such imprecise knowledge could be characterized by an appropriate prior. With no prior information, and being able to maximize the likelihood that can involve two unknown parameters, we obtain the same results as with the more usual one-parameter CRM. This is due to the parameter orthogonality. There is therefore no efficiency gain although there is the advantage of learning about the relationship between the different toxicity types. For more details about the simulation study refer to Iasonos and Zohar (2011).

## 2.7   COMBINED TOXICITY-EFFICACY STUDIES

An interesting aspect of clinical trial design is the definition of composite endpoints. In the context of Phase I/II trials, investigators are interested in finding a dose that is safe and, in addition, meets some threshold for efficacy. Information on efficacy is obtained during the trial and may be as important as that relating to toxicity. Thall et al. (2001) have used the CRM framework to identify a feasible MTD based on infusibility and toxicity in the context of T-cell infusion trials. Braun (2002) has also illustrated the bivariate CRM in the presence of two competing outcomes. The designs proposed by O'Quigley et al. (2001) incorporate a bivariate outcome since they aim to control toxicity and viral reduction at the recommended dose level for early dose finding studies in HIV. The ideas extend immediately to the cancer setting in which, instead of viral reduction, we have some other objective measure of response. Initial doses are given, from some fixed range of dose regimens. The doses are ordered in terms of their toxic potential. At any dose, a patient can have one of three outcomes: toxicity (whether or not the treatment is otherwise effective), nontoxicity together with an insufficient response, and, thirdly, nontoxicity in the presence of an adequate response. The goal of the study is the identification of the dose leading to the greatest percentage of successes. This dose is called the MSD (most successful dose).

One simple approach with encouraging results was the following. A CRM design is used to target some low toxicity level. Information is simultaneously accrued on efficacy. Whenever efficacy is deemed too low at the target toxicity level, that level and all levels lower than it are removed from investigation. The target toxicity is then increased. Whenever efficacy is sufficiently high for the treatment to be considered successful, the trial is brought to a close. Rules for making decisions on efficacy are based on the sequential probability ratio test. This class of designs has great flexibility. Starting with the inclusion of the first patient, information on the rate of successes among those patients not suffering toxic side effects is gathered. A true rate of success of $p_0$ or lower is considered unsatisfactory. A rate $p_1$ or higher of successes is considered a promising treatment. A model free approach would allow us to determine, on the basis of empirical observations, which of the aforementioned rates is more likely. This is expensive in terms of patient numbers required. A strong modeling approach uses under-parameterized models. These create a structure around which we can home in quickly on the best level. This parallels the use of the CRM for the simpler situation of Phase I toxicity studies. Failure to distinguish between the previous two hypotheses leads to further experimentation. The experimentation is carried out at a level guided by the toxicity criterion. A conclusion in favor of a success rate greater than $p_1$ at some level brings the trial to a close with a recommendation for that level. A conclusion in favor of a success rate lower than $p_0$, at some level, leads to that level, and all lower levels, being removed from further study. At the same time we increase the target "acceptable toxicity" from $\theta$ to $\theta + \Delta\theta$. The trial then continues at those remaining levels. Values for the target toxicity level will start out low, for example, $\theta = 0.1$, and this value may be increased subsequently. The amount $\Delta\theta$ by which $\theta$ increases and the highest value that is allowed are parameters that can be fixed by the investigator. A special case would be $\Delta\theta = 0$.

Specifically, consider a trial in which $j = 1,\ldots,n$ patients may be entered and $n$ is the greatest number of patients that we are prepared to enter. As before, $Y_j$ is a binary random variable (0.1) where 1 denotes a toxic response. Let $V_j$ be a binary random variable (0.1) where 1 denotes a response to treatment for the $j$th patient ($j = 1,\ldots,n$). The probability of acceptable treatment response, given no toxicity, at $X_j = x_j$ is given by

$$Q(x_j) = \Pr(V_j = 1 | X_j = x_j, Y_j = 0) \tag{2.5}$$

so that $P(d_i) = Q(d_i)\{1 - R(d_i)\}$ is the probability of success at dose $d_i$. The goal of the experiment is to identify the dose level $\ell$ such that $P(d_\ell) > P(d_i)$ for all $i$ not equal to $\ell$.

As for toxicity only experiments, we take $R(x_j) = \Pr(Y_j = 1 | X_j = x_j) = \psi(x_j, a)$. We introduce an additional modeling assumption which concerns the conditional probability of success given absence of toxic side effects. We express this as

$$Q(x_j) = \Pr(V_j = 1 | X_j = x_j, Y_j = 0) = E(V_j | x_j, Y_j = 0) = \phi(x_j, b) \tag{2.6}$$

where $\phi(x,b)$ is a one-parameter working model. Thus, we assume that $Q(x)$ is also monotonic in $x$. Since it is possible to construct, relatively plausible, counterexamples to this assumption, in contrast to the monotonicity assumption for $\psi(x)$, we should consider this to be a stronger assumption. Nonetheless such an assumption may often be reasonable, at least as an approximation. Under these models the success rate can be expressed, in terms of the parameters $a$ and $b$, as

$$P(d_i) = \phi(d_i, b)\{1 - \psi(d_i, a)\} \tag{2.7}$$

Once we have at least one toxicity and one nontoxicity together with at least one success and one nonsuccess, then we are in a position to estimate the parameters $a$ and $b$. The next dose to be used is the one which maximizes $P(d_i)$, $i = 1,...,k$.

## 2.8   ADDED FLEXIBILITY BASED ON BAYESIAN MODEL CHOICE

Extra flexibility can be obtained by relaxing some of the model's rigidity. Useful gains can be made but care is needed. For example, our usual intuition might lead us to believe that the simple added flexibility provided by a two-parameter model, for example, a logistic model, would improve performance when compared to a one-parameter model. This is not so (see Section 2.3) and, in general, we can only increase the dimension of the parameter space when we wish to include some added information of an orthogonal nature, such as group heterogeneity for which we have available an indicator variable designating the different groups. However, rather than making the full step of increasing the parameter space from, say, $\mathcal{R}^1$ to $\mathcal{R}^2$, we could, instead, choose a small finite set of models to work with, choosing the one that "best fits" the observations. Such an approach can be formalized under the heading of Bayesian model choice (Gelfand and Ghosh 1998) so that large sample theory, for example, becomes available to us. Suppose that instead of the single model of Equation 2.1, we have some class of models of interest and we denote these models as $\psi_m(x_j, a)$ for $m = 1,..., M$ where there are a total of $M$ possible models. In particular, we might consider

$$\psi_m(d_i, a) = \alpha_{mi}^{\exp(a)}, \quad (i = 1,...,k; m = 1,...,M) \tag{2.8}$$

where $0 < \alpha_{m1} < \cdots < \alpha_{mk} < 1$ and $-\infty < a < \infty$, as an immediate generalization of the single model described in Section 2.3.1. Further, we may wish to take account of any prior information concerning the plausibility of each model and thus introduce $\pi(m)$, $m = 1,..., M$ where $\pi(m) \geq 0$ and where $\Sigma_m \pi(m) = 1$. In the simplest case where each model is weighted equally, we would take $\pi(m) = 1/M$. Here, we consider some examples.

### 2.8.1   PATIENT HETEROGENEITY

Since patients differ in the way they may react to a treatment, we may sometimes be in a position to specifically address the issue of patient heterogeneity. One example occurs in patients with acute leukemia where it has been observed that children will better tolerate more aggressive doses (standardized by their weight) than adults. Likewise, heavily pretreated patients are often more likely to suffer from toxic side effects than lightly pretreated patients. In such situations we may wish to carry out separate trials for the different groups in order to identify the appropriate MTD for each group. Otherwise we run the risk of recommending an "average" compromise dose level, too toxic for a part of the population and suboptimal for the other. Usually, clinicians carry out two separate trials or split a trial into two arms after encountering the first DLT when it is believed that there are two distinct prognostic groups. This has the disadvantage of failing to utilize information common to both

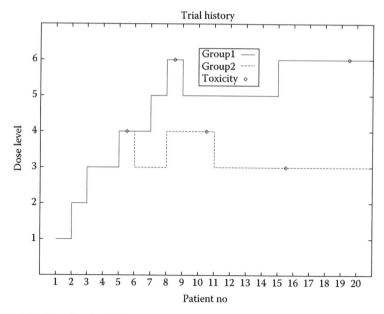

**FIGURE 2.2**    Simulated trial for two groups.

groups. A two-sample CRM, essentially two separate CRM designs, joined by an association parameter, has been developed so that only one trial is carried out based on information from both groups (see Figure 2.2 for illustration). A multi-sample CRM is a direct generalization although we must remain realistic in terms of what is achievable in the light of the available sample sizes.

Let $z$ be the binary indicator variable for the two groups. Otherwise, we use the same notation as previously defined. For clarity, we suppose that the targeted probability is the same in both groups and is denoted by $\theta$, although this assumption is not essential to our conclusions. The papers by O'Quigley et al. (1999) and O'Quigley and Paoletti (2003) focus mostly on models for the two-group case, since this case is the most common and there are not usually enough resources, in terms of patient numbers, to deal with more complex structures. Elaborating higher dimensional models, at least conceptually, is straightforward. The dose toxicity model is written as

$$\Pr(Y = 1 \mid d_i, z) = \psi(d_i, a, b) \tag{2.9}$$

where the parameter $b$ measures to some extent the difference between the groups. An obvious example which has been used successfully is

$$\psi(d_i, a, b) = \alpha_i^{\exp(a+bz)}, \quad (i = 1, \ldots, k) \tag{2.10}$$

where, again, $0 < \alpha_1 < \cdots < \alpha_k < 1$; $-\infty < a < \infty$, $-\infty < b < \infty$ and $z$ is a binary group indicator. Asymptotic theory is cumbersome for these models but consistency can be shown under restrictive assumptions as shown by O'Quigley et al. (1999).

An alternative approach, in harmony with the underlying CRM idea of exploiting under-parameterized models, is to be even more restrictive than allowed by the aforementioned regression models. Rather than allow for a large, possibly infinite, range of potential values for the second parameter $b$, measuring differences between the groups, the differences themselves are taken from a very small finite set.

If the recommended MTD for the first group is some level, say, $d_0$, then the other group will be recommended either the same level or some level, one, two, or more, steps away from it. The idea is to parameterize these steps directly. The indices themselves are modeled and the model is less cluttered if we work with $\log \psi(d_i, a)$ rather than $\psi(d_i, a)$ writing

$$\log \psi(d_i, a) = \exp(a) \log \alpha_{\phi(i)}; \quad \phi(i) = i + z h_i(t) \tag{2.11}$$

where

$$h_i(t) = t I(1 \leq i + t \leq k) + k I(i + t > k) + I(i + t < 1), \quad t = 0, 1, 2, \ldots, \tag{2.12}$$

the second two terms in the previous expression taking care of edge effects. It is easy to put a discrete prior on $t$, possibly giving the most weight to $t = 0$ and only allowing one or two dose level shifts if the evidence of the accumulating data points strongly in that direction. For example, the following formulation allows up to a single difference in dose levels between the groups:

1. Model 1: $m = 1$

$$\Pr(Y = 1 \mid d_i, z = 0) = \psi(d_i, a), \quad i = 1, \ldots, k$$
$$\Pr(Y = 1 \mid d_i, z = 1) = \psi(d_i, a), \quad i = 1, \ldots, k$$

2. Model 2: $m = 2$

$$\Pr(Y = 1 \mid d_i, z = 0) = \psi(d_i, a), \quad i = 1, \ldots, k$$
$$\Pr(Y = 1 \mid d_i, z = 1) = \psi(d_{i+1}, a), \quad i = 1, \ldots, k - 1$$
$$\Pr(Y = 1 \mid d_i, z = 1) = \psi(d_k, a), \quad i = k$$

3. Model 3: $m = 3$

$$\Pr(Y = 1 \mid d_i, z = 0) = \psi(d_i, a), \quad i = 1, \ldots, k$$
$$\Pr(Y = 1 \mid d_i, z = 1) = \psi(d_{i-1}, a), \quad i = 2, \ldots, k$$
$$\Pr(Y = 1 \mid d_i, z = 1) = \psi(d_1, a), \quad i = 1$$

This difference can be in either direction, corresponding to a situation in which we do not know, or we are not certain which of the two groups is likely to fare the worst. At the same time we rule out the possibility that any difference, should one exist, be greater than a single level. It is obviously very straightforward to construct models which would allow for differences up to two or more levels, again in either direction. Also, we can allow differences in one direction to be limited to one level at most whereas, in the other direction, we may allow greater differences than one level. We could even decide that we allow differences of one or more levels in only one direction, and no differences at all in the other direction. This would correspond to the case where we know that should any difference exist it can only be in a given direction. In practice this is likely to be the most common situation, a well known example being heavily pretreated and lightly pre-treated patients. The MTD for the heavily pretreated patients will be no higher than that for the lightly pretreated patients. Given the specifics of the particular study, and whatever information we have on orderings, or group spacings, we then can write down the model, following which we use Bayesian model choice to select that model which is "closest" to the observations. The number of potential models is small and, in practice, we work through the indices $m$, maximizing, for each value of $m$, the likelihood or the posterior density as a function of $a$. The overall maximum is the one we choose.

## 2.8.2 PARTIAL ORDERING IN DOSE LEVELS

A fundamental assumption thus far is the monotonicity of the dose–toxicity curve. This is a reasonable assumption for single agent trials in which the administration of greater doses of the agent is expected to produce a higher proportion of patients with dose-limiting toxicities. When studying multiple agents or a combination of agents this assumption may not hold since some of the orderings of the toxicity probabilities between combinations of agents are not known prior to the study. Conaway et al. (2004) and Wages et al. (2011) proposed methods for Phase I trials involving multiple agents in which some of the orderings are unknown. As an example, these papers cite a study by Patnaik et al. (2000) involving paclitaxel and carboplatin administered in the combinations shown in Table 2.7. The ordering for combinations 3 and 5 is not known since combination 3 has a greater dose of paclitaxel but a lower dose of carboplatin than combination 5. Many of the orderings are known. For example, combination 2 has a greater probability of a toxicity than combination 1 because combination 2 has the same dose of paclitaxel and the same dose of carboplatin as combination 1.

The papers by Conaway et al. (2004) and Wages et al. (2011) consider all possible "simple orders" consistent with the known orderings. A simple order is one in which

**TABLE 2.7**

**Illustrating Drug Combinations**

| | Combination | | | | | |
|---|---|---|---|---|---|---|
| Agent | 1 | 2 | 3 | 4 | 5 | 6 |
| Paclitaxel | 54 | 67.5 | 81 | 94.5 | 67.5 | 67.5 |
| Carboplatin | 6 | 6 | 6 | 6 | 7.5 | 9 |

all orderings between pairs of treatment combinations are known. In the Patnaik et al. (2000) study, there are six possible simple orders for the toxicity probabilities associated with the treatment combinations:

$$m = 1 : R(x_1) \leq R(x_2) \leq R(x_3) \leq R(x_4) \leq R(x_5) \leq R(x_6)$$

$$m = 2 : R(x_1) \leq R(x_2) \leq R(x_3) \leq R(x_5) \leq R(x_6) \leq R(x_4)$$

$$m = 3 : R(x_1) \leq R(x_2) \leq R(x_5) \leq R(x_6) \leq R(x_3) \leq R(x_4)$$

$$m = 4 : R(x_1) \leq R(x_2) \leq R(x_5) \leq R(x_3) \leq R(x_4) \leq R(x_6)$$

$$m = 5 : R(x_1) \leq R(x_2) \leq R(x_3) \leq R(x_5) \leq R(x_4) \leq R(x_6)$$

$$m = 6 : R(x_1) \leq R(x_2) \leq R(x_5) \leq R(x_3) \leq R(x_6) \leq R(x_4)$$

Each of the simple orders can be thought of as one of $M = 6$ possible models.

Using the accumulated data from $j$ patients, $\Omega_j$, the maximum likelihood estimate $\hat{a}_m$ of the parameter $a_m$ in Equation 2.8 can be computed for each ordering $m$, $m = 1, \ldots, M$, along with the value of the log-likelihood at $\hat{a}_m$. Wages et al. (2011) propose an escalation method that first chooses the ordering with the largest maximized log-likelihood value, $\mathcal{L}_m(\hat{a}_m)$. If we denote this ordering by $m^*$, the authors use the estimate of $a_{m^*}$ to estimate the toxicity probabilities for each treatment combination under ordering $m^*$, $\hat{R}(d_i) = \psi_m^*(d_i, \hat{a}_m^*)$, $(i = 1, \ldots, k)$. The next patient is then allocated to the dose combination with the estimated toxicity probability closest to the target. Wages et al. (in press) investigate several variations of this basic design, including two-stage designs and designs that incorporate randomization among the different possible orderings and describe the operating characteristics of their proposed design.

### 2.8.3 BAYESIAN AVERAGING AND MAXIMIZATION FOR WORKING MODEL SELECTION

The choice of the working model, that is, the $\alpha_i$ in the setting up of any CRM design is largely arbitrary. Cheung and Chappell (2002) describe how operating characteristics can be less sensitive to certain working model choices. O'Quigley and Zohar (2010) indicate that an "unreasonable" choice may have a negative impact on operating characteristics. Unfortunately it is not easy to provide a sharp and precise definition as to what we mean by "reasonable" and the only operationally useful definition of a reasonable model would be one that exhibits good robustness properties. Some working models, while respecting the constraints of Shen and O'Quigley (1996) required for convergence, might be anticipated to be not reasonable in this sense. Lee and Cheung (2009) provide algorithms which can furnish a satisfactory, if not optimal, working model. Their approach is based on that of indifference intervals described in Cheung and Chappell (2002). A somewhat different strategy for tackling the same question was adopted by Yin and Yuan (2009). These authors suggested that, rather than identify a single working model, we work with a class of working models and make progress by appealing to the technique of Bayesian model averaging (BMA). This technique makes use of the posterior estimates for the relevant toxic probabilities and these are then weighted with respect to the corresponding posterior model probabilities. Daimon et al. (2011) also considered making use of several working models, selecting one model via an adaptive technique based on different criteria. Yin and Yuan (2009) showed that their approach leads to some gains in robustness and can therefore provide some added assurance that the results of a study are not unduly influenced by arbitrary design features.

## 2.9  DISCUSSION

The CRM is often referred to as the Bayesian alternative to the classic up and down designs used in Phase I studies. This is quite an inaccurate description since, as seen here, there is nothing particularly Bayesian about the CRM. Furthermore, the driving ideas and algorithms are very different from those behind the standard up and down design. In O'Quigley et al. (1990), for the sake of simplicity, Bayesian estimators and vague priors were proposed. However, there is nothing to prevent us working with other estimators, in particular the maximum likelihood estimator as described in Section 2.3.

More fully Bayesian approaches, and not simply a Bayesian estimator, have been suggested for use in the context of Phase I trial designs. By more fully we mean more in the Bayesian spirit of inference, in which we quantify prior information, observed from outside the trial as well as that solicited from clinicians and/or pharmacologists. Decisions are made more formally using tools from decision theory. Any prior information can subsequently be incorporated via the Bayesian formula into a posterior density that also involves the actual current observations. Given the typically small sample sizes often used, a fully Bayesian approach has some appeal in that we would not wish to waste any relevant information at hand. Gatsonis and Greenhouse (1992) consider two-parameter probit and logit models for dose response and study the effect of different prior distributions.

Whitehead and Williamson (1998) carried out similar studies but with attention focusing on logistic models and beta priors. Whitehead and Williamson (1998) worked with some of the more classical notions from optimal design for choosing the dose levels in a bid to establish whether much is lost by using suboptimal designs. O'Quigley et al. (1990) ruled out criteria based on optimal design due to the ethical criterion of the need to attempt to assign the sequentially included patients at the most appropriate level for the patient. This same point was also emphasized by Whitehead and Williamson (1998) where they suggest that the CRM could be viewed as a special case of their designs with their second parameter being assigned a degenerate prior and thereby behaving as a constant. This view is technically correct but does not give the full story in that, for the single sample case, two-parameter CRM and one-parameter CRM have a more important difference relating to consistency.

Two-parameter CRM was seen to behave poorly (O'Quigley et al. 1990) and is generally inconsistent (Shen and O'Quigley 1996). We have to view the single parameter as necessary in the homogeneous case because, unless we violate the allocation rule (for example, by introducing some randomization into the design), the model is otherwise overspecified. Two parameters are not identifiable.

A quite different Bayesian approach has been proposed by Babb et al. (1998). The context is fully Bayesian. Rather than aim to concentrate experimentation at some target level as does CRM, the aim here is to escalate as fast as possible toward the MTD, while sequentially safeguarding against overdosing. This is interesting in that it could be argued that the aim of the approach translates in some ways more directly the clinician's objective than does CRM. Model mis-specification within the context of overdose control was further investigated by Chu et al. (2009). The approach appears promising and the methodology may be a useful modification of CRM when primary concern is on avoiding overdosing and we are in a position to have a prior on a two-parameter function.

## REFERENCES

Ahn C. (1998). An evaluation of phase I cancer clinical trial designs. *Statistics in Medicine*, 17(14): 1537–1549.

Babb J, Rogatko A, Zacks S. (1998). Cancer phase I clinical trials: Efficient dose escalation with overdose control. *Statistics in Medicine*, 17: 1103–1120.

Braun TM. (2002). The bivariate continual reassessment method. Extending the CRM to phase I trials of two competing outcomes. *Control Clinical Trials*, 23(3): 240–256.

Cheung YK, Chappell R. (2002). A simple technique to evaluate model sensitivity in the continual reassessment method. *Biometrics*, 58: 671–674.

Chevret S. (1993). The continual reassessment method in cancer phase I clinical trials: A simulation study. *Statistics in Medicine*, 12(12): 1093–1108.

Chu P, Lin Y, Shih WJ. (2009). Unifying CRM and EWOC designs for phase I cancer clinical trials. *Journal of Statistical Planning and Inference*, 139(3): 1146–1163.

Conaway M, Dunbar S, Peddada S. (2004). Designs for single-or multiple-agent phase I trials. *Biometrics*, 45: 661–669.

Daimon S, Zohar S, O'Quigley J. (2011). Bayesian adaptive model-selecting continual reassessment methods in phase I dose-finding clinical trials. *Statistics in Medicine*, 30(13): 1563–1573.

Garrett-Mayer E. (2006). The continual reassessment method for dose-finding studies: A tutorial. *Clinical Trials*, 3(1): 57–71.

Gatsonis C, Greenhouse JB. (1992). Bayesian methods for phase I clinical trials. *Statistics in Medicine*, 11: 1377–1389.

Gelfand A, Ghosh S. (1998). Model choice: A minimum posterior predictive loss approach. *Biometrika*, 85: 1–11.

Goodman S, Zahurak ML, Piantadosi S. (1995). Some practical improvements in the continual reassessment method for phase I studies. *Statistics in Medicine*, 14: 1149–1161.

Gooley TA, Martin PJ, Fisher LD, Pettinger M. (1994). Simulation as a design tool for phase I/II clinical trials: An example from bone marrow transplantation. *Control Clin Trials*, 15(6): 450–462.

Iasonos A, Wilton AS, Riedel ER, Seshan VE, Spriggs DR. (2008). A comprehensive comparison of the continual reassessment method to the standard 3 + 3 dose escalation scheme in phase I dose-finding studies. *Clinical Trials*, 5:465–477.

Iasonos A, Zohar S, O'Quigley J. (2011). Incorporating lower grade toxicity information into dose finding designs. *Clinical Trials*, 8(4): 370–379.

Korn EL, Midthune D, Chen TT, Rubinstein LV, Christian MC, Simon R. (1994). A comparison of two phase I trial designs. *Statistics in Medicine*, 18: 1799–1806.

Lee SM, Cheung YK. (2009). Model calibration in the continual reassessment method. *Clinical Trials*, 6(3): 227–238.

Moller S. (1995). An extension of the continual reassessment method using a preliminary up and down design in a dose finding study in cancer patients in order to investigate a greater number of dose levels. *Statistics in Medicine*, 14: 911–922.

Natarajan L, O'Quigley J. (2003). Interval estimates of the probability of toxicity at the maximum tolerated dose for small samples. *Statistics in Medicine*, 22: 1829–1836.

O'Quigley J. (1992). Estimating the probability of toxicity at the recommended dose following a phase I clinical trial in cancer. *Biometrics*, 48: 853–862.

O'Quigley J. (1999). Another look at two phase I clinical trial designs (with commentary). *Statistics in Medicine*, 18: 2683–2692.

O'Quigley J. (2002). Continual reassessment designs with early termination. *Biostatistics,* 3(1): 87–99.

O'Quigley J. (2006). Theoretical study of the continual reassessment method. *Journal of Statistical Planning and Inference,* 136(6): 1765–1780.

O'Quigley J, Chevret S. (1991). Methods for dose finding studies in cancer clinical trials: A review and results of a Monte Carlo study. *Statistics in Medicine*, 10: 1647–1664.

O'Quigley J, Hughes MD, Fenton T. (2001). Dose-finding designs for HIV studies. *Biometrics*, 57(4): 1018–1029.

O'Quigley J, Paoletti X, Maccario J. (2002). Non-parametric optimal design in dose finding studies. *Biostatistics,* 3(1): 51–56.

O'Quigley J, Hughes MD, Fenton T, Pei L. (2010). Dynamic calibration of pharmacokinetic parameters in dose-finding studies. *Biostatistics*, 11(3): 537–545.

O'Quigley J, Paoletti X. (2003). Continual reassessment method for ordered groups. *Biometrics*, 59: 430–440.

O'Quigley J, Pepe M, Fisher L. (1990). Continual reassessment method: A practical design for phase I clinical trials in cancer. *Biometrics*, 46: 33–48.

O'Quigley J, Reiner E. (1998). A stopping rule for the continual reassessment method. *Biometrika*, 85(3): 741–748.

O'Quigley J, Shen LZ. (1996). Continual reassessment method: A likelihood approach. *Biometrics*, 52: 673–684.

O'Quigley J, Shen L, Gamst A. (1999). Two sample continual reassessment method. *Journal of Biopharmaceutical Statistics*, 9: 17–44.

O'Quigley J, Zohar S. (2010). Retrospective robustness of the continual reassessment method. *Journal of Biopharmaceutical Statistics*, 20(5): 1013–1025.

Patnaik A, Warner E, Michael M, Egorin M, Moore M, Siu L, Fracasso P et al. (2000). Phase I dose-finding and pharmacokinetic study of paclitaxel and carboplatin with oral valspodar in patients with advanced solid tumors. *Journal of Clinical Oncology*, 18: 3677–3689.

Piantadosi S, Fisher JD, Grossman S. (1998). Practical implementation of a modified continual reassessment method for dose-finding trials. *Cancer Chemotheraphy and Pharmacology*, 41(6): 429–436.

Piantadosi S, Liu G. (1996). Improved designs for dose escalation studies using pharmacokinetic measurements. *Statistics in Medicine*, 15(15): 1605–1618.

Reiner E, Paoletti X, O'Quigley. (1998). Operating characteristics of the standard phase I clinical trial design. *Computational Statistics and Data Analysis*, 30: 303–315.

Shen LZ, O'Quigley J. (1996). Consistency of continual reassessment method in dose finding studies. *Biometrika*, 83: 395–406.

Shu J, O'Quigley J. (2008). Dose-escalation designs in oncology: ADEPT and the CRM. *Statistics in Medicine*, 27(26): 5345–5353; discussion 5354–5355.

Silvapulle MJ. (1981). On the existence of maximum likelihood estimators for the binomial response models. *Journal of the Royal Statistical Society: Series B*, 3: 310–313.

Storer BE. (1989). Design and analysis of phase I clinical trials. *Biometrics*, 45: 925–937.

Storer BE. (1993). Small-sample confidence sets for the MTD in a phase I clinical trial. *Biometrics*, 49: 1117–1125.

Storer BE. (1998). Phase I clinical trials. In *Encyclopedia of Biostatistics*, Wiley, New York.

Thall PF, Sung H, Choudhury A. (2001). Dose-finding based on feasibility and toxicity in T-cell infusion trials. *Biometrics*, 57: 914–921.

Wages N, Conaway M, O'Quigley J. (2011). Continual reassessment method for partial ordering. *Biometrics*. doi: 10.1111/j.1541–0420.2011.01560.x.

Wages N, Conaway M, O'Quigley J. (2011). Dose-finding design for multi-drug combinations. *Clinical Trials*, 8(4): 380–389.

Whitehead J, Williamson D. (1998) Bayesian decision procedures based on logistic regression models for dose-finding studies. *Journal of Biopharmaceutical Statistics*, 8: 445–467.

Yin G, Yuan Y. (2009). Bayesian model averaging continual reassessment method in phase I clinical trials. *Journal of the American Statistical Association*, 104: 954–968.

Zohar S, Chevret S. (2001). The continual reassessment method: Comparison of Bayesian stopping rules for dose-ranging studies. *Stat Med.*, 20(19): 2827–2843.

# 3 Pharmacokinetics in Clinical Oncology
## *Statistical Issues*

*Gary L. Rosner, Peter Müller, Simon Lunagomez, and Patrick A. Thompson*

## CONTENTS

## 3.1 INTRODUCTION

All drugs share the feature that they are formulated to have an effect on some body system. In oncology, that effect may be to shrink the size of a tumor, reduce the growth rate of the tumor, or protect noncancer cells from potentially harmful effects of the chemotherapy, to name a few examples. Pharmacokinetics (PK) is the study of what happens to drugs once they enter the body. The study of a drug's PK will often entail drawing blood samples to measure the concentration of the compound, possibly along with metabolites, over time. In some instances, it is even possible to measure the amount of the drug or metabolite in the tumor tissue itself, such as in leukemia, or in the microenvironment in which the cancer resides, such as through the use of microdialysis (Brunner and Müller 2002).

It is generally not enough to know the PK of the drug, since we are most interested in the clinical effect of the drug. Pharmacodynamics (PD) is the study of how

PK relates to measured outcomes, such as clinical response, risk of toxicity, or even some in vitro measure of cellular response to a drug. A perhaps overly simplistic, though useful, characterization of PK and PD is that PK measures what happens to the drug after it enters the body and PD measures what happens to the body after the introduction of the drug.

As with other aspects of biomedical science and clinical research in the beginning of the twenty-first century, researchers have begun to look into genetic variation and associations with the PK and PD of drugs. Although there do not yet appear to be firm definitions, the terms pharmacogenetics and pharmacogenomics describe such studies. We will differentiate these two areas of study with the following definitions. Pharmacogenetics studies the heritable factors that contribute to PK and PD variation in a population. That is, how does genetic variation within and between populations contribute to clinical differences in how individuals react or respond to drugs? Pharmacogenomics, on the other hand, examines how mutations and other differences at the level of the genome might provide useful targets for drug development. The National Institutes of Health of the United States is supporting a large effort to aid research into pharmacogenetics and pharmacogenomics (Klein et al. 2001).

The statistical issues that arise in pharmacogenetic studies are similar to the issues that arise in most genetic epidemiology studies. For example, if one has identified a gene associated with the metabolism of an anticancer drug and one wishes to see if genetic variation at this allele is associated with different risks of toxicity, one may wish to carry out a study prospectively or retrospectively. The prospective study design might call for blood samples at entry to the study, with genotyping. Then one would look for associations between genotype and whether or not a patient experienced toxicity. For a retrospective study, one might identify patients who have experienced toxicity and find an appropriate control group, perhaps with matching. Then one would only have to genotype this subset of the study's patients for analysis of the association between toxicity and genotype. Obviously, if some genetic variants put the patient at risk of fatal toxicity, the retrospective design may well miss these patients without banked blood samples.

Some of the other statistical issues that arise in pharmacogenetic studies include single nucleotide polymorphism (SNP) studies and determination of haplotypes. With the many variants at specific loci within a gene, there exists the potential for carrying out many hypothesis tests and declaring false positive associations. Furthermore, many SNPs are in linkage disequilibrium, meaning they tend to move together and be highly correlated. One can gain some extra power by grouping SNPs together if they are highly correlated with each other. Statistical techniques to group SNPs into such groups, called haplotype blocks, are an endeavor carried out in pharmacogenetic studies, as well as other genetic-based studies. More information is contained in the chapter on haplotypes in this volume. Also, information about pharmacogenomics, in general, and oncology-specific issues are contained in recent edited volumes (Licinio and Wong 2002; Innocenti 2008).

In this chapter, we will explore some of the main statistical issues in the study of PK and PD in clinical oncology. Most of these same issues arise in clinical research relating to other diseases, but our focus is cancer.

## 3.2 PHARMACOKINETICS AND PHARMACODYNAMICS OF ANTICANCER AGENTS

The most common basis for determining a drug's PK is measured drug concentration in the blood. PK studies call for drawing blood samples during and/or after an infusion and assaying the concentration of the compound in the blood. The relationship between the drug's concentrations and time is characterized by a system of differential equations that defines a pharmacokinetic model (Gibaldi and Perrier 1982). Quite often, the differential equations incorporate the so-called compartments to allow for changes in the loglinear decay of the drug after the end of the infusion. These differential equations describe the instantaneous change in concentration of the drug or its metabolites within each compartment, with direct or indirect communication between compartments.

We often use compartmental models to characterize the relationship between plasma concentration and time, primarily because they seem to fit and have a physiologic interpretation. The compartments in these models are based on the notion that the drug circulates through the body in the blood stream and may visit other parts of the body before it is eliminated. The plasma or blood compartment may be considered the central compartment for a drug that is infused intravenously, but the drug will likely pass through the liver, kidneys, and, hopefully, the tumor. Eventually, most of the drug returns to the compartment from which it is eliminated, which may be the central compartment. The transit between the plasma and these other organs or "compartments" forms part of the system of differential equations characterizing the change in concentration over time. Figure 3.1 illustrates a simple two-compartment model.

Depending on the form of the differential equation describing the instantaneous rate of change of a compartment's concentration, the kinetics may be linear or nonlinear. A drug is said to have linear kinetics if, for two different doses, the concentrations that result from each dose are proportional to the doses. If, however, the

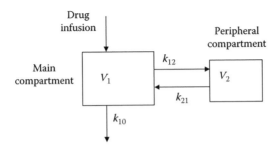

**FIGURE 3.1** Simple two-compartment model characterizing the disposition of a drug given by continuous infusion.

concentrations arising from different doses are not proportional to doses, then the drug exhibits nonlinear kinetics. Nonlinear kinetics can occur if a process gets saturated, so that no matter what the concentration, the rate of change remains constant. At the risk of over simplification, the drug exhibits linear kinetics if one can take the concentration–time curve associated with one dose of the drug, rescale and, perhaps, shift it and end up with the concentration–time curve associated with another dose. Modeling nonlinear kinetics is more difficult computationally, because there is no analytic solution to the differential equations. Instead, one has to find the solution numerically.

Generally, one has to use a nonlinear regression package, such as the nls() function in $R$, to estimate an individual's PK model parameters. When analyzing a series of data for individuals in a study, one has to use more specialized computer programs to deal with the nonlinear repeated measurements. Discovering algorithms for fitting nonlinear repeated-measurements data continues to be an area of active research, with some development relating to modeling HIV dynamics (Delyon et al. 1999; Huang et al. 2006; Samson et al. 2006). There are software packages specifically for fitting PK models. Please see the end of this chapter for a list of several noncommercial packages for fitting pharmacokinetic models. In the compartmental model, the unknown parameters to estimate include the volumes of the compartments and the rate constants for the movement of drug between compartments and out of the body. The volume of distribution, labeled $V_1$ in Figure 3.1, is the hypothetical volume of the main compartment from which we measure the concentrations over time. Being a parameter in the PK model, the volume of distribution is hypothetical in the sense that it is generally not interpretable as the volume of plasma, say, in the body. Patient-specific estimates of volumes of distribution often exhibit greater variability and sometimes much larger values than one would expect for the volume of blood in human bodies. In essence, the compartment-specific volumes of distribution and rate parameters are model parameters that have a theoretical interpretation loosely based on physiologic considerations.

Some of the basic parameters that describe the PK of a drug include clearance, area-under-the-concentration–time curve (AUC), steady-state concentration ($C_{ss}$), the elimination half-life, volume of distribution, the elimination rate parameter, and bioavailability for drugs administered via a route other than directly into the blood stream. These characteristics of the PK of a drug are either explicit parameters in the concentration–time function or are functions of the model parameters. Clearance, measured in volume per unit time (e.g., L/h), is most often used to characterize a drug or to compare a drug's PK in different populations. By clearance, one generally means *total body clearance*, that is, the sum of the individual clearances of the drug from all organs. Another important measure is the AUC, which is a measure of systemic exposure to the drug. The AUC is usually given in units of concentration times time (e.g., $\mu g \times h/mL$). If a drug is given by intravenous infusion, clearance (CL) and AUC are inversely proportional, with the proportionality being the infused dose. That is, $CL = d_{i.v.}/AUC$, where $d_{i.v.}$ is the administered dose.

Many anticancer drugs are given by constant continuous intravenous infusion over an extended period of time. During the infusion, plasma concentrations of the drug increase but eventually reach a constant value if the infusion lasts long enough. The $C_{ss}$ is, as the name implies, the plateau concentration reached in the plasma during continuous infusion at a constant rate. Steady-state concentration and clearance are inversely proportional to each other. The proportionality constant is the infusion rate, that is, $CL = InfRate/C_{ss}$.

The elimination half-life is the time it takes for half of the administered dose to be eliminated from the body. Usually, the plasma concentration is within 10% of the $C_{ss}$ after an infusion lasting four half-lives of the drug.

These PK-derived parameters are functions of the compartmental model's parameters. Thus, once one has fit the model, one can estimate these derived parameters. One can estimate some PK parameters without fitting a compartmental model. As indicated earlier, one can estimate total-body clearance if one has an estimate of the $C_{ss}$ during a continuous infusion at a constant infusion rate. Another example is a so-called noncompartmental estimate of the AUC. If one has enough concentration–time pairs for a patient, one can use the trapezoidal rule to compute the area under the concentration–time curve. If the final concentration is not zero, a reasonable approximation might be a simple exponential decay with slope based on the logarithm of the last two concentrations. This estimate for the AUC is attractive, since it does not depend on any model assumptions. Usually, however, authors report the estimated AUC without any attempt to attach a measure of uncertainty to the estimate.

Many anticancer drugs are available in oral form, which is more convenient in case of chronic dosing or for patients who may find it difficult to get to a clinic. When drugs are taken orally, they pass through and are disseminated from the gut. Ultimately, the drug reaches the circulation system, from which it will get to the rest of the body. Bioavailability relates to the biological availability of the active compound in the drug. Estimation often derives from individual estimates of PK relating the amount of drug or active metabolite in the blood stream after oral administration to the amount of the drug in the blood stream after intravenous administration. Bioavailability will typically be between 0 and 1. Variation in bioavailability, which has to be estimated, contributes to PK and PD variability. Estimates of bioavailability derive from PK studies in which each subject receives the drug via different administration, usually in a crossover study. Bioequivalence, a related concept, refers to the evaluation of two different formulations of the same drug, such as comparing a generic formulation to the original formulation. If two formulations are bioequivalent, then one assumes they will act the same way and have the same effectiveness. Statistical issues include designing crossover studies and modeling within-subject and between-subject sources of variation (Chow and Liu 2009).

The disposition of a drug in the plasma or tissue may be affected by many factors, including genetic factors, environmental factors, diet, age, and other drugs being taken or foods being digested at the same time the drug is in the body. As part of the learning about a drug's PK, one will often look for associations between patient characteristics and patient-specific PK parameters. A common approach is to fit separate models to each patient's concentration–time data and then carry out statistical inference on the patient-specific PK model parameter estimates. This two-stage approach ignores uncertainty in the parameter estimates, and may thereby lead to false declarations of significant differences. For example, one might regress each patient-specific AUC or clearance on age or smoking status or genotype to look for patterns or potentially significant differences. Analyses of patient-specific model estimates and covariates are exploratory, since they typically ignore the uncertainty in the PK-derived parameters. Inference that accounts for all sources of uncertainty is preferable.

PK modelers have long realized that there is heterogeneity between individuals in terms of subject-specific model parameters. This realization led to the use of mixed-effects models and hierarchical modeling, allowing for between and within variation. Sheiner et al. (1972, 1977, 1979a) were among the first to recognize the usefulness of these models for predicting the time course of a drug's concentration for individuals. Other researchers followed up on these ideas, and this research led to a general approach to studying variation of the PK of a drug in a population, called population modeling (Racine-Poon and Smith 1990). Population modeling is, essentially, a hierarchical model, as in Equation 3.1:

$$y_{ij} = f\left(t_{ij}, \theta_i\right) + e_{ij}, e_{ij} \sim F \quad \text{with } E\left[e_{ij}\right] = 0$$

$$\theta_i \mid \theta_0 \sim G\left(\theta\right) \quad \text{with } E\left[\theta_i\right] = \theta_0 \tag{3.1}$$

$$\theta_0 \sim H\left(\bullet\right)$$

In this equation, $y_{ij}$ is the $j$th concentration of the drug at time $t_{ij}$ for the $i$th patient. The patient's own model parameters are denoted by $\theta_i$, which are assumed randomly distributed in the population. The population distribution of these individual parameters $\theta_i$ is characterized by $G$ and indexed by parameter $\theta_0$, corresponding to the mean of the $\theta_i$ in Equation 3.1. The population distribution, $G$, may involve other unknown parameters, such as the variance or regression-type parameters relating subject-specific means to covariates. We express our uncertainty about the mean parameter value in the population through the hyperprior distribution denoted $H$. The residual difference between the measured concentrations for the $i$th patient at time $t_{ij}$ and the modeled concentrations is a random variable $e_{ij}$ having zero mean and distribution $F$.

Typically, the distribution of the residuals is considered normal or lognormal. The variance may be a function of the mean concentration level, such as when one wishes to fit a constant coefficient of variation model. The distribution of subject-specific model parameters is also often treated as normal or lognormal. A frequentist analysis would typically stop at the level of the population distribution. A Bayesian analysis, on the other hand, will also specify a distribution for the parameters in the population distribution via a hyperprior distribution. The inclusion of a hyperprior and hyperparameters allows for between-individual variation while learning about the distribution of subject-specific parameters. A Bayesian hierarchical model also makes prediction for a new patient straightforward. The book by Davidian and Giltinan describes well many of the frequentist and Bayesian methods for analyzing repeated measures having a nonlinear relationship with time (Davidian and Giltinan 1995).

### 3.2.1 EXAMPLE

As an example, we consider the analysis of the anticancer agent methotrexate in infants (children less than 1 year old) with leukemia. The clinical prognosis for children younger than 1 year old who are diagnosed with acute lymphoblastic leukemia (ALL) is worse than for older children. It may be that the disease is different or, perhaps, the infant's organs, particularly the kidneys, are not yet fully developed, causing the PK of anticancer drugs to be different in the infants.

Children with ALL often receive methotrexate as part of their chemotherapeutic treatment regimen. Methotrexate is cleared from the body by the kidneys, and variability in the drug's PK may be associated with key measures of renal function, such as glomerular filtration rate (GFR), tubular secretion, and renal blood flow. Each of these characteristics of renal function change as the kidneys mature during the first few months after birth. Additionally, the liver may continue to develop after birth, leading to altered drug metabolism during the first few months of life. Thus, as infants develop, there may be changes in the drug's absorption, distribution, metabolism, and elimination.

Little is known about the PK of methotrexate in very young children. Therefore, pediatric oncologists were interested to learn what they could by collecting data as part of a larger study carried out by the Children's Oncology Group (COG). In this study, infants with ALL received methotrexate as a high-dose infusion ($4\,g/m^2$) over 24h on weeks 4, 5, 11, and 12 from the start of the treatment regimen. The infusion was divided into an initial $200\,mg/m^2$ loading dose given over 20min, followed by $3.8\,g/m^2$ infused over 23h and 40min, the remainder of the 24h infusion duration. The patients received 24h infusions of methotrexate a week apart and again 7 and 8 weeks after the first infusion of the drug.

The PK study combined data from two sources. As part of routine monitoring of the infants on the study, some blood samples allowed the measurement of methotrexate concentration levels. The patient charts held these data, allowing for retrospective collection. The remaining patients in our sample underwent more extensive sampling. Aside from the dose of methotrexate actually received and concentration–time data, the dataset also included patient characteristics, such as age, height, weight, body-surface area, and serum creatinine. The protocol called for measuring methotrexate levels within each course of therapy at the end of the 24h infusion and every 24h following the end of the infusion until the concentration was less than $0.18\,\mu M$. The 18 patients who underwent more extensive sampling had their additional blood draws during their first methotrexate infusion. Sample collection for this subset of the patients was at 1, 6, 12, and 23h after the start of the first methotrexate infusion.

Altogether, the dataset included 70 patients with enough information to model at least one course of methotrexate. We could analyze data during the first course of therapy for 62 patients. The dataset contained a total of 686 methotrexate concentration–time pairs measured during 199 doses of methotrexate given to the 70 infants.

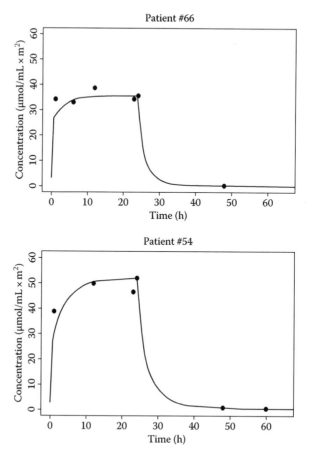

**FIGURE 3.2** Observed and fitted methotrexate concentrations for two infants in the study. The lines are based on point-wise posterior means.

The primary measure of kidney function in the dataset was an estimate of the GFR. The estimate is a function of the infant's length and the creatinine measured in the infant's plasma (Schwartz et al. 1984, 1987).

Figure 3.2 shows the concentration–time data for two of the more extensively sampled patients during their first course of methotrexate. One sees in the figures how the concentrations approach a plateau corresponding the $C_{ss}$ over the course of the 24 h infusion. The figures also show that these two patients have quite different $C_{ss}$ (around 52 $\mu$mol/(mL $\times$ m$^2$) versus around 35 $\mu$mol/(mL $\times$ m$^2$)).

As indicated earlier, one can estimate the total-body clearance of a drug from the $C_{ss}$ and the infusion rate. Even though the infusion rate was not constant over the 24 h infusion, it was constant after the first 20 min. Therefore, it seemed reasonable to estimate the clearance at steady state from these data.

If one estimates clearance from the end-of-infusion or 23 and 24 h concentrations and uses these estimates in a regression analyses with patient covariates, then one is ignoring the uncertainty associated with these estimates. Ignoring this uncertainty may result in a false-positive finding of an association between clearance and patient characteristics. Instead, we chose to fit a population or hierarchical model. We used the program PKBugs (Lunn et al. 1999), which runs in WinBUGS (Lunn et al. 2000). We fit a model for the log concentrations having a normal residual, with the subject-specific parameters also being lognormal. The full hierarchical model is

$$\log\left(y_{i,j}\right) \sim N\left(\log\left(C\left[t_{i,j},\theta_i,d_i\right]\right),\tau\right)$$

$$\theta_i \sim \text{MVN}\left(X_i\psi,\Omega\right)$$

$$\psi \sim \text{MVN}\left(\psi_0,C\right)$$

$$\tau^{-1} \sim \text{Gamma}\left(0.001,0.001\right), \Omega^{-1} \sim \text{Wishart}\left(R,\rho\right)$$

Here, $y_{i,j}$ is the concentration measured on patient $i$ at time $t_{i,j}$. In the model, $N(\mu, \tau)$ denotes a normal distribution with mean $\mu$ and variance $\tau$, while a multivariate normal distribution with mean vector $\mathbf{m}$ and variance–covariance matrix $\Omega$ is denoted MVN($\mathbf{m}, \Omega$). The compartmental model is denoted $C(t_{i,j}, \theta_i, d_i)$, which is a function of time, model parameters, and dose $d_i$. The function relating concentration to time, parameters, and dose for a two-compartment model (see Figure 3.1) can be written as a sum of two exponential functions (Gibaldi and Perrier 1982; Lunn et al. 1999).

$$C\left(t_{i,j},\theta_i,d_i\right) = A_1 e^{-\lambda_1 t}\left(1 - e^{\lambda_1 t^*}\right) + A_2 e^{-\lambda_2 t}\left(1 - e^{\lambda_2 t^*}\right)$$

$$T = \text{infusion duration}$$

$$t^* = \min\left(t,T\right)$$

$$A_i = \frac{k_0\left(k_{21} - \lambda_i\right)}{V_1\lambda_i\left(\lambda_{3-i} - \lambda_i\right)}, \quad i = 1,2$$

$$k_0 = \text{infusion rate} = \text{dose/infusion duration}$$

The two parameters $\lambda_1$ and $\lambda_2$ are functions of the rate parameters shown in Figure 3.1. They satisfy the following two equations, in terms of the rate constants:

$$\lambda_1 + \lambda_2 = k_{10} + k_{12} + k_{21} \text{ and } \lambda_1\lambda_2 = k_{10}k_{21} \quad \text{with } \lambda_1 > \lambda_2 \text{ by definition}$$

The patient-specific model parameters are $\theta_i$. This vector includes the four parameters in the pharmacokinetic model, namely, log(CL), log(Q), log($V_1$), and log($V_2$), recalling that each patient has his or her own set of parameters. Here, $V_1$ and $V_2$ are the respective volumes of the central and peripheral compartments shown in

Figure 3.1. The CL equals $V_1$ times $k_{10}$. The parameter $Q$ is called the distributional clearance between the two compartments, which is assumed to be the same. That is, $Q$ satisfies $Q = k_{12}V_1 = k_{21}V_2$.

Returning to the hierarchical model, the hyperparameters had the following values. The variance matrix for the patient-specific parameters ($\Omega$) had an inverse-Wishart prior with $\rho = 4$ degrees of freedom and scale matrix $R$ corresponding to 50% coefficient of variation for each parameter. The parameters, in turn, may depend on patient characteristics $X_i$ (e.g., the age or GFR for child $i$) through a linear regression with coefficients $\psi$. These regression coefficients had a multivariate normal prior with variance matrix $C$ equal to $10^4$ times the identity matrix. The hypermean $\psi_0$ for the regression coefficients was a vector with nonzero values for the PK parameter-specific intercepts and zero for the covariate effects. The nonzero hypermeans came from an analysis of related data.

Figure 3.2 shows the PKBugs fits to the data as the solid line. These are the piecewise posterior mean concentrations for the patients over time. Having fit the model, we examined potential relationships with covariates by plotting the posterior means of the parameters or functions of the parameters against the potential covariates (Wakefield 1996). We did not find a strong relationship between age (0 and 12 months) and clearance, given the large amount of noise in these data. Nevertheless, since the primary question motivating this study concerned an association between age and clearance among the infants, we modeled the logarithm of clearance as a function of age in the population PK (hierarchical) model. The posterior mean of the coefficient was 0.034 (posterior standard deviation = 0.038). We did not find any strong associations between the covariates available to us and PK in this dataset. Further modeling based on exploratory plots mentioned in the previous paragraph suggested an association between the model-derived parameters GFR and clearance.

### 3.2.2 NONPARAMETRIC MODEL

In the previous example, we assumed a parametric distribution for the subject-specific parameters in the model. Assuming a normal or lognormal distribution may be restrictive in some cases. Some investigators have sought to incorporate nonparametric estimation of the population distribution (Mallet 1986; Mallet et al. 1988b; Schumitzky 1991, 1993). Bayesian nonparametric modeling removes the assumption that subject-specific PK parameters vary in a population according to a normal distribution. In particular, knowledge that potential effect modifiers exist, such as genetics, different diets, etc., means that there might be multi-modal distributions of the PK parameters in a study population. The earliest attempts to be nonparametric in the population distribution built up mass at discrete locations, according to the data. In this approach (Mallet 1986), the distribution of $\theta_i$ in Equation 3.1 is left completely unspecified (i.e., $\theta_i \sim F$). The likelihood function becomes a function of the unknown distribution function $F$, and the problem becomes one of maximum likelihood estimation of a mixing distribution (Laird 1978; Lindsay 1983). One can show that the maximum likelihood estimate is a discrete distribution with support on at most $n$ points, where $n$ is the number of patients in the sample (Laird 1978; Mallet 1986).

If one wants to include continuous covariates in the population model, one has to finesse the problem a bit to make it work with the nonparametric approaches discussed in the previous paragraph (Mallet et al. 1988a). Furthermore, one would typically consider modeling the model parameters with a continuous distribution. Davidian and Gallant used smooth nonparametric maximum likelihood to allow for a family of continuous distributions that can incorporate continuous covariates explicitly. The smooth nonparametric maximum likelihood solution to the problem estimates the underlying distribution of a k-variate random vector from a class of densities that are at least $k/2$ times differentiable. A density in the specified class may be represented for all practical purposes as a series expansion of a polynomial times a normal density function (Gallant and Nychka 1987; Davidian and Gallant 1993).

None of these nonparametric or semi-parametric methods are Bayesian, however. Instead, they are mixed-effects models with unspecified distributions for the random effects. One can, however, carry out full Bayesian inference in a hierarchical model with nonlinear regression functions and still be nonparametric. Wakefield and Walker (1997) used a Dirichlet process (Ferguson 1973) prior for the distribution of the subject-specific parameters in a hierarchical model with a nonlinear regression, such as a compartmental PK model. The Dirichlet process (DP) is a distribution on the space of distributions, allowing inference on the underlying distribution of parameters and, thereby, greater flexibility. With a DP prior for the subject-specific parameters, however, the posterior is necessarily discrete.

We have found that a Dirichlet process mixture allows for nonparametric and semiparametric modeling for these problems (West et al. 1994; Escobar and West 1995; Müller and Rosner 1998). Instead of the subject-specific parameters having a DP prior, they have a parametric prior (e.g., normal or other distributional family) with a DP prior on the parameters of that distribution. Simply put, with a normal prior at the population level with random subject-specific means and a DP prior on those means, the prior model for the subject-specific parameters becomes a mixture of normals, with the weights and locations coming from a Dirichlet process hyperprior. The distribution of subject-specific parameters in the population is a mixture of continuous densities, such as normal densities, with mixing (i.e., random weights) over the random locations (means). The Dirichlet process is the prior mixing measure. The discrete nature of the posterior from a Dirichlet process prior is not a problem, since this prior is on the locations of a continuous density. Thus, the posterior distribution is continuous with this model. Covariates are incorporated via the conditional distribution of the parameters, given the covariates. The result is a semi-parametric regression yielding a smooth curve as a weighted mixture of linear regressions over the range of the covariates.

### 3.2.2.1  Nonparametric Example

We first applied a Dirichlet process mixture model to a dataset consisting of white blood cell counts measured while patients are receiving increasing doses of a chemotherapeutic drug in a phase I study (Müller and Rosner 1997, 1998; Rosner and Müller 1997). For cytotoxic cancer chemotherapy, myelosuppression (lowered blood counts) is a common side effect, getting more severe as doses increase. Thus, there is great interest in monitoring patients' blood counts as a pharmacodynamic end point, especially when escalating doses in a phase I study.

The analysis of blood count data for cancer patients receiving myelosuppressive doses of chemotherapy is an example of a pharmacodynamic analysis of a nonlinear model for repeated measurement data. We implemented the Dirichlet process mixture model to analyze these data, with the dose of the drug serving as the pharmacologic covariate. The model can also be fit to other repeated measurements, including drug concentrations measured over time.

Non-Bayesian analyses of the time-course of blood count data using nonlinear models for repeated measurements data have also appeared in the pharmacodynamics literature. Karlsson et al. (1995) used a spline-based model to analyze similar data, although with splines they had to constrain each patient's profile to return to baseline at the end of the course of chemotherapy. There are also models that incorporate PK and PD simultaneously by hypothesizing an "effect" compartment (Sheiner et al. 1979b; Unadkat et al. 1986; Verotta and Sheiner 1987). These analyses via a so-called indirect-response model have not yet been much studied in the statistical literature. Minami et al. (1998, 2001) used this approach to model blood count data collected on cancer patients receiving different chemotherapeutic drugs. Recently, a mechanistic model based on physiologic considerations of neutrophil formation has found application in modeling myelosuppression by anticancer agents (Friberg et al. 2002; Friberg and Karlsson 2003).

### 3.2.2.2  Combining Data

Another statistical issue in studies of population PK of drugs concerns combining data from multiple sources. Combining analyses across different population pharmacokinetic or pharmacodynamic studies would seem to be a good way to learn more about the distribution of PK parameters in the general population, or to allow for more precise inference on the effects of patient characteristics on PK. With mixture priors, it is not at all obvious how to combine data in a sensible way that leads to borrowing strength across the studies but still allows for each study to maintain its own idiosyncrasies as characterized through the flexible mixture model. We have developed a method for use with finite mixtures, allowing for a common measure and study-specific mixtures (Lopes et al. 2003). We have also developed an ANOVA-like decomposition of the random locations in a Dirichlet process via the dependent Dirichlet process (De Iorio et al. 2004). This appears to be a useful modeling strategy for such meta-analyses, since they maintain flexibility in the inference and allow for different degrees of exchangeability.

### 3.2.2.3  Dose Individualization

With the ability to model a drug's PK and, simultaneously account for between-individual variation, came the realization of the potential to predict a person's individual PK if given the drug. This realization then led to the possibility of PK-guided dosing, meaning that physicians and clinical pharmacologists can tailor the dose of a drug for an individual to that individual's own ability to handle the drug. Other areas of clinical medicine benefited from the use of PK-guided dosing, including the use of antibiotics (Jelliffe 1986; Jelliffe et al. 1991, 1993). Several researchers called for PK-guided dosing in medical oncology, recognizing that the of ten narrow therapeutic window (i.e., the narrow range of doses that are neither too toxic nor too low to allow for clinical efficacy) might be made wider if patients received doses that would be expected to lead to systemic exposure in some target range. Attempts to use PK to guide dosing in cancer have also appeared but have not yet been put into practice (Collins 1990; Ratain et al. 1991; D'Argenio and Rodman 1993).

### 3.2.2.4 Dose Individualization Example

An example of a fully Bayesian design for pharmacologically guided dosing in cancer is given by a study from the University of Texas MD Anderson Cancer Center. Our clinical collaborator treats patients with leukemia using bone marrow transplantation. With this form of anticancer therapy, the patient receives ultrahigh doses of chemotherapy. The drugs are highly toxic, and at these doses, the patient's blood cells are virtually wiped out. Without circulating white blood cells, people are subject to potentially fatal infection from pathogens that would otherwise not cause much of a reaction. In order to help the patient's body recover its ability to produce white blood cells, the transplant oncologist infuses either bone marrow or peripheral blood stem cells. An allogeneic transplant is one in which the patient receives cells from a donor, one who matches the patient in some way. Autologous transplants reinfuse cells removed from the patient prior to the ultrahigh-dose chemotherapy.

In transplant therapy, the medical oncologist seeks to treat the patient with doses that are high enough to kill any and all cancer cells but not so high that the drugs kill the patient. Most transplant regimens give the drugs at fixed doses that are a function of body size as measured by the body-surface area (Chabner and Collins 1990). If there are sources of pharmacokinetic and pharmacodynamic variation beyond body size, some patients may well receive a dose that is either too high or too low.

One might instead define a target range of exposure to the drug, such as via the area-under-the-concentration–time curve or AUC. In fact, our clinical collaborator told us that he had a target range for the AUC of the drug busulfan when given intravenously. He wanted to design a study in which patients first received a small, nontherapeutic dose of the drug, with blood draws to allow pharmacokinetic analysis. With the pharmacokinetic model fit to the concentration–time data for the test dose, he thought that one could predict the dose that would achieve the desired AUC. We agreed and set about to design this study.

We chose to determine a fully Bayesian design for the study. There was clearly a loss function, namely, achieving an AUC that is either too low or too high, with greater loss as the AUC was farther away from the ends of the target interval. Furthermore, the study called for prediction, for which the Bayesian approach excels. Among other advantages, Bayesian modeling offers the ability to incorporate sources of uncertainty in the algorithm. Finally, we already had data from earlier studies without the test dose. Thus, we could incorporate historical information as prior information to improve precision.

We did not assume that the patients in the two historical studies were fully exchangeable, choosing instead to keep the studies separate in a hierarchical model.

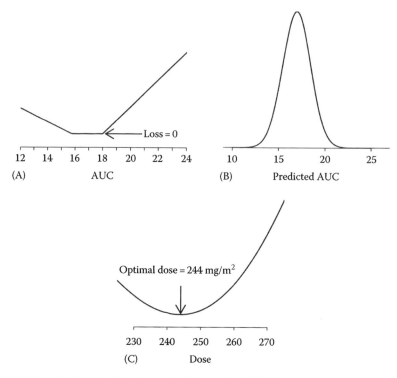

**FIGURE 3.3** (A) The loss function as it relates to the AUC. (B) An example predictive distribution for the AUC if the next patient receives a particular dose. (C) The expected utility as a function of dose, allowing one to determine the optimal dose while incorporating the many sources of uncertainty.

We did, however, want to allow for a Bayesian nonparametric prior distribution in our inference. Therefore, we chose to use the so-called dependent Dirichlet process prior in our model (De Iorio et al. 2004). This model allows for some borrowing of strength across the studies, while still retaining study-specific differences within a larger nonparametric model.

Our utility function consisted of two straight lines on either end of the target AUC range (Figure 3.3A). The slopes of the two lines differed, in that the loss would rise more steeply for exceeding the range than for falling short of it. The reason for the lack of symmetry is that too high a dose might lead to death, whereas too low a dose might still provide some therapeutic benefit to the patient.

Based on the results of the PK analysis of the test dose, along with the information contained in the previous studies, we computed the posterior predictive distribution of the AUC for a host of possible doses. Figure 3.3B shows an example predictive distribution for a hypothetical new patient receiving some fixed dose. The utility function $u(d, y, \theta)$ in this study is minus the loss associated with a given AUC and is a function of the dose of the drug ($d$), the concentrations over time ($y$), and the patient's

PK parameters ($\theta$). Integrating the utility function with respect to the posterior predictive distribution of the AUC for a fixed dose gives the expected loss for that dose. That is, the optimal dose $d^*$ satisfies

$$d^* = \underbrace{\arg\max}_{d} \iint u(d, y, \theta) p_d(y|\theta) p(\theta|\text{Data}) \, dy \, d\theta,$$

where $p_d(y|\theta)$ is the sampling distribution of the future concentrations as a function of dose ($d$) and the PK parameters. Of course, the calculations would refer to a specific patient, but we have suppressed the subscripts for ease of presentation. Over a range of doses and associated expected utilities, one can pick the dose with the highest expected utility (or, in our case, the lowest expected loss), as illustrated in Figure 3.3C. The study we designed will use the patient's test data to tailor the dose of the high-dose chemotherapy to the specific patient. This study is ongoing.

### 3.2.2.5 Design

Another important aspect of designing population studies of PK and PD concerns the timing of measurements. Quite often, pharmacologists choose sampling times based on D-optimality criteria or similar criteria relating to minimizing some function of the variance–covariance matrix. Bayesian optimal design has generally been Bayesian versions of D-optimality and the like (Merlé et al. 1994; Chaloner and Verdinelli 1995; Merlé and Mentré 1995). An early example of using information theory to design a PK study is given by D'Argenio (1990). For a recent review, see Ogungbenro et al. (2009).

### 3.2.2.6 Design Example

We have proposed a fully Bayesian design with a loss function that incorporates inconvenience to the patient (Stroud et al. 2001). The Cancer and Leukemia Group B (CALGB) was preparing to carry out a large study of 3 h infusions of paclitaxel to treat women with metastatic breast cancer. The proposed sample size was large, and the study provided an excellent opportunity to study the pharmacology of this important anticancer drug among a large group of women. Investigators had reported that the PK parameter with the greatest association with myelosuppression, the primary toxicity, was the time during which the concentration of the drug is above some threshold level (Gianni et al. 1995). Therefore, the CALGB was interested in having a good estimate of the time above the threshold concentration and wanted the sampling times to provide for a good estimate.

Estimating the time above some threshold concentration requires drawing samples around the time when one might expect the concentration to drop below the threshold. This requirement means that women would potentially have to stay in the clinic longer than clinically necessary, or even return the next day, in order to ensure that one gets a sample with the most information about when the concentration drops below a threshold. A collaborating clinical pharmacologist suggested, in fact, that the study require a blood sample 24 h after the start of the infusion.

The treating clinicians did not want to require that the women return to the clinic the day after the infusion, arguing that such a requirement would be too disruptive for the women participating in the study. We decided to approach the design question from a decision-theoretic standpoint, by including an increasing cost for times after 7 h from the start of the infusion, which is the length of time the women would be asked to remain in the clinic for routine surveillance. That is, we wanted to find the optimal times in order to maximize the precision of estimated PK parameters (in particular, AUC and the time above a threshold concentration), accounting for the potential cost of requiring women to wait around or even return to the clinic the next day. The utility also included a gain as the posterior precision (inverse of the variance) of the PK characteristic of interest ($S(\theta)$, such as AUC or time above a threshold concentration) increased. Equation 3.2 shows the utility as a function of the times ($t$) and the data ($y$). The cost associated with a set of possible sampling times is the sum of each time's cost, and each time's cost is zero or the squared difference between that sampling time and 7 h. The parameter $c$ calibrates a change in cost because of a sampling time with improved precision:

$$u(t, y) = \mathrm{var}\left(S(\theta)|t, y\right)^{-1} - c \sum_{i=1}^{k} (t_i - 7)^2 \tag{3.2}$$

Of course, it is not straightforward to decide how to weigh estimation precision with the cost of waiting to draw samples, since these are not on a common metric. Our approach called for working with the clinicians to calibrate the relative weights when it came time to implement the study design.

We used historical PK data for a prior distribution in our design. Because of the nonlinear nature of the mean function, we had to use Markov chain Monte Carlo (MCMC) methods for inference (Gamerman 1998). We also used MCMC methods to determine the utility surface, treating the problem as one in which we generate random samples from some probability distribution known up to a constant of proportionality (Müller and Parmigiani 1995; Müller 1999). In the end, we found that the utility surface was relatively flat, and we had to work with a numerically exaggerated transformation of the surface to find the times associated with the peak utility. Of course, it was highly informative for the clinical pharmacologists to know that the utility surface was relatively flat over some range of potential sampling times, since this meant that there would not be much loss in using sampling times that might be *suboptimal* yet be appealing for other reasons not captured by the utility function.

## 3.3   SUMMARY

In this chapter, we have highlighted some of the statistical issues that arise in studies of the PK and PD of a drug. We used case studies when available to illustrate methods. The field is a fascinating one and has the potential to individualize therapy for patients, thereby maximizing the chance of clinical benefit while minimizing the risk of serious toxicity.

## 3.4  SOFTWARE

There are software packages available commercially for fitting pharmacokinetic models. There are also some programs that are available free to academic institutions. Here are four software packages in alphabetical order, along with the addresses of the associated websites.

ADAPT (http://bmsr.usc.edu/Software/Adapt/adptmenu.html): A suite of programs for fitting pharmacokinetic and pharmacodynamic models. The website also includes user-supplied functions for fitting complex models. Work on a version of the package that will allow population or hierarchical modeling is underway.

MCSIM (http://toxi.ineris.fr/activites/toxicologie_quantitative/mcsim/mcsim.php): A package that allows one to fit one's own statistical or simulation models and carry out Bayesian inference via Markov chain Monte Carlo simulations. It is useful for physiologically based pharmacokinetic (or toxicokinetic) modeling.

MONOLIX (http://software.monolix.org/sdoms/software/): Monolix is free software that one can use to fit nonlinear repeated measures data. Model fitting is based on a stochastic approximation to the EM algorithm. One can download related research papers from the website, where one can also find some demos and tutorials.

PKBUGS (http://www.med.ic.ac.uk/divisions/60/pkbugs_web/home.html): An add-on program for carrying out fully Bayesian pharmacokinetic analyses within WinBUGS (http://www.mrc-bsu.cam.ac.uk/bugs/welcome.shtml). One can modify the code generated by the program for problem-specific analyses.

## ACKNOWLEDGMENTS

We thank the Children's Oncology Group and Dr. Lisa Bomgaars for permission to discuss the infant methotrexate study. This work was partially supported by grants CA75984, CA75984, and GM 61393.

## REFERENCES

Brunner, M. and M. Müller. 2002. Microdialysis: An in vivo approach for measuring drug delivery in oncology. *European Journal of Clinical Pharmacology* 58(4):227–234.

Chabner, B. A. and J. M. Collins. 1990. *Cancer Chemotherapy: Principles and Practice*. Philadelphia, PA: J. B. Lippincott Company.

Chaloner, K. and I. Verdinelli. 1995. Bayesian experimental design: A review. *Statistical Science* 10(3):273–304.

Chow, S.-C. and J.-P. Liu. 2009. *Design and Analysis of Bioavailability and Bioequivalence Studies*, 3rd edn. Boca Raton, FL: Chapman & Hall/CRC.

Collins, J. M. 1990. Pharmacokinetics and clinical monitoring. In *Cancer Chemotherapy: Principles and Practice*, eds. B. W. Chapner and J. M. Collins, pp. 16–31. Philadelphia, PA: Lippincott.

D'Argenio, D. Z. 1990. Incorporating prior parameter uncertainty in the design of sampling schedules for pharmacokinetic parameter estimation experiments. *Mathematical Biosciences* 99(1):105–118.

D'Argenio, D. Z. and J. H. Rodman. 1993. Targeting the systemic exposure of teniposide in the population and the individual using a stochastic therapeutic objective. *Journal of Pharmacokinetics and Biopharmaceutics* 21(2):223–251.

Davidian, M. and A. R. Gallant. 1993. The nonlinear mixed effects model with a smooth random effects density. *Biometrika* 80(3):475–488.

Davidian, M. and D. M. Giltinan. 1995. *Nonlinear Models for Repeated Measurement Data.* London, U.K.: Chapman & Hall.

De Iorio, M., P. Müller, G. L. Rosner, and S. N. MacEachern. 2004. An ANOVA model for dependent random measures. *Journal of the American Statistical Association* 99:205–215.

Delyon, B., M. Lavielle, and E. Moulines. 1999. Convergence of a stochastic approximation version of the EM algorithm. *Annals of Statistics* 27(1):94–128.

Escobar, M. D. and M. West. 1995. Bayesian density estimation and inference using mixtures. *Journal of the American Statistical Association* 90(430):577–588.

Ferguson, T. S. 1973. A Bayesian analysis of some nonparametric problems. *Annals of Statistics* 1:209–230.

Friberg, L. E., A. Henningsson, H. Maas, L. Nguyen, and M. O. Karlsson. 2002. Model of chemotherapy-induced myelosuppression with parameter consistency across drugs. *Journal of Clinical Oncology* 20(24):4713–4721.

Friberg, L. E. and M. O. Karlsson. 2003. Mechanistic models for myelosuppression. *Investigational New Drugs* 21(2):183–194.

Gallant, A. R. and D. W. Nychka. 1987. Semi-nonparametric maximum likelihood estimation. *Econometrica* 55(2):363–390.

Gamerman, D. 1998. *Markov Chain Monte Carlo: Stochastic Simulation for Bayesian Inference.* Boca Raton, FL: CRC Press.

Gianni, L., C. M. Kearns, A. Giani, et al. 1995. Nonlinear pharmacokinetics and metabolism of paclitaxel and its pharmacokinetic/pharmacodynamic relationships in humans. *Journal of Clinical Oncology* 13(1):180–190.

Gibaldi, M. and D. Perrier. 1982. *Pharmacokinetics,* 2nd edn. New York: Marcel Dekker, Inc.

Huang, Y., D. Liu, and H. Wu. 2006. Hierarchical Bayesian methods for estimation of parameters in a longitudinal HIV dynamic system. *Biometrics* 62(2):413–423.

Innocenti, F. ed. 2008. *Genomics and Pharmacogenomics in Anticancer Drug Development and Clinical Response.* Totowa, NJ: Humana Press.

Jelliffe, R.W. 1986. Clinical applications of pharmacokinetics and control theory: Planning, monitoring, and adjusting dosage regimens of aminoglycosides, lidocaine, digitoxic, and digoxin. In *Selected Topics in Clinical Pharmacology,* ed. R. Maronde, pp. 26–82. New York: Springer-Verlag.

Jelliffe, R. W., T. Iglesias, A. K. Hurst, K. A. Foo, and J. Rodriguez. 1991. Individualising gentamicin dosage regimens. A comparative review of selected models, data fitting methods, and monitoring strategies. *Clinical Pharmacokinetic Concepts* 21(6):461–478.

Jelliffe, R. W., A. Schumitzky, M. Van Guilder, et al. 1993. Individualizing drug dosage regimens: Roles of population pharmacokinetic and dynamic models, Bayesian fitting, and adaptive control. *Therapeutic Drug Monitoring* 15(5):380–393.

Karlsson, M. O., R. E. Port, M. J. Ratain, and L. B. Sheiner. 1995. A population model for the leukopenic effect of etoposide. *Clinical Pharmacology and Therapeutics* 57:325–334.

Klein, T. E., J. T. Chang, M. K. Cho et al. 2001. Integrating genotype and phenotype information: An overview of the PharmGKB project. *The Pharmacogenomics Journal* 1:167–170.

Laird, N. 1978. Nonparametric maximum likelihood estimation of a mixing distribution. *Journal of the American Statistical Association* 73:805–811.

Licinio, J. and M.-L. Wong, eds. 2002. *Pharmacogenomics: The Search for Individualized Therapies.* Weinheim, Germany: Wiley-VCH.

Lindsay, B. G. 1983. The geometry of mixture likelihoods: A general theory. *Annals of Statistics* 11:86–94.

Lopes, H. F., P. Müller, and G. L. Rosner. 2003. Bayesian meta-analysis for longitudinal data models using multivariate mixture priors. *Biometrics* 59(1):66–75.

Lunn, D. J., A. Thomas, N. Best, and D. Spiegelhalter. 2000. WinBUGS—A Bayesian modelling framework: Concepts, structure, and extensibility. *Statistics and Computing* 10:325–337.

Lunn, D. J., J. Wakefield, A. Thomas, N. Best, and D. Spiegelhalter. 1999. *PKBugs User Guide, Version 1.1.* London, U.K.: Department of Epidemiology & Public Health, Imperial College of Science, Technology and Medicine.

Mallet, A. 1986. A maximum likelihood estimation method for random coefficient regression models. *Biometrika* 73(3):645–656.

Mallet, A., F. Mentré, J. Gilles, et al. 1988a. Handling covariates in population pharmacokinetics, with an application to gentamicin. *Biomedical Measurement and Information Control* 2:138–146.

Mallet, A., F. Mentré, J.-L. Steimer, and F. Lokiec. 1988b. Nonparametric maximum likelihood estimation for population pharmacokinetics, with application to cyclosporine. *Journal of Pharmacokinetics and Biopharmaceutics* 16(3):311–327.

Merlé, Y. and F. Mentré. 1995. Bayesian design criteria: Computation, comparison, and application to a pharmacokinetic and a pharmacodynamic model. *Journal of Pharmacokinetics and Biopharmaceutics* 23(1):101–125.

Merlé, Y., F. Mentré, A. Mallet, and A. H. Aurengo. 1994. Designing an optimal experiment for Bayesian estimation: Application to the kinetics of iodine thyroid uptake. *Statistics in Medicine* 13(2):185–196.

Minami, H., Y. Sasaki, N. Saijo, et al. 1998. Indirect-response model for the time course of leukopenia with anticancer drugs. *Clinical Pharmacology and Therapeutics* 64(5):511–521.

Minami, H., Y. Sasaki, T. Watanabe, and M. Ogawa. 2001. Pharmacodynamic modeling of the entire time course of leukopenia after a 3-hour infusion of paclitaxel. *Japanese Journal of Cancer Research* 92(2):231–238.

Müller, P. 1999. Simulation-based optimal design. In *Bayesian Statistics 6: Proceedings of the Sixth Valencia International Meeting*, eds. J. M. Bernardo, J. O. Berger, A. P. Dawid, and A. F. M. Smith, pp. 459–474. Oxford, U.K.: Oxford University Press.

Müller, P. and G. Parmigiani. 1995. Optimal design via curve fitting of Monte Carlo experiments. *Journal of the American Statistical Association* 90:1322–1330.

Müller, P. and G. L. Rosner. 1997. A Bayesian population model with hierarchical mixture priors applied to blood count data. *Journal of the American Statistical Association* 92:1279–1292.

Müller, P. and G. Rosner. 1998. Semiparametric PK/PD models. In *Practical Nonparametric and Semiparametric Bayesian Statistics*, eds. D. Dey, P. Miller, and D. Sinha, pp. 323–337. New York: Springer-Verlag.

Ogungbenro, K., A. Dokoumetzidis, and L. Aarons. 2009. Application of optimal design methodologies in clinical pharmacology experiments. *Pharmaceutical Statistics* 8(3):239–252.

Racine-Poon, A. and A. F. M. Smith. 1990. Population models. In *Statistical Methodology in the Pharmaceutical Sciences*, ed. D. A. Berry, pp. 139–162. New York: Marcel Dekker, Inc.

Ratain, M. J., R. Mick, R. L. Schilsky, N. J. Vogelzang, and F. Berezin. 1991. Pharmacologically based dosing of etoposide: A means of safely increasing dose intensity. *Journal of Clinical Oncology* 9(8):1480–1486.

Rosner, G. L. and P. Müller. 1997. Bayesian population pharmacokinetic and pharmacodynamic analyses using mixture models. *Journal of Pharmacokinetics and Biopharmaceutics* 25(2):209–233.

Samson, A., M. Lavielle, and F. Mentré. 2006. Extension of the SAEM algorithm to left-censored data in nonlinear mixed-effects model: Application to HIV dynamics model. *Computational Statistics and Data Analysis* 51(3):1562–1574.

Schumitzky, A. 1991. Nonparametric EM algorithms for estimating prior distributions. *Applied Mathematics and Computation* 45:141–157.

Schumitzky, A. 1993. The nonparametric maximum likelihood approach to pharmacokinetic population analysis. In *Proceedings of the 1993 Western Simulation Mulitconference—Simulation in Health Care*, pp. 95–100. San Diego, CA: Society for Computer Simulation.

Schwartz, G. J., L. P. Brion, and A. Spitzer. 1987. The use of plasma creatinine concentration for estimating glomerular filtration rate in infants, children, and adolescents. *Pediatric Clinics of North America* 34(3):571–590.

Schwartz, G. J., L. G. Feld, and D. J. Langford. 1984. A simple estimate of glomerular filtration rate in full-term infants during the first year of life. *Journal of Pediatrics* 104(6):849–854.

Sheiner, L. B., S. Beal, B. Rosenberg, and V. V. Marathe. 1979a. Forecasting individual pharmacokinetics. *Clinical Pharmacology and Therapeutics* 26(3):294–305.

Sheiner, L. B., B. Rosenberg, and V. Marathe. 1977. Estimation of population characteristics of pharmacokinetic parameters from routine clinical data. *Journal of Pharmacokinetics and Biopharmaceutics* 5:445–479.

Sheiner, L. B., B. Rosenberg, and K. L. Melmon. 1972. Modelling of individual pharmacokinetics for computer-aided drug dosage. *Computers and Biomedical Research* 5(5):411–459.

Sheiner, L. B., D. R. Stanski, S. Vozeh, R. D. Miller, and J. Ham. 1979b. Simultaneous modeling of pharmacokinetics and pharmacodynamics: Application to *d*-tubocurarine. *Clinical Pharmacology and Therapeutics* 25:358–371.

Stroud, J. R., P. Müller, and G. L. Rosner. 2001. Optimal sampling times in population pharmacokinetic studies. *Applied Statistics* 50(3):345–359.

Unadkat, J. D., F. Bartha, and L. B. Sheiner. 1986. Simultaneous modeling of pharmacokinetics and pharmacodynamics with nonparametric kinetic and dynamic models. *Clinical Pharmacology and Therapeutics* 40(1):86–93.

Verotta, D. and L. B. Sheiner. 1987. Simultaneous modeling of pharmacokinetics and pharmacodynamics: An improved algorithm. *Computer Applications in the Biosciences* 3(4):345–349.

Wakefield, J. 1996. The Bayesian analysis of population pharmacokinetic models. *Journal of the American Statistical Association* 91(433):62–75.

Wakefield, J. and S. Walker. 1997. Bayesian nonparametric population models: Formulation and comparison with likelihood approaches. *Journal of Pharmacokinetics and Biopharmaceutics* 25(2):235–253.

West, M., P. Müller, and M. D. Escobar. 1994. Hierarchical priors and mixture models, with applications in regression and density estimation. In *Aspects of Uncertainty: A Tribute to D. V. Lindley*, eds. A. F. M. Smith and P. Freeman, pp. 363–386. New York: John Wiley & Sons.

# 4 Statistics of Phase 0 Trials

*Larry Rubinstein*

## CONTENTS

## 4.1 INTRODUCTION AND STATEMENT OF THE CONCEPT: MEASURING BIOLOGICAL EFFECTIVENESS (WITH A PD ENDPOINT) AS A VERY EARLY SCREENING AND DRUG DEVELOPMENT TOOL

Currently only 5% of investigational new drug (IND) applications to the Food and Drug Administration (FDA) in oncology result in clinically approved agents [1,2]. This is a very serious problem, since the development of a new agent is a lengthy and expensive process and many of these agents fail relatively late in that process. The fact that an increasing proportion of IND anticancer agents are molecularly targeted suggests testing the agent for effectiveness against the target by means of a PD assay very early in the drug development process. This is particularly useful and important since the pre-clinical tests of such effectiveness are often misleading, yielding both false-positive and false-negative results. For this reason, the FDA issued a new Exploratory IND (expIND) Guidance in 2006, to allow for such studies as small first-in-man trials, conducted at dose levels and administration schedules not expected to result in significant clinical toxicity, and generally restricted to at most approximately 1 week per patient [1,2]. Conducting studies under this guidance requires substantially less pre-clinical toxicology work than is required for standard IND phase 1 studies [1,2]. Therefore, phase 0 studies can be administered while the toxicology studies preparatory to filing a standard IND are being conducted, and they will not postpone the time until the phase 1 trial can be initiated.

Phase 0 studies can be very effective tools for determining very early in the drug development process whether an agent has the anticipated biologic effect. They can also be used to prioritize among analogs or agents designed to have the same molecular target by means of comparing pharmacokinetic (e.g., oral bioavailability) and/ or PD characteristics (although we will not deal explicitly with such comparative designs). They are an opportunity for developing and validating clinical PD assays very early in the drug development process, to enable more reliable usage of such assays in phase 1 and phase 2 trials [3]. Finally, they can contribute to better defining the appropriate dose range or administration schedule to take into phase 1 and phase 2 testing.

## 4.2 STATISTICAL DESIGN OF A PHASE 0 TRIAL

The challenge presented by the PD-driven phase 0 study is to assess the change in the PD endpoint effected by the agent, with very few patients, each treated over a short period of time, but to maintain a certain amount of statistical rigor. Kummar et al. [1] and Murgo et al. [2] give several statistical designs to address this challenge in different clinical contexts, three of which we present here, as well as giving a general approach to the design of such trials. Typically, a phase 0 trial will encompass several escalating dose levels for the experimental agent. In general, the approach taken is to mimic the design of a phase 2 study [4], and to design the phase 0 study as a phase 2 study in miniature for each separate dose level. Thus, the first step is to define what is meant by a PD "response" for each individual patient, which is analogous to defining what constitutes an objective tumor response for a patient in a phase 2 trial. The second step is to define what constitutes a promising observed PD response rate for each dose level—in other words, how many patients must demonstrate a PD response for the dose level to be declared biologically effective. This is analogous to setting a threshold for observed response rate in a phase 2 trial, in order that the agent be deemed sufficiently promising for further testing [4]. Further details of this approach are given in the following sections.

### 4.2.1 DETERMINING STATISTICAL SIGNIFICANCE OF A PD EFFECT AT THE PATIENT LEVEL: DEFINING A PD RESPONSE

In oncology, generally, the PD endpoint is assessed both in tumor tissue and in an easily assayed surrogate tissue such as blood (peripheral blood mononuclear cells [PBMCs]). The tumor tissue assay is considered to be more reliable with respect to reflecting the biological effect of the agent in what is generally the target tissue of interest [1,3]. However, the number of tumor biopsies per patient usually is severely limited for ethical reasons [1,2]. Therefore, the PBMC assay, for example, is used as a surrogate, since multiple PBMC assays can be performed both pre-treatment and post-treatment, thus allowing for assessment of both the pre-treatment variability at the patient level and the post-treatment PD effect over time [1–3]. Generally, there are only two tumor biopsies, one taken shortly before treatment with the agent, and one taken at the post-treatment time point of greatest interest, often when the PD effect is anticipated to be at its maximum. The measure of treatment effect for the tumor PD assay is the difference between the pre-treatment and post-treatment values (often measured on the log scale rather than on the original). Generally, there are multiple PBMC assays both pre-treatment and post-treatment. The primary measure of treatment effect for the PBMC assay is the one that corresponds in time to that of the tumor assay—the difference between the most immediately pre-treatment PBMC assay and the post-treatment PBMC assay closest in time to that of the tumor biopsy. The other pre-treatment PBMC assays should, ideally, cover a time span comparable to that of the pre-treatment vs. post-treatment biopsies. In that way, they provide a measure of the natural variation of the assay, for an individual patient, over that time span. The other post-treatment PBMC assays provide a means of assessing the post-treatment PD effect over time, as a secondary set of PD endpoints.

Defining a PD "response," both for the tumor assay and for the PBMC assay, usually involves both a biologic criterion and a statistical criterion for what is significant. The biologic criterion generally depends upon characteristics of the biologic target of the agent. For example, in the recent National Cancer Institute (NCI) phase 0 trial of ABT-888 [5,6], the criterion chosen was that the reduction in the assay value had to be at least twofold. The statistical criterion may be either 90% confidence or 95% confidence (generally one sided, since the anticipated treatment effect is generally in one direction) that the observed treatment effect is not a result of the sort of natural random variation in the assay, for an individual patient, that would be seen in the absence of a true treatment effect. For the PBMC assay, this natural variation can be assessed by the pooled intra-patient standard deviation (SD) of the pre-treatment values. However, for the tumor assay, multiple pre-treatment assays per patient will generally not be available. Therefore, the inter-patient SD of the pre-treatment values must be used instead. Details concerning the definition of a PD response are illustrated in Figure 4.1. The thresholds for declaring the PD effect (pre-treatment value minus post-treatment value, for the case where the agent is anticipated to reduce the assay value, as in the NCI phase 0 trial [5,6]) statistically significant (at the one-sided .10 or .05 significance levels) are calculated from the variance of the difference of two normally distributed variables. (If the number of samples from which to estimate the pre-treatment variability of the assay is very limited (under 20), consideration should be given to using t-distribution, rather than normal distribution, cut-off values.)

## 4.2.2 Determining Statistical Significance of a PD Effect for a Given Dose Level

For each dose level, the investigators may set a threshold for the number of patients, among the total, that must demonstrate a PD response, in order for the dose level to be judged as yielding a promising biologic effect. Since the false-positive rate for a

**Defining PD Response at the Patient Level**

Calculate the baseline variance and standard deviation (SD) of the PD value
(In surrogate tissue, the baseline variance is the pooled intra-patient baseline
variance determined by calculating the baseline variances for each patient,
separately, and then averaging the separate variances across patients. In tumor
tissue, the baseline variance is the inter-patient baseline variance calculated across
patients. In either case, the baseline SD is the square root of the baseline variance.)

⇓

Measure PD effect as pre-treatment value minus post-treatment value

⇓

If the PD effect is greater than 1.8 (2.3) times the baseline SD, then it is statistically
significant at the .10 (.05) significance level

⇓

A statistically significant PD effect, at the patient level, is called a PD response

**FIGURE 4.1**    This figure illustrates the defining of PD "response" for an individual patient. Multipliers of the baseline SD are derived from asymptotic normal distribution theory. Significance levels are one sided.

PD response, for an individual patient, has been determined (as given previously), the false-positive rate for declaring a dose level effective, for each assay separately and for the two combined, can be calculated from the binomial distribution. (As indicated earlier, the tumor tissue assay is generally considered to be more reliable than a PBMC, or other surrogate tissue, assay, but the number of biopsies per patient is limited for ethical reasons; therefore, PBMC assays are generally used, in addition. If the PBMC assay has been established as a reliable surrogate for the tumor assay, or if biopsies are impracticable, the PBMC assay may be the only one available.) Likewise, for a targeted PD response rate, across patients, the power to declare the dose level effective, for each of the two assays, can be calculated. The investigators may employ a one-stage or two-stage design to assess the PD response rate at each dose level, just as in phase 2 studies [4], and the calculations of power and false-positive rate are done in an identical fashion. If a dose level proves unpromising, in general, escalation to the next dose level will occur. If a dose level proves promising, escalation to the next dose level may or may not occur, according to the judgment of the investigators. Toxicity may also be a factor in the dose escalation; this will be discussed further. Examples of designs to target 80%, 60%, or 40% PD response rates, across patients are given later. More generally, one may use available online software to determine the "Simon optimal" and "minimax" designs [4] (e.g., that supplied by the Biometric Research Branch, NCI at http://linus.nci.nih.gov/brb/samplesize/otsd. html), to be used at each dose level. Likewise, one may use available online software to construct a trial design, to be used at each dose level, that is not strictly optimal or minimax, or to precisely evaluate such designs (e.g., that supplied by CRAB and the SWOG http://www.swogstat.org/stat/public/twostage.htm). We will discuss this further in Section 4.2.4.

### 4.2.3 THREE PHASE 0 TRIAL DESIGNS: DESIGNS TO DETECT AN 80%, 60%, OR 40% PD RESPONSE RATE ACROSS PATIENTS

To target a true 80% PD response rate at each dose level, a one-stage design may be used. Three patients are treated and the dose level is declared effective with respect to either PD assay if at least two of the patients demonstrate a PD response which is significant at the .10 level. This design yields 90% power to detect a true 80% PD response rate, across patients, for either assay, with an overall 6% false-positive rate for the two assays combined, under the null hypothesis that the agent has no biologic effect. This is the design that was used in the NCI phase 0 trial of ABT-888 [5,6], and it is illustrated in Figure 4.2.

To target a true 60% PD response rate at each dose level, a two-stage design may be used. Three patients are treated and the cohort is expanded to five patients if exactly one patient, for either PD assay, demonstrates a PD response which is significant at the .05 level. The dose level is declared effective with respect to either PD assay if at least two of the patients demonstrate a PD response which is significant at the .05 level. This design yields 89% power to detect a true 60% PD response rate, across patients, for either assay, with an overall 4% false-positive rate for the two assays combined, under the null hypothesis that the agent has no biologic effect. This design is illustrated in Figure 4.3.

To target a true 40% PD response rate at each dose level, a similar two-stage design may be used. Five patients are treated and the cohort is expanded to eight patients if exactly one patient, for either PD assay, demonstrates a PD response which is significant at the .05 level. The dose level is declared effective with respect to either PD assay if at least two of the patients demonstrate a PD response which is significant at the .05 level. This design yields 87% power to detect a true 40% PD response rate, across patients, for either assay, with an overall 10% false-positive rate for the two assays combined, under the null hypothesis that the agent has no biologic effect. This design is illustrated in Figure 4.4.

**Design 1: Defining a Significant PD Effect at the Dose Level when the Target PD Response Rate Is 80% Across Patients**

Treat three patients

⇓

Declare the PD effect statistically significant at the dose level, for either endpoint, if at least two of the three patients demonstrate a PD response at the .10 significance level

⇓

This yields, for either endpoint, 90% power, at the dose level, to detect an 80% PD response rate across patients, with an overall 6% false-positive rate for both endpoints combined

**FIGURE 4.2** This figure illustrates the defining of what constitutes a promising observed response rate for a dose level. The target (true) PD response rate, across patients, is 80%. Power and false-positive rate are derived from the binomial distribution.

**Design 3: Defining a Significant PD Effect at the Dose Level when
the Target PD Response Rate Is 60% Across Patients**

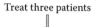

Treat three patients

⇓

Treat an additional two patients if exactly one of the three patients (for
either endpoint) demonstrates a PD response at the .05 significance level

⇓

Declare the PD effect statistically significant at the dose level, for either
endpoint, if at least two of the three (or five) patients demonstrate a PD
response at the .05 significance level

⇓

This yields, for either endpoint, 89% power, at the dose level, to detect a
60% PD response rate across patients, with an overall 4% false-positive
rate for both endpoints combined

**FIGURE 4.3**    This figure illustrates the defining of what constitutes a promising observed response rate for a dose level with a two-stage design. The target (true) PD response rate, across patients, is 60%. Power and false-positive rate are derived from the binomial distribution.

**Design 3: Defining a Significant PD Effect at the Dose Level when
the Target PD Response Rate Is 40% Across Patients**

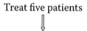

Treat five patients

⇓

Treat an additional three patients if exactly one of the five patients (for
either endpoint) demonstrates a PD response at the .05 significance level

⇓

Declare the PD effect statistically significant at the dose level, for
either endpoint, if at least two of the eight patients demonstrate a PD
response at the .05 significance level

⇓

This yields, for either endpoint, 87% power, at the dose level, to detect
a 40% PD response rate across patients, with an overall 10% false-
positive rate for both endpoints combined

**FIGURE 4.4**    This figure illustrates the defining of what constitutes a promising observed response rate for a dose level with a two-stage design. The target (true) PD response rate, across patients, is 40%. Power and false-positive rate are derived from the binomial distribution.

## 4.2.4  CONSTRUCTING PHASE 0 TRIAL DESIGNS

As mentioned earlier, phase 0 trials can be constructed as a series of miniature phase 2 trials, one for each dose level, as the dose levels escalate. Across the dose levels, the investigators must determine what PD response rate is sufficiently promising that it should be detected with high probability (generally, at least .90). At each dose level, the design must be capable of distinguishing between that target response rate and the "null rate" associated with the likelihood of a false-positive PD measure for an individual patient (generally, .05–.10). In Section 4.2.3 we gave designs to distinguish between PD response rates of 10% vs. 80%, 5% vs. 60%, and 5% vs. 40%, each with approximately 90% power to detect the target PD response rate and declare the agent promising at a particular dose level, according to either of the two assays (tumor and surrogate tissue), and each with overall false-positive rate of 4%–10%. These designs, although reasonable, are neither "Simon optimal" nor minimax [4]. It would be reasonable to use an optimal design if the dose level (or the agent, in general) was unlikely to be effective, to minimize the patients expended for that situation. On the other hand, it would be reasonable to use a minimax design if the dose level was likely to be effective, to minimize the patients expended for that situation.

In Table 4.1, we give optimal and minimax designs for various combinations of $p_0$ (the null PD response rate) and $p_1$ (the target PD response rate), along with their statistical operating characteristics. These designs are all identical in structure to those of Simon [4], except that accrual is terminated at stage 1 if the number of responses is at least $r + 1$, meaning that the dose level has already been proven effective (this is consistent with the objective to keep the phase 0 trial as small as possible). For purposes of comparison, we also give the design examples of Section 4.2.3 (including the one-stage design used in the NCI phase 0 trial, designated as ** in the table), which compare quite favorably to their corresponding optimal and minimax counterparts. In putting these individual dose-level designs together into a phase 0 trial with escalating dose levels, the investigators may choose to halt the trial, or not, when an effective dose level has been reached (the observed PD rate is adequate). Likewise, they may choose to continue dose escalation, or not, until such an effective dose level has been reached.

It is interesting to note that the standard $3 + 3$ phase 1 dose escalation design can also be viewed as a series of miniature phase 2 trials constructed so as to test the rate of absence of dose-limiting toxicity (the "DLT-free rate") at each successive dose level, and escalate on that basis. Thus, a phase 0 trial could be designed to test the "toxicity-free" rate along with the PD response rate. Here, we are using the term toxicity-free somewhat loosely, since, by definition, phase 0 trials should not involve clinical toxicity; however, it is possible that the investigators might have a separate assay for an unfavorable PD response, which is a biomarker for potential clinical toxicity at a higher dose level, along with the assay for the target PD response, which is a biomarker for potential clinical benefit at a higher dose level. It is also possible that an analog of an effective, but overly toxic, agent would be tested in phase 0, where reduction of that toxicity was the primary concern. In Table 4.2, we give examples of "Simon optimal" phase 0 trial designs to discriminate between unsatisfactory toxicity-free rates $p_0$ (.40–.50), for which we would want to halt the dose escalation with high probability (at least .90), and target toxicity-free rates $p_1$ (.80–.90), for which we would want to halt the dose escalation with low probability (at most .10), along with their statistical operating characteristics. As it happens, these designs are also all minimax. All are identical in structure to those of Simon [4], except that accrual is terminated at stage 1 if the number of toxicity-free patients is at least $r + 1$, meaning that the dose level has already been proven adequate. For comparison, we also give

## TABLE 4.1
## Simon Optimal and Minimax Designs (Designed to Have $\alpha = .05$ and $(1 - \beta) = .9$) to Evaluate PD Response for Individual Dose Levels in a Phase 0 Trial

| False Positive and Target Response Rates | | Dose Level Activity Judged Inadequate if Response Rate | | Probability of Positive Result for $p_0$ and $p_1$ | | Prob. of Stage 1 Determ. of Activity for $p_0$ and $p_1$ | |
|---|---|---|---|---|---|---|---|
| $p_0$ | $p_1$ | $\leq r_1/n_1$ | $\leq r/n$ | $\alpha$ | $1 - \beta$ | $PET_0$ | $PET_1$ |
| .05 | .40 | 0/5 | 2/14 | .024 | .900 | .775 | .395 |
|  |  | 0/7 | 2/12 | .019 | .908 | .702 | .608 |
| *.05 | .40 | 0/5 | 1/8 | .052 | .866 | .797 | .741 |
| .05 | .50 | 0/4 | 1/7 | .038 | .906 | .829 | .751 |
|  |  | Same | Same | Same | Same | Same | Same |
| .05 | .60 | 0/3 | 1/6 | .027 | .918 | .864 | .712 |
|  |  | 0/4 | 1/5 | .023 | .913 | .829 | .847 |
| *.05 | .60 | 0/3 | 1/5 | .020 | .890 | .864 | .712 |
| .10 | .70 | 0/2 | 2/8 | .025 | .905 | .810 | .090 |
|  |  | 0/3 | 2/6 | .015 | .920 | .730 | .370 |
| .10 | .80 | 0/2 | 1/4 | .019 | .951 | .820 | .680 |
|  |  | Same | Same | Same | Same | Same | Same |
| ** .10 | .80 | — | 1/3 | .028 | .896 | — | — |

$p_0$ = The false-positive rate associated with determining a PD response for an individual patient.

$p_1$ = The target PD response rate, for a dose level, minimally necessary to establish promise.

$r_1/n_1$ (for stage 1) and $r/n$ (for stage 2) are the maximum number of [responses]/ [the number of patients] for declaring the dose level response rate inadequate.

* These rows correspond to examples given in Section 4.2.3 and are neither optimal nor minimax, but compare favorably to them.

** This row corresponds to the one-stage "Design 1" (Figure 4.2), used in the NCI phase 0 trial, which is neither optimal nor minimax, but compares favorably to them.

In each row, except * and **, upper numbers relate to the optimal and lower numbers to the minimax design. These designs are all identical in structure to those of Simon [4] (excluding design **, which has only one stage), except that accrual is terminated at stage 1 if the number of responses is at least $r + 1$, meaning that the dose level has already been proven effective.

**TABLE 4.2**

**Simon Optimal (and Minimax) Designs (Designed to have $\alpha = .1$ and $(1 - \beta) = .9$) to Continue Dose Escalation Based on Toxicity-Free Rate in a Phase 0 Trial**

| Lower and Upper Target Toxicity-Free Rates | | Halt Dose Escalation if Toxicity-Free Rate | | Probability of Dose Escalation for $p_0$ and $p_1$ | | Prob. of Stage 1 Determ. of Escalation for $p_0$ and $p_1$ | |
|------|------|------|------|------|------|------|------|
| $p_0$ | $p_1$ | $\leq r_1/n_1$ | $\leq r/n$ | For $p_0$ | For $p_1$ | $PET_0$ | $PET_1$ |
| * .40 | .90 | 1/3 | 4/6 | .082 | .906 | .712 | .757 |
| .40 | .90 | 1/3 | 3/5 | .087 | .919 | .648 | .028 |
| .45 | .85 | 1/3 | 6/10 | .087 | .908 | .575 | .061 |
| .50 | .80 | 3/7 | 10/16 | .099 | .905 | .500 | .033 |

$p_0$ = The target toxicity-free rate, for a dose level, for which one wants a low (<.10) probability of dose escalation.

$p_1$ = The target toxicity-free rate, for a dose level, for which one wants a high (>.90) probability of dose escalation.

$r_1/n_1$ (for stage 1) and $r/n$ (for stage 2) are the maximum number of [patients with toxicity] /[the number of patients] for declaring the toxicity-free rate inadequate.

* This row corresponds to the standard 3 + 3 dose escalation design, which is neither optimal nor minimax, and includes the additional stipulation that dose escalation will occur after stage 1 if all three patients are toxicity-free (even though that does not guarantee that, if three additional patients were accrued to the dose level, at least four of the six would be toxicity-free).

The rows other than * give two-stage designs, based on toxicity-free rate, which are both optimal and, as it happens, minimax. All are identical in structure to those of Simon [4], except that accrual is terminated at stage 1 if the number of patients toxicity-free is at least $r + 1$, meaning that the dose level has already been proven adequate.

the statistical operating characteristics of the standard 3 + 3 phase 1 dose escalation design, which can be seen as discriminating between a $p_0$ of .40 and a $p_1$ of .90.

## 4.3  EXAMPLE OF A PHASE 0 TRIAL—THE NCI PARP INHIBITOR TRIAL—AND FURTHER DISCUSSION OF PHASE 0 STATISTICAL ISSUES

The NCI selected ABT-888, an inhibitor of the DNA repair enzyme poly (ADP-ribose) polymerase (PARP), for the first ever phase 0 trial for two reasons [5,6]. First, it was anticipated to have a wide margin of safety relative to target modulating doses in pre-clinical models. This is an essential characteristic for a phase 0 agent. Phase 0 trials cannot promise any benefit for the patients who participate, so there must be reasonable assurance that toxicity will be minimal. Second, it was anticipated to have wide therapeutic applicability if demonstrated effective. Elevated PARP levels are characteristic of tumors and can result in resistance to both chemotherapy (CT) and radiotherapy (RT). Therefore, PARP inhibitors hold promise of wide applicability as CT and RT sensitizers. The NCI trial demonstrated statistically significant reduction in PAR levels (a surrogate for PARP inhibition) in both tumor and PBMCs [5,6].

There are a number of statistical issues relating to phase 0 trials that deserve further mention:

1. In the NCI phase 0 trial it was found that the variance of the pre-treatment PD assay values was reduced if the logs of the values were used instead. It is often appropriate to log-transform PD assay values since geometric, rather than arithmetic, changes in value are thought to be qualitatively similar along the assay scale.

2. It will often be the case that assessing the PD treatment effect can be done with greater statistical power if the mean effect is measured across patients and then a test applied of the null hypothesis that the mean effect is equal to 0. Analogously, there have been proposals that phase 2 trials be assessed by testing whether the mean tumor shrinkage is statistically significant [7]. The problem with this approach is that a statistically significant mean treatment effect does not necessarily imply a biologically relevant treatment effect for a meaningful proportion of the patients [8]. For this reason, the NCI phase 0 trial investigators chose to impose the additional criterion of a biologically relevant level of PAR reduction for the individual patients. Likewise, it was felt appropriate to determine, for the individual patients, whether the PAR reduction observed was statistically significant. This follows the standard phase 2 model of determining what would constitute a response, for the individual patient, suggestive of benefit for that patient, and then assess the proportion of patients demonstrating such a response [8]. There may be phase 0 situations where this approach is too statistically demanding, and it is appropriate to resort to assessing the mean treatment PD effect.

3. For the tumor biopsy assay, multiple pre-treatment assays per patient will generally not be available, for ethical reasons. Therefore, the inter-patient SD of the pre-treatment values must be used instead of the intra-patient SD, which cannot be determined. The inter-patient variability will often be substantially greater than the intra-patient variability. This can seriously limit the ability to declare an observed treatment effect measured by the tumor assay to be statistically significant. For example, in the NCI phase 0 trial, an observed 95% post-treatment reduction in the tumor assay value was required for statistical significance, while an observed 55% post-treatment reduction was sufficient for the PBMC assay [2].

## 4.4   CONCLUSIONS

Phase 0 trials provide an excellent opportunity to establish feasibility and further refine target or biomarker assay methodology in a limited number of human samples before initiating larger trials involving patients receiving toxic doses of the study agent. We have demonstrated that, despite the small sample size, the nature of the PD assay values allow for a reasonable degree of statistical rigor and, especially in the case of the surrogate assays (which can be repeated multiple times), a reasonable degree of statistical power. We have shown how phase 0 trials, with reasonable statistical operating characteristics, can be constructed, to determine PD responses associated with either potential clinical benefit or potential clinical toxicity. Phase 0 trials do not replace phase 1 trials conducted to establish dose-limiting toxicities and define a recommended phase 2 dose. On the other hand, data from phase 0 trials allow phase 1 studies to begin at a higher, potentially more efficacious dose, use a more limited and rationally focused schedule for PD sampling, and use a qualified PD analytic assay for assessing target modulation. Likewise, phase 0 trials, with PD endpoints, will not eliminate the need for phase 2 trials to establish the agent's ability to yield tumor response or clinical benefit; but they will allow for early termination of development of agents that fail to yield the anticipated biologic effect. Therefore, the effort expended to conduct rationally designed phase 0 trials should conserve resources in the long run by improving the efficiency and success of subsequent clinical development.

## REFERENCES

1. Kummar S, Kinders R, Rubinstein L, Parchment RE, Murgo AJ, Collins J, Pickeral O, et al. Compressing drug development timelines in oncology using 'phase 0' trials. *Nature Reviews/Cancer* 2007; **7**: 131–139.
2. Murgo AJ, Kummar S, Rubinstein L, Gutierrez M, Collins J, Kinders R, Parchment RE, et al. Designing phase 0 cancer clinical trials. *Clinical Cancer Research* 2008; **14**: 3675–3682.
3. Kinders R, Parchment RE, Ji J, Kummar S, Murgo AJ, Gutierrez M, Collins J, et al. Phase 0 clinical trials in cancer drug development: From FDA guidance to clinical practice. *Molecular Interventions* 2007; **7**: 325–334.
4. Simon R. Optimal two-stage designs for phase II clinical trials. *Controlled Clinical Trials* 1989; **10**: 1–10.
5. Kummar S, Gutierrez M, Kinders R, Rubinstein L, Parchment RE, Philips L, Ji J, et al. Phase 0 pharmacodynamic, pharmacokinetic study of ABT-888, an inhibitor of poly (ADP-ribose) polymerase (PARP), in patients with advanced malignancies. *Annals of Oncology* 2008; **19** (Suppl. 3): 20.
6. Kummar S, Kinders R, Gutierrez M, Rubinstein L, Parchment RE, Phillips LR, Ji J, et al. Phase 0 clinical trial of the poly (ADP-ribose) polymerase (PARP) inhibitor ABT-888 in patients with advanced malignancies. *Journal of Clinical Oncology* 2009; **27**: 2705–2711.
7. Karrison TG, Maitland ML, Stadler WM, Ratain MJ. Design of phase II cancer trials using a continuous endpoint of change in tumor size: Application to a study of sorafenib and erlotinib in non–small-cell lung cancer. *Journal of the National Cancer Institute* 2007; **99**: 1455–1461.
8. Rubinstein L, Dancey J, Korn E, Smith M, Wright J. Early average change in tumor size in a phase 2 trial: Efficient endpoint or false promise. *Journal of the National Cancer Institute* 2007; **99**: 1422–1423.

# 5 CRM Trials for Assessing Toxicity and Efficacy

*Sumithra J. Mandrekar and Daniel J. Sargent*

## CONTENTS

## 5.1 INTRODUCTION

Historically, dose-seeking clinical trial designs have geared toward establishing the maximum tolerated dose (MTD) of a therapeutic regimen, with safety as the primary outcome. A fundamental assumption of these designs is that of a monotone increasing dose–toxicity and dose–efficacy relationship. Based on this assumption, the highest dose found to be safe is also assumed to be the dose most likely to be efficacious (Storer, 1989). As such, determining the MTD of a new agent (or combination) was the sole goal of phase I trials. While this paradigm has been successful in oncology for cytotoxic agents, it is not always appropriate for molecularly targeted therapies, vaccines, and/or immunotherapy. Targeted therapies including monoclonal antibodies have become a major focus of oncology drug development. Agents like imatinib, bevacizumab, and trastuzumab have demonstrated clinical benefit in several cancers, whereas others like R115777, ISIS 3521, and ZD1839 have produced negative results (Gelmon et al., 1999; Harris, 2004; Parulekar and Eisenhauer, 2004). The proposed mechanisms of action for these agents during the phase I testing are not straightforward in that (1) the dose–efficacy curves are usually unknown and (2) dose–toxicity relationships are expected to be minimal. The dose–efficacy curves for these novel therapies may follow a nonmonotone pattern such as a quadratic curve or an increasing curve with a plateau. Figure 5.1 depicts three possible dose–efficacy curves for such agents, specifically a monotonically increasing dose–efficacy curve, an increasing dose–efficacy curve with a plateau,

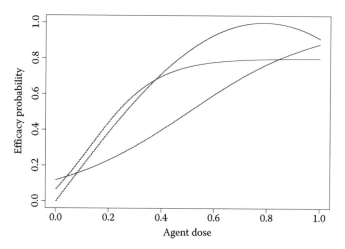

**FIGURE 5.1**    Dose–efficacy curves for targeted agents and novel therapies.

and a unimodal or parabolic dose–efficacy curve. Consider, for example, a therapeutic approach based on immunotherapy where an agent is given to a patient in an
attempt to stimulate the patient's own immune system to fight the tumor. In such
cases, overstimulation of the immune system could in fact interfere with efficacy or
even prove to be harmful (toxic) for the patient (Linsley, 2005). Ideally, dose-finding
studies for such agents should incorporate both measures of efficacy and toxicity,
and the primary aim should be to identify the biologically optimal dose (BOD)
instead of the MTD.

In the setting of combination therapies, there is a further added complexity
involved with the determination of the MTD (or the BOD). Ideally, an understanding of the underlying biologic rationale for the combination would be available, for
example, are the toxicity profiles of the agents overlapping or additive? Is the efficacy
of the two agents' additive, complementary, or synergistic? Typically, a set of predetermined combination dose levels are explored that are based on the single agent
MTD or preclinical cell lines experiment demonstrating synergy, where the dose of
one agent under investigation is escalated while the dose of the second agent remains
constant until a tolerable combination dose level is achieved. Clearly, not all possible
combination levels can be feasibly tested. In reality, preclinical or clinical data to
define the optimal dose combination exploration is however lacking, and an efficient
dose-seeking algorithm thus highly desirable. Despite the increased testing of such
combination treatments in oncology, few designs for dose escalation of two or more
agents have been proposed (Simon and Korn, 1991; Thall et al., 2003; Conaway et
al., 2004; Wang and Ivanova, 2005; Yin and Yuan, 2009; Hamberg et al., 2010).
A majority of these designs base their dose-finding algorithm on the dose–toxicity
relationships (with a goal to identify the MTD of the combination), again based on
the assumption that higher dose level combinations will provide the maximal therapeutic efficacy. Designs for dose-finding studies to establish the BOD of two or more

agents utilizing both toxicity and efficacy are limited (Huang et al., 2007; Dragalin et al., 2008), as the dose–toxicity and dose–efficacy surfaces for combination therapies are inherently more complex.

In this chapter, we review model-based designs that assist with the identification of the BOD of a single or dual agent combinations in a phase I setting utilizing both toxicity and efficacy data. An obvious requirement for such BOD-based designs is the existence of a direct or surrogate measure of efficacy. Some possible efficacy endpoints include the minimum effective blood concentration level of the agent, percent target inhibition of a marker, minimum expression level of a molecular target (targeted biologic response), tumor response, or pharmacokinetic endpoints in addition to toxicity (Gelmon et al., 1999; Parulekar and Eisenhauer, 2004; Hamberg et al., 2010). The existence of such a surrogate marker of efficacy, particularly one that has been properly validated, is a nontrivial issue. For the purposes of the designs considered in this chapter, we will assume that such a marker (of efficacy) exists. Thus, this chapter is organized into the following sections: Section 5.2 provides a brief overview of the framework of the standard continual reassessment method (CRM) as well as some of the extensions to the traditional CRM, Section 5.3 reviews the model-based trivariate CRM (TriCRM) designs for single and dual agent drug combinations, Section 5.4 discusses a hypothetical example of a dual agent TriCRM design, and Section 5.5 ends with some concluding remarks.

## 5.2  CONTINUAL REASSESSMENT METHOD (CRM)

The CRM design introduced the concept of dose–toxicity models to guide the dose-finding process (O'Quigley et al., 1990; O'Quigley, 2011). The dose–toxicity model represents the investigator's a priori belief in the likelihood of dose limiting toxicity (DLT) according to delivered dose, which thereafter is updated sequentially using cumulative patient toxicity data. While the choice of the prior distribution is always a concern in the Bayesian framework, CRM designs have proven to be robust to model mis-specification (Shen and O'Quigley, 1996) as long as the models themselves are selected based upon clinical knowledge. The original version of the CRM allowed for skipping of dose levels during escalation, which had the consequence that a large proportion of patients could be exposed to unacceptably toxic doses if the prespecified model were incorrect. Several modifications to the original CRM have been proposed to address these safety concerns, such as starting the trial at the lowest dose level, not allowing for skipping of dose levels during escalation, and requiring at least three patients at each dose level prior to escalation (Goodman et al., 1995; Piantadosi et al., 1998; Heyd and Carlin, 1999). The classical and modified CRMs are all model-based adaptive designs that have demonstrated superior operating characteristics compared to algorithm-based designs (such as the traditional 3 + 3 design) in simulation settings: A higher proportion of patients are treated at levels closer to the optimal dose level, and fewer numbers of patients are required to complete the trial.

### 5.2.1 Extensions to the CRM Design

Current statistical approaches have extended the standard CRM design discussed earlier in two directions to allow the modeling of toxicity and efficacy outcomes in a phase I setting. The first approach maintains the bivariate structure of outcomes through a joint modeling of toxicity and efficacy, whereas the second approach collapsed the combination of toxicity and efficacy outcomes into an ordinal trinary variable that follows a sequential order: acceptable toxicity (i.e., no DLTs) and no efficacy, acceptable toxicity (i.e., no DLTs) but with efficacy, or unacceptable toxicity (i.e., DLTs) that renders any efficacy irrelevant. Examples of the first approach include the following: the bivariate CRM that utilizes a marginal logit dose–toxicity curve and a marginal logit dose–disease progression curve with a flexible bivariate distribution of toxicity and progression (Braun, 2002), a dose-finding algorithm based on the efficacy–toxicity trade-offs (Thall and Cook, 2004), a dose-finding design using toxicity and efficacy odds ratios (Yin et al., 2006), and bivariate probit models for toxicity and efficacy (Bekele and Shen, 2005; Dragalin et al., 2008). In terms of the second approach of collapsing the combination of toxicity and efficacy outcomes into an ordinal outcome, simple models with a power function were explored by O'Quigley et al. (2001) and Wang and Ivanova (2005); more sophisticated models such as the proportional odds (PO) model (Thall and Russell, 1998) or continuation ratio (CR) models (Zhang et al., 2006; Mandrekar et al., 2007) have also been explored. Here, we review the theoretical model framework, the design specifics, and the simulation results of the CR model-based trivariate CRM (TriCRM) designs for single and dual agent drug combinations in the next section.

## 5.3 TRIVARIATE CRM (TriCRM) DESIGNS

### 5.3.1 Theoretical Framework

Let $y = (y_0, y_1, y_2)$ denote a trinary ordinal variable representing the three possible outcomes of acceptable toxicity without efficacy, acceptable toxicity with efficacy, and severe toxicity, respectively, with corresponding probabilities denoted by $\psi(x, \theta) = \{\psi_0(x, \theta), \psi_1(x, \theta), \psi_2(x, \theta)\}$. The probability of each outcome is a function of the dose of the agent ($x$) together with the parameter vector ($\theta$), with the following assumptions:

- $\psi_0(x, \theta)$, the probability of acceptable toxicity without efficacy is a decreasing function of the dose ($x$).
- $\psi_2(x, \theta)$, the probability of severe toxicity is an increasing function of the dose.
- The probability of acceptable toxicity with efficacy, that is, treatment success, $\psi_1(x, \theta)$ can be a nonmonotone function of the dose ($x$).

Extending this framework to the dual agent setting, $x = (x_1, x_2)$ is now an indicator of dose levels for each agent, and $\theta$ is the set of parameters that characterize the true toxicity and efficacy curves for each agent, with "no response" as no efficacy and acceptable toxicity, "success" as efficacy and acceptable toxicity, and "toxicity" as unacceptable toxicity, defined for each agent, respectively. The probability of no response, $\psi_0(x, \theta)$, is assumed to decrease monotonically with increase in dose level of each agent, the probability of toxicity, $\psi_2(x, \theta)$, is assumed to increase monotonically with increase in dose level of each agent, and when dose level of one agent is fixed, the success probability, $\psi_1(x, \theta)$, is unimodal (monotone increasing or monotone decreasing or parabolic) in the dose levels of the other agent.

Zhang et al. (2006) proposed the continuation ratio (CR) regression model for a single agent TriCRM model as given in the following:

$$\log\left(\frac{\psi_1}{\psi_0}\right) = \mu + \alpha + \beta_1 \cdot x \tag{5.1}$$

$$\log\left(\frac{\psi_2}{\psi_0 + \psi_1}\right) = \alpha + \beta_2 \cdot x \tag{5.2}$$

where $\theta = (\mu, \alpha, \beta)$, $\beta_1 > 0$, and $\beta_2 > 0$ to ensure the monotonic relationships of $\psi_1(x, \theta)/\psi_0(x, \theta)$ and $\psi_2(x, \theta)$ with dose $(x)$. If $n$ is the number of cohorts treated at the current time, $x$ is an $n \times 1$ dose vector with element $x_i$, and $y$ is an $n \times 3$ outcome matrix with $y_i$ as the $i$th row, for $i = 1, 2, 3, \ldots n$; then given the dose-outcome model and current data $(x; y)$, the likelihood function is given by

$$L(\theta \mid x, y) = \prod_{i=1}^{n} \psi_0(x_i, \theta)^{y_{0i}} \cdot \psi_1(x_i, \theta)^{y_{1i}} \cdot \psi_2(x_i, \theta)^{y_{2i}} \tag{5.3}$$

where
  $x_i$ is the dose administered to the $i$th cohort
  $y_i = (y_{0i}; y_{1i}; y_{2i})$ is the trinomial outcome of the $i$th cohort with size $c_i = (y_{0i} + y_{1i} + y_{2i})$ at dose $x_i$
  $\psi_j (\cdot), j = 0, 1, 2$, are the probabilities as defined earlier

This likelihood function is updated as data from each successive cohort become available. If only a binary toxicity outcome measure (toxic versus nontoxic) is available, then this likelihood function is essentially the same as that for the standard CRM model based on a two parameter logistic model using only the dose–toxicity relationship. Mandrekar et al. (2007) extended the single agent CR model to accommodate two agents by including two additional slope parameters for the second agent as given in the following:

$$\log\left(\frac{\psi_1}{\psi_0}\right) = \mu + \alpha + \beta_1 \cdot x_1 + \beta_3 \cdot x_2 \tag{5.4}$$

$$\log\left(\frac{\psi_2}{\psi_0 + \psi_1}\right) = \alpha + \beta_2 \cdot x_1 + \beta_4 \cdot x_2 \tag{5.5}$$

where $\beta_1 > 0$, $\beta_2 > 0$, $\beta_3 > 0$, and $\beta_4 > 0$ to ensure the monotonic relationship for each agent marginally. The likelihood function is constructed similarly to the single agent scenario (Equation 5.3), where $x \in R^{n \times 2}$ is the dose matrix with rows $x_i$ for each agent, and $y \in R^{n \times 3}$ is the outcome matrix, where $n$ is the number of patient cohorts already treated in the trial. To facilitate numerical computation within the Bayesian framework, both models utilize independent broad uniform priors for the parameter $\theta$ to account for potential uncertainties.

## 5.3.2 Decision Functions and Dose-Finding Algorithm

Let $\pi_0$ be the maximum tolerable toxicity probability, which is prespecified prior to trial initiation. The decision functions $\delta_1(x;\theta)$ and $\delta_2(x;\theta)$ are considered jointly with the accumulated toxicity and efficacy data for decision making of dose escalation or de-escalation, as outlined in the following:

$$\delta_1(x;\theta) = I\left[\psi_2(x;\theta) < \pi_0\right]$$

$$\delta_2(x;\theta) = \max_{x \in c(x)}\left\{\psi_1(x;\theta)\right\} \tag{5.6}$$

Specifically, the toxicity criterion requires $\delta_1(x;\theta) = 1$, that is, the toxicity probability at the single agent or combination dose levels is smaller than the pre-specified limit of $\pi_0$. Given that the toxicity criterion is satisfied, the success criterion $\delta_2(x;\theta) = \max_{x \in c(x)}\left\{\psi_1(x;\theta)\right\}$ seeks to maximize the probability of success, that is, among all the possible dose levels or dose level combinations, it selects the dose level or the combination dose level with the highest estimated success probability. In the single agent setting, $\delta_2(x;\theta)$ can also be specified to maximize the difference between the success probability and toxicity probability instead of just maximizing the success probability as given in (3.5) (Zhang et al., 2006). Specifically,

$$\delta_2(x;\theta) = \psi_1(x;\theta) - \lambda\psi_2(x;\theta); \quad 0 \le \lambda \le 1$$

$$\delta_2(x^*;\theta) = \max_{x \in c(x)} \delta_2(x;\theta) \tag{5.7}$$

Thus, the success criterion seeks to maximize either the difference between the success probability and toxicity probability if $\lambda = 1$, or the success probability if $\lambda = 0$. The value of $\lambda$ can be varied between 0 and 1 to include toxicity in the efficacy criterion.

A step-by-step approach to conducting a trial using the model-based TriCRM designs for single or dual agent combination is given in the following:

1. Treat a cohort of $k$ patients at a time, starting from the lowest dose level in the case of a single agent, or to the three lowest dose level combinations for the dual agent.

2. Skipping of dose levels is not recommended; thus, doses are escalated only by one level at a time but dose de-escalation is not necessarily restricted. For a trial with dual agents, the proposed level for the next cohort must be a neighbor of one of the combination levels already tested, where a neighbor refers to a change in dose level of at most one agent by at most one level.

3. At each interim point, $\hat{\theta}$ is updated and the decision functions given by (3.6) are evaluated using the accumulated toxicity and efficacy data.

4. If $\delta_1(x;\hat{\theta})=0$ for all dose levels (or combinations), and the current dose level is the lowest dose level (or combination), the trial is terminated and no dose level is recommended.

5. If $\delta_1(x;\hat{\theta})=0$ for all dose levels, but the current level is not the lowest, then treat the next cohort of patients at the lowest dose level (or combination).

6. Otherwise, the next dose level at which $\delta_2(x;\hat{\theta})$ is maximized among those with $\delta_1(x;\hat{\theta})=1$ is chosen for the next cohort of patients.

7. The trial is terminated after at least a minimum number of patients (say $n_1$) have been treated, provided at least a prespecified number of patients (say $m$) have been treated at the proposed combination dose level, or until a maximum number of patients (say $n_2$) are treated, whichever occurs first. As a default, $n_1$ is chosen as 18, $m$ is chosen as 9, and $n_2$ is chosen as 30 and 45 for the single and dual agent settings.

Extensive simulation studies were carried out to evaluate the performance of the TriCRM designs. While the dose–toxicity curves were monotone increasing in all the scenarios, the dose–efficacy curves were monotone increasing, monotone decreasing, or unimodal. In the single agent setting, the average sample size ranged from 16 to 25 patients depending on the location of the BOD, the percentage of patients treated at the optimal dose level varied from 25% (unimodal dose-efficacy case) to as high as 75%, and the no-recommendation rate was high when the starting dose is too toxic. Zhang et al. (2006) also showed that the TriCRM design is more efficient in identifying the optimal dose compared to a design where patients are randomly assigned to dose levels, which has been proposed as an approach for dose finding for nontoxic agents. The scenarios for the dual agent TriCRM design were complicated by the fact that each agent had a different dose–efficacy or a dose–toxicity curve of its own. In this setting, a dose success region was also defined, in addition to the optimal dose combination that included all those dose levels with acceptable toxicity that have a success probability within 15% of the highest success probability (Mandrekar et al., 2007). The percentages of patients treated at the optimal dose level combinations (region) varied from 57% to 71%, with a high non-recommendation rate for toxic combinations. The average sample size ranged from 21 to 34 for the six scenarios considered in their simulations. For further details on the simulation settings, and the results, refer to Zhang et al. (2006), Mandrekar et al. (2007, 2010).

## 5.4 ILLUSTRATION OF THE TRICRM DESIGN FOR A SINGLE AGENT DOSE-FINDING TRIAL

Here, we consider the implementation of a TriCRM design in a mock trial in the setting of head and neck cancer. Patients with head and neck cancer have a global cancer predilection throughout the oropharyngeal mucosa. Oral leukoplakia is an established precursor lesion to oropharyngeal cancer. Current management options include watchful waiting, laser ablation, or aggressive surgical resection. Photodynamic therapy (PDT) coupled with a photosensitizing agent (Aminolevulinic Acid HCL, ALA) could potentially permit a targeted therapy approach to high-risk mucosal lesions. Typically, extremely high energies with spot sizes of 1–2 mm are used to coagulate blood vessels in the vocal cord, with no adjuvant drug. In this mock trial, assume that equivalent or superior clinical outcomes at much lower laser energy densities could potentially be obtained through the introduction of the photosensitizing agent, ALA. We describe here a dose-finding clinical trial design that attempts to determine the safety and tolerability of the optimal laser dose (PDT) needed to activate ALA in the oral cavity among subjects with premalignant oral lesions.

Let the dose levels to be experimented be ALA ($60 \, mg/kg$) + $4 \, J/cm^2$, ALA ($60 \, mg/kg$) + $6 \, J/cm^2$, ALA ($60 \, mg/kg$) + $7 \, J/cm^2$, and ALA ($60 \, mg/kg$) + $8 \, J/cm^2$, where a higher dose may not necessarily improve efficacy, but could result in increased toxicity. Unacceptable adverse events will be defined as third degree burn in the treated region as well as any significant side effects (tissue damages) from ALA following the common toxicity criteria (CTC). Efficacy is measured in terms of response rate defined as either a complete or partial response. A complete response is defined as complete regression of treated lesions by clinical imaging, a partial response (PR) is defined as 50% or greater regression of the treated lesion area in clinical imaging, and no response (NR) is defined as no clinical change or less than 50% regression of the treated lesion. The proposed design would then use the continuation ratio (CR) model incorporating both adverse events and efficacy to estimate the optimal laser dose needed to activate ALA in the oral cavity. The dose-finding algorithm of the TriCRM design will use two decision functions: an adverse events criterion that requires that the unacceptable adverse events probability at each dose level is less than a prespecified rate (say 30%), and an efficacy criterion that maximizes the success probability among the dose levels that meet the adverse events criterion. The trial would then proceed as follows: (1) assign three patients to the lowest starting dose level; (2) based on the accumulated data at any point in the trial, update the parameter estimates of the CR model and evaluate the adverse events criterion for the dose range to be explored; (3) within the dose ranges that satisfy the adverse events criterion, identify the dose level that has the maximum estimated success probability; (4) assign the next cohort of three patients to the dose level that has the maximum estimated success probability; and (5) repeat the previous steps until at least 9 patients are treated at the optimal dose level combination or until a maximum of 18 patients are treated, whichever occurs first. In the event that the entire dose range does not satisfy the adverse event criterion, and the current dose level is not the starting dose level, this design has the flexibility to start the trial all over again by assigning the next three patients to the starting dose level instead of terminating the trial based on the premise that additional data might be needed at each dose level for a more accurate estimation of the true toxicity and efficacy curves. The trial could be designed to allow (or not allow) skipping of dose levels in the dose escalation process. An advantage of this design is that it summarizes patient outcomes in terms of both adverse events and efficacy. Moreover, the trial would be terminated early if all dose levels to be explored are determined to have an unacceptable adverse event rate.

## 5.5   CONCLUDING REMARKS

The failure of promising agents in randomized studies has prompted a reconsideration of the standard dose-finding paradigm, with the recognition that improved drug development strategies for both single agent and dual agent combinations are required. While the assumption of a monotonically increasing dose–toxicity curve is almost always appropriate from a biological standpoint, a monotonically increasing relationship between dose and efficacy has been challenged by the recent development of molecularly targeted therapies, vaccines, and immunotherapy. Model-based designs are certainly not perfect or recommended for every dose-finding study, but they provide an attractive alternative (notwithstanding the previously mentioned challenges) compared to the traditional algorithm-based up and down methods when one or both of the following is true: (1) Number of dose levels for escalation/de-escalation is large, that is, six or higher, for example, and (2) agent(s) being tested is(are) expected to have unknown dose efficacy outcomes. In the first case, the traditional designs would typically require a larger number of patients to be treated if indeed the optimal dose level is near the highest dose level. In the second case, the dose escalation/de-escalation decisions are based not only on safety but also a measure of efficacy that is quick and reliable to assess. Despite the favorable characteristics of CRM-based designs for dose-finding studies of targeted therapies from a theoretical standpoint, there exists significant scientific and pragmatic reasons for why these designs are not yet "popular" choices for dose-finding studies (Rogatko et al., 2007; Zohar and Chevret, 2007; Mandrekar et al., 2010). Some of the scientific reasons for not relying on model-based designs for early phase studies include (1) lack of validated biomarkers for efficacy, (2) lack of validated assays, (3) real-time assessment of the biomarker outcome not possible, (4) dichotomous efficacy outcomes inaccurate and suboptimal (model-based designs for time to event or other continuous endpoints are limited/nonexistent), and (5) inability of some of the designs to accommodate categorical (as opposed to a continuum) dose level combinations. Several pragmatic issues have limited the use of these designs in early phase clinical trials, including (1) lack of familiarity with the design, (2) fear of the "black-box" decision-making framework in comparison to the straightforward decision process with the traditional non-model-based designs, (3) perceived loss of control of the data and relying on the statistical model to decide where to treat the next cohort of patients, (4) fear of lack of regulatory acceptance, and (5) finally, and most importantly, resistance to change and unwilling to be the "first" to try a new approach. The challenge of determining an optimal dose for biologic and molecularly targeted agents is considerable from both a clinical and statistical standpoint in early phase trials. The model-based designs we present have been shown to have considerable promise, at least from a theoretical standpoint, in improving the ability to identify the BOD.

## REFERENCES

Bekele BN, Shen Y. A Bayesian approach to jointly modeling toxicity and biomarker expression in a phase I/II dose-finding trial. *Biometrics* 2005; 61(2):343–354.
Braun T. The bivariate continual reassessment method: Extending the CRM to phase I trials of two competing outcomes. *Controlled Clinical Trials* 2002; 23(3):240–256.
Conaway MR, Dunbar S, Peddada SD. Designs for single or multiple-agent phase I trials. *Biometrics* 2004; 60:661–669.
Dragalin V, Fedorov VV, Wu Y. Adaptive designs for selecting drug combinations based on efficacy-toxicity response. *Journal of Statistical Planning and Inference* 2008; 138:352–373.
Gelmon KA, Eisenhauer EA, Harris AL, Ratain MJ, Workman P. Anticancer agents targeting signaling molecules and cancer cell environment: Challenges for drug development. *Journal of the National Cancer Institute* 1999; 91(15):1281–1287.
Goodman SN, Zahurak ML, Piantadosi S. Some practical improvements in the continual reassessment method for phase I studies. *Statistics in Medicine* 1995; 14(11):1149–1161.
Hamberg P, Ratain MJ, Lesaffre E, Verweij J. Dose-escalation models for combination phase I trials in oncology. *European Journal of Cancer* 2010; 46(16):2870–2878.
Harris M. Monoclonal antibodies as therapeutic agents for cancer. *The Lancet Oncology* 2004; 5:292–302.
Heyd JM, Carlin BP. Adaptive design improvements in the continual reassessment method for phase I studies. *Statistics in Medicine* 1999; 18(11):1307–1321.
Huang X, Biswas S, Oki Y, Issa JP, Berry DA. A parallel phase I/II clinical trial design for combination therapies. *Biometrics* 2007; 63(2):429–436.
Linsley PS. New look at an old costimulator [comment]. *Nature Immunology* 2005; 6(3):231–232.
Mandrekar SJ, Cui Y, Sargent DJ. An adaptive phase I design for identifying a biologically optimal dose for dual agent drug combinations. *Statistics in Medicine* 2007; 26(11):2317–2330.
Mandrekar SJ, Qin R, Sargent DJ. Model-based phase I designs incorporating toxicity and efficacy for single and dual agent drug combinations: Methods and challenges. *Statistics in Medicine* 2010; 29(10):1077–1083.
O'Quigley J. Dose-finding using continual re-assessment method. In *Handbook of Statistics in Clinical Oncology*, 3rd edn., eds. J. Crowley, D. P. Ankerst, and A. Hoering. Chapman & Hall/CRC: Taylor & Francis, Boca Raton, FL, 2011.
O'Quigley J, Hughes MD, Fenton T. Dose-finding designs for HIV studies. *Biometrics* 2001; 57(4):1018–1029.
O'Quigley J, Pepe M, Fisher L. Continual reassessment method: A practical design for phase 1 clinical trials in cancer. *Biometrics* 1990; 46:33–48.
Parulekar WR, Eisenhauer EA. Phase I trials design for solid tumor studies of targeted, non-cytotoxic agents: Theory and practice. *Journal of the National Cancer Institute* 2004; 96(13):990–997.

Piantadosi S, Fisher JD, Grossman S. Practical implementation of a modified continual reassessment method for dose-finding trials. *Cancer Chemotheraphy and Pharmacology* 1998; 41(6):429–436.

Rogatko A, Schoeneck D, Jonas W, Tighiouart M, Khuri FR, Porter A. Translation of innovative designs into phase I trials. *Journal of Clinical Oncology* 2007; 25(31):4982–4986.

Shen LZ, O'Quigley J. Consistency of continual reassessment method under model misspecification. *Biometrika* 1996; 83(2):395–405.

Simon R, Korn EL. Selecting combinations of chemotherapeutic drugs to maximize dose intensity. *Journal of Biopharmaceutical Statistics* 1991; 1:247–258.

Storer BE. Design and analysis of phase I clinical trials. *Biometrics* 1989; 45(3):925–937.

Thall PF, Cook JD. Dose-finding based on efficacy-toxicity trade-offs. *Biometrics* 2004; 60(3):684–693.

Thall PF, Millikan RE, Mueller P, Lee SJ. Dose-finding with two agents in phase I oncology trials. *Biometrics* 2003; 59:487–496.

Thall PF, Russell KE. A strategy for dose-finding and safety monitoring based on efficacy and adverse outcomes in phase I/II clinical trials. *Biometrics* 1998; 54:251–264.

Wang K, Ivanova A. Two-dimensional finding in discrete dose space. *Biometrics* 2005; 61:217–222.

Yin G, Li Y, Ji Y. Bayesian dose-finding in phase I/II clinical trials using toxicity and efficacy odds ratios. *Biometrics* 2006; 62(3):777–784.

Yin G, Yuan Y. Bayesian dose-finding in oncology for drug combinations by copula regression. *Journal of the Royal Statistical Society: Series C (Applied Statistics)* 2009; 58:211–224.

Zhang W, Sargent DJ, Mandrekar SJ. An adaptive dose-finding design incorporating both toxicity and efficacy. *Statistics in Medicine* 2006; 25(14):2365–2383.

Zohar S, Chevret S. Recent developments in adaptive designs for phase I/II dose-finding studies. *Journal of Biopharmaceutical Statistics* 2007; 17(6):1071–1083.

# 6 Seamless Phase I/II Trial Design for Assessing Toxicity and Efficacy for Targeted Agents

*Antje Hoering, Michael LeBlanc,*
*and John J. Crowley*

## CONTENTS

## 6.1   INTRODUCTION

The main goal in phase I trials for traditional cytotoxic agents is to determine the maximal tolerated dose (MTD). The underlying premise is that both efficacy and toxicity increase monotonically with increasing dose levels. Only toxicity, not efficacy, is monitored during a traditional phase I trial. The standard $3+3$ design accrues three to six patients at a time to a given dose level and then increases the dose level until dose limiting toxicity (DLT) is observed. If two or more DLTs are observed in a group of six patients at that dose level, dose escalation ceases and the MTD has been exceeded. The highest dose where no more than one DLT in six subjects is observed is the MTD. Storer reviews the performance of this and other traditional phase I trial designs in the first chapter of this handbook [9].

The premise for phase I trials for cytostatic or targeted agents is generally different. Since the targeted agent is designed to specifically interfere with a molecular pathway directly related to specific characteristics of the tumor, it is hypothesized to be less toxic than a traditional cytotoxic agent. Toxicity does not necessarily increase with increasing dose levels. Efficacy does not necessarily increase monotonically with increasing dose levels either, but may plateau after it reaches maximal efficacy; higher dose levels past this point may no longer yield higher efficacy.

Thus, the goal for dose-finding trials for targeted agents should be to determine the dose level that provides highest efficacy while assuring the safety of that dose level. We refer to this dose as the best dose. A variety of continual reassessment models (CRMs) have been proposed for this purpose. These are summarized in Chapter 5 of this handbook [7]. Hunsberger et al. [4] recently proposed a dose escalation trial for targeted therapies similar to the traditional 3 + 3 phase I trial, but with dose escalation solely based on biomarker response, assuming that no significant toxicity will occur. These proposed trial designs address the issue of finding such a dose and have good statistical properties. None of these trial designs appears to have found widespread acceptance in the clinical trials community yet. Here we propose a phase I / II trial design to assess both toxicity and efficacy to find the best dose as well as a good dose. In this context the *best* dose is defined as the dose level that maximizes efficacy while assuring safety and a *good* dose is defined as a dose level where efficacy is above a predefined boundary while maintaining safety. Targeted agents are often difficult and expensive to manufacture in larger quantities and a smaller dose provides economic benefit. Thus under some circumstances a *good* dose may even be preferable to the *best* dose. Jain et al. [5] recently evaluated several phase I trials for targeted agents and found evidence that patients on lower dose levels do not necessarily fare worse.

This phase I/II design can easily be implemented and interpreted. It allows for extended cohorts of patients at dose levels close to the best dose to more precisely determine toxicity and efficacy of the new agent. In addition, different patient populations may be enrolled to the phase I and phase II portion. Traditionally the patient population for assessing toxicity is broader than the patient population for the first efficacy trials.

## 6.2 PHASE I/II TRIAL DESIGN FOR TARGETED AGENTS

We recently investigated the operating statistics of this two-step dose-finding trial for assessing both toxicity and efficacy for a new targeted agent [3]. Both steps are implemented in the same protocol to insure seamless continuation. For the first step we use a traditional phase I trial design, such as the 3 + 3, the accelerated titration, or the CRM model. This step only assesses toxicity and finds the MTD. This step insures that the dose levels at and below the MTD are safe in humans. Even if a new agent is not anticipated to have toxicity and has been shown to be safe in animal models, it is important to be certain of that fact before exposing a large number of humans to a new agent [2].

The goal of the second step is to determine the best dose in terms of efficacy and toxicity as a dose level no larger than the MTD. Great care has to be taken in determining the best efficacy endpoint for this part of the trial. Defining an early efficacy endpoint based on tumor biology for these agents is often difficult. In addition, some of these targeted agents are not necessarily expected to yield sufficient tumor shrinkage to achieve a clinical response by standard response criteria (e.g., RECIST). One possibility is to use progression-free survival at a single time point or disease control rate (clinical response of stable or better).

For this second step we propose a phase II modified selection design [6] for two or three dose levels at and below the MTD to determine efficacy and evaluate a dose level for both efficacy and toxicity. We assume that a binary endpoint for efficacy such as the ones discussed previously has been determined. We suggest accruing approximately 15–20 patients per dose level and assess both toxicity and efficacy for those patients. Each dose level is an arm in our phase II trial. We first evaluate each arm independently for both efficacy and toxicity. We perform a simple hypothesis test to determine efficacy and assess the power of the test statistic by determining the probability of passing the efficacy boundary independently in each arm. We also determine how many patients experience a DLT and define a toxicity boundary, which is traditionally 33%. If the percentage of patients experiencing a DLT at a specific dose level (arm) is larger than or equal to the toxicity boundary, this dose level is considered to be too toxic and is not pursued any further. On the other hand, if the percentage of patients experiencing a DLT in a specific arm is lower than the toxicity boundary, we consider this arm having acceptable toxicity. We next determine the probability of picking the arm with the largest efficacy while assuring acceptable toxicity and a minimal efficacy level as defined earlier using a slightly modified methodology of selection designs. This expanded cohort of 15–20 patients for two or three dose levels allows us to get a more precise estimate of toxicity and efficacy and thus a higher probability of correctly determining the best dose before launching into a larger trial.

## 6.3 UNDERLYING MODEL ASSUMPTIONS AND SIMULATION STUDIES

We assume that toxicity and efficacy are binary measures. In general, toxicity and efficacy are closely linked. Each dose level has a specific average toxicity and efficacy associated with it. We thus simulate the toxicity and efficacy data using a correlated bivariate logistic regression model. The correlation can be measured by a correlation coefficient or an odds ratio relating the two endpoints. We chose the odds ratio as a means to measure the correlation as it has better numerical properties and there exists a readily available R-package (VGAM) [10].

Let the marginal probabilities (for toxicity and efficacy) be logistic and depend on the parameter $\beta$. For an observation with covariate vector x the marginal probabilities are then given by

$$Pr(Y = 1) = \frac{\exp(x\beta)}{1 + \exp(x\beta)}$$

Let $p_{ij}$ be the joint probability for toxicity $i = (0,1)$ and efficacy $j = (0,1)$. The odds ratio $\psi$ is defined by $\psi = p_{11} p_{00}/p_{10} p_{01}$. For a description of bivariate odds ratio models see Ref. [8]. The joint probability $p_{11}$ can be expressed in terms of the marginal probabilities $p_1$ and $p_2$ as follows [1]:

$$p_{11} = \begin{cases} 1/2(\psi-1)^{-1}\left(a-\sqrt{a^2+b}\right) & \text{for} \quad \psi \neq 0 \\ p_1 p_2 & \quad\quad \psi = 0 \end{cases}$$

where

$a = 1+(p_1+p_2)(\psi-1)$ and $b = -4\psi(\psi-1)p_1 p_2$

$p_1$ and $p_2$ denote the marginal probabilities for toxicity and efficacy, respectively

For our simulation studies we use six dose levels, which is a commonly used number of dose levels for early therapeutic studies. We assume that the dose–response curve is monotonically increasing with increasing dose and remains constant after a critical dose is reached. The window of the six dose levels examined may include different parts of that dose–response curve. We distinguish three types of efficacy scenarios. As discussed earlier, efficacy may be measured in different ways depending on the underlying mechanism of the agent of interest. Here we refer to all the efficacy measures loosely as response measures, keeping in mind, however, that the actual efficacy measure may be different from the traditionally defined response. Figure 6.1a depicts the three response scenarios as a function of dose level. Response scenario R1: This scenario assumes a continuous increase in response with increasing dose level within the dose levels considered. In this case the leveling-off could occur outside the dose ranges considered. Response scenario R2: In scenario 2 we assume an increase in response for the first four dose levels after which it levels off. Response scenario R3: Scenario 3 describes the scenario where the response is independent of the dose level within the range considered.

Similarly, we assume three types of toxicity scenarios; for the scenario with monotone increase in toxicity we consider two different slopes, so that there is a total of 4 toxicity scenarios. More specifically, these scenarios are as follows: Toxicity scenario T1: Scenario 1 assumes that toxicity increases until a maximum toxicity is achieved after which it levels off. Toxicity scenario T2 and T3: Scenarios T2 and T3 assume that toxicity increases monotonically with dose level, where the increase is steeper for T2 than T3. Toxicity scenario T4: Finally, scenario 4 assumes negligible toxicity. Those scenarios are illustrated in Figure 6.1b.

Based on these four toxicity scenarios and three response scenarios there are twelve possible combinations of scenarios. The *best* dose is defined as the one that maximizes efficacy while maintaining acceptable toxicity and a minimal efficacy, that is, the rate of DLTs is below the toxicity limit and efficacy passes the efficacy boundary. In addition, we define a *good* dose level as a dose level with acceptable toxicity and efficacy passing the efficacy boundary. For each of the response and toxicity scenario combinations the best dose levels and good dose levels by efficacy and toxicity are summarized in Table 6.1.

In our simulation studies we determined the probability of correctly identifying the MTD in the phase I trial using a traditional "3+3" trial design. A CRM or accelerated titration design could also be used for this step. We used 1000 simulations.

For the phase I trial 3 different outcomes for each of the toxicity scenarios can be distinguished: The MTD is correctly determined, the MTD is too large, or the MTD

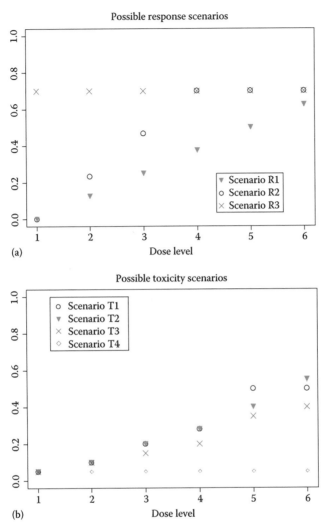

**FIGURE 6.1** (a) Possible response scenarios as a function of dose level. Plotted are the marginal probabilities as a function of dose level. (b) Possible toxicity scenarios as a function of dose level. Plotted are the marginal probabilities as a function of dose level.

is too low. In our simulation studies for the phase II portion we determined the power of the efficacy test, the probability of the doses being tested to be too toxic, and the probability of correctly determining the best dose. We randomized 40 patients to two dose levels, the dose level determined by the phase I part (arm 1) and the dose level immediately below the MTD (arm 2). The hypothesis test for response used in this example tests H0: $p = 0.05$ versus HA: $p = 0.30$. The toxicity limit in our simulations is defined to be 33%. In our simulation studies, arm 1 is chosen if the toxicity is below the toxicity boundary, if the efficacy is above the efficacy boundary, and if the observed efficacy is larger than the efficacy in arm 2. Arm 2 is chosen if the toxicity

**TABLE 6.1**

**Overall Probability of Selecting the *Best* or *Good* Dose Level**

| Efficacy Scenario | Toxicity Scenario | Best Dose Level | Good Dose Level | Probability of Picking *Best* Dose with Our Proposed Design | Probability of Picking *Good* Dose with Our Proposed Design | Probability of Picking *Best* Dose with Traditional Ph I/II Design | Probability of Picking *Good* Dose with Traditional Ph I/II Design |
|---|---|---|---|---|---|---|---|
| R1 | T1 | 4 | 4 | 0.16 | 0.16 | 0.21 | 0.21 |
| R1 | T2 | 4 | 4 | 0.15 | 0.15 | 0.18 | 0.18 |
| R1 | T3 | 4 | 4 | 0.29 | 0.29 | 0.30 | 0.30 |
| R1 | T4 | 6 | 4–6 | 0.61 | 0.88 | 0.84 | 0.89 |
| R2 | T1 | 4 | 3, 4 | 0.20 | 0.55 | 0.21 | 0.51 |
| R2 | T2 | 4 | 3, 4 | 0.20 | 0.52 | 0.19 | 0.46 |
| R2 | T3 | 4 | 3, 4 | 0.38 | 0.58 | 0.31 | 0.48 |
| R2 | T4 | 4–6 | 3–6 | 0.89 | 0.93 | 0.89 | 0.93 |
| R3 | T1 | 1–4 | 1–4 | 0.93 | 0.93 | 0.86 | 0.86 |
| R3 | T2 | 1–4 | 1–4 | 0.90 | 0.90 | 0.80 | 0.80 |
| R3 | T3 | 1–4 | 1–4 | 0.85 | 0.85 | 0.78 | 0.78 |
| R3 | T4 | 1–6 | 1–6 | 0.97 | 0.97 | 0.97 | 0.97 |

Compared are the properties of a traditional phase I design followed by a traditional phase II trial design and the seamless phase I/II trial design proposed in this chapter.

is below the toxicity boundary, if the efficacy is above the efficacy boundary, and if the observed efficacy is larger than or equal to the efficacy in arm 1. These two probabilities do not add up to one as neither arm is chosen if the toxicity is too high or the efficacy is not large enough.

We also compared our results with a combination of the same phase I trial and a traditional single-arm phase II trial at the dose level determined by the phase I trial. We used the same total sample size and determine the probability of correctly picking the best dose level and a good dose level using the previous definitions. We evaluated the overall probability of picking a good and best dose level using our proposed design as a sum of the probabilities of the different possible ways to select a *good* or *best* dose level (Figure 6.2).

## 6.4   RESULTS AND DISCUSSION

The first four columns of Table 6.1 summarize the twelve toxicity and efficacy scenario combinations and their respective MTD, *best* and *good* dose levels as defined earlier. For some scenarios there is only one *best* dose and one *good* dose, whereas for others several or even all dose levels can be considered *good*. In the scenarios R1T1, R1T2, and R1T3, level 4 is the MTD and the only level that crosses the efficacy

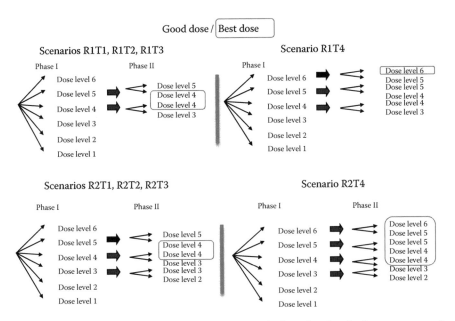

**FIGURE 6.2**  Possible ways to select a good dose or the best dose level using our proposed design for response scenarios R1 and R2. Good dose levels as defined by toxicity and efficacy are listed below the phase II portion. The best dose levels are circled.

boundary. On the other extreme is scenario R3T4 where all levels are considered safe and all levels cross the efficacy boundary.

Detailed results of our simulations of the phase I part of the trial can be found in [3]. We chose a high correlation or odds ratio between efficacy and toxicity for simulating the efficacy and toxicity data. The log odds ratio we chose for all our simulation studies is 4.6. The 3 + 3 design is very conservative. The probability of reaching the level above the MTD is in general small. In the scenarios with dose level 4 being the MTD, the probability of correctly identifying the MTD or the dose level below is similar and in general somewhere between 20% and 30%. Scenarios T2 and T3 both assume a monotone increase in toxicity with dose level 4 being the MTD. The only difference is that scenario T2 has a steeper increase than scenario T3; dose level 5 for T2 is set at 40%, well above the MTD whereas dose level 5 for T3 is set at 35%, just slightly above the MTD. As a result, the mass of the probability distribution for T3 is moved to the right compared to T2 and the probability of correctly reaching the MTD (level 4) or the level above the MTD (level 5) is higher than for T2.

Figure 6.2 illustrates the possible ways to reach a good dose or the best dose for response scenarios R1 and R2. Again, a good dose is defined as any dose achieving efficacy above a predefined boundary while maintaining safety, and a best dose achieves maximum efficacy while maintaining safety. The schema for scenarios R1T1, R1T2, and R1T3 on the top left side of Figure 6.2 illustrates the two possible ways to reach dose level 4 (the only level with acceptable toxicity and efficacy). If the MTD is correctly identified in phase I, the patients will be randomized between dose levels 4 and 3 and there is the possibility to end up with the best dose level. If the phase I trial picks level 5 (the dose level right above the MTD), patients will be randomized between level 5 and 4 in the phase II portion of the trial and again there is the possibility to select the best dose level. The more "best" dose levels there are the more ways there are to correctly identify the best dose. For scenario R3T4 (not shown) all dose levels are considered "best" levels.

Details of our phase II simulation results for the phase I trial can be found in Ref. [3]. In the case that the phase I trial correctly identifies the MTD, patients are being randomized to two dose levels: the MTD (arm 1) and the dose level immediately below the MTD (arm 2). Similar simulation studies were performed for the case that the phase I trial identifies the dose level above or below the MTD as the correct dose. In addition to evaluating the power, the probability of more than 33% of patients experiencing an MTD in each arm was determined. Finally, we determined the probability of selecting the better dose level (in our example arm 1) by using our modified selection design taking into account both efficacy and toxicity.

We also evaluated the influence of the correlation of efficacy and toxicity. As mentioned earlier, we chose a large odds ratio for simulating our data as in general efficacy and toxicity are highly correlated. To explore the influence of this correlation we did simulation studies for the case that the phase I trial identifies the MTD correctly, but unlike Table 6.1, the odds ratio was chosen to be 1 (log odds = 0), which corresponds to no correlation of toxicity and efficacy. The probability of an arm being too toxic is slightly lower in the case of no correlation, and thus the probability of picking the best dose by efficacy and toxicity is slightly higher compared to the same probability calculated using a large correlation.

Table 6.1 compares our results to the traditional sequence of a phase I trial followed by a single-arm phase II trial at the dose level determined by the phase I trial using the same total sample size. We have to keep in mind that due to the discreteness of the binomial distribution, the alpha levels which are determined by the efficacy boundary in the two examples (single arm with 40 patients versus two-arm with 20 patients each) are not identical. It is 0.05 for the traditional single-arm trial and 0.07 for each of the arms in the phase II selection design.

In general, the probability of picking a good or best dose is similar or larger in our proposed design than in the traditional design. The traditional design fares better if the true efficacy is close to the alternative hypothesis for the MTD (scenario R1). In that case doubling the sample size in the phase II portion yields a considerably higher power and thus higher probability of the phase II portion having a positive outcome. If the underlying toxicity is not uniformly low relative to the maximum toxicity cutoff (i.e., excluding T4 in our examples), the difference in probability of picking a good or best dose is at most 5% higher than in our proposed design. The only occasion where the traditional design fares considerably better is in determining the best dose for the scenario where the true efficacy is close to the alternative hypothesis for the MTD (R1) and toxicity is negligible (T4). In all other response scenarios our proposed design performs better than the traditional design. This is particularly true for finding a good dose in the efficacy scenario R2 and the toxicity scenarios T1–T3 where toxicity is not negligible.

The 3 + 3 phase I trial design is designed to be very conservative. For the toxicity scenarios T1 and T2, the probability of determining the dose level above the MTD as the correct dose level is 8% or lower. Thus, it is very unlikely for efficacy scenarios R1 and R2 to eventually arrive at the best dose level by reaching the dose level above the MTD first. On the other hand, the probability of reaching the dose level right below the MTD as the correct dose level in a phase I trial is often as high as that of reaching the MTD. A possible consideration that would greatly increase the probability of reaching the best dose level with our seamless phase I/II trial design would be to randomize patients to three dose levels, the dose level determined to be the MTD by the phase I trial and the dose levels right below and right above that dose. This would be a possibility if there was strong evidence in animal studies and the understanding of the pathways of activity that this new agent was not toxic. This would obviously require continuous toxicity monitoring in the phase II portion and appropriate toxicity stopping rules for the higher dose levels. Three dose levels would also allow simple logistic regression modeling under the assumption of smooth dose and toxicity profiles to reduce variance of estimates of response or toxicity at a given toxicity level.

In summary, this seamless phase I/II trial design performs in most cases better than a traditional design using the same overall sample size. We chose a 3 + 3 trial design for the simulation studies of the phase I portion of the trial; other phase I trial designs such as a CRM or accelerated titration could have been used instead. A possibility would be to slightly increase the sample size in the phase II portion of the proposed design and thus assuring the highest probability of finding the most efficacious and least toxic dose level. This design allows assessing a few dose levels more closely for both efficacy and toxicity and greater certainty of having correctly determined the best dose level before launching into a large efficacy trial. It should thus be considered even in the scenarios where a slightly larger sample size may be required.

## ACKNOWLEDGMENT

This work was supported in part by grants #CA038926 and #CA90998 from the National Cancer Institute.

## REFERENCES

1. Dale JR. (1986). Global cross-ratio models for bivariate, discrete, ordered responses. *Biometrics*, 42: 909–917.
2. Hanrahan EO, Heymach JV. (2007). Vascular endothelial growth factor receptor tyrosine kinase inhibitors vandetanib (ZD6474) and AZD2171 in lung cancer. *Clinical Cancer Research*, 13: 4617s–4622s.
3. Hoering A, LeBlanc M, Crowley J. (2011) Seamless phase I/II trial design for assessing toxicity and efficacy for targeted agents. *Clinical Cancer Research*, 17:640–646.
4. Hunsberger S et al. (2005). Dose escalation trial designs based on a molecularly targeted endpoint. *Statistics in Medicine*, 24: 2171–2181.
5. Jain RK et al. (2010). Phase I oncology studies: Evidence that in the era of targeted therapies patients on lower doses do not fare worse. *Clinical Cancer Research*, 16: 1289–1297.

6. Liu PY, Moon J, LeBlanc M. (2011). Phase II selection designs. In Chapter 10: *Handbook of Statistics in Clinical Oncology*, 3rd edn., eds. Crowley J and Hoering A, Seattle, WA: Cancer Research & Biostatistics.

7. Mandrekar S, Sargent D. (2011). CRM trials assessing toxicity and efficacy. In Chapter 5: *Handbook of Statistics in Clinical Oncology*, 3rd edn., eds. Crowley J and Hoering A, Seattle, WA: Cancer Research & Biostatistics.

8. McCullagh P, Nelder JA. (1989). *Generalized Linear Models*, 2nd edn., Chapman & Hall.

9. Storer BE. (2011). Choosing a phase I design. In Chapter 1: *Handbook of Statistics in Clinical Oncology*, 3rd edn., eds. Crowley J and Hoering A, Seattle, WA: Cancer Research & Biostatistics.

10. Yee TW. (2009). The VGAM R-package: Vector generalized linear and additive models.

# Part II

**Phase II Trials**

# 7 Overview of Phase II Clinical Trials

*Stephanie Green*

## CONTENTS

## 7.1  DESIGN

Standard phase II studies are used to screen new regimens for activity and to decide which ones should be tested further. To screen regimens efficiently, the decisions generally have been based on single-arm studies using short-term endpoints, typically tumor response in cancer studies, in limited numbers of patients. The problem is formulated as a test of the null hypothesis $H_0$: $p = p_0$ versus the alternative hypothesis $H_A$: $p = p_A$, where $p$ is the probability of response, $p_0$ is the probability that if true would mean that the regimen was not worth studying further, and $p_A$ is the probability that if true would mean it would be important to identify the regimen as active and to continue studying it. Typically, $p_0$ is a value at or somewhat below the historical probability of response to standard treatment for the same stage of disease, and $p_A$ is typically somewhat above.

For ethical reasons, studies of new agents usually are designed with two or more stages of accrual allowing early stopping due to inactivity of the agent. A variety of approaches to early stopping have been proposed. Although several of these include options for more than two stages, only the two-stage versions are discussed in this chapter. In typical clinical settings, it is difficult to manage more than two stages. An early approach due to Gehan (1961) suggested stopping if $0/N$ responses were observed, where the probability of $0/N$ was less than 0.05 under a specific alternative (for $p_0 = 0.2$, $N = 14$). Otherwise, accrual was to be continued until the sample size was large enough for estimation at a specified level of precision.

Fleming (1982) proposed stopping when results are inconsistent either with $H_0$ or $H_{AA}: p=p'$, where $H_0$ is tested at level $\alpha$ and $p'$ is the alternative for which the procedure has power $1-\alpha$. The bounds for stopping after the first stage of a two-stage design are the nearest integer to $N_1 p' - Z_{1-\alpha}\{Np'(1-p')\}^{1/2}$ for concluding early that the regimen should not be tested further, and the nearest integer to $N_1 p_0 + Z_{1-\alpha}\{Np_0(1-p_0)\}^{1/2}+1$ for concluding early that the regimen is promising, where $N_1$ is the first stage sample size and $N$ is the total after the second stage. At the second stage, $H_0$ is accepted or rejected according to the normal approximation for a single-stage design. Since then, other authors, rather than proposing tests, have proposed choosing stopping boundaries to minimize the expected number of patients required, subject to level and power specifications. Chang et al. (1987) proposed minimizing the average expected sample size under the null and alternative hypotheses. Simon (1989), recognizing the ethical imperative of stopping when the agent is inactive, recommended stopping early only for unpromising results and minimizing the expected sample size under the null or, alternatively, minimizing the maximum sample size. A problem with these designs is that sample size has to be accrued exactly for the optimality properties to hold, so in practice they cannot be carried out faithfully in many settings. Particularly, in multi-institution settings, studies cannot be closed after a specified number of patients have been accrued. It takes time to send out and process a closure notice, and, during this time, more patients will have been approached to enter the trial. Patients who have been asked and have agreed to participate in a trial should be allowed to do so, and this means that there is a period of time during which institutions can continue registering patients even though the study is closing. Furthermore, some patients may be found to be ineligible after the study is closed. It is rare to end up with precisely the number of patients planned, making application of fixed designs problematic.

To address this problem, Green and Dahlberg (1992) proposed designs allowing for variable attained sample sizes. The approach is to accrue patients in two stages to have level approximately 0.05 and power approximately 0.9 and to stop early if the agent appears unpromising. Specifically, the regimen is concluded unpromising, and the trial is stopped early if the alternative $H_A: p=p_A$ is rejected in favor of $p<p_A$ at the 0.02 level after the first stage of accrual. The agent is concluded promising if $H_0: p=p_0$ is rejected in favor of $p>p_0$ at the 0.055 level after the second stage of accrual. The level 0.02 was chosen to balance the concern of treating the fewest possible patients with an inactive agent against the concern of rejecting an active agent due to treating a chance series of poor risk patients. Level 0.05 and power 0.9 are reasonable for solid tumors due to the modest percent of agents found to be active in this setting (Simon, 1987); less conservative values might be appropriate in more responsive diseases.

The design has the property that stopping at the first stage occurs when the estimate of the response probability is less than approximately $p_0$, the true value that would mean the agent would not be of interest. At the second stage, the agent is concluded to warrant further study if the estimate of the response probability is greater than approximately $(p_A+p_0)/2$, which typically would be equal to or somewhat above the historical probability expected from other agents and a value at which one might be expected to be indifferent to the outcome of the trial. However, there are no optimality properties. Chen and Ng (1998) proposed a different approach to flexible design by optimizing with respect to expected sample size under $p_0$ across possible attained sample sizes. They assumed a uniform distribution over sets of eight consecutive $N_1$s; presumably, if information is available on the actual distribution in a particular setting, then the approach could be used for a better optimization. To address the problem of temporary closure of studies, Herndon (1998) proposed an alternative approach that allows patient accrual to continue while results of the first stage are reviewed. Temporary closures are disruptive, so this approach might be reasonable for cases where accrual is relatively slow with respect to submission of information. If too rapid, the ethical aim of stopping early due to inactivity is lost.

Table 7.1 illustrates several of the design approaches mentioned earlier for level 0.05 and power 0.9 tests including Fleming designs, Simon minimax designs, Green and Dahlberg designs, and Chen and Ng optimal design sets. Powers and levels are reasonable for all approaches. Chen and Ng designs have the correct level on average, although individual realizations have levels up to 0.075 among the tabled designs. Of the four approaches, Green and Dahlberg designs are the most conservative with respect to early stopping for level 0.05 and power 0.9, whereas Chen and Ng designs are the least.

In another approach to phase II design, Storer (1992) suggested a procedure similar to two-sided testing instead of the standard one-sided test. In this approach, two hypothesis tests, one for $H_0$ and one for $H_A$ are performed. The phase II is considered negative ($H_A$: $p=p_A$ is rejected) if the number of responses is sufficiently low, positive ($H_0$: $p=p_0$ is rejected) if sufficiently high, and equivocal if intermediate (neither hypothesis rejected). For a value $p_m$ between $p_0$ and $p_A$, upper and lower rejection bounds are chosen such that the probability of concluding the trial is positive is less than $\gamma$ when $p=p_m$, and the probability of concluding the trial is negative is also less than $\gamma$ when $p=p_m$. The sample size and $p_m$ are chosen to have adequate power to reject $H_A$ under $p_0$ or $H_0$ under $p_A$. When $p_0=0.1$ and $p_A=0.3$, an example of a Storer design is to test $p_m=0.193$ with $\gamma=0.33$ and power 0.8 under $p_0$ and $p_A$. For a two-stage design, $N_1$, $N$, $r_{L1}$, $r_{U1}$, $r_{L2}$, and $r_{U2}$ are 18, 29, 1, 6, 4, and 7, respectively, where $N_1$ is the sample size for the first stage, $N$ is the total sample size, and $r_{Li}$ and $r_{Ui}$ are upper and lower rejection bounds for stage $i$, $i=1, 2$. If the final result is equivocal (5 or 6 responses in 29 for this example), the conclusion is that other information is necessary to make the decision. Hong and Wang (2007) discuss a three conclusion approach for small randomized phase IIs.

Other proposals for single-arm phase II studies include designs with multinomial outcomes. Zee et al. (1999) and Chang et al. (2007) consider three possible outcomes—response, stability, and early progression—with a goal of recommending further testing if the number of responses is sufficiently high and number of early progressions is sufficiently low. Following Chang et al., the null hypothesis is $H_0$: $p_R \leq p_{R0}$ or $p_F \geq p_{F0}$, where R refers to response and failure F refers to early progression, and the study is designed to have power for the alternative $p_R = p_{R0} + \Delta_R$ and $p_F = p_{F0} - \Delta_F$. The rejection region for a single-stage design of fixed sample size is of the form $R \geq r$ and $F \leq f$, where $R$ and $F$ are the number of responses and early progressions, respectively. The sample size will be larger than that required for individual binomial tests of response or failure since both the response and failure nulls

**TABLE 7.1**

**Examples of Designs**

| | $H_0$ versus $H_A$ | $N_1$ | $a_1$ | $b_1$ | $N$ | $a_2$ | $b_2$ | Level (Average and Range for Chen) | Power (Average and Range for Chen) |
|---|---|---|---|---|---|---|---|---|---|
| Fleming | 0.05 versus 0.2 | 20 | 0 | 4 | 40 | 4 | 5 | 0.052 | 0.92 |
| | 0.1 versus 0.3 | 20 | 2 | 6 | 35 | 6 | 7 | 0.053 | 0.92 |
| | 0.2 versus 0.4 | 25 | 5 | 10 | 45 | 13 | 14 | 0.055 | 0.91 |
| | 0.3 versus 0.5 | 30 | 9 | 16 | 55 | 22 | 23 | 0.042 | 0.91 |
| Simon | 0.05 versus 0.2 | 29 | 1 | — | 38 | 4 | 5 | 0.039 | 0.90 |
| | 0.1 versus 0.3 | 22 | 2 | — | 33 | 6 | 7 | 0.041 | 0.90 |
| | 0.2 versus 0.4 | 24 | 5 | — | 45 | 13 | 14 | 0.048 | 0.90 |
| | 0.3 versus 0.5 | 24 | 7 | — | 53 | 21 | 22 | 0.047 | 0.90 |
| Green | 0.05 versus 0.2 | 20 | 0 | — | 40 | 4 | 5 | 0.047 | 0.92 |
| | 0.1 versus 0.3 | 20 | 1 | — | 35 | 7 | 8 | 0.020 | 0.87 |
| | 0.2 versus 0.4 | 25 | 4 | — | 45 | 13 | 14 | 0.052 | 0.91 |
| | 0.3 versus 0.5 | 30 | 8 | — | 55 | 22 | 23 | 0.041 | 0.91 |
| Chen | 0.05 versus 0.2 | 17–24 | 1 | — | 41–46 | 4 | 5 | 0.046 | 0.90 |
| | | | | | 47–48 | 5 | 6 | 0.022–0.069 | 0.845–0.946 |
| | 0.1 versus 0.3 | 12–14 | 1 | — | 36–39 | 6 | 7 | 0.050 | 0.90 |
| | | 15–19 | 2 | | 40–43 | 7 | 8 | 0.029–0.075 | 0.848–0.938 |
| | 0.2 versus 0.4 | 18–20 | 4 | — | 48 | 13 | 14 | 0.050 | 0.90 |
| | | 21–24 | 5 | | 49–51 | 14 | 15 | 0.034–0.073 | 0.868–0.937 |
| | | 25 | 6 | | 52–55 | 15 | 16 | | |
| | 0.3 versus 0.5 | 19–20 | 6 | — | 55 | 21 | 22 | 0.050 | 0.90 |
| | | 21–23 | 7 | | 56–58 | 22 | 23 | 0.035–0.064 | 0.872–0.929 |
| | | 24–26 | 8 | | 59–60 | 23 | 24 | | |
| | | | | | 61–62 | 24 | 25 | | |

$N_1$ is the sample size for the first stage of accrual, $N$ is the total sample size after the second stage of accrual, $a_i$ is the bound for accepting $H_0$ at stage $i$, and $b_i$ is the bound for rejecting $H_0$ at stage $i$ for $i = 1, 2$. Designs are listed for Fleming (1982), Simon (1989), Green and Dahlberg (1992); the optimal design set is listed for Chen and Ng (1998).

must be rejected. For example, if $\Delta$ is 0.2 for each of response and early progression, $p_{R0}$ is 0.3, $p_{F0}$ is 0.4, level is 0.05, and power is 0.8, then a sample size of 49 patients is required. For a positive trial, at least 21 responses and at most 13 early progressions must be observed. For a trial with only response as the endpoint, 39 patients would be required. Optimal two-stage designs are also described in the Chang et al. article; for the same example, 48 patients are accrued in two stages of 24, and the trial is stopped early if $R \geq 14$ and $F \leq 4$ ($H_0$ rejected) or if either $R \leq 8$ or $F \geq 9$ ($H_0$ accepted). However, it is noted that some of these designs optimized for minimum sample size may not be ideal for other reasons (e.g., early stopping rule insufficiently conservative) so some adjustment might be in order.

Panageas et al. (2002) address a similar design, where both complete response and partial response are of interest. For this setting, the hypotheses of interest are $H_0$: $p_{CR} \leq p_{0CR}$ and $p_{PR} \leq p_{0PR}$ versus $H_0$: $p_{CR} > p_{0CR}$ or $p_{PR} > p_{0PR}$. As for Chang et al. (2007) designs, the outcome is multinomial (CR, PR, and No Response); but, in this case, the number of CRs and PRs are the statistics of interest rather than CRs and failures (no response). Lin et al. (2008) consider a similar trinomial outcome consisting of response, prolonged stable, and failure. Here, the hypotheses of interest are $H_0$: $p_R \leq p_{0R}$ and $p_C \leq p_{0C}$ versus $H_0$: $p_R > p_{0R}$ or $p_C > p_{0C}$, where C is clinical benefit response (objective response or prolonged stable; note $p_{0R}$ must be $< p_{0C}$). In this case, the statistics of interest are $R$ and $R + S$ ($R$ is the number of responses and $S$ is the number of prolonged stable disease). This arises in settings where it is thought a new agent might provide benefit through long term disease control not fully reflected by response.

Window designs are another option of recent interest. These involve treatment of newly diagnosed patients with a new regimen for a short period prior to start of standard therapy. This allows testing in patients not compromised by prior treatment so may improve the chance of identifying active regimens. On the other hand, delay of standard treatment may put patients at risk so settings in which such trials are used should be considered carefully. Another potential concern with window designs is that the short-term endpoint chosen (4–12 weeks) may not be sufficiently predictive of the longer term outcomes of primary interest. Trinomial outcomes (response, stable, and early failure) are common for these designs (Chang et al., 2007).

Stratified designs addressing the issue of heterogeneity in phase II populations have also gained recent interest. If subpopulations of patients have different underlying response probabilities, the usual approach of specifying a single value for the null may not be applicable to the population accrued. If the subpopulations are well understood, then designs that depend on the mix of patient types accrued may be advantageous. London and Chang (2005) propose the following single-stage statistic conditional on the number of patients accrued in each stratum. Here, $p_{i0}$ is the null probability of response for stratum $i$ and $N_i$ is the sample size accrued to stratum $i$, $i = 1 - k$:

$$T = \frac{R - \sum_{i=1}^{k} N_i p_{i0}}{\sqrt{\sum_{i=1}^{k} N_i p_{i0}(1 - p_{i0})}}$$

The rejection region will be equivalent to $R = \sum_{i=1}^{k} R_i > r_0$, where $r_0$ is such that $P(R > r_0 | N_i, p_{i0}, i = 1 \ldots k)$ is approximately equal to $\alpha$. Sample size calculations require estimates of the relative accrual rates of the strata. If the estimates are off, then power might be different from the calculation. For instance, if there are three strata with $p_0$s of 0.4, 0.2, and 0.1, $\Delta$s for the alternative are 0.2 for each stratum, level and power are specified as 0.05 and 0.8, and the expected proportion of patients from the three strata are 50%, 30%, and 20%, then 36 patients are sufficient. If the final sample sizes are 18, 10, and 8, then 14 responses are required to reject the null, and conditional level and power are on target at 0.04 and 0.82; if 24, 8 and 4 are accrued, then 16 responses are required and power drops to 0.78; while if 12 are accrued in each, then 12 responses are required and power is 0.86. Two-stage designs in this setting are discussed in the article and in more detail in Sposto and Gaynon (2009). A caveat with this approach is that conclusions cannot be drawn for each subpopulation. A different approach should be used if an answer in each group is of primary interest. See also Chapters 11, 28, and 32.

## 7.2  ANALYSIS OF STANDARD PHASE II DESIGNS

As noted in Storer (1992), the hypothesis testing framework typically used in phase II studies is useful for developing designs and determining sample size. The resulting decision rules are not always meaningful, however, except as tied to hypothetical follow-up trials that in practice may or may not be done. Thus, it is important to present confidence intervals for phase II results that can be interpreted appropriately regardless of the nominal decision made at the end of the trial as to whether further study of the regimen is warranted. The main analysis issue is estimation after a multistage trial, since the usual estimation procedures assuming a single-stage design are biased. Various approaches to generating confidence intervals have been proposed. These involve ordering the outcome space and inverting tail probabilities or test acceptance regions, as in estimation following single-stage designs; however, with multistage designs, the outcome space does not lend itself to any simple ordering.

Jennison and Turnbull (1983) order the outcome space by which boundary is reached, by the stage stopped at, and by the number of successes. Stopping at stage $i$ is considered more extreme than stopping at stage $i+1$ regardless of the number of successes. A value $p$ is not in the $1-2\alpha$ confidence interval if the probability under $p$ of the observed result or one more extreme according to this ordering is less than $\alpha$ in either direction. Chang and O'Brien (1986) order the sample space instead based on the likelihood principle. For each $p$, the sample space for a two-stage design is ordered according to $L(x,N^*) = [(x/N^*)^x(1-p)^{N^*-x}]/[p^x\{(N^*-x)/N^*\}^{N^*-x}]$, where $N^*$ is $N_1$ if the number of responses $x$ can only be observed at the first stage and $N$ if at the second. A value $p$ is in the confidence interval if one half of the probability of the observed outcome plus the probability of a more extreme outcome according to this ordering is $\alpha$ or less. The confidence set is not always strictly an interval, but the authors state that the effect of discontinuous points is negligible. Chang and O'Brien intervals are shorter than those of Jennison and Turnbull, although this in part would be because Jennison and Turnbull did not adjust for discreteness by assigning only one half of the probability of the observed value to the tail as Chang and O'Brien did. Duffy and Santner (1987) recommend ordering the sample space by success percent and also develop intervals of shorter length than Jennison and Turnbull intervals. Koyama and Chen (2008) describe methods for testing, estimation, and confidence intervals for two-stage Simon (1989) designs assuming the first stage sample size is fixed but allowing for the second stage to be variable. The method involves specifying conditional testing levels given results at the first stage. If the second stage is fixed, the confidence interval is based on ordering the sample space by number of successes, while for a sample size not equal to planned number, ordering of the sample space is defined to be consistent with the testing procedure.

Although they produce shorter intervals, Chang and O'Brien and Duffy and Santner approaches have the major disadvantage of requiring knowledge of the final sample size in order to calculate an interval for a study stopped at the first stage; as noted earlier, this typically will be random. The Jennison and Turnbull approach can be used, because it only requires knowledge up to the stopping time. The Koyama and Chen approach has the disadvantage of not using all of the information from the first stage if this stage over-accrues, but advantages in controlling conditional level and in allowing for variable second-stage accrual.

However, it is not entirely clear how important it is to adjust confidence intervals for the multistage nature of the design. From the point of view of appropriately reflecting the activity of the agent tested, the usual interval assuming a single-stage design may be sufficient. In this setting, the length of the confidence interval is not of primary importance because sample sizes are small and all intervals are long. Similar to Storer's idea, it is assumed that if the confidence interval excludes $p_0$, the regimen is considered active, and if it excludes $p_A$, the regimen is considered insufficiently active. If it excludes neither, results are equivocal. This seems reasonable whether or not continued testing is recommended for the better equivocal results.

For Green and Dahlberg designs, the differences between Jennison and Turnbull and unadjusted tail probabilities are 0 if the trial stops at the first stage, and are

$$-\sum_{0}^{a_1} \mathrm{bin}(i, N_1, P) \sum_{x-i}^{N-N_1} \mathrm{bin}(j, N-N_1, P)$$

for the upper tail if stopped at the second stage

and

$$+\sum_{0}^{a_1} \mathrm{bin}(i, N_1, P) \sum_{x-i+1}^{N-N_1} \mathrm{bin}(j, N-N_1, P)$$

for the lower tail if stopped at the second stage

where $a_1$ is the stopping bound for accepting $H_0$ at the first stage. Both the upper and lower confidence bounds are shifted to the right for Jennison and Turnbull intervals. These therefore will more often appropriately exclude $p_0$ when $p_A$ is true and inappropriately include $p_A$ when $p_0$ is true compared to the unadjusted interval. However, the tail differences are generally small resulting in small differences in the intervals. Based on the normal approximation, the absolute value of the upper tail difference is less than approximately 0.003 when the lower bound of the unadjusted interval is $p_0$, whereas the lower tail difference is constrained to be <0.02 for $p > p_A$ due to the early stopping rule. Generally, the shift in a Jennison and Turnbull interval is noticeable only for small $x$ at the second stage. As Rosner and Tsiatis (1998) note, such results, indicating activity in the first stage and no activity in the second, are unlikely, possibly suggesting the independent identically distributed assumption was incorrect.

For example, consider a common design for testing $H_0$: $p=0.1$ versus $H_A$: $p=0.3$: stop in favor of $H_0$ at the first stage if 0 or 1 responses are observed in 20 patients and otherwise continue to a total of 35. Of the 36 possible trial outcomes if planned sample sizes are achieved, the largest discrepancy in the 95% confidence intervals occurs if two responses are observed in the first stage and none in the second. For this outcome, the Jennison and Turnbull 95% confidence interval is from 0.02 to 0.25, while the unadjusted interval is from 0.01 to 0.19. Although not identical, both intervals lead to the same conclusions: the alternative is ruled out. For the Fleming and Green and Dahlberg designs listed in Table 7.1, Table 7.2 lists the probabilities that the 95% confidence intervals lie above $p_0$ (evidence the regimen is active), below $p_A$ (evidence the agent has insufficient activity to pursue), or cover both $p_0$ and $p_A$ (inconclusive). In no case are $p_0$ and $p_A$ both excluded. Probabilities are calculated for $p=p_A$ and $p=p_0$, both for unadjusted and for Jennison and Turnbull adjusted intervals. For the Green and Dahlberg designs considered, probabilities for the unadjusted and for the Jennison and Turnbull adjusted intervals are the same in most cases. The only discrepancy occurs for the 0.2 versus 0.4 design when the final outcome is 11/45 responses. In this case, the unadjusted interval is from 0.129 to 0.395, while the Jennison and Turnbull interval is from 0.131 to 0.402. There are more differences between adjusted and unadjusted probabilities for Fleming designs, the largest for ruling out $p_A$ in the 0.2 versus 0.4 and 0.1 versus 0.3 designs. In these

**TABLE 7.2**

**Probabilities under $p_0$ and $p_A$ for Unadjusted and Jennison–Turnbull (J–T) Adjusted 95% Confidence Intervals**

|  |  | Probability 95% CI is above $p_0$ When $p =$ | | Probability 95% CI is below $p_A$ When $p =$ | | Probability 95% CI Includes $p_0$ and $p_A$ When $p =$ | |
|---|---|---|---|---|---|---|---|
|  |  | $p_0$ | $p_A$ | $p_0$ | $p_A$ | $p_0$ | $p_A$ |
| 0.05 versus 0.2 | Green J–T | 0.014 | 0.836 | 0.704 | 0.017 | 0.282 | 0.147 |
|  | Unadjusted | 0.014 | 0.836 | 0.704 | 0.017 | 0.282 | 0.147 |
|  | Fleming J–T | 0.024 | 0.854 | 0.704 | 0.017 | 0.272 | 0.129 |
|  | Unadjusted | 0.024 | 0.854 | 0.704 | 0.017 | 0.272 | 0.129 |
| 0.1 versus 0.3 | Green J–T | 0.020 | 0.866 | 0.747 | 0.014 | 0.233 | 0.120 |
|  | Unadjusted | 0.020 | 0.866 | 0.747 | 0.014 | 0.233 | 0.120 |
|  | Fleming J–T | 0.025 | 0.866 | 0.39 | 0.008 | 0.583 | 0.126 |
|  | Unadjusted | 0.025 | 0.866 | 0.515 | 0.011 | 0.460 | 0.123 |
| 0.2 versus 0.4 | Green J–T | 0.025 | 0.856 | 0.742 | 0.016 | 0.233 | 0.128 |
|  | Unadjusted | 0.025 | 0.856 | 0.833 | 0.027 | 0.142 | 0.117 |
|  | Fleming J–T | 0.023 | 0.802 | 0.421 | 0.009 | 0.556 | 0.189 |
|  | Unadjusted | 0.034 | 0.862 | 0.654 | 0.022 | 0.312 | 0.116 |
| 0.3 versus 0.5 | Green J–T | 0.022 | 0.859 | 0.822 | 0.020 | 0.156 | 0.121 |
|  | Unadjusted | 0.022 | 0.859 | 0.822 | 0.020 | 0.156 | 0.121 |
|  | Fleming J–T | 0.025 | 0.860 | 0.778 | 0.025 | 0.197 | 0.115 |
|  | Unadjusted | 0.025 | 0.860 | 0.837 | 0.030 | 0.138 | 0.110 |

designs, no second-stage Jennison and Turnbull interval excludes the alternative, making this probability unacceptably low under $p_0$.

The examples presented suggest that adjusted confidence intervals do not necessarily result in more sensible intervals in phase II designs and, in some cases, are worse than not adjusting.

## 7.3 OTHER PHASE II DESIGNS

### 7.3.1 MULTIARM PHASE II DESIGNS

Occasionally, the aim of a phase II study is not to decide whether a particular regimen should be studied further but to decide which of several new regimens should be taken to the next phase of testing. In these cases, selection designs are used, often formulated as follows: take on to further testing the treatment arm observed to be best by any amount, where the number of patients per arm is chosen to be large enough such that if one treatment is superior by $\Delta$ and the rest are equivalent, the probability of choosing the superior treatment is $p$. Simon et al. (1985) published sample sizes for selection designs with response endpoints, and Steinberg and Venzon (2002) proposed an approach to early selection in this setting. After the first stage of accrual for a two-arm trial, one of the treatments is chosen for further study if the number of responses is higher by at least a specified amount $d_E$, where $d_E$ is chosen such that the probability of choosing an arm inferior by $\Delta$ is small. The procedure can be extended to three or more arms.

Liu et al. (1993) provide sample sizes for selection designs with survival endpoints. For survival, the approach is to choose the arm with the smallest estimated $\beta$ in a Cox model. Sample size is chosen such that if one treatment is superior with $\beta = \ln(1 + \Delta)$ and the others have the same survival, then the superior treatment will be chosen with probability $p$.

Theoretically, selection designs are reasonable, but, in reality, the designs are not strictly followed. If response is poor in all arms, the conclusion should be to pursue none of the regimens, which is not an option for these designs. If a striking difference is observed, then the temptation is to bypass the confirmatory phase III trial. In a follow-up to the survival selection paper, Liu et al. (1999) noted that the probability of an observed $\beta$ better than $\ln(1.7)$, which cancer investigators consider striking, is not negligible. With two to four arms, the probabilities are 0.07–0.08 when, in fact, there are no differences in the treatment arms. See also Chapter 10, which includes a discussion of selection designs with a minimum efficacy bounds.

With treatment advancements and more segmentation of patient populations, historical control estimates may be unreliable and preliminary comparative information may be necessary. Thus, randomized phase II trials with control arms have become substantially more common over the last several years. These are sometimes described as "non-comparative" but this is disingenuous; an informal comparison is always done and acted upon, with no way of judging the suitability of the conclusion. It is best to understand the properties of the design, so that results are less likely to be overinterpreted.

Although small randomized phase IIs with high level and low power have been suggested (e.g., Rubinstein et al., 2005), it should be kept in mind that a small randomized controlled phase II does not necessarily provide better conclusions than a single arm trial if the null is well characterized. Consider a trial of a new regimen for which the control probability is estimated to be 0.4. A single arm trial requires about 40 patients to test $H_0: p = 0.4$ versus the alternative hypothesis $H_A: p = 0.65$ with level 0.05 and power 0.9. A randomized trial with level 0.2 and power 0.8 for a difference of 0.25 requires about 60. If the null of 0.4 is correct, the single-arm trial will have a substantially lower chance of false-positive and false-negative results than the randomized trial despite requiring fewer patients. If the null was incorrectly specified and should have been in the range of 0.36 to 0.47, the single arm trial still will have a lower chance of false-positive and false-negative errors than the randomized trial. Outside of this range, the single-arm trial will be better with respect to one type of error and worse with respect to the other. If a randomized phase II is judged necessary, then to have the same level and power as a single arm study, a standard two-arm randomized trial will need to be about four times the size of the single-arm trial. See also Chapter 9.

Randomized discontinuation designs are a variation on a standard randomized controlled phase II. For discontinuation designs, patients are treated with standard of care plus a new agent and after a specified time on treatment patients who have not progressed are randomized to continue with the new agent or to receive standard of care only. If randomized patients who do not continue with the new agent do worse than those who do continue, then the new agent is concluded active. Although this approach has been used successfully, the number of patients required to start on treatment in order to have a reasonable number of randomized patients on trial is often prohibitively large. In addition, Capra (2004) notes that for realistic situations, power is better if all patients are randomized. He also notes it may be of concern that half of patients doing well on treatment will be required to stop.

### 7.3.2 PHASE II DESIGNS WITH MULTIPLE ENDPOINTS

The selected primary endpoint of a phase II trial is just one consideration in the decision to pursue a new regimen. If response is primary, secondary endpoints such as survival and toxicity must also be considered. For instance, a trial with a sufficient number of responses to be considered active may still not be of interest if too many patients experience life-threatening toxicity or if they all die quickly. On the other hand, a trial with an insufficient number of responses but a good toxicity profile and promising survival might still be considered for future trials.

Designs have been proposed to incorporate multiple endpoints explicitly into phase II studies. Bryant and Day (1995) proposed an extension of Simon's approach, identifying designs that minimize the expected accrual when the regimen is unacceptable either with respect to response or toxicity. Their designs are terminated at the first stage if either the number of responses is $C_{R1}$ or less, or the number of patients without toxicity is $C_{T1}$ or less, or both. The regimen is concluded useful if the number of patients with responses, and the number without toxicity are greater than $C_{R2}$ and $C_{T2}$, respectively, at the second stage. $N_1$, $N$, $C_{R1}$, $C_{T1}$, $C_{R2}$, and $C_{T2}$ are chosen such that the probability of recommending the regimen when the probability of no toxicity is acceptable ($p_T \geq p_{T1}$) but response is unacceptable ($p_R \leq p_{R0}$) is less than or equal to $\alpha_R$, the probability of recommending the regimen when response is acceptable ($p_R \geq p_{R1}$) but toxicity is unacceptable ($p_T \leq p_{T0}$) is less than or equal to $\alpha_T$, and the probability of recommending the regimen when both are acceptable is $1 - \beta$ or better. The constraints are applied either uniformly over all possible correlations between toxicity and response or assuming independence of toxicity and response. Minimization is done subject to the constraints. For many practical situations, minimization assuming independence produces designs that perform reasonably well when the assumption is incorrect.

Conaway and Petroni (1995) proposed similar designs assuming a particular relationship between toxicity and response, an optimality criterion, and a fixed total sample size are all specified. Design constraints proposed include limiting the probability of recommending the regimen to $\alpha$ or less when both response and toxicity are unacceptable and to $\gamma$ or less anywhere else in the null region (response or toxicity unacceptable but not both). The following year, Conaway and Petroni (1996) proposed boundaries allowing for tradeoffs between toxicity and response. Instead of dividing the parameter space as in Figure 7.1a, it is divided according to investigator specifications, as in Figure 7.1b, allowing for fewer patients with no toxicity when the response probability is higher and the reverse.

Their proposed test accepts $H_0$ when a statistic $T(\mathbf{x})$ is less than $c_1$ at the first stage or is less than $c_2$ at the second, subject to maximum level $\alpha$ over the null region and power at least $1 - \beta$ when $p_R = p_{R1}$ and $p_T = p_{T1}$ for an assumed value for the association between response and toxicity. The statistic $T(\mathbf{x})$ is $\sum P_{ij}^* \ln\left(P_{ij}^* / \hat{P}_{ij}\right)$, where $ij$ indexes the cells of the $2 \times 2$ response-toxicity table, $\hat{P}_{ij}$s are the usual probability estimates, and $P_{ij}^*$s are the values achieving $\inf \sum P_{ij} \ln(P_{ij} / \hat{P}_{ij})$.

$T(\mathbf{x})$ can be interpreted in some sense as a distance from the result to $H_0$. Interim stopping bounds are chosen to satisfy optimality criteria. The authors' preference is minimization of the expected sample size under the null. See also Chapter 8.

Thall and Cheng (2001) proposed another approach to multiendpoint design. Parameters of interest are $\Delta = (\Delta_R, \Delta_T)$, where $\Delta_R = g(p_{R1}) - g(p_{R0})$ is the difference between probability of response on experimental treatment ($p_{R1}$) and probability of historical response ($p_{R0}$), and $\Delta_T = g(p_{T1}) - g(p_{T0})$ is the difference between the

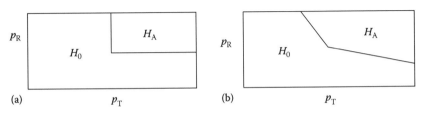

**FIGURE 7.1** Division of parameter space for two approaches to bivariate phase II design. (a) An acceptable probability of response and an acceptable probability of no toxicity are each specified. (b) Acceptable probabilities are not fixed at one value for each but instead allow for trade-off between toxicity and response. $p_R$ is the probability of response and $p_T$ is the probability of acceptable toxicity.

probability of acceptable toxicity on experimental treatment ($p_{T1}$) and the probability of acceptable toxicity historically ($p_{T0}$), after arcsine square square root transformation. Target parameters ($\xi_R$, $\xi_T$) are identified and the alternative region is the set of all $\Delta$s at least as desirable as the target, that is, {$\Delta$: $\Delta_R \geq \xi_R$ and $\Delta_T \geq \xi_T$}. If multiple targets are identified, the alternative $\Omega_A$ is the convex hull of these regions. Trial outcome is $\hat{\Delta} = (g(\hat{p}_{R1}) - g(\hat{p}_{R0}), g(\hat{p}_{T1}) - g(\hat{p}_{T0}))$. The rejection region $R(x)$ is {$(y-x, z-x)|(y, z) \in \Omega_A$}, where the sample size $n$ and a number $x$ are chosen such that $\Pr\{\hat{\Delta} \in R(x)|\Delta = (0, 0)\} \leq \alpha$ and $\Pr\{\hat{\Delta} \in R(x)|\Delta = (\xi_R, \xi_T)\} \geq 1 - \beta$ for each target. The test is based on approximate bivariate normality of $\sqrt{4n}(\hat{\Delta} - \Delta)$. Interim stopping boundaries are based on optimality criteria.

There are a number of practical problems with these designs. As for other designs relying on optimality criteria, they generally cannot be done faithfully in realistic settings. Even when they can be carried out, defining toxicity as a single yes–no variable is problematic, because typically several toxicities of various grades are of interest. Perhaps the most important issue is that of the response-toxicity trade-off. Any function specified is subjective and cannot be assumed to reflect the preferences of either investigators or patients in general.

### 7.3.3 BAYESIAN PHASE II DESIGNS

Bayesian approaches provide another formulation of phase II designs. As described in Estey and Thall (2003), prior probability distributions are assigned to $\pi_H$, the true historical probability of response, and to $\pi_E$, the true probability of response of the regimen under study. The prior for $\pi_H$ is informative, whereas the prior for $\pi_E$ generally is not. After each specified interim analysis time the posterior distribution of $\pi_E$, which also serves as the prior for the next stage of accrual, is calculated given the data. The distribution of $\pi_H$ is also updated if there is a randomized control arm, which the authors recommend. Accrual is stopped if the posterior probability that $\pi_E$ is greater than $\pi_H$ is small. The maximum sample size is chosen such that the final posterior distribution for $\pi_E$ if accrual completes is sufficiently precise, and the regimen under study is considered worth further study if there is a reasonable probability that $\pi_E$ is better than $\pi_H$. As with any Bayesian designs, care must be taken that the a priori assumptions do not unduly influence the conclusion and that stopping criteria are sufficiently conservative.

The Bayesian framework has been used to address other phase II issues. For example, Cheung and Thall (2002) addressed the problem of temporary study closure for certain types of response endpoints by proposing an adaptive Bayesian method. At each interim analysis time, an approximate posterior distribution is calculated using all of the event time data available including data from patients still on treatment for whom final endpoint determination is unknown. Nuisance parameters in the likelihood are replaced by consistent estimates. The design may reduce trial duration, but practical difficulties include the need for current follow-up and the numerous analyses. Case and Morgan (2003) describe a non-Bayesian two-stage approach to this problem when the outcome is survival status at $X$ months.

Other examples of Bayesian applications include Sambucini (2010) who describes an adaptive two-stage phase II, where the second-stage sample size is not chosen until results from the first stage are known and Ding et al. (2008), who suggest that combining information across several related single-arm phase II trials done in sequence using Bayesian decision theoretic methods has potential for more efficient screening of new agents than the usual one at a time approach.

## 7.4 DISCUSSION

Despite the precise formulation of decision rules, phase II trials are not as objective as we would like. The small sample sizes used cannot support decision-making based on all aspects of interest in a trial. Trials combining more than one aspect, such as toxicity and response, are fairly arbitrary with respect to the relative importance placed on each endpoint, including the 0 weight placed on the endpoints not included, and so are subject to about as much imprecision in interpretation as results of single endpoint trials. Furthermore, a phase II trial would rarely be considered on its own. By the time a regimen is taken to phase III testing, multiple phase II trials have been done and the outcomes of the various trials weighed and discussed.

For practical reasons, optimality considerations both with respect to design and confidence intervals are not particularly compelling in phase II trials. Sample sizes in the typical clinical setting are small and variable, making it more important to use procedures that work reasonably well across a variety of circumstances rather than optimally in one. Also, there are various characteristics that it would be useful to optimize; compromise is usually in order. Perhaps statistical considerations in a phase II design are most useful in keeping investigators realistic about how limited such designs are.

Randomization in itself does not guarantee a phase II will be reliable. Small sample sizes will still mean the probability of error is high. If a new population is being studied a larger randomized phase II may be worth the investment, both for learning about the new target population and to better assess the potential of the new regimen.

As a final note, keep in mind that for many cancers phase II studies with tumor response as the primary endpoint have not proven to be reliable in predicting success in phase III. For instance, Zia et al. (2005) describe 43 phase III trials done after the ideal case of phase IIs with the same regimen in the same population—with only a 28% success rate in phase III. Although response may be useful for demonstrating biologic activity, the primary endpoint used to assess efficacy should be considered carefully to best reflect potential for long-term benefit.

Detailed discussion of various phase II design issues introduced in this chapter are discussed in following chapters.

## REFERENCES

Bryant, J. and Day, R. 1995. Incorporating toxicity considerations into the design of two-stage phase II clinical trials. *Biometrics* 51:1372–1383.

Capra, W. 2004. Comparing the power of the discontinuation design to that of the classic randomized design on time-to-event endpoints. *Controlled Clinical Trials* 25:168–177.

Case, L.D. and Morgan, T. 2003. Design of phase II cancer trials evaluating survival probabilities. *BMC Medical Research Methodology* 3:6.

Chang, M., Devidas, M., and Anderson, J. 2007. One- and two-stage designs for phase II window studies. *Statistics in Medicine* 26:2604–2614.

Chang, M. and O'Brien, P. 1986. Confidence intervals following group sequential tests. *Controlled Clinical Trials* 7:18–26.

Chang, M., Therneau, T., Wieand H.S. et al. 1987. Designs for group sequential phase II clinical trials. *Biometrics* 43:865–874.

Chen, T. and Ng, T.-H. 1998. Optimal flexible designs in phase II clinical trials. *Statistics in Medicine* 17:2301–2312.

Cheung, Y.K. and Thall, P.F. 2002. Monitoring the rates of composite events with censored data in phase II clinical trials. *Biometrics* 58:89–97.

Conaway, M. and Petroni, G. 1995. Bivariate sequential designs for phase II trials. *Biometrics* 51:656–664.

Conaway, M. and Petroni, G. 1996. Designs for phase II trials allowing for a trade-off between response and toxicity. *Biometrics* 52:1375–1386.

Ding, M., Rosner, G., and Müller, P. 2008. Bayesian optimal design for phase II screening trials. *Biometrics* 64:886–894.

Duffy, D. and Santner, T. 1987. Confidence intervals for a binomial parameter based on multistage tests. *Biometrics* 43:81–94.

Estey, E.H. and Thall, P.F. 2003. New designs for phase 2 clinical trials. *Blood* 102:442–448.

Fleming, T. 1982. One sample multiple testing procedures for phase II clinical trials. *Biometrics* 38:143–151.

Gehan, E. 1961. The determination of number of patients in a follow-up trial of a new chemotherapeutic agent. *Journal of Chronic Diseases* 13:346–353.

Green, S. and Dahlberg, S. 1992. Planned vs attained design in phase II clinical trials. *Statistics in Medicine* 11:853–862.

Herndon, J. 1998. A design alternative for two-stage, phase II, multicenter cancer clinical trials. *Controlled Clinical Trials* 19:440–450.

Hong, S. and Wang, Y. 2007. A three-outcome design for randomized comparative phase II clinical trials. *Statistics in Medicine* 26:3525–3534.

Jennison, C. and Turnbull, B. 1983. Confidence intervals for a binomial parameter following a multistage test with application to MIL-STD 105D and medical trials. *Technometrics* 25:49–58.

Koyama, T. and Chen, H. 2008. Proper inference from Simon's two-stage designs. *Statistics in Medicine* 27:3145–3154.

Lin, X., Allred, A., and Andrews, G. 2008. A two-stage phase II trial design utilizing both primary and secondary endpoints. *Pharmaceutical Statistics* 7:88–92.

Liu, P.Y., Dahlberg, S., and Crowley, J. 1993. Selection designs for pilot studies based on survival endpoints. *Biometrics* 49:391–398.

Liu, P.Y., LeBlanc, M., and Desai, M. 1999. False positive rates of randomized phase II designs. *Controlled Clinical Trials* 20:343–352.

London, W. and Chang, M. 2005. One- and two-stage designs for stratified phase II clinical trials. *Statistics in Medicine* 24:2597–2611.

Panageas, K., Smith, A., Gönen, M. et al. 2002. An optimal two-stage phase II design utilizing complete and partial response information separately. *Controlled Clinical Trials* 23:367–379.

Rosner, G. and Tsiatis, A. 1988. Exact confidence intervals following a group sequential trial: A comparison of methods. *Biometrika* 75:723–729.

Rubinstein, L., Korn, E., Freidlin, B. et al. 2005. Design issues of randomized phase II trials and a proposal for phase II screening trials. *Journal of Clinical Oncology* 23:7199–7206.

Sambucini, V. 2010. A Bayesian predictive strategy for an adaptive two-stage design in phase II clinical trials. *Statistics in Medicine* 29:1430–1442.

Simon, R. 1987. How large should a phase II trial of a new drug be? *Cancer Treatment Reports* 71:1079–1085.

Simon, R. 1989. Optimal two-stage designs for phase II clinical trials. *Controlled Clinical Trials* 10:1–10.

Simon, R., Wittes, R., and Ellenberg, S. 1985. Randomized phase II clinical trials. *Cancer Treatment Reports* 69:1375–1381.

Sposto, R. and Gaynon, P. 2009. An adjustment for patient heterogeneity in the design of two-stage phase II trials. *Statistics in Medicine* 28:2566–2579.

Steinberg, S. and Venzon, D. 2002. Early selection in a randomized phase II clinical trial. *Statistics in Medicine* 21:1711–1726.

Storer, B. 1992. A class of phase II designs with three possible outcomes. *Biometrics* 48:55–60.

Thall, P.F. and Cheng, S.-C. 2001. Optimal two-stage designs for clinical trials, based on safety and efficacy. *Statistics in Medicine* 20:1023–1032.

Zee, B., Melnychuk, D., Dancey, J. et al. 1999. Multinomial phase II cancer trials incorporating response and early progression. *Journal of Biopharmaceutical Statistics* 9:351–363.

Zia, M., Siu, L., Pond, G. et al. 2005. Comparison of outcomes of phase II studies and subsequent randomized control studies using identical chemotherapy regimens. *Journal of Clinical Oncology* 23:6982–6991.

# 8 Designs Based on Toxicity and Response

*Gina R. Petroni and Mark R. Conaway*

## CONTENTS

## 8.1 INTRODUCTION

In principle, phase II trials evaluate whether a new agent is sufficiently promising to warrant a comparison with the current standard of treatment. An agent is considered sufficiently promising based on the proportion of patients who "respond," that is, experience some objective measure of disease improvement. The toxicity of the new agent, usually defined in terms of the proportion of patients experiencing severe side effects, has been established in a previous phase I trial.

In practice, the separation between establishing the toxicity of a new agent in a phase I trial and establishing the response rate in a phase II trial is artificial. Most phase II trials are conducted not only to establish the response rate, but also to gather additional information about the toxicity associated with the new agent. Conaway and Petroni[1] and Bryant and Day[2] cite several reasons why toxicity considerations are important for phase II trials:

1. *Sample sizes in phase I trials.* The number of patients in a phase I trial is small and the toxicity profile of the new agent is estimated with little precision. As a result, there is a need to gather more information about toxicity rates before proceeding to a large comparative trial.
2. *Ethical considerations.* Most phase II trials are designed to terminate the study early if it does not appear that the new agent is sufficiently promising to warrant a comparative trial. These designs are meant to protect patients from receiving substandard therapy. Patients should be protected also from receiving agents with excessive rates of toxicity and consequently, phase II trials should be designed with the possibility of early termination of the study if an excessive number of toxicities are observed. This consideration

is particularly important in studies of intensive chemotherapy regimens, where it is hypothesized that a more intensive therapy induces a greater chance of a response but also a greater chance of toxicity.

3. The characteristics of the patients enrolled in the previous phase I trials may be different than those of the patients to be enrolled in the phase II trial. For example, phase I trials often enroll patients for whom all standard therapies have failed. These patients are likely to have a greater extent of disease than patients who will be accrued to the phase II trial.

With these considerations, several proposals have been made for designing phase II trials that formally incorporate both response and toxicity endpoints. Conaway and Petroni[1] and Bryant and Day[2] propose methods that extend the two-stage designs of Simon.[3] In each of these methods, a new agent is considered sufficiently promising if it exhibits both a response rate that is greater than that of the standard therapy and a toxicity rate that does not exceed that of the standard therapy. Examples of these designs used in practice include Artz et al.,[4] Meropol et al.,[5] and Foon et al.[6] Jin,[7] and Wu and Liu[8] propose modifications to the procedure of Conaway and Petroni.[1]

Conaway and Petroni[9] present designs that allow for a trade-off between response and toxicity rates. In these designs, a new agent with a greater toxicity rate might be considered sufficiently promising if it also has a much greater response rate than the standard therapy. Thall et al.,[10,11] Thall and Sung,[12] Chen and Smith,[13] and Thall[14] propose Bayesian methods for monitoring response and toxicity that can also incorporate a trade-off between response and toxicity rates.

## 8.2 DESIGNS FOR RESPONSE AND TOXICITY

Conaway and Petroni[1] and Bryant and Day[2] present multi-stage designs that formally monitor response and toxicity. As a motivation for the multi-stage designs, we first describe the methods for a fixed sample design, using the notation in Conaway and Petroni.[1] In this setting, binary variables representing response and toxicity are observed in each of $N$ patients. The data are summarized in a $2 \times 2$ table where $X_{ij}$ is the number of patients with response classification $i$ and toxicity classification $j$ (Table 8.1). The observed number of responses is $X_R = X_{11} + X_{12}$ and the observed number of patients experiencing a severe toxicity is $X_T = X_{11} + X_{21}$. It is assumed that the cell counts in this table ($X_{11}, X_{12}, X_{21}, X_{22}$) have a multinomial distribution with underlying probabilities ($p_{11}, p_{12}, p_{21}, p_{22}$). That is, in the population of patients to be treated with this new agent, a proportion, $p_{ij}$, would have response classification $i$ and toxicity classification $j$ (Table 8.2). With this notation, the probability of a response is $p_R = p_{11} + p_{12}$ and the probability of a toxicity is $p_T = p_{11} + p_{21}$.

The design is based on having sufficient power to test the null hypothesis that the new treatment is "not sufficiently promising" to warrant further study against the alternative hypothesis that the new agent is sufficiently promising to warrant a comparative trial. Conaway and Petroni[1] and Bryant and Day[2] interpret the term "sufficiently promising" to mean that the new treatment has a greater response rate than the standard and that the toxicity rate with the new treatment is no greater than that of the standard treatment. Defining $p_{R0}$ as the response rate with the standard

**TABLE 8.1**

**Classification of Patients by Response and Toxicity**

|                |       | Toxicity |          |           |
|----------------|-------|----------|----------|-----------|
|                |       | **Yes**  | **No**   | **Total** |
| Response       | Yes   | $X_{11}$ | $X_{12}$ | $X_R$     |
|                | No    | $X_{21}$ | $X_{22}$ | $N - X_R$ |
|                | Total | $X_T$    | $N - X_T$| $N$       |

**TABLE 8.2**

**Population Proportions for Response and Toxicity Classifications**

|                |       | Toxicity |          |           |
|----------------|-------|----------|----------|-----------|
|                |       | **Yes**  | **No**   | **Total** |
| Response       | Yes   | $p_{11}$ | $p_{12}$ | $p_R$     |
|                | No    | $p_{21}$ | $p_{22}$ | $1 - p_R$ |
|                | Total | $p_T$    | $1 - p_T$| $1$       |

treatment and $p_{T0}$ as the toxicity rate for the standard treatment, the null hypothesis can be written as

$$H_0 : p_R \leq p_{R0} \text{ or } p_T \geq p_{T0}$$

$$H_a : p_R > p_{R0} \text{ and } p_T < p_{T0}$$

The null and alternative regions are displayed in Figure 8.1.

A statistic for testing $H_0$ versus $H_a$ is $(X_R, X_T)$, with a critical region of the form $C = \{(X_R, X_T) : X_R \geq c_R \text{ and } X_T \leq c_T\}$. We reject the null hypothesis and declare the treatment sufficiently promising if we observe many responses and little toxicity. We do not reject the null hypothesis if we observe too few responses or too much toxicity. Conaway and Petroni[1] choose the sample size, $N$, and critical values $(c_R, c_T)$ to constrain three error probabilities to be less than pre-specified levels $\alpha$, $\gamma$, and $\beta$, respectively. The three error probabilities are as follows:

1. The probability of incorrectly declaring the treatment promising when the response and toxicity rates for the new therapy are the same as those of the standard therapy.
2. The probability of incorrectly declaring the treatment promising when the response rate for the new therapy is no greater than that of the standard or the toxicity rate for the new therapy is greater than that of the standard therapy.

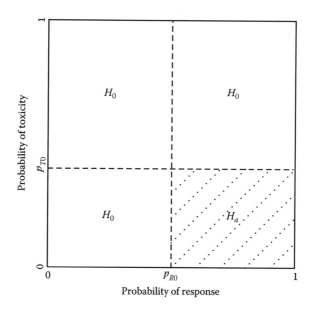

**FIGURE 8.1**  Null and alternative regions for a bivariate design.

3. The probability of declaring the treatment not promising at a particular point in the alternative region. The design should yield sufficient power to reject the null hypothesis for a specific response and toxicity rate, where the response rate is greater than that of the standard therapy and the toxicity rate is less than that of the standard therapy.

Mathematically, these error probabilities are expressed as

1. $P(X_R \geq c_R, X_T \leq c_T | p_R = p_{R0}, p_T = p_{T0}, \theta) \leq \alpha$

2. $\displaystyle \sup_{p_R \leq p_{R0} \text{ or } p_T \geq p_{T0}} P(X_R \geq c_R, X_T \leq c_T | p_R, p_T, \theta) \leq \gamma$

3. $P(X_R \geq c_R, X_T \leq c_T | p_R = p_{Ra}, p_T = p_{Ta}, \theta) > \beta$

where these probabilities are computed for a pre-specified value of the odds ratio, $\theta = (p_{11} p_{22})/(p_{12} p_{21})$, in Table 8.2. The point $(p_{Ra}, p_{Ta})$ is a pre-specified point in the alternative region, with $p_{Ra} > p_{R0}$ and $p_{Ta} < p_{T0}$.

Conaway and Petroni[1] compute the sample size and critical values by enumerating the distribution of $(X_R, X_T)$ under particular values for $(p_R, p_T, \theta)$. As an example, Conaway and Petroni[1] present a proposed phase II trial of high-dose chemotherapy for patients with non-Hodgkin's lymphoma. Results from earlier studies for this patient population have indicated that standard therapy results in an estimated response rate of 50% with approximately 30% of patients experiencing life-threatening toxicities. In addition, previous results indicated that approximately 35%–40% of the patients who experienced a complete response also experienced life-threatening toxicities. The odds ratio, $\theta$, is determined by the assumed response rate, toxicity rate, and the conditional probability of experiencing a life-threatening toxicity given that patient had a complete response. Therefore, $(p_{R0}, p_{T0})$ is assumed to be (0.50, 0.30) and the odds ratio is assumed to be 2.0. Conaway and Petroni[1] chose values $\alpha = 0.05$, $\gamma = 0.30$ and $\beta = 0.10$. The trial is designed to have approximately 90% power at the alternative determined by $(p_{Ra}, p_{Ta}) = (0.75, 0.15)$.

The extension to multi-stage designs is straightforward. The multi-stage designs allow for the early termination of a study if early results indicate that the treatment is not sufficiently effective or is too toxic. Although most phase II trials are carried out in at most two stages, for the general discussion, Conaway and Petroni[1] assume that the study is to be carried out in $K$ stages. At the end of the $k$th stage, a decision is made whether to enroll patients for the next stage or to stop the trial. If the trial is stopped early, the treatment is declared not sufficiently promising to warrant further study. At the end of the $k$th stage, the decision to continue or terminate the study is governed by the boundaries $(c_{Rk}, c_{Tk})$, $k = 1,\ldots, K$. The study continues to the next stage if the total number of responses observed up to and including the $k$th stage is at least as great as $c_{Rk}$ and the total number of toxicities up to and including the $k$th stage is no greater than $c_{Tk}$. At the final stage, the null hypothesis that the treatment is not sufficiently promising to warrant further study is rejected if there are a sufficient number of observed responses (at least $c_{RK}$) and sufficiently few observed toxicities (no more than $c_{TK}$).

In designing the study, the goal is to choose sample sizes for the stages $m_1, m_2,\ldots,$ $m_K$ and boundaries $(c_{R1}, c_{T1})$, $(c_{R2}, c_{T2}),\ldots, (c_{RK}, c_{TK})$ satisfying the error constraints listed earlier. For a fixed total sample size, $N = \Sigma_k m_k$, there may be many designs that satisfy the error requirements. An additional criterion, such as one of those proposed by Simon[3] in the context of two-stage trials with a single binary endpoint, can be used to select a design. The stage sample sizes and boundaries can be chosen to give the minimum expected sample size at the response and toxicity rates for the standard therapy $(p_{R0}, p_{T0})$ among all designs that satisfy the error requirements. Alternatively, one could choose the design that minimizes the maximum expected sample size over the entire null hypothesis region. Conaway and Petroni[1] compute the "optimal" designs for these criteria for two-stage and three-stage designs using a fixed pre-specified value for the odds ratio, $\theta$. Through simulations, they evaluate the sensitivity of the designs to a misspecification of the value for the odds ratio.

Bryant and Day[2] also consider the problem of monitoring binary endpoints representing response and toxicity. They present "optimal" designs for two-stage trials that extend the designs of Simon.[3] In the first stage, $N_1$ patients are accrued and classified by response and toxicity; $Y_{R1}$ patients respond and $Y_{T1}$ patients do not experience toxicity. At the end of the first stage, a decision to continue to the next stage or to terminate the study is made according to the following rules, where $N_1$, $C_{R1}$, and $C_{T1}$ are parameters to be chosen as part of the design specification:

1. If $Y_{R1} \leq C_{R1}$ and $Y_{T1} > C_{T1}$, terminate due to inadequate response.
2. If $Y_{R1} > C_{R1}$ and $Y_{T1} \leq C_{T1}$, terminate due to excessive toxicity.
3. If $Y_{R1} \leq C_{R1}$ and $Y_{T1} \leq C_{T1}$, terminate due to both factors.
4. If $Y_{R1} > C_{R1}$ and $Y_{T1} > C_{T1}$, continue to the second stage.

In the second stage, $N_2-N_1$ patients are accrued. At the end of this stage, the following rules govern the decision whether or not the new agent is sufficiently promising, where $N_2$, $C_{R2}$, and $C_{T2}$ are parameters to be determined by the design:

1. If $Y_{R2} \leq C_{R2}$ and $Y_{T2} > C_{T2}$, "not promising" due to inadequate response
2. If $Y_{R2} > C_{R2}$ and $Y_{T2} \leq C_{T2}$, "not promising" due to excessive toxicity
3. If $Y_{R2} \leq C_{R2}$ and $Y_{T2} \leq C_{T2}$, "not promising" due to both factors
4. If $Y_{R2} > C_{R2}$ and $Y_{T2} > C_{T2}$, "sufficiently promising"

The principle for choosing the stage sample sizes and stage boundaries is the same as in Conaway and Petroni.[1] The design parameters are determined from pre-specified error constraints. Although the papers differ in the particular constraints considered, the motivation for these error constraints is the same. One would like to limit the probability of recommending a treatment that has an insufficient response rate or excessive toxicity rate. Similarly, one would like to constrain the probability of failing to recommend a treatment that is superior to the standard treatment in terms of both response and toxicity rates. Finally, among all designs meeting the error criteria, the optimal design is the one that minimizes the average number of patients treated with an ineffective therapy.

In choosing the design parameters, $Q=(N_1, N_2, C_{R1}, C_{R2}, C_{T1}, C_{T2})$, Bryant and Day[2] specify an acceptable $(P_{R1})$ and an unacceptable $(P_{R0})$ response rate along with an acceptable $(P_{T1})$ and unacceptable $(P_{T0})$ rate of non-toxicity. Under any of the four combinations of acceptable or unacceptable rates of response and non-toxicity, Bryant and Day[2] assume that the association between response and toxicity is constant. The association between response and toxicity is determined by the odds ratio, $\varphi$, in the $2 \times 2$ table cross-classifying response and toxicity,

$$\varphi = \frac{P(\text{no response, toxicity}) * P(\text{response, no toxicity})}{P(\text{no response, no toxicity}) * P(\text{response, toxicity})}$$

Bryant and Day[2] parameterize the odds ratio in terms of response and no toxicity so $\varphi$ corresponds to $1/\theta$ in the notation of Conaway and Petroni.[1] For a design, $Q$, and an odds ratio, $\varphi$, let $\alpha_{ij}(Q, \varphi)$ be the probability of recommending the treatment, given that the true response rate equals $P_{Ri}$ and the true non-toxicity rate equals $P_{Tj}$, $i=0, 1; j=0, 1$. Constraining the probability of recommending a treatment with an insufficient response rate leads to $\alpha_{01}(Q, \varphi) \leq \alpha_R$, where $\alpha_R$ is a pre-specified constant. Constraining the probability of recommending a treatment with an insufficient response rate leads to $\alpha_{10}(Q, \varphi) \leq \alpha_T$, and ensuring a sufficiently high probability of recommending a truly superior treatment requires $\alpha_{11}(Q, \varphi) \geq 1 - \beta$, where $\alpha_T$ and $\beta$ are pre-specified constants. Bryant and Day[2] note that $\alpha_{00}(Q, \varphi)$ is less than either $\alpha_{01}(Q, \varphi)$ or $\alpha_{10}(Q, \varphi)$, so that an upper bound on $\alpha_{00}(Q, \varphi)$ is implicit in these constraints.

There can be many designs that meet these specifications. Among these designs, Bryant and Day[2] define the optimal design to be the one that minimizes the expected number of patients in a study of a treatment with an unacceptable response or toxicity rate. Specifically, Bryant and Day[2] choose the design, $Q$, that minimizes the maximum of $E_{01}(Q, \varphi)$ and $E_{10}(Q, \varphi)$, where $E_{ij}$ is the expected number of patients accrued when the true response rate equals $P_{Ri}$ and the true non-toxicity rate equals $P_{Tj}$, $i = 0, 1; j = 0, 1$. The expected value $E_{00}(Q, \varphi)$ does not play a role in the calculation of the optimal design because it is less than both $E_{01}(Q, \varphi)$ and $E_{10}(Q, \varphi)$.

The stage sample sizes and boundaries for the optimal design depend on the value of the nuisance parameter, $\varphi$. For an unspecified odds ratio, among all designs that meet the error constraints, the optimal design minimizes the maximum expected patient accruals under a treatment with an unacceptable response or toxicity rate, $\max_{\varphi}\{\max(E_{01}(Q, \varphi), E_{10}(Q, \varphi))\}$. Assumptions about a fixed value of the odds ratio lead to a simpler computational problem; this is particularly true if response and toxicity are assumed to be independent ($\varphi = 1$). Bryant and Day[2] provide bounds that indicate that the characteristics of the optimal design for an unspecified odds ratio do not differ greatly from the optimal design found by assuming that response and toxicity are independent. By considering a number of examples, Conaway and Petroni[1] came to a similar conclusion, although they did note that the properties of the design, particularly the overall type I error, can be affected by a poor specification of the odds ratio. They suggested that a number of odds ratio values be considered in creating the design.

Jin[7], and Wu and Liu[8] propose methods to limit the dependence of the Conaway and Petroni[1] design on the specification of the odds ratio. Jin[7] shows that the type I error criteria used by Conaway and Petroni[1]:

$$\sup_{p_R \leq p_{R0} \text{ or } p_T \geq p_{T0}} P(X_R \geq c_R, X_T \leq c_T | p_R, p_T, \theta) \leq \gamma$$

is equivalent to $\max\{P(X_R \geq c_R | p_R = p_{R0}), P(X_T \leq c_T | p_T = p_{T0})\} \leq \gamma\}$. The design of Jin[7] controls each of these probabilities separately, constraining $P(X_R \geq c_R | p_R = p_{R0}) \leq \gamma_R$ and $P(X_T \leq c_T | p_T = p_{T0}) \leq \gamma_T$. In addition to giving additional flexibility in the specification of type I error control for response or toxicity, the properties of this design depend on the assumed odds ratio only through the type II error, making the design more robust against misspecification of the odds ratio. The cost of the additional flexibility and protection against misspecification is a greater sample size requirement.

Wu and Liu[8] use an adaptive approach which reestimates the sample size based on an estimated odds ratio. Specifically, they set a maximum sample size, $n_{max}$, and choose a sample size $n_1 \leq n_{max}$ from which the odds ratio will be estimated. From this estimated odds ratio, a new sample size, $n$, will be computed. Wu and Liu[8] outline several choices that can be made depending on $n$, $n_1$, and $n_{max}$. The study might be stopped if the recomputed sample size, $n$, is less than the number of patients already enrolled, or the investigators may choose to continue enrolling up to $n_{max}$ patients. If $n_1 < n < n_{max}$, the investigators can use either the recomputed sample size, $n$, or the maximum sample size, $n_{max}$. Wu and Liu[8] note that with either of these cases, with $n < n_{max}$, the error requirements are preserved. If the recomputed sample size $n$ exceeds $n_{max}$, the investigators can use a sample size of $n$ or $n_{max}$. Choosing a sample size of $n$ preserves the error requirements, but it may not be feasible to enroll these many patients.

## 8.3 DESIGNS THAT ALLOW A TRADE-OFF BETWEEN RESPONSE AND TOXICITY

The designs for response and toxicity proposed by Conaway and Petroni[1] and Bryant and Day[2] share a number of common features, including the form for the alternative region. In these designs, a new treatment must show evidence of a greater response rate and a lesser toxicity rate than the standard treatment. In practice, a trade-off could be considered in the design, since one may be willing to allow greater toxicity to achieve a greater response rate, or be willing to accept a slightly lower response rate if lower toxicity can be obtained. Conaway and Petroni[9] propose two-stage designs for phase II trials that allow for early termination of the study if the new therapy is not sufficiently promising and allow for a trade-off between response and toxicity.

The hypotheses are the same as those considered for the bivariate designs of the previous section. The null hypothesis is that the new treatment is not sufficiently promising to warrant further study, either due to an insufficient response rate or excessive toxicity. The alternative hypothesis is that the new treatment is sufficiently effective and safe to warrant further study. The terms "sufficiently safe" and "sufficiently effective" are relative to the response rate, $p_{R0}$, and the toxicity rate, $p_{T0}$, for the standard treatment.

One of the primary issues in the design is how to elicit the trade-off specification. Ideally, the trade-off between safety and efficacy would be summarized as a function of toxicity and response rates that defines a treatment as "worthy of further study." In practice, this can be difficult to elicit. A simpler method for obtaining the trade-off information is for the investigator to specify the maximum toxicity rate, $p_{T,max}$, that would be acceptable if the new treatment were to produce responses in all patients. Similarly, the investigator would be asked to specify the minimum response rate, $p_{R,min}$, that would be acceptable if the treatment produced no toxicities.

Figure 8.2 illustrates the set of values for the true response rate ($p_R$) and true toxicity rate ($p_T$), which satisfy the null and alternative hypotheses. The values chosen for Figure 8.2 are $p_{R0}=0.5$, $p_{T0}=0.2$, $p_{R,min}=0.4$, and $p_{T,max}=0.7$. The line connecting the point ($p_{R0}, p_{T0}$) and (1, $p_{T,max}$) is given by the equation $p_T=p_{T0}+\tan(\psi_T)(p_R - p_{R0})$, where $\tan(\psi_T)=(p_{T,max} - p_{T0})/(1 - p_{R0})$. Similarly, the equation of the line connecting ($p_{R0}, p_{T0}$) and (1, $p_{R,min}$) is given by the equation

$$p_T = p_{T0} + \tan(\psi_R)(p_R - p_{R0})$$

where $\tan(\psi_R)=p_{T0}/(p_{R0} - p_{R,min})$. With $\psi_T \leq \psi_R$ the null hypothesis is

$$H_0: p_T \geq p_{T0} + \tan(\psi_T)(p_R - p_{R0}) \text{ or } p_T \geq p_{T0} + \tan(\psi_R)(p_R - p_{R0})$$

and the alternative hypothesis is

$$H_a: p_T < p_{T0} + \tan(\psi_T)(p_R - p_{R0}) \text{ and } p_T < p_{T0} + \tan(\psi_R)(p_R - p_{R0})$$

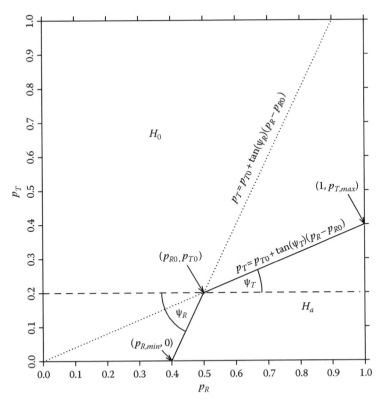

**FIGURE 8.2**  Null and alternative regions for a trade-off design.

The forms of the null and alternative are different for the case where $\psi_T \geq \psi_R$, although the basic principles in constructing the design and specifying the trade-off information remain the same (cf. Conaway and Petroni[9]). Special cases of these hypotheses have been used previously: $\psi_T=0$ and $\psi_R=\pi/2$ yield the critical regions of Conaway and Petroni[1] and Bryant and Day[2]; $\psi_R=\psi_T=0$ yield hypotheses in terms of toxicity alone; and $\psi_R=\psi_T=\pi/2$ yield hypotheses in terms of response alone.

To describe the trade-off designs for a fixed sample size, we use the notation and assumptions for the fixed sample size design described in Section 8.2. As in their earlier work, Conaway and Petroni[9] determine sample size and critical values under an assumed value for the odds ratio between response and toxicity. The sample size calculations require a specification of a level of type I error, $\alpha$, and power, $1-\beta$, at a particular point $p_R=p_{Ra}$ and $p_T=p_{Ta}$. The point $(p_{Ra}, p_{Ta})$ satisfies the constraints defining the alternative hypothesis and represents the response and toxicity rates for a treatment considered to be superior to the standard treatment. The test statistic is denoted by $T(\hat{p})$, where $\hat{p}=(1/N)(X_{11}, X_{12}, X_{21}, X_{22})$ is the vector of sample proportions in the four cells of Table 8.1, and is based on computing an "I-divergence measure" (cf. Robertson et al.[15]).

The test statistic has the intuitively appealing property of being roughly analogous to a "distance" from $\hat{p}$ to the region $H_0$. Rejection of the null hypothesis results when the observed value of $T(\hat{p})$ is "too far" from the null hypothesis region. A vector of observed proportions $\hat{p}$ leads to rejection of the null hypothesis if $T(\hat{p}) \geq c$. For an appropriate choice of sample size ($N$), significance level ($\alpha$) and power ($1 - \beta$), the value $c$ can be chosen to (1) constrain the probability of recommending a treatment that has an insufficient response rate relative to the toxicity rate and (2) ensure that there is a high probability of recommending a treatment with response rate $p_{Ra}$ and toxicity rate $p_{Ta}$. The critical value $c$ is chosen to meet the error criteria:

1. $$\sup_{(p_R, p_T) \in Ho} P(T(\hat{p}) \geq c | p_R, p_T, \theta) \leq \alpha$$

2. $P(T(\hat{p}) \geq c | p_{Ra}, p_{Ta}, \theta) \geq 1 - \beta$

These probabilities are computed for a fixed value of the odds ratio, $\theta$, by enumerating the value of $T(\hat{p})$ for all possible realizations of the multinomial vector ($X_{11}$, $X_{12}$, $X_{21}$, $X_{22}$).

The trade-off designs can be extended to two-stage designs that allow for early termination of the study if the new treatment does not appear to be sufficiently promising. In designing the study, the goal is to choose the stage sample sizes ($m_1$, $m_2$) and decision boundaries ($c_1$, $c_2$) to satisfy error probability constraints similar to those in the fixed sample size trade-off design:

1. $$\sup_{(p_R, p_T) \in Ho} P(T_1(\hat{p}_1) \geq c_1, T_2(\hat{p}_1, \hat{p}_2) \geq c_2 | p_R, p_T, \theta) \leq \alpha$$

2. $P(T_1(\hat{p}_1) \geq c_1, T_2(\hat{p}_1, \hat{p}_2) \geq c_2 | p_{Ra}, p_{Ta}, \theta) \geq 1 - \beta$

where

$T_1$ is the test statistic computed on the stage 1 observations
$T_2$ is the test statistic computed on the accumulated data in stages 1 and 2

As in the fixed sample size design, these probabilities are computed for a fixed value of the odds ratio and are found by enumerating all possible outcomes of the trial.

In cases where many designs meet the error requirements, an "optimal" design is found according to the criterion in Bryant and Day[2] and Simon.[3] Among all designs that meet the error constraints, the chosen design minimizes the maximum expected sample size under the null hypothesis. Through simulations, Conaway and Petroni[9] investigate the effect of fixing the odds ratio on the choice of the optimal design. They conclude that unless the odds ratio is badly misspecified, the choice of the odds ratio has little effect on the properties of the optimal design.

The critical values for the test statistic are much harder to interpret than the critical values in Conaway and Petroni[1] or Bryant and Day,[2] which are counts of the number of observed responses and toxicities. We recommend two plots, similar to Figures 2 and 3 in Conaway and Petroni,[9] to illustrate the characteristics of the trade-off designs. The first is a display of the power of the test, so that the investigators can see the probability of recommending a treatment with true response rate $p_R$ and true toxicity rate $p_T$. The second plot displays the rejection region, so that the investigators can see the decision about the treatment that will be made for specific numbers of observed responses and toxicities. With these plots, the investigators can better understand the implications of the trade-off being proposed.

The trade-off designs of Conaway and Petroni[9] were motivated by the idea that a new treatment could be considered acceptable even if the toxicity rate for the new treatment is greater than that of the standard treatment, provided the response rate improvement is sufficiently large. This idea also motivated the Bayesian monitoring method of Thall et al.,[10,11] They note that, for example, a treatment that improves the response rate by 15% points might be considered promising, even if its toxicity rate is 5% points greater than the standard therapy. If, however, the new therapy increases the toxicity rate by 10% points, it might not be considered an acceptable therapy.

Thall et al.[10,11] outline a strategy for monitoring each endpoint in the trial. They define, for each endpoint in the trial, a monitoring boundary based on pre-specified targets for an improvement in efficacy and an unacceptable increase in the rate of adverse events. In the example given earlier for a trial with a single response endpoint and a single toxicity endpoint, the targeted improvement in response rate is 15% and the allowance for increased toxicity is 5%.

Thall et al.[10,11] take a Bayesian approach that allows for monitoring each endpoint on a patient by patient basis. Although their methods allow for a number of efficacy and adverse event endpoints, we will simplify the discussion by considering only a single efficacy event (response) and a single adverse event endpoint (toxicity). Before the trial begins, they elicit a prior distribution on the cell probabilities in Table 8.2. Under the standard therapy, the cell probabilities are denoted $P_S = (p_{S11}, p_{S12}, p_{S21}, p_{S22})$; under the new experimental therapy, the cell probabilities are denoted $P_E = (p_{E11}, p_{E12}, p_{E21}, p_{E22})$. Putting a prior distribution on the cell probabilities $(p_{G11}, p_{G12}, p_{G21}, p_{G22})$ induces a prior distribution on $p_{GR} = p_{G11} + p_{G12}$ and on $p_{GT} = p_{G11} + p_{G21}$, where $G$ stands for either $S$ or $E$. A Dirichlet prior for the cell probabilities is particularly convenient in this setting, since this induces a Beta prior on $p_{GR}$ and $p_{GT}$, for $G = S$ or $E$.

In addition to the prior distribution, Thall et al.[10,11] specify a target improvement, $\delta(R)$, for response, and a maximum allowable difference, $\delta(T)$, for toxicity. The monitoring of the endpoints begins after a minimum number of patients, $m$, have been observed. It continues until either a maximum number of patients, $M$, have been accrued, or a monitoring boundary has been crossed.

In a typical phase II trial, in which only the new therapy is used, the distribution on the probabilities under the standard therapy remains constant throughout the trial, while the distribution on the probabilities under the new therapy is updated each time a patient's outcomes are observed. After the response and toxicity classification on $j$ patients, $X_j$, have been observed, there are several possible decisions one could make. If there is strong evidence that the new therapy does not meet the targeted improvement in response rate, then the trial should be stopped and the new treatment declared "not sufficiently promising." Alternatively, if there is strong evidence that the new treatment is superior to the standard treatment in terms of response the targeted improvement for response, the trial should be stopped and the treatment declared "sufficiently promising." In terms of toxicity, the trial should be stopped if there is strong evidence of an excessive toxicity rate with the new treatment. Thall et al.[10,11] translate these rules into statements about the updated (posterior) distribution $[p_E|X_j]$ and the prior distribution $p_S$, using pre-specified cut-off for what constitutes "strong evidence." For $m \leq j \leq M$, the monitoring boundaries are as follows:

1. $P[p_{ER} - p_{SR} > \delta(R)|X_j] \leq p_L(R)$
2. $P[p_{ER} > p_{SR}|X_j] \geq p_U(R)$
3. $P[p_{ET} - p_{ST} > \delta(T)|X_j] \geq p_U(T)$

where $p_L(R)$, $p_U(R)$, and $p_U(T)$ are pre-specified probability levels. Numerical integration is required to compute these probabilities, but the choice of the Dirichlet prior makes the computations relatively easy. Extensions to the method that allows for mixture priors and monitoring cohorts of size greater than one are given in Thall and Sung.[12]

Thall and Russell[16] present Bayesian methods for combined phase I/II trials. These designs can be used for dose finding based on response and toxicity criteria. The models impose an ordering on a combined response–toxicity endpoint and monitor the trial by updating the probability of response and toxicity.

Thall[14] proposes a design in which contours of "equally desirable outcomes" in terms of the probability of response and toxicity are specified in advance of the trial. To illustrate, Thall[14] gives a numerical example where the historical probabilities of response and toxicity with the standard treatment are represented by the ordered pair $(p_R, p_T) = (0.4, 0.3)$. Examples of "equally desirable outcomes" might be (0.55, 0.4), (0.60, 0.45), and (0.40, 0.15). The pair (0.55, 0.4) trades a 10% point increase in the toxicity probability for an improvement of 15% points in the response probability. Thall[14] describes two ways of eliciting families of contours. One way is for the investigators to specify a set of pairs, $\{(p_{R1}, p_{T1}), (p_{R2}, p_{T2}),..., (p_{RK}, p_{TK})\}$ along with numerical values $\{\delta_1, \delta_2,..., \delta_K\}$ for the desirability of the $k$th pair, $k=1,..., K$. The other is for the investigators to specify pairs of response and toxicity probabilities that are equally desirable. These contours are then used to define a region, $E$, such that each pair of response and toxicity probabilities, $(p_R, p_T)$, in the region are more desirable than points outside the region, which includes the response and toxicity probabilities associated with the current standard. Decisions about the treatment are made from the posterior probability, $P[(p_R, p_T) \in E|\text{data}]$, with sufficiently large values of this posterior probability indicative of a treatment with response and toxicity probabilities that are more desirable than the current standard.

Chen and Smith[13] use a Bayesian theoretic decision approach to design trials for correlated binary endpoints for response and toxicity. They define a "zone of trade-off" by specifying a rectangle defined by the response probability in the interval $(p_{R0} - \delta_{R-}, p_{R0} + \delta_{R+})$, and the toxicity probability in the interval $(p_{T0} - \delta_{T-}, p_{T0} + \delta_{T+})$, where $p_{R0}$ and $p_{T0}$ are the response and toxicity rates for the current standard treatment, and $\delta_{R-}$, $\delta_{R+}$, $\delta_{T-}$ and $\delta_{T+}$ are pre-specified constants. Inside this rectangle, the new therapy is considered inferior to the standard therapy if $\theta_E < \theta_s$, where $\theta_E = p_R * (1 - p_T)/[(1 - p_R) * p_T]$ and $\theta_s = p_{R0} * (1 - p_{T0})/[(1 - p_{R0}) * p_{T0}]$. In a single-arm phase II study, $\theta_s$ is assumed known. At any interim evaluation, the Bayes risk is computed for each of three possible decisions: (1) stop the trial and declare the new therapy not worthy of further study, (2) stop the trial and recommend the new therapy for evaluation in a phase III trial, or (3) continue to enroll patients in the phase II trial. The Bayes risk is computed from a loss function that incorporates the loss in conducting the current trial and the loss in making an incorrect decision about the new therapy.

## 8.4 SUMMARY

All of the methods discussed in this chapter have advantages in monitoring toxicity in phase II trials. None of the methods use asymptotic approximations for distributions and are well-suited for the small sample sizes encountered typically in phase II trials. The bivariate designs of Conaway and Petroni,[1] Bryant and Day,[2] Jin,[7] and Wu and Liu[8] have critical values that are based on the observed number of responses and the observed number of toxicities; these statistics are easily calculated and interpreted by the investigators.

The trade-off designs of Conaway and Petroni[9] have a trade-off strategy that permits the allowable level of toxicity to increase with the response rate. In contrast, in the trade-off example of Thall et al.[10,11] a 5% increase in toxicity would be considered acceptable for a treatment with a 15% increase in response. Because the allowance in toxicity is pre-specified, this means that only a 5% increase in toxicity is allowable even if the response rate with the new treatment is as much as 30%. With the trade-off of Conaway and Petroni,[9] the standard for "allowable toxicity" is greater for a treatment with a 30% improvement than for one with a 15% improvement. The methods of Thall et al.[10,11] have advantages in terms of being able to monitor outcomes on a patient-by-patient basis. At each monitoring point, the method can provide graphical representations of the probability associated with each of the decision rules. The designs of Thall,[14] and Chen and Smith[13] give additional flexibility in how response and toxicity are traded.

Although the methods presented are discussed in terms of toxicity and response, where toxicity is a predefined measure of adverse events related to protocol treatment and response is a predefined measure of efficacy, the designs apply to any bivariate endpoints. For example, in vaccine trials assessing immune response, the efficacy response parameter could be replaced with an earlier measure of immune response.

## REFERENCES

1. Conaway MR and Petroni GR. Bivariate sequential designs for phase II trials. *Biometrics*. 1995; 51:656–664.
2. Bryant J and Day R. Incorporating toxicity considerations into the design of two-stage phase II clinical trials. *Biometrics*. 1995; 51:1372–1383.
3. Simon R. Optimal two-stage designs for phase II clinical trials. *Controlled Clinical Trials*. 1989; 10:1–10.
4. Artz A, Stadler W, Vogelzang N, Zimmerman T, and Ryan C. A phase II trial of sequential chemotherapy with docetaxel and methotrexate followed by gemcitabine and cisplatin for metastatic urothelial cancer. *American Journal of Clinical Oncology*. 2005; 28:109–113.

5. Meropol N, Niedzwiecki D, Shank B, Colacchio T, Ellerton J, Valone F, Budinger S et al. Induction therapy for poor-prognosis anal canal carcinoma: A phase II study of the cancer and leukemia group B (CALGB 9281). *Journal of Clinical Oncology*. 2008; 26:3229–3234.
6. Foon K, Boyiadzis M, Land S, Marks S, Raptis A, Pietragallo L, Meisner D et al. Chemoimmunotherapy with low-dose fludarabine and cyclophosphamide and high dose rituximab in previously untreated patients with chronic lymphocytic leukemia. *Journal of Clinical Oncology*. 2008; 27:498–503.
7. Jin H. Alternative designs of phase II trials considering response and toxicity. *Contemporary Clinical Trials*. 2007; 28:525–531.
8. Wu C and Liu A. An adaptive approach for bivariate phase II clinical trial designs. *Contemporary Clinical Trials*. 2007; 28:482–486.
9. Conaway MR and Petroni GR. Designs for phase II trials allowing for trade-off between response and toxicity. *Biometrics*. 1996; 52:1375–1386.
10. Thall PF, Simon RM, and Estey EH. Bayesian sequential monitoring designs for single-arm clinical trials with multiple outcomes. *Statistics in Medicine*. 1995; 14:357–379.
11. Thall PF, Simon RM, and Estey EH. New statistical strategy for monitoring safety and efficacy in single-arm clinical trials. *Journal of Clinical Oncology*. 1996; 14:296–303.
12. Thall PF and Sung HG. Some extensions and applications of a Bayesian strategy for monitoring multiple outcomes in clinical trials. *Statistics in Medicine*. 1998; 17:1563–1580.
13. Chen Y and Smith B. Adaptive group sequential design for phase II clinical trials: A Bayesian decision theoretic approach. *Statistics in Medicine*. 2009; 28:3347–3362.
14. Thall P. Some geometric methods for constructing decision criteria based on two-dimensional parameters. *Journal of Statistical Planning and Inference*. 2008; 138:516–527.
15. Robertson T, Dykstra RL, and Wright FT. *Order Restricted Statistical Inference*. Chichester, U.K.: John Wiley & Sons, Ltd., 1988.
16. Thall PF and Russell KE. A strategy for dose-finding and safety monitoring based on efficacy and adverse outcomes in phase I/II clinical trials. *Biometrics*. 1998; 54:251–264.

# 9 Designs Using Time-to-Event Endpoints/Single-Arm versus Randomized Phase II Designs

*Catherine M. Tangen and John J. Crowley*

## CONTENTS

The objective of a phase II study is to evaluate whether a particular regimen has enough biologic activity in a given disease to warrant further investigation. We would like to have a mechanism in which the candidate agents or regimens can be screened relatively quickly, and for practical and ethical reasons, we would like to expose the minimal number of patients in order to evaluate activity. To plan an efficient phase II trial, there need to be at least three key considerations: What is the most appropriate endpoint? What is the optimal patient population, and what is the most reasonable statistical design?

## 9.1  CHOOSING AN APPROPRIATE ENDPOINT

Previously, phase II cancer clinical trials predominantly used response rate as the primary endpoint, where in the solid tumor setting, response usually involves a reduction in the dimensions of the measurable disease. However, there are shortcomings to using response rate as the primary endpoint for evaluating efficacy: (1) Response has not been shown to be strongly correlated with survival across a number of disease sites (Forastiere et al. 1992, Durie et al. 2004), (2) there are challenges to evaluating response (Kimura and Tominaga 2002, Erasmus et al. 2003, McHugh and Kao 2003), and (3) there are new classes of agents that are being tested which are not expected to be cytotoxic (tumor reducing), but instead they are cytostatic; that is, the agents may delay disease progression but not reduce the tumor size. For these reasons, other endpoints such as survival and progression-free survival (PFS) are more frequently becoming the primary endpoint of choice for evaluating phase II drugs (Markham 1997).

One endpoint that has drawn some attention in the cytostatic era is disease control rate (DCR). DCR is the proportion of patients who have a best response of stable disease or better with a particular regimen. The DCR has been shown to be more strongly correlated with survival that response rate in some disease settings (Lara et al. 2008).

### 9.1.1  PROGRESSION-FREE SURVIVAL

PFS is defined as the interval from start of the trial to date of progression, or in the absence of progression, death due to any cause. Using PFS as the primary endpoint of a phase II study has appeal because it measures (or more closely measures) a clinically meaningful endpoint that impacts a patient's life. It also provides consistency with planned phase III trials that would also use survival or PFS as the primary endpoint. Two arguments that have been made in support of using response as an endpoint are that (1) subsequent treatments do not impact it and (2) response status is evaluated more quickly than progression or survival status. However, by using PFS as the primary endpoint, it is not necessary to wait until all patients have progressed or died or even until the median has been estimated. It is possible to specify the null and alternative hypotheses in terms of a shorter interval of time, such as the expected event rate at a landmark such as 6 months; thus, the interval needed to assess the PFS endpoint is in line with that needed for response, and like response, PFS should not be impacted by subsequent treatments.

There are some drawbacks to using PFS as the primary endpoint. PFS can be difficult to measure reliably and is sensitive to the timing of disease assessment (Panageas et al. 2007). Any variation in disease assessment schedule between arms can make PFS look artificially different. Infrequent disease assessment can cause an overestimation of the progression-free interval. Secondly, PFS is not always predictive of survival, that is, PFS may not be an adequate surrogate marker for survival in many disease settings. Showing an improvement in PFS without an improvement in survival may also not be clinically relevant, particularly if the experimental regimen is more toxic or expensive than the current standard. Finally, in some disease settings, the definition of progression is not standardized. For example, in hormone refractory prostate cancer, which is primarily a disease of the bone, the role of PSA kinetics, pain, and the optimal measure of bone progression is unclear (Scher et al. 2008).

It is interesting to note that some clinical trialists feel that using response or DCR as the primary endpoint allows one to design a phase II trial with a single-arm, whereas the specification of PFS as the endpoint requires randomization. However, DCR and PFS at a fixed landmark are essentially the complement of each other. In the absence of progression or death, the best response must be stable or better disease.

### 9.1.2 Overall Survival

Overall survival (OS) has also been considered as a phase II endpoint. However, it also has drawbacks. Subsequent therapies may affect OS and confound the interpretation of treatment effect, and time to death takes longer to obtain, thus requiring a longer trial than one which employs PFS, disease control, or response. Using OS in a randomized phase II trial can also complicate the ability to mount a randomized phase III trial using survival, as some may perceive the treatment comparison already answered. For diseases with very short median OS and lack of effective salvage treatment, or where PFS cannot be reliably measured, OS may be a preferred endpoint for phase II trials (Rubinstein et al. 2009).

## 9.2 CHOOSING THE TARGET POPULATION

The study population should be the one to which we wish to generalize the results of the trial when it is completed. It has been hypothesized that common tumors may be common because many mutations can cause them, and a targeted agent may only work against tumors with specific mutations. Depending on how well understood the mechanism of action is for a study regimen, enriching the trial population for those with the hypothesized target of interest may increase the likelihood of observing activity if the agent is active (Stewart 2010). An argument for randomized phase II trials is that the design allows for the distinction between prognostic factors and predictive factors. Additionally, there may not be good historical data for the relevant subsets of patients, and so a one-arm trial may be difficult to design. However, unless the marker is quite prevalent, there is no statistical power to evaluate a marker by treatment interaction for the endpoint of interest in a randomized phase II trial. Despite the logic of enriching the patient population with those most likely to respond, prospective enrichment based upon molecular markers has rarely been used in cancer drug development. Often there are not credentialed assays for evaluating individual patients prior to enrollment into the phase II trial. However, the situation might be different by the time the phase III trial is ready for enrollment. Chapter 17 deals with phase III study designs using targeted agents.

## 9.3   STUDY DESIGN

There are strong and diverging opinions about the use of single-arm versus random-ized phase II trials. However, most would agree that it depends on the circumstances of the trial. With the shift in phase II endpoints away from response and more toward PFS, there has been concern raised that prognostic factors may impact these end-points in a way that was not thought to impact response. This has led to a concern that the outcome of a small phase II trial may be highly dependent on the patient population selected and the mix of prognostic factors in a given study population. To address such concerns, there has been a trend toward the use of randomized phase II trials to better ensure a less biased comparison between a standard and experimen-tal treatment group. However, introducing a second arm as a comparator also adds substantial variability to the comparison. Essentially, that is the quandary—concern about bias or concern about variability.

### 9.3.1   Single-Arm Phase II Designs

#### 9.3.1.1   Comparisons with Historical Experience

This strategy is typically used for phase II studies that have response as the primary endpoint, but as previously mentioned this design can also be used for time-to-event measures like PFS. Based on previous experience, one would specify the level at which there would not be interest in an agent (null hypothesis) versus the alternative hypoth-esis which is the level at which one would consider pursuing an agent in a phase III study. For example, one might specify a 20% versus 40% response rate for an agent where there was some modest level of activity using standard treatment. A two-stage design is then typically employed where, if adequate activity is observed in the first group of patients, the study will continue to the second stage of accrual (Fleming 1982, Simon 1989); see also Chapter 7. If the regimen being studied consists of agents already shown to be active, a single-stage (or pilot) design may be appropriate. Because there is already experience with the agents being studied there is less concern about exposing patients to an ineffective treatment, so a one-stage design is usually used with a sample size of typically 50–100 patients, avoiding the delays of a multi-stage design.

A similar design strategy could be used in the phase II setting by substituting PFS or survival for response rate. One could specify a 6 month PFS estimate of 20% ver-sus 40%, for example, where if only 20% of the patients are alive and free of progres-sion at 6 months, there would be no interest in the regimen, whereas if 40% or more of the patients are free of progression, then there would be considerable interest in pursuing the agent if other considerations such as toxicity were also favorable. This could be tested in a one- or two-stage design.

One design that has been proposed to avoid temporary closure was proposed by Herndon (1998), where a slight over-accrual to the first stage is allowed while assess-ing the endpoint on patients in the first cohort. In a similar vein, it may be reason-able to conduct an interim analysis of a phase II study in order to avoid temporary closure. The alternative hypothesis is tested at the alpha 0.005 level or at some other appropriate level at the approximate mid-point, and the study would be closed only for the case where there is lack of adequate activity.

One straightforward design option for conducting a pilot study would be to specify the null and alternative hypothesis in terms of median PFS or OS. For example, in the advanced disease setting, a median survival of 9 months might not be of interest while a median survival of 12 months or greater would be of further interest. By assuming uniform accrual and an exponential distribution, it is straightforward to calculate the sample size needed. If a study is to have 90% power and take 2 years of accrual with one additional year of follow-up and a one-sided $\alpha = 0.05$, then 134 patients or 67 per year would be needed. With this one-stage design, it is also possible to specify an interim analysis to test for lack of biologic activity.

One of the challenges of implementing a historical control phase II trial is choosing the appropriate null and alternative hypothesis levels. As recommended by Korn et al. (2001), there must be sufficient historical data on a patient population, untreated or treated with active agents that are similar to the patient population being considered for treatment with the experimental agent. The historical data would need to be the survival or PFS experience for a group of patients with the same stage of disease and amount of prior treatment, similar organ function and performance status, and the procedures used for monitoring progression should be the same. Another important recommendation is that patients should come from the same type of institutions with the same referral patterns in a recent era so diagnostic measures and supportive care would be similar. For example, using the results of a single institution study in order to define the level of interest and disinterest in a regimen might not be readily translatable to a large, diverse cooperative group phase II trial. These considerations are not unique to trials using a PFS endpoint as these are essentially the same factors that need to be considered when designing a phase II *response* study using historical experience as a comparison.

Even if historical control outcome data are known to vary, that does not necessitate a randomized trial design. If there are known risk factors that are strongly correlated with the endpoint of interest and they explain a substantial portion of the variability of the outcome (e.g., response, PFS), then an algorithm can be developed to predict what the historical outcome level would have been for a current cohort of patients. This would serve as the historical control null hypothesis. Activity beyond that would be attributable to the experimental treatment regimen. This statistical method was recently applied to metastatic melanoma (Korn et al. 2008), and algorithms for other cancer populations are also being explored. However, this modeling approach cannot be employed in settings in which strong prognostic factors have yet to be identified.

### 9.3.1.2 Each Patient as His Own Control

With this type of design, in a single group of patients who have progressive disease, we want to evaluate whether an agent is able to slow down the rate of progression relative to their pretreatment rate of progression.

Mick et al. (2000) have proposed a methodology for evaluating time-to-progression as the primary endpoint in a one-stage design. Typically, patients being offered phase II studies of new agents have failed a previous regimen. The prior time to progression interval is referred to as $TTP_1$ and is not censored; that is, all progressions are observed. Time to progression after the experimental agent, $TTP_2$, may or may not be censored at analysis. They propose that the "growth modulation index" ($TTP_2/TTP_1$) will have a null ratio value ($HR_0$) of 1.0, and the index needs to be greater than 1.33 if a new regimen is to be considered effective at delaying progression. The degree of correlation between the paired failure times is a key feature of this design since the patient serves as his own historical control, a concept that was originally suggested by Von Hoff (1998). The authors note that in some cases it may be reasonable to hypothesize that, by the natural history of the disease, one would expect $TTP_2$ to be shorter than $TTP_1$, which would indicate a null value less than 1.0. Hypothesis tests about the hazard ratio from paired data may be conducted under a log-linear model.

Von Hoff (2010) employed a similar design for their pilot study. They used a sign test to evaluate whether ($TTP_2/TTP_1$) $> 1.3$ in 15% of patients as the null hypothesis.

One can propose a range of null and alternative hypotheses based on disease and treatment considerations. However, this design approach can be difficult to implement because patients must be enrolled for both intervals of progression; that is, patients are enrolled prior to their first-line treatment for a trial of second-line treatment. As pointed out by Korn et al. (2001), enrolling patients after they progress on first-line treatment avoids these problems but leads to potential bias in the selection of the patients included in the trial.

### 9.3.2 MULTIARM DESIGNS

#### 9.3.2.1 Randomized Selection Designs

In some cases, the aim of a phase II trial is not to identify whether an agent has biologic activity, but instead to select which agent of several should be chosen to be tested in the phase III setting. This is known as a selection trial. The intent is not to definitively compare each of the regimens with one another, but to pick the most promising agent to carry forward. The endpoint can be based on response rates, but also survival or PFS is typically used as the criterion for picking the best arm. Selection designs are covered in detail in Chapter 10.

#### 9.3.2.2 Randomized Phase II: Comparison of Regimen with a Control Group

There have been a number of review papers published on the merits and shortcomings of randomized phase II comparison trial designs (Van Glabbeke et al. 2002, Wieand 2005, Taylor et al. 2006, Redman and Crowley 2007, Gan et al. 2010, Mandrekar and Sargent 2010, Seymour et al. 2010). Newer drugs are expected to prolong the progression-free interval but not necessarily result in disease response. PFS is perceived to be a more heterogeneous outcome, which is more dependent on the mix of prognostic factors in the patient pool than is the case with tumor response. If the endpoint has not been assessed consistently over time or is not available from historical trials, there may be a compelling reason to conduct a randomized trial. Several statisticians have published their take on designing randomized phase II

**TABLE 9.1**

**Approximate Number of Total Events for a Randomized Phase II Trial with PFS as an Endpoint**

| Error Rates ($\alpha$, $\beta$) | Hazard Ratios ($\Delta$) | | |
|---|---|---|---|
| | $\Delta = 1.3$ | $\Delta = 1.5$ | $\Delta = 1.7$ |
| 10%, 10% | 384 | 161 | 94 |
| 10%, 20%, or 20%, 10% | 264 | 110 | 64 |
| 20%, 20% | 166 | 69 | 41 |

Using the formula: $L = \{(Z1 - \alpha + Z1 - \beta)/(0.5 * \ln(\Delta))\}2$ where $L$ is the total number of events and which assumes a logrank test with a one-sided $\alpha$ (Fleming and Harrington 1991).

trials (Korn et al. 2001, Rubinstein et al. 2005). The goal is to assess activity of a new regimen compared to a standard in a preliminary fashion by specifying effect sizes and statistical error rates which keep the sample size in the range of an expected phase II trial. Table 9.1 illustrates the total number of events that must be observed in the combined arms with the specified treatment effect size and statistical error rates when the logrank test is used. In this example, we are specifying PFS endpoints but the same holds true for a survival endpoint as well. The total sample size will be impacted by the accrual and event rate.

A typical trial might involve a standard regimen as the control and a standard + a new targeted agent as the experimental treatment. This design can only be conducted successfully if patients are willing to accept being randomized to either arm. Korn et al. (2001) recommend a moderate one-sided alpha of 0.10 or 0.20, which reduces the required sample size. Conducting a randomized design in the phase II setting with a control arm establishes some legitimacy for comparison between the arms. Hence, there is a great temptation to interpret the results literally and not carry the agent forward to proper phase III testing. Liu et al. (1999) calculated the probabilities of observing a hazard ratio greater than 1.3, 1.5, and 1.7 when the true hazard ratio is 1 between all treatments in a randomized phase II trial. In a two-arm trial with 40 patients per arm, the probabilities were 0.37, 0.17, and 0.07 for detecting the respective hazard ratios. Thus, the false-positive rates are very high if one treats randomized phase II trial results as conclusive.

Randomized trials have been viewed favorably because they tend to reduce the bias between the control and experimental treatment groups. However, in small randomized studies with significant patient heterogeneity, fairly large imbalances can still occur by chance. Careful selection of stratification factors can help to ensure balance of important prognostic variables. However, small studies can support only minimal stratification, and there may also be important unmeasured prognostic factors that are not balanced in small randomized trials.

### 9.3.2.3   Randomization Discontinuation Design

There can be substantial heterogeneity of tumor growth rates in patient populations. Some patients' tumors will grow slowly naturally. In order to distinguish anti-proliferative activity of a novel agent from indolent disease, Rosner et al. (2002) proposed what they call a "randomized discontinuation design" (RDT). A generic study schema can be seen in Figure 9.1. All patients are initially treated with the experimental agent (part I of trial), and these patients can be thought of as coming from a target population of patients with a given disease and stage. Patients without progression are randomized in a double-blind fashion to continuing therapy or placebo (part II). Patients who are non-compliant or experience adverse events are also typically not randomized. This allows the investigators to assess if apparent slow tumor growth is attributable to the drug or to the selection of patients with slow-growing tumors. By selecting a more homogeneous population, the randomized portion of the study may require fewer patients than would a study randomizing all patients.

Kopec et al. (1993) have reviewed the advantages and limitations of discontinuation studies, and compared the RDT design to the classic randomized clinical trial (RCT) design in terms of clinical utility and efficiency (sample size). What they found is that one sees the greatest gain in efficiency with the RDT design when the placebo response rate is low and the relative response rate is modest. They concluded that the RDT design is quite useful for studying the effect of long-term, non-curative therapies, when the definition of "clinically important effect" is relatively small, and the use of a placebo should be minimized for ethical or feasibility reasons. On the other hand, the RDT design is limited if the objective of the study is to estimate the treatment effect and toxicity within the target population of patients with the disease of interest, or if the treatment is potentially curative. The relative efficiency of the RDT design depends on the accuracy of the selection criteria with respect to identifying true treatment responders and to some degree those with good compliance and lack of limiting toxicities. As pointed out by Friedman et al. (1985), because the RDT evaluates a highly selected sample, this design can overestimate benefit and underestimate toxicity. The RDT design, which can end up requiring a fairly large sample size, may be answering an irrelevant hypothesis; namely, given that one initially responds to a new agent, is more of the drug better than stopping at the time of response?

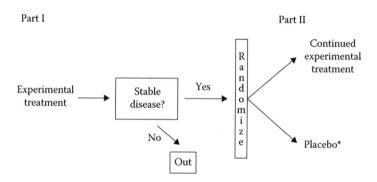

**FIGURE 9.1**   RDT schema.

## 9.4 DESIGNING INFORMATIVE PHASE II TRIALS

It is not uncommon for results from a positive phase II trial not to be confirmed with a subsequent phase III trial. There can be a number of reasons why two trials provide conflicting conclusions. The phase II trial may have used an intermediate endpoint that did not adequately capture treatment effect relative to survival, the patient population may differ with regard to known (or unknown) predictive factors, or the phase II trial results may have been a false positive (Table 9.2).

There are two ways that a phase II trial can be declared positive at its conclusion. Either it is a truly active regimen that has been correctly identified or it is an inactive regimen that has been incorrectly identified as being active (i.e., false positive). Table 9.3 shows the fraction of positive trials that are expected to be "false positives" depending on the assumed underlying prevalence of truly active regimens. In this example, we are assuming that 10% (or 20%) of all regimens studied in phase II trials are active. Simon (1987) estimated that 10% of phase II agents are active. Here, the term "active" means that the treatment under investigation has the level of activity specified by the alternative hypothesis if it could be measured perfectly.

By specifying small error rates like what are typically used in phase III trials and single-arm phase II trials ($\alpha=0.05$, $\beta=0.10$), for every three-phase II trials that are concluded to be positive, on average one of them would be a false positive. As error rates are relaxed in order to reduce the sample size, the chance that a trial concluded

### TABLE 9.2
### Statistical Error Rates

| Conclusion Based on Trial | Truth | |
| --- | --- | --- |
| | **Agent is Not Active** | **Agent is Active** |
| Agent is not active | Correct conclusion | Type II error=$\beta$, "false negative" $1-\beta$=statistical power |
| Agent is active | Type I error=$\alpha$, "false positive" | Correct conclusion |

### TABLE 9.3
### Impact of Error Rates on the False-Positive Rate among Phase II Trials Concluded to be Positive

| Error Rates, $\alpha$ and $\beta$ | Percentage of Active Agents Correctly Identified $(1-\beta)$ (%) | Percentage False Positive Assuming 10% of Regimens Are Truly Active (%) | Percentage False Positive Assuming 20% of Regimens Are Truly Active (%) |
| --- | --- | --- | --- |
| 0.05, 0.10 | 90 | 33 | 18 |
| 0.10, 0.10 | 90 | 50 | 31 |
| 0.10, 0.20 | 80 | 53 | 33 |
| 0.20, 0.20 | 80 | 69 | 50 |

to be positive is actually a false positive increases. If the type I error rate is doubled from 5% to 10% (typical of randomized phase II trials) and the statistical power remains 90% ($\beta = 0.10$), then half of positive phase II trials would be expected to be false positives. If a greater proportion of truly active regimens are tested as is shown in the last column, the chance of a false positive decreases from 50% to 31%. Based on this table, it should not come as a surprise that a significant number of phase III trials will not confirm the results of a positive phase II trial. Randomization does not solve the problem. Both one-arm and randomized two-arm trials require the specification of type I and II error rates, and in fact, randomized phase II trials typically allow error rates to be larger than their single-arm counterpart in order to keep sample size at an attainable level.

The best way to increase the chance of making the correct conclusion at the end of a phase II trial is to design the trial with smaller error rates (which also means increasing the sample size). This is often not feasible or desirable, and researchers are willing to make a trade-off between making an incorrect conclusion and having a smaller trial. The other way to reduce false positives in phase II trials is to test better drugs.

## 9.5  CONCLUDING COMMENTS

With the development of cytostatic agents, attention has been given to developing new phase II trial designs to address the expected lack of cytoreductive activity with these regimens. Endpoints that incorporate information about progression or survival are reasonable choices that can be straightforward to conduct. There is no single phase II study design that fits all situations. In settings where adequate historical controls exist, historically controlled phase II trials are more efficient. In other cases where there is substantial heterogeneity and a lack of good historical control data, a randomized design is likely the better design choice. Identification of the appropriate study population is just as important as the actual study design, particularly in the setting of targeted study drugs.

## ACKNOWLEDGMENT

This work was supported in part by grant #CA038926 from the National Cancer Institute.

## REFERENCES

Durie BGM, Jacobson J, Barlogie B, Crowley J. 2004. Magnitude of response with myeloma frontline therapy does not predict outcome: Importance of time to progression in Southwest Oncology Group chemotherapy trials. *J Clin Oncol* 22:1857–1863.

Erasmus JJ, Gladish GW, Broemeling L et al. 2003. Interobserver and intraobserver variability in measurement of non-small-cell carcinoma of the lung lesions: Implications for assessment of tumor response. *J Clin Oncol* 21(13):2574–2582.

Fleming TR. 1982. One sample multiple testing procedures for phase II clinical trials. *Biometrics* 38:143–151.

Fleming TR, Harrington DP. 1991. *Counting Processes and Survival Analysis*. New York: John Wiley & Sons, Inc.

Forastiere AA, Metch B, Schuller DE et al. 1992. Randomized comparison of cisplatin plus fluorouracil and carboplatin plus fluorouracil versus methotrexate in advanced squamous-cell carcinoma of the head and neck: A Southwest Oncology Group study. *J Clin Oncol* 10:1245–1251.

Friedman LM, Furberg CD, DeMets DL. 1985. *Fundamentals of Clinical Trials*, 2nd edn. Littleton, MA: PSG Publishing Company.

Gan HK, Grothey A, Pond GR et al. 2010. Randomized phase II trials: Inevitable or inadvisable? *J Clin Oncol* 28:2641–2647.

Herndon JE. 1998. A design alternative for two-stage phase II, multicenter cancer clinical trials. *Control Clin Trials* 19:440–450.

Kimura M, Tominaga T. 2002. Outstanding problems with response evaluation criteria in sold tumors (RECIST) in breast cancer. *Breast Cancer* 9(2):153–159.

Kopec JA, Abrahamowicz M, Esdaile JM. 1993. Randomized discontinuation trials: Utility and efficacy. *J Clin Epidemiol* 46(9):959–971.

Korn EL, Arbuck SG, Pluda JM et al. 2001. Clinical trial designs for cytostatic agents: Are new approaches needed? *J Clin Oncol* 19(1):265–272.

Korn EL, Liu PY, Lee SJ et al. 2008. Meta-analysis of phase II cooperative group trials in metastatic stage IV melanoma to determine progression-free and overall survival benchmarks for future phase II trials. *J Clin Oncol* 26:527–534.

Lara PN, Jr., Redman MW, Kelly K et al. 2008. Disease control rate at 8 weeks predicts clinical benefit in advanced non-small-cell lung cancer: Results from Southwest Oncology Group randomized trials. *J Clin Oncol* 26:463–467.

Liu PY, LeBlanc M, Desai M. 1999. False positive rates of randomized phase II designs. *Control Clin Trials* 20:343–352.

Mandrekar SJ, Sargent DJ. 2010. Randomized phase II trials: Time for a new era in clinical trial design. *J Thorac Oncol* 5:932–934.

Markham M. 1997. Challenges associated with evaluating the clinical utility of noncytotoxic pharmaceutical agents in oncology. *J Cancer Res Clin Oncol* 123:581–582.

McHugh K, Kao S. 2003. Response evaluation criteria in solid tumors (RECIST): Problems and need for modifications in paediatric oncology? *Br J Radiol* 76(907):433–436.

Mick R, Crowley JJ, Carroll RJ. 2000. Phase II clinical trial design for noncytotoxic anticancer agents for which time to disease progression is the primary endpoint. *Control Clin Trials* 21:343–359.

Panageas KS, Ben-Porat L, Dickler MN et al. 2007. When you look matters: The effect of assessment schedule on progression-free survival. *J Natl Cancer Inst* 99:428–432.

Redman M, Crowley J. 2007. Small randomized trials. *J Thorac Oncol* 2:1–2.

Rosner GL, Stadler W, Ratain MJ. 2002. Randomized discontinuation design: Application to cytostatic antineoplastic agents. *J Clin Oncol* 20(22):4478–4484.

Rubinstein L, Crowley J, Ivy P et al. 2009. Randomized phase II designs. *Clin Cancer Res* 15:1883–1890.

Rubinstein LV, Korn EL, Freidlin B et al. 2005. Design issues of randomized phase II trials and a proposal for phase II screening trials. *J Clin Oncol* 23:7199–7206.

Scher HI, Halabi S, Tannock I et al. 2008. Design and end points of clinical trials for patients with progressive prostate cancer and castrate levels of testosterone: Recommendations of the Prostate Cancer Clinical Trials Working Group. *J Clin Oncol* 26:1148–1159.

Seymour L, Ivy SP, Sargent D et al. 2010. The design of phase II clinical trials testing cancer therapeutics: Consensus recommendations from the clinical trial design task force of the national cancer institute investigational drug steering committee. *Clin Cancer Res* 16:1764–1769.

Simon R. 1987. How large should a phase II trial of a new drug be? *Cancer Treat Rep* 71:1079–1085.

Simon R. 1989. Optimal two-stage designs for phase II clinical trials. *Control Clin Trials* 10:1–10.

Stewart DJ. 2010. Randomized phase II trials: Misleading and unreliable. *J Clin Oncol* 28(31):e649–e650.

Taylor JM, Braun TM, Li Z. 2006. Comparing an experimental agent to a standard agent: Relative merits of a one-arm or randomized two-arm Phase II design. *Clin Trials* 3:335–348.

Van Glabbeke M, Steward W, Armand JP. 2002. Non-randomised phase II trials of drug combinations: Often meaningless, sometimes misleading. Are there alternative strategies? *Eur J Cancer* 38:635–638.

Von Hoff DD. 1998. There are no bad anticancer agents, only bad clinical trial designs. *Clin Cancer Res* 4:1079–1086.

Von Hoff DD. 2010. Pilot study using molecular profiling of patients' tumors to find potential targets and select treatments for their refractory cancers. *J Clin Oncol* 28:4877–4883.

Wieand HS. 2005. Randomized phase II trials: What does randomization gain? *J Clin Oncol* 23:1794–1795.

# 10 Phase II Selection Designs

*P.Y. Liu, James Moon, and Michael LeBlanc*

## CONTENTS

## 10.1 BASIC CONCEPT

When there are multiple promising new therapies in a disease setting, it may not be feasible to test all of them against the standard treatment in a definitive phase III trial. The sample sizes required for a phase III study with more than three arms could be prohibitive [1]. In addition, the analysis can be highly complex and prone to errors due to the large number of possible comparisons in a multi-arm study. An alternative strategy is to screen the new therapies first in a phase II setting and choose one to test against a standard treatment in a simple two-arm phase III trial. Selection designs can be used in such circumstances.

Simon et al. [2] first introduced statistical methods for ranking and selection to the oncology literature. In a selection design, patients are randomized to treatments involving new combinations or schedules of known active agents, or new agents for which activity against the disease in question has already been demonstrated in some setting. In other words, the regimens under testing have already shown promise. Now the aim is to narrow down the choice for formal comparisons to the standard therapy. With this approach, one always selects the observed best treatment for further study, however small the advantage over the others may appear to be. Hypothesis tests are not performed. Sample size requirements are established so that, should there exist a superior treatment, it will be selected with a high probability. The necessary sample sizes are usually similar to those associated with pilot phase II trials before phase III testing.

Before proceeding further, it is important to note that although the statistical principles for selection designs are simple, its proper application can be slippery. Falsely justified by the randomized treatment assignment, the major pitfall of the design is to treat the observed ranking as conclusive and forego the required phase III testing. This practice is especially dangerous when a control arm is included as the basis for selection, or when all treatment arms are experimental but a standard treatment does not exist for the particular disease. A "treatment of choice" can be declared with false justifications in these situations. If such a conclusion is desired, phase III studies with appropriately planned type I and type II errors should be conducted. Regarding a two-arm selection design, Sargent and Goldberg [3–5] states the following: "The goal of the randomized phase II trial is to ensure that if one treatment is clearly inferior to the other, there is a small probability that the inferior treatment will be carried forward to a phase III trial." Because of the design's moderate sample sizes and lack of type I error control for false positive findings, the results are error prone when treated as ends in themselves [6]. There must be a plan for a definitive Phase III study following the phase II selection study. Prior to embarking on a selection study, it is vital that the investigators understand the design's limitations and the proper interpretation of upcoming results.

## 10.2   SAMPLE SIZE REQUIREMENTS

### 10.2.1   BINARY OUTCOMES

Table 10.1 is reproduced from Simon et al. [2] for binary outcomes with K = 2, 3, and 4 groups.

The sample sizes were presumably derived by normal approximations to binomial distributions. With the listed N per group and true response rates, the correct selection probability should be approximately 0.90. A check by exact probabilities indicates that the actual correct selection probability ranges from 0.88 in most cases down to 0.86 when N is small. Increasing the sample size per group by six raises the correct selection probability to 0.90 in all cases and may be worth considering when N is less than 30.

Except in extreme cases, Table 10.1 indicates the sample size to be relatively insensitive to baseline response rates (i.e., response rates of groups 1 through K − 1). Since precise knowledge of the baseline rates is often not available, a conservative approach is to use always the largest sample size for each K, that is, 37, 55, and 67 patients per group for K = 2, 3, and 4, respectively. While a total N of 74 for two groups is in line with large phase II studies, the total number of patients required for four groups, that is, close to 270, could render the design impractical for many applications. Obviously the sample size can be reduced for differences greater than the 15% used for Table 10.1. However, if tumor response rate is the outcome of interest, it is generally low (e.g., 10%–20%) for many types of cancer and an absolute 15%

**TABLE 10.1**

**Sample Size per Treatment for Binary Outcomes and 0.90 Correct Selection Probability**

| Response Rates | | N per Group | | |
|---|---|---|---|---|
| $P_1,...,P_{K-1}$ | $P_K$ | K = 2 | K = 3 | K = 4 |
| 10% | 25% | 21 | 31 | 37 |
| 20% | 35% | 29 | 44 | 52 |
| 30% | 45% | 35 | 52 | 62 |
| 40% | 55% | 37 | 55 | 67 |
| 50% | 65% | 36 | 54 | 65 |
| 60% | 75% | 32 | 49 | 59 |
| 70% | 85% | 26 | 39 | 47 |
| 80% | 95% | 16 | 24 | 29 |

*Source:* Simon, R. et al., *Cancer Treat. Rep.*, 69, 1375, 1985.

increase would certainly indicate a superior response rate. Such a treatment should not be missed in the selection process by inadequate sample sizes. Similarly, a correct selection probability of 0.90 should also be treated as the standard since a lower probability would result in too many false negative trials.

## 10.2.2 SURVIVAL OUTCOMES

For censored survival data, Liu et al. [7] suggested fitting the Cox proportional hazards model, $h(t, z) = h_0(t)\exp(\beta'z)$, to the data where z is the $(K-1)$ dimensional vector of treatment group indicators and $\beta = (\beta_1, K, \beta_{K-1})$ is the vector of log hazard ratios. We proposed selecting the treatment with the smallest $\hat{\beta}_1$ (where $\hat{\beta}_K \equiv 0$) for further testing. Sample sizes for 0.90 correct selection probability were calculated based on the asymptotic normality of the $\hat{\beta}$. The requirements for exponential survival and uniform censoring are reproduced in Table 10.2. Simulation studies of robustness of the proportional hazards assumption found the correct selection probabilities to be above 0.80 for moderate departures from the assumption.

As with binary outcomes, the sample sizes become less practical when there are more than three groups or the hazard ratio between the worst and the best groups is smaller than 1.5.

Table 10.2 covers scenarios where the patient enrollment period is similar to the median survival of the worst groups. It does not encompass situations where these two quantities are quite different. Since the effective sample size for exponential survival distributions is the number of uncensored observations, the actual numbers of expected events are the same for the different rows in Table 10.2. For a 0.90 correct selection probability, Table 10.3 gives the approximate number of events needed per group for the worst groups. With ∫I dF as the proportion of censored observations, where I and F

**TABLE 10.2**

**Sample Size per Treatment for Exponential Survival Outcomes with 1 Year Accrual and 0.90 Correct Selection Probability**

|        |        | K = 2 | | | K = 3 | | | K = 4 | | |
|--------|--------|-------|-------|-------|-------|-------|-------|-------|-------|-------|
| Median | Follow | HR = 1.3 | HR = 1.4 | HR = 1.5 | HR = 1.3 | HR = 1.4 | HR = 1.5 | HR = 1.3 | HR = 1.4 | HR = 1.5 |
| 0.5    | 0      | 115 | 72  | 51  | 171 | 107 | 76  | 206 | 128 | 91  |
|        | 0.5    | 71  | 44  | 31  | 106 | 66  | 46  | 127 | 79  | 56  |
|        | 1      | 59  | 36  | 26  | 88  | 54  | 38  | 106 | 65  | 46  |
| 0.75   | 0      | 153 | 96  | 69  | 229 | 143 | 102 | 275 | 172 | 122 |
|        | 0.5    | 89  | 56  | 40  | 133 | 83  | 59  | 160 | 100 | 70  |
|        | 1      | 70  | 44  | 31  | 104 | 65  | 46  | 125 | 78  | 55  |
| 1      | 0      | 192 | 121 | 87  | 287 | 180 | 128 | 345 | 216 | 153 |
|        | 0.5    | 108 | 68  | 48  | 161 | 101 | 72  | 194 | 121 | 86  |
|        | 1      | 82  | 51  | 36  | 122 | 76  | 54  | 147 | 92  | 65  |

*Source:*  Liu, P.Y. et al., *Biometrics*, 49, 391, 1993.

Median = Median survival in years for groups 1 through K − 1; Follow = Additional follow-up in years after accrual completion; HR = Hazard ratio of groups 1 through K − 1 vs. group K.

**TABLE 10.3**

**Expected Event Count per Group for the Worst Groups for Exponential Survival and 0.90 Correct Selection Probability**

|   | HR | | |
|---|------|------|------|
| K | 1.3 | 1.4 | 1.5 |
| 2 | 54 | 34 | 24 |
| 3 | 80 | 50 | 36 |
| 4 | 96 | 60 | 43 |

HR = Hazard ratio of groups 1 through K − 1 vs. group K.

are the respective cumulative distribution functions for censoring and survival times, readers may find the expected event count more flexible for planning purposes.

## 10.3   VARIATIONS OF THE DESIGN

### 10.3.1   Designs with Minimum Activity Requirements

Though the selection design is most appropriate when adequate therapeutic effect is no longer in question, the idea of selection is sometimes applied to randomized phase

II trials when anti-cancer activities have not been previously established for the treatments involved. Alternatively, the side effects of the treatments could be substantial that a certain activity level must be met in order to justify the therapy. In such cases, each treatment arm is designed as a stand-alone phase II trial with the same acceptance criterion for all arms. When more than one treatment arms are accepted, the observed best arm is selected for further study [8,9]. The design typically specifies a null activity level which does not justify the further pursuit of a treatment, and an alternative activity level that would definitely render a treatment worthy of more investigation. The sample size and an end-of-study acceptance criterion signifying rejection of the null hypothesis are then specified, with the one-sided type I error rate and power often set at 0.05 and 0.90, respectively. When there are K arms with selection as the end goal, we recommend Bonferoni adjustment of the individual arm's type I error rate in order to maintain the study-wide type I error at 0.05. In the following sections, we examine the correct selection probability from these designs.

### 10.3.1.1 Binary Outcomes

For binary outcomes, standard designs without a selection component have been well developed; see overview of phase II designs by Green in Chapters 7 and 16. Table 10.4 lists three such designs.

Designs B1 and B2 represent typical situations in new agent testing for cancer treatment, where moderate tumor response rates in the 20%–30% range already warrant further investigations. Design B3 is more for theoretical interest when response rates are near 50%.

### TABLE 10.4
### Three Phase II Designs for Binary Data

| K | Nominal $\alpha$ per Arm | N per Arm | Acceptance Level[a] | Exact $\alpha$ | Exact Power |
|---|---|---|---|---|---|
| **Design B1: Null level = 5%, alternative level = 20%** | | | | | |
| 2 | 0.025 | 45 | ≥6/45 | 0.0239 | 0.91 |
| 3 | 0.0167 | 50 | ≥7/50 | 0.0118 | 0.90 |
| 4 | 0.0125 | 50 | ≥7/50 | 0.0118 | 0.90 |
| **Design B2: Null level = 10%, alternative level = 30%** | | | | | |
| 2 | 0.025 | 36 | ≥8/36 | 0.0235 | 0.89 |
| 3 | 0.0167 | 40 | ≥9/40 | 0.0155 | 0.89 |
| 4 | 0.0125 | 45 | ≥10/45 | 0.0120 | 0.91 |
| **Design B3: Null level = 40%, alternative level = 60%** | | | | | |
| 2 | 0.025 | 62 | ≥33/62 | 0.0239 | 0.89 |
| 3 | 0.0167 | 69 | ≥37/69 | 0.0151 | 0.89 |
| 4 | 0.0125 | 75 | ≥40/75 | 0.0133 | 0.90 |

[a] Response rates signifying treatment worthy of further investigation.

Assume the same true response rate configuration as in Table 10.1, that is, $P_1 = \ldots = P_{K-1} < P_K$, for designs B1–B3. Table 10.5 indicates that, when the true $P_1$ and $P_K$ values are the same as the null and alternative design parameters respectively, that is, 5%/20% for Design B1, 10%/30% for Design B2, and 40%/60% for Design B3, the chance of a correct selection result is approximately the same as the design power, 0.90, in all three cases. In other words, the operating characteristics of the phase II design dominate in this case and the chance of an inferior arm's passing the acceptance level and further surpassing the best arm is negligible. When the true $P_1$ and $P_K$ are far higher than the null and alternative levels of the phase II design, all arms will

**TABLE 10.5**

**Correct Selection Probabilities for Binary Data Designs with Minimum Acceptance Level[a] (3000 Simulations)**

Design B1, testing 5% vs. 20%, true $P_K - P_1 = 15\%$

| True $P_1/P_K$[b] | 5%/20% | 10%/25% | 15%/30% | 20%/35% | 30%/45% |
|---|---|---|---|---|---|
| K=2 | 0.91 | 0.96 | 0.95 | 0.94 | 0.91 |
| K=3 | 0.89 | 0.95 | 0.92 | 0.90 | 0.87 |
| K=4 | 0.90 | 0.92 | 0.90 | 0.88 | 0.84 |

Design B2, testing 10% vs. 30%, true $P_K - P_1 = 15\%$

| True $P_1/P_K$ | 10%/25% | 15%/30% | 20%/35% | 30%/45% | 40%/55% |
|---|---|---|---|---|---|
| K=2 | 0.71 | 0.86 | 0.90 | 0.89 | 0.88 |
| K=3 | 0.69 | 0.85 | 0.87 | 0.83 | 0.82 |
| K=4 | 0.71 | 0.85 | 0.85 | 0.80 | 0.80 |

Design B2, testing 10% vs. 30%, true $P_K - P_1 = 20\%$

| True $P_1/P_K$ | 10%/30% | 15%/35% | 20%/40% | 30%/50% | 40%/60% |
|---|---|---|---|---|---|
| K=2 | 0.89 | 0.95 | 0.96 | 0.95 | 0.94 |
| K=3 | 0.88 | 0.94 | 0.94 | 0.91 | 0.93 |
| K=4 | 0.90 | 0.95 | 0.93 | 0.93 | 0.92 |

Design B3, testing 40% vs. 60%, true $P_K - P_1 = 15\%$

| True $P_1/P_K$ | 40%/55% | 45%/60% | 50%/65% | 55%/70% | 60%/75% |
|---|---|---|---|---|---|
| K=2 | 0.66 | 0.88 | 0.95 | 0.95 | 0.96 |
| K=3 | 0.62 | 0.86 | 0.92 | 0.92 | 0.94 |
| K=4 | 0.65 | 0.88 | 0.90 | 0.93 | 0.93 |

Design B3, testing 40% vs. 60%, true $P_K - P_1 = 20\%$

| True $P_1/P_K$ | 40%/60% | 45%/65% | 50%/70% | 55%/75% | 60%/80% |
|---|---|---|---|---|---|
| K=2 | 0.88 | 0.97 | 0.98 | 0.99 | 0.99 |
| K=3 | 0.88 | 0.96 | 0.98 | 0.98 | 0.99 |
| K=4 | 0.90 | 0.97 | 0.98 | 0.99 | 0.99 |

[a] Probability of the true best arm passing the acceptance level and being the observed best arm.

[b] $P1 = \ldots = P_{K-1}$

meet the acceptance requirement and selection design properties take over. When $P_K - P_1 = 15\%$, Table 10.1 results can be used as a general guide for correct selection probability. For example, when $K = 2$, the per arm sample sizes of 45, 36, and 62 in Table 10.4 compare favorably with the highest N of 37 from Table 10.1; therefore, the correct selection probabilities are generally 0.88 or higher when minimum acceptance level is easily met by the best arm. However, when $P_1 = 30\%$, $P_K = 45\%$, and $K = 4$, per Table 10.1, the N required per arm is 62 for an approximate 0.90 correct selection probability. The corresponding N for $K = 4$ in Designs B1 and B2 are 50 and 45, respectively; therefore, the correct selection probabilities in Table 10.5 are less than 0.90. When $P_K - P_1 = 20\%$, as is the distance between the alternative and null values for Designs B2 and B3, correct selection probabilities are approximately 0.90 or higher in all cases examined.

In general, applying Bonferoni adjustment to per-arm type I errors performs adequately with respect to correct selection probabilities in the situations examined, of which the parameter ranges cover most cancer trial applications. The approach is appropriate when the emphasis is on the initial step of screening the treatments for minimum acceptable anti-tumor activities. If meeting the minimum activity level is relatively assured and the emphasis is on selection, it would be more appropriate to design the trial with the larger sample size between what is required for the phase II and the selection portions.

### 10.3.1.2   Survival Outcomes

The approach for binary outcomes can be applied to survival outcomes as well. With Bonferoni adjustment for type I errors, phase II designs with null and alternative hypotheses are used first to test the minimum acceptance level. Selection ensues when two or more arms are accepted. Assuming exponential survival and uniform censoring, Table 10.6 lists correct selection probabilities for one scenario from Table 10.2. The results are generalizable to other accrual and follow-up length combinations since the event count, hazard ratio, and the number of arms, which are represented here, are the determinants for power or selection probability under the exponential assumption.

Similar to binary data results, when the null median $m_1 = 0.75$ and $m_K/m_1 = 1.5$ as designed, the phase II operating characteristics dominate and the correct selection probability is approximately 0.90—the same as the individual arm's planned power. The correct selection probability is poor when $m_1 = 0.75$ and $m_K/m_1 = 1.3$. When the worst median is higher than the null level of 0.75, selection properties begin to apply. For example, for Design S3, $K = 4$, $N = 147$ per arm and the worst median is 0.95, the expected exponential event count is 75 with 1 year accrual and an additional 0.5 year follow-up. Compared to Table 10.3, the event count required for 0.90 correct selection probability is 96, 60, and 43 for $m_K/m_1 = 1.3$, 1.4, and 1.5, respectively, thus explaining the corresponding correct selection probabilities of 0.86, 0.93, and 0.97 in Table 10.6.

### 10.3.2   DESIGNS WITH MINIMUM ADVANTAGE REQUIREMENTS

Some authors propose changing the selection criterion so that the observed best treatment will be further studied only when its minimum advantage over all other treatments

**TABLE 10.6**

**Correct Selection Probabilities for Exponential Survival Design[a] with 1 Year Accrual, 0.5 Year Follow-Up and Minimum Acceptance Level (3000 Simulations)**

| True $m_1$ | Correct Selection Probability for $m_K/m_1$[b] = | | |
| --- | --- | --- | --- |
| | 1.3 | 1.4 | 1.5 |
| Design S1: K=2, N=124 per arm, observed median acceptable if >0.95 | | | |
| 0.75 | 0.57 | 0.78 | 0.91 |
| 0.85 | 0.84 | 0.94 | 0.97 |
| 0.95 | 0.90 | 0.96 | 0.98 |
| Design S2: K=3, N=137 per arm, observed median acceptable if >0.96 | | | |
| 0.75 | 0.53 | 0.77 | 0.89 |
| 0.85 | 0.84 | 0.93 | 0.97 |
| 0.95 | 0.88 | 0.95 | 0.98 |
| Design S3: K=4, N=147 per arm, observed median acceptable if >0.96 | | | |
| 0.75 | 0.54 | 0.77 | 0.90 |
| 0.85 | 0.83 | 0.93 | 0.97 |
| 0.95 | 0.86 | 0.93 | 0.97 |

[a] All designs are for detecting a hazard ratio of 1.5 over the null median of 0.75 with one-sided 0.05/K type I error and 0.90 power for each arm.

[b] $m_1 = \ldots = m_{K-1} < m_K$.

is greater than some positive $\Delta$; otherwise, the selection will be based on other factors. Table 10.7 gives some binary data sample size requirements [3–5] for $\Delta = 0.05$.

While this approach is appealing because the decision rule is easier to carry out in practice, the sample sizes required generally more than double those in Table 10.1. For example, for K=2, $P_1 = 35\%$, $P_2 = 50\%$, and 0.90 correct selection probability, it can be interpolated from Table 10.1 that 36 patients per treatment are required for $\Delta = 0$. With the same configuration, the required number of patients is 75 per group for $\Delta = 5\%$. Clearly when $\Delta > 5\%$, the sample size requirement would be impractical. Even with $\Delta = 5\%$ and 75 patients per group, the results are by no means definitive when a greater than 5% difference is seen. When $P_1 = P_2 = 35\%$ and N=75, the chance of observing $|p_1 - p_2| > 5\%$ is approximately 52% (where $p_1$ and $p_2$ are the observed proportions; $P_1$ and $P_2$ are the true proportions). On the other hand, with $\Delta = 0$ and N=36 per Table 10.1, the chance of observing $|p_2 - p_1| > 5\%$ is approximately 0.81 when the true $P_1 = 35\%$ and $P_2 = 50\%$. Therefore, with an incremental gain in the probability of correctly observing a $\Delta > 5\%$ but double the sample size, this approach may only be practical when patient resource is plentiful. While precision is improved with the larger sample sizes, the results are nevertheless non-definitive.

### 10.3.3 DESIGNS IN WHICH ONE OR MORE ARMS ARE FAVORED

In some situations, it might not be appropriate to allow all of the arms an equal chance of being selected. An example might be a selection between two experimental arms

**TABLE 10.7**

**Sample Size per Treatment for Binary Outcomes and 0.90 Correct Selection Probability When Requiring an Absolute 5% Minimum Advantage for Selection**

| Response Rates (%) | | N per Group | | |
|---|---|---|---|---|
| $P_1,..., P_{K-1}$ | $P_K$ | K = 2 | K = 3 | K = 4 |
| 5 | 20 | 32 | 39 | 53 |
| 15 | 30 | 53 | 77 | 95 |
| 25 | 40 | 71 | 98 | 119 |
| 35 | 50 | 75 | 115 | 147 |

*Sources:* Sargent, D.J. and Goldberg, R.M., *Stat. Med.,* 20, 1051, 2001; Lui, K.J., *Stat. Med.,* 21, 625, 2002; Sargent, D.J., *Stat. Med.,* 21, 628, 2002.

where one of the arms is known to have much more severe side effects. In such a case, a variation on the design with a minimum advantage requirement as described earlier could be utilized. Although this design can be applied to more than two arms, for the sake of simplicity this discussion will be limited to the two-arm case. In this design, one arm is favored over the other. That arm is always chosen unless the non-favored arm has an observed positive advantage $\geq \Delta$. That is, to be selected, the non-favored arm must not only perform better but also "beat the point spread." This is not to be confused with a randomized phase II design, in which a formal hypothesis test between the two arms is performed.

### 10.3.4 DESIGNS FOR ORDERED TREATMENTS

When the K ($\geq 3$) treatments under consideration consist of increasing dose schedules of the same agents, the design can take advantage of this inherent order. A simple method is to fit regression models to the outcomes with treatment groups coded in an ordered manner. Logistic regression for binary outcomes and the Cox model for survival are obvious choices. A single independent variable with equally spaced scores for the treatments could be included in the regression. If the sign of the observed slope is in the expected direction, the highest dose with acceptable toxicity is selected for further study. Otherwise, the lowest dose schedule would be selected.

Compared to the non-ordered design, this approach should require smaller sample sizes for the same correct selection probability. Limited simulations were conducted with the following results. For binary data with K=3, $P_1 = 40\%$, $P_3 = 55\%$, $P_1 \leq P_2 \leq P_3$, approximately N=35 per arm is needed for a 0.90 chance that the slope from the logistic regression is positive. Compared to N=55 given in Table 10.1, this is a substantial reduction in sample size. Similarly, for K=4, $P_1 = 40\%$, $P_4 = 55\%$, $P_1 \leq P_2 \leq P_3 \leq P_4$, 40 patients per arm are needed instead of 67. For exponential survival data with a 1.5 hazard ratio between the worst groups and the best group, approximately 28 and 32 events per group are needed for the worst groups for $K = 3$ and 4, respectively, as compared to 36 and 43 given in Table 10.3.

## 10.4 CONCLUDING REMARKS

The statistical principles of selection design are simple and adaptable to various situations in cancer clinical research. Applied correctly, the design can serve a useful function in the long and arduous process of new treatment discovery. However, as mentioned in the beginning, the principal misuse of the design is to treat the results as ends in themselves without the required phase III investigations. We previously published the false positive rates of this misapplication [6]. It was shown that impressive looking differences arise with high frequencies purely by chance with selection design sample sizes. We also pointed out that performing hypothesis tests post-hoc changes the purpose of the design. If the goal is to reach definitive answers, then a phase III comparison should be designed with appropriate analyses and error rates. Testing hypotheses with selection sample sizes can be likened to conducting the initial interim analysis for phase III trials. It is well known that small sample type I error assessments are unstable and extremely stringent p-values are required to "stop the trial" at this early stage.

Finally, when historical benchmarks are not available for setting a minimum acceptance activity level, the inclusion of a standard or control treatment in a selection design should be utilized with caution. Without a control arm, any comparison between the current standard and the observed best treatment from a selection trial is recognized as informal because the limitations of historical comparisons are widely accepted. When a control arm is included for randomization, the legitimacy for comparison is established and there can be great temptation to interpret the results literally and "move on." If there are no efficacy differences between treatments, the chance of observing an experimental treatment better than the control is $(K-1)/K$, that is, 1/2 for $K = 2$, 2/3 for $K = 3$, etc. Again, an observed advantage for an experimental treatment simply means its substantial inferiority is unlikely so that further testing may be warranted and must be conducted for definitive comparisons.

## ACKNOWLEDGMENT

This work was supported in part by grant #CA038926 from the National Cancer Institute.

## REFERENCES

1. Liu PY, Dahlberg S. Design and analysis of multiarm clinical trials with survival endpoints. *Controlled Clinical Trials* 1995; 16:119–130.
2. Simon R, Wittes RE, Ellenberg SS. Randomized phase II clinical trials. *Cancer Treatment Reports* 1985; 69:1375–1381.
3. Sargent DJ, Goldberg RM. A flexible design for multiple armed screening trials. *Statistics in Medicine* 2001; 20:1051–1060.

4. Lui KJ. Letter to the editor: A flexible design for multiple armed screening trials. *Statistics in Medicine* 2002; 21:625–627.

5. Sargent, DJ. Author's reply to letter to the editor. *Statistics in Medicine* 2002; 21:628.

6. Liu PY, LeBlanc M, Desai M. False positive rates of randomized phase II designs. *Controlled Clinical Trials* 1999; 20: 343–352.

7. Liu PY, Dahlberg S, Crowley J. Selection designs for pilot studies based on survival. *Biometrics* 1993; 49:391–398.

8. Herbst RS, Kelly K, Chansky K, Mack PC, Franklin WA, Hirsch FR, Atkins JN et al. Phase II selection design trial of concurrent chemotherapy and cetuximab versus chemotherapy followed by cetuximab in advanced-stage non-small-cell lung cancer: Southwest Oncology Group study S0342. *Journal of Clinical Oncology* 2010; 28(31):4747–4754.

9. Hoering A, LeBlanc M, Crowley J. Seamless phase I/II trial design for assessing toxicity and efficacy for targeted agents. *Clinical Cancer Research* 2010; 17(4):1–7.

# 11 Phase II with Multiple Subgroups
## Designs Incorporating Disease Subtype or Genetic Heterogeneity

*Michael LeBlanc, Cathryn Rankin,*
*and John J. Crowley*

## CONTENTS

## 11.1 INTRODUCTION

Patients registered to a Phase II study often are heterogeneous and may not be expected to respond equally to a new treatment. Tumors can consist of multiple subtypes diagnosed either histologically or by molecular methods. For example, soft tissue sarcomas or non-Hodgkin lymphomas have multiple subtypes that can be identified by microscopic inspection of the tumor sample. Similarly, newer genomic measurements such as gene expression or comparative genomic hybridization on these tumors can now lead to refinement or regrouping of patients for clinical studies. For instance, expression of measures of HER2, EGFR, VEGF may influence the expectation of response by certain drugs in some tumors. While we are specifically interested in Phase II studies in oncology, our ideas relate more broadly to the use of biomarker or subtype information in the design of clinical experiments.

In this chapter we present a simple strategy for dealing with tumors with multiple subgroups or histologies. We build our proposal on a traditional design for simple one-arm study in oncology. For such studies, activity is often not fully understood, and for ethical and patient resource reasons the designs have multiple stages (often two stages) where one can stop earlier and declare futility if insufficient activity is seen (Simon 1989; Green and Dahlberg 1992; Green et al. 2002). At the end of the first stage, typically accrual is halted until sufficient data have been submitted and analyzed at the statistical office to determine if the study should be re-opened to accrue to the next stage.

A problem with a single stratum Phase II study is that it uses the overall response rate (or another summary statistic), and if efficacy truly varies among subgroups of patients, strata with good efficacy will be combined with those with limited or no activity and may falsely lead to an overall negative conclusion. A schematic of single-arm study that includes multiple subtypes of disease, A, B, or C, is included in Figure 11.1. Alternatively, one can conduct multiple strata specific studies, with each strata having its own accrual goal and efficacy estimate with no mechanism for "joint learning" across the strata. However, it may be clear that there is overall limited activity in all strata at some point, but separate individual analyses may not lead to enough evidence to stop each stratum and hence accrual will continue. An example of a published clinical study for soft tissue sarcoma in the literature using a "joint learning" via Bayesian methods is Chugh et al. (2009).

Our goal is to present flexible frequentist Phase II strategies that are inclusive with respect to the patient population, but with appropriate subgroups acknowledged in the designed hypothesis testing and subsequent analyses. Figure 11.2 shows two options. Where the relative expected activity is not known between the strata, we would run a Phase II study with multiple subgroups, but with testing that includes both the subgroups and a combined test. This is represented by the left panel. In the situation where there is an expected ordering, for instance decreasing expression of some tumor based on a drug target, we propose an alternative testing strategy, represented by a sequence of nested sets or circles in the right panel of Figure 11.2.

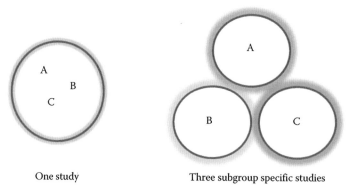

One study                    Three subgroup specific studies

**FIGURE 11.1**    Representation of a single phase II study versus several subgroup specific studies.

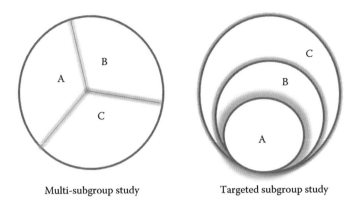

Multi-subgroup study          Targeted subgroup study

**FIGURE 11.2** Representation of a multiple disjoint subgroup phase II study versus nested targeted study.

We demonstrate the properties of our multiple subgroup Phase II method in terms of simulations motivated by a multi-histology sarcoma study with clinical response as the primary endpoint. While we choose to implement the design with multiple interim futility analyses, the strategy is more general; the essential idea is that for Phase II studies there are potential gains (in expected sample size or power) for using a combination of subgroup and overall analyses while appropriately characterizing the overall design statistical error rates. While much of our proposal appeared in LeBlanc et al. (2009), here we clarify the futility testing and $p$-value calculations and provide additional simulations to better understand the properties of the strategy.

## 11.2 PHASE II DESIGN WITH MULTIPLE SUBTYPES

We consider a strategy that tests both within each subtype and combined across subtypes. The design is presented in terms of binary response data or disease control rate at some specific time point, but the same methods could easily be extended to time-to-event patient outcomes. For instance, the parameter estimates given in Section 11.2.1 could be hazard estimates or non-parametric estimates appropriate for survival data.

Denote a clinical response model for the outcome of interest for $K$ subgroups or disease subtypes $R_k: k = 1, \ldots, K$, where individuals in subgroup $k$ with outcomes (responses) are modeled as

$$Y_{ik} = 1 \text{ with probability } \theta_k$$

$$0 \text{ with probability } 1 - \theta_k$$

We assume that that different subtypes of patients register to the study at a rate proportional to the frequencies of the subtypes of the disease $\upsilon_k$. Simple estimates of the response rates for each stratum are estimated proportions (fraction of patients with response $Y_{ik} = 1$ for each stratum $\hat{\theta}_k$) and the overall estimate is the fraction of patients with $Y_{ik} = 1$ over all $k$ strata $\hat{\theta}$.

We propose a sequential design, motivated by traditional two-stage Phase II designs, and assume that at least $n_s^{min}$ patients will be accrued to any stratum before considering testing for futility against the alternative hypothesis $\theta_A$ and that a maximum number of patients, $n_s^{max}$, can be accrued to any stratum. In addition to the subgroup analysis, the patients on study as a whole are combined and the design tests for futility when a minimum $n^{min}$ patients have been accrued. The maximum size of the study is $n^{max}$ patients, where $n^{max}$ is less than or equal to the number of patients which would be accrued at full accrual for all strata, $Kn_s^{max}$.

As a practical issue, even in a single-arm study, a temporary closure while waiting for patient outcome (response) information to be forwarded to the statistical office can lead to diminished enthusiasm and subsequent accrual rates. Given the assumption of multiple strata, we focus on the case where responses are assumed to be available relatively quickly, as temporary closures on multiple strata would likely exacerbate the problems seen in single stratum studies. Therefore, we will also propose to analyze the data when each group of $q$ (say 5 or 10 patients) is registered to the study after achieving some minimum sample size. An alternative would be to analyze after each fixed number of patients are evaluated for response (say 4 months after registration) rather than just based on accrual. We note that this idea works with response, short-term disease control rates or short-term ($\leq 4$ month) progression-free survival. Furthermore, even if multiple interim analyses are not feasible for a given disease, a design with a single interim analysis using the combined and subgroup testing would still have some attractive sample size and power properties relative to separate Phase II studies for each subtype of the disease.

## 11.2.1   Unordered Subgroups

We test the alternative hypothesis within each subgroup. The $p$-value for the alternative hypothesis is the chance of observing success rate as small as or smaller than the observed rate under the alternative hypothesis $\theta_A$

$$p_k^A = \Pr\left(\widehat{\theta^*}_{jk} \leq \hat{\theta}_{jk} \mid \theta_A\right)$$

The success proportion is defined as $\hat{\theta}_{jk} = r_{jk}/n_{jk}$ where $r_{jk}$ is the number of successes when $n_{jk}$ patients are assessed for response at analysis time $j$ where $n_{jk} \geq n_s^{min}$. If the subgroup test is rejected at an analysis, $p_k^A < \alpha_A$, testing at level $\alpha_A$, then accrual to that stratum is discontinued, but continues for the remaining strata. To improve the probability of stopping early in the event of limited (or no) activity, the data are also combined across the subtypes and we test the overall alternative hypothesis. The $p$-value for the overall test is calculated, as the chance or probability the combined rate would be as small as or smaller than the observed success rate

$$p^A = \Pr\left(\widehat{\theta^*}_j \leq \hat{\theta}_j \mid \bar{\theta}_A\right)$$

where $r_j$ is the total number of successes across all strata when $n_j$ patients are assessed for response at analysis time $j$. As in the subgroup tests, the alternative overall test is calculated only after a prespecified number of patients are accrued, $n^{min}$. Therefore, all overall tests of the alternative are conducted with sample sizes, $n_j \geq n^{min}$. If the overall test of the alternative is rejected, $p^A < \alpha_A$, then accrual to the entire study is terminated. We think it is sensible for the overall alternative to be set closer to the null hypothesis than the alternative of interest for a subgroup or histology, $\bar{\theta}_A < \theta_A$. For instance, while a subgroup alternative value for response probability could be $\theta_A = 0.3$ (for a null response probability $\theta_0 = 0.1$), a smaller treatment activity may be of interest for the study as a whole; hence, in this case, an alternative of $\bar{\theta}_A = 0.2$ may be appropriate. Therefore, one could pick the $\bar{\theta}_A = \gamma \theta_A + (1 - \gamma) \theta_0$ where $\gamma$ is a fraction between 0 and 1 where that is thought of as the minimum fraction of patients achieving the subgroup alternative to be of interest in an overall comparison. For example, if we choose $\gamma = 0.5$ or moving 50% of patients to the subgroup, this motivates the $\bar{\theta}_A = 0.2$ alternative hypothesis ($0.2 = 0.5 \times 0.3 + (1 - 0.5) \times 0.1$.

After completing accrual, the $p$-value corresponding to the test of the null hypothesis is

$$p_k^0 = \Pr\left(\widehat{\theta}^*_{jk} \geq \hat{\theta}_{jk} \mid \theta_0\right)$$

for each stratum and the $p$-value of the null hypothesis test is

$$p^0 = \Pr\left(\widehat{\theta}^*_j \geq \hat{\theta}_j \mid \theta_0\right)$$

for the combined group. The subgroup null hypothesis would be rejected if $p_k^0 < \alpha_{0s}$ or the overall patient group rejected if $p^0 < \alpha_0$; we think it will usually be sufficient to keep the subgroup and overall Type 1 specification equal, $\alpha_{0s} = \alpha_0$ if one sets $\alpha_0 = 0.05$, leading to a larger overall experiment-wise Type 1 error rate greater than $\alpha_0$; but we calculate it for a given design.

An important aspect of the design is the selection of sample sizes per stratum, $n_s^{min}$ and $n_s^{max}$, corresponding to a possible first test of the alternative hypothesis and maximum stratum sample size for each stratum $s$, and similar sample sizes for the entire study, $n^{min}$ and $n^{max}$. We propose using a standard two-stage design to pick $n_s^{min}$ and $n_s^{max}$ as done by Green and Dahlberg (1992), or Green et al. (2002). The same strategy is used to pick the overall sizes based on null and alternative hypotheses $\theta_0$ and $\bar{\theta}_A$.

We think a desirable property of the method is that a single stratum is stopped only for futility outcome data associated with that stratum. Negative results in one stratum lead to stopping accrual of patients to other strata only if the combined results cause rejection of the alternative hypothesis. However, more complex borrowing or learning could potentially reduce variance and lead to greater savings in sample size. This has been done in the literature using Bayesian methods such as those implemented by Thall et al. (2003) and Thall and Wathen (2008). The posterior probability of the stratum specific response rates can be used to guide stopping accrual. However, we believe non-Bayesian borrowing strategies could also be utilized. For instance, simple ridge regression shrinkage could be used as a bridge between the single stratum analysis and combined analysis. One could replace the aforementioned individual stratum estimates with

$$\tilde{\theta}_{jk} = \gamma \hat{\theta}_j + (1 - \gamma)\hat{\theta}_{jk}$$

for each subgroup and the $p$-values for futility testing could be evaluated as done previously. While the shrinkage factor $\gamma$ needs to be chosen, one or a small number of values (say 0.2 and 0.5) might be reasonable to encourage borrowing for futility testing. While ad hoc, the full frequentist properties can be evaluated.

### 11.2.2 ORDERED OR TARGETED SUBGROUP

For some drug and disease combinations, it is strongly suspected that the drug will have greatest activity within a subtype of disease or a group of patients expressing a marker or combination of markers. In that case, a special subgroup and overall design can be used. Of course there still needs some belief of the potential efficacy for the drug outside the targeted subgroup to make it appropriate to include a broader group of patients. Targeted or nested subgroup design and analyses in the Phase III setting were developed by Hoering et al. (2008).

In this case, one may focus on accrual both within the subgroup and total for the study. Consider the target test of the alternative hypothesis

$$p_t^A = \Pr\left(\widehat{\theta^*}_{jt} \le \hat{\theta}_{jt} \mid \theta_{At}\right)$$

where $\hat{\theta}_{jt}$ is the success or response estimate in the targeted subgroup consisting the $n_{jt}$ patients in the strata $k \in S$, where $S$ is the set of strata indicating the target or most promising biologic group. In this case, the alternative hypothesis of interest, $\theta_{At}$, corresponds to the targeted subgroup. Once sufficient patients are accrued to the target group, the test of the targeted subgroup alternative hypothesis is conducted. If the target test is rejected, then entire study is closed. There is an important difference between this study design and the unordered subgroup case described in the previous section. Here, given sufficient understanding or of the target and drug, one may be willing to infer that lack of efficacy for the targeted subgroup implies overall futility, and not just for a subgroup of patients. Given that ordered hypothesis, the design will lead to smaller sample sizes under the null than the unordered design. At the end of accrual, there are tests of the null hypothesis for both the targeted group:

$$p_t^0 = \Pr\left(\widehat{\theta^*}_{jt} \ge \hat{\theta}_{jt} \mid \theta_0\right)$$

and the test for the overall group with $p$-value defined as $p^0$. The overall experimental null hypothesis is rejected if either of the two $p$-values is less than $\alpha$. This leads to the potential for improved power when there is substantial activity in the targeted subgroup but little or no improved activity in the other strata. The sample size for testing the null hypothesis in targeted group can be set using (Green and Dahlberg 1992); however, if the targeted null hypothesis is rejected (and drug assumed to be promising), one would likely want to have reasonable stratum specific estimates of response rates. Therefore, one may also want to allow the targeted group to accrue to the total of the stratum specific sample sizes, unless there is a decision to stop early for futility.

## 11.3  SIMULATIONS BASED ON SOFT TISSUE SARCOMA

### 11.3.1  UNORDERED SUBGROUPS

We will use simulations based on a prior SWOG cooperative group soft tissue sarcoma study (von Mehrun et al. 2011). The study was conducted to test sorafenib, which is an agent with multiple molecular targets that may be of relevance in soft tissue sarcomas. The drug was potentially interesting because several subtypes of adult high-grade soft tissue sarcomas were known to express VEGFR and PDGFR in these tumor types.

The primary objective of the Phase II study was to assess the clinical response probability (confirmed complete response and partial response) in patients soft tissue sarcoma, with the most frequent histologies assumed to be high-grade leiomyosarcoma or high-grade liposarcoma, and several other histologies (angiosarcoma, hemangiosarcoma, and hemangiopericytoma) combined into the third stratum. Our design-specified response would be assessed within histologic subtypes as well as combined over all subtypes. We note that the design actually used in the SWOG study only assessed clinical responses at a limited number of times.

Each hypothetical Phase II multi-subtype clinical trial was generated with subtype frequencies: Subgroup 1 leiomyosarcoma (50%), Subgroup 2 liposarcoma (30%), and Subgroup 3 angiosarcoma/hemangiosarcoma/hemangiopericytoma (20%). We assumed that the probability of response for all three strata was $\theta_0 = 0.05$ under the null hypothesis and the alternative hypothesis of subgroup alternative response probability was $\theta_A = 0.25$. The overall alternative hypothesis response rate was set at $\bar{\theta}_A = 0.15$.

We generated simulated data where each of the three strata had a maximum sample size of 25 patients. Futility testing is first conducted after 15 patients have been accrued to any stratum. Overall futility testing (testing the alternative hypothesis) is first done after 30 patients have been accrued in total. An overall maximum of 75 patients that can be accrued was set for the study design. The Type 1 error for the futility analyses based on testing of the alternative hypotheses was $\alpha_A = 0.02$, similar to that of Green and Dalhberg (1992), and testing of the null was specified with $\alpha_0 = 0.05$. To encourage a smaller overall expected sample size when there is limited activity, futility analyses were conducted after every five patients accrued. In practice, this will be done after five patients are assessable for response rather than accrued. To estimate properties of the design, we generated 5000 simulated clinical trials and we evaluated following four hypothetical scenarios:

1. *No improved activity*: $\theta_1 = \theta_2 = \theta_3 = 0.05$.
2. *Improved activity in frequent subtype*: $\theta_1 = 0.25$, $\theta_2 = \theta_3 = 0.05$.
3. *Improved activity in infrequent subtype*: $\theta_1 = \theta_2 = 0.05$, $\theta_3 = 0.25$.
4. *Limited activity in all subtypes* $\theta_1 = \theta_2 = \theta_3 = 0.15$.

We evaluated some important aspects of Phase II designs, the expected sample size for the new design N(SubT), the expected sample size for the simple Phase II study in each stratum N(Simple), power for stratum specific studies Power(Simple), and power for new design Power(SubT). Therefore, N(SubT) is the sample size using subgroup efficacy testing but with combined or overall group futility testing and Power(SubT) is power for subgroup efficacy test with combined futility testing. An additional piece of information provided in the tables is the conditional probability of rejecting the null hypothesis for the specific stratum, given either the overall or the stratum-specific hypotheses have been rejected. We include the target accrual and the experiment-wise power in the individual figure captions.

Under the null hypothesis that the response rate is 5% in all three strata, as presented in Table 11.1, there is considerable reduction in the expected sample size by using the additional combined futility testing. Overall, the reduction is approximately 18% with the biggest reductions in expected sample size observed for the infrequent histologies. Table 11.1 shows that the Type 1 error for each stratum is less than $\alpha_0 = 0.05$ due to the futility testing. While one could modify the individual stratum tests to control the overall Type 1 error, we choose to just report the overall error. The experiment-wise Type 1 error is inflated due to the multiple strata, with the separate stratum analysis of 10% and with the combined (SubT) strategy 8.4%. The slightly smaller Type 1 error is due to combined group futility testing.

The second scenario (Table 11.2) investigates the case where the compound was only effective in the frequent subgroup (which we assume to be 50% of the patients with soft tissue sarcoma). The strategy of using multiple strata specific Phase IIs and the combined strategy yield similar expected sample sizes. Importantly, under the alternative, the conditional probability of rejecting the null hypothesis for that stratum

---

**TABLE 11.1**

**No Improved Activity**

| Stratum | Accrual | Rate | N(Simp) | Power(Simp) | N(SubT) | Power(SubT) | Cond. Prob. |
|---------|---------|------|---------|-------------|---------|-------------|-------------|
| 1 | 0.50 | 0.05 | 20.10 | 0.04 | 18.74 | 0.03 | 0.31 |
| 2 | 0.30 | 0.05 | 20.10 | 0.03 | 16.69 | 0.03 | 0.37 |
| 3 | 0.20 | 0.05 | 20.69 | 0.04 | 14.70 | 0.02 | 0.28 |

Min stratum = 15, max stratum = 25, min combined = 30, max combined = 75. Experiment-wise power (Simp) = 0.0996, experiment-wise power (SubT) = 0.0842.

## TABLE 11.2
### Improved Activity in the Frequent Subtype

| Stratum | Accrual | Rate | N(Simp) | Power(Simp) | N(SubT) | Power(SubT) | Cond. Prob. |
|---------|---------|------|---------|-------------|---------|-------------|-------------|
| 1 | 0.50 | 0.25 | 24.86 | 0.89 | 24.66 | 0.89 | 0.99 |
| 2 | 0.30 | 0.05 | 19.94 | 0.04 | 19.82 | 0.03 | 0.04 |
| 3 | 0.20 | 0.05 | 20.53 | 0.03 | 20.19 | 0.04 | 0.05 |

Min stratum=15, max stratum=25, min combined=30, max combined=75. Experiment-wise power (Simp)=0.8998, experiment-wise power (SubT)=0.903.

## TABLE 11.3
### Improved Activity in the Infrequent Subtype

| Stratum | Accrual | Rate | N(Simp) | Power(Simp) | N(SubT) | Power(SubT) | Cond. Prob. |
|---------|---------|------|---------|-------------|---------|-------------|-------------|
| 1 | 0.50 | 0.05 | 19.97 | 0.03 | 19.73 | 0.03 | 0.06 |
| 2 | 0.30 | 0.05 | 19.99 | 0.03 | 19.55 | 0.03 | 0.05 |
| 3 | 0.20 | 0.25 | 24.89 | 0.90 | 23.27 | 0.83 | 0.99 |

Min stratum=15, max stratum=25, min combined=30, max combined=75. Experiment-wise power (Simp)=0.8998, Experiment-wise power (SubT)=0.903.

## TABLE 11.4
### Limited Improved Activity in All Subtypes

| Stratum | Accrual | Rate | N(Simp) | Power(Simp) | N(SubT) | Power(SubT) | Cond. Prob. |
|---------|---------|------|---------|-------------|---------|-------------|-------------|
| 1 | 0.50 | 0.15 | 24.00 | 0.53 | 23.94 | 0.53 | 0.62 |
| 2 | 0.30 | 0.15 | 24.11 | 0.54 | 23.81 | 0.53 | 0.60 |
| 3 | 0.20 | 0.15 | 24.05 | 0.53 | 23.79 | 0.52 | 0.58 |

Min stratum=15, max stratum=25, min combined=30, max combined=75. Experiment-wise power (Simp)=0.897, Experiment-wise power (SubT)=0.9076.

given any rejection of the null for the combined method is 99%. In Table 11.3, the case where the improvement is limited to the infrequent subtype (20% frequency), the experiment-wise power for the combined strategy is 90% which is again approximately the same as the individual subgroup trials strategy. The false study terminations for overall futility also lead to a smaller sample size for the infrequent group. While the comparisons for the simple method and new strategies are quite close for these two scenarios, the comparison to a single combined study is striking. Even with sample size equal to the total sample size of the study (75 patients), a single combined analysis for improved activity in an infrequent histology would only have power of 39%.

Finally, Table 11.4 shows that if sorafinib were approximately equally effective in all subgroups, the combined strategy yields a power of 91% which is only slightly higher than the probability of rejecting at least one of the individual strata (90%). However, for a given stratum there is only an approximately 53%–54% chance of rejecting the null hypothesis, potentially leading to falsely concluding negative results for one or more subgroups. In summary, for the sarcoma study, the subgroup/combined Phase II strategy leads to smaller sample sizes under the null and improved power when there was limited efficacy across subtypes.

## 11.3.2 ORDERED OR TARGETED SUBGROUP

We also used the same trial characteristics to study the impact of a design where efficacy is expected to be best within one or more subtypes. We assumed that the most frequent and most infrequent subgroups were combined to make a targeted subgroup containing about 70% of patients. Such a design would be useful if it were known (or strongly believed) that those histologies or genetically defined subgroups were most biologically suited to a particular treatment. For instance, tumors in those subgroups might express the target molecule most highly among all histologies. Under this design, given that we assume that the efficacy will be greatest in the targeted group, evidence of a lack of efficacy for the targeted group implies overall futility, not just subgroup futility. Therefore, the entire study would be closed if the targeted subgroup alternative hypothesis is rejected. Note, while one could limit the total sample size of the subgroups or combined subgroups expected to have greatest efficacy, we choose only to focus on futility testing. Therefore, the targeted test of the null will be based on full accrual to the stratum or strata representing the targeted group. A motivation for not stopping for the potentially smaller sample size is that would likely still want to have good response rates estimates within each of the subtype strata if the targeted null hypothesis is rejected.

Testing of the alternative hypothesis within the subgroup was conducted as described in Section 11.2.2, with alternative response probability of $\theta_{Ar} = 0.20$. Under the null hypothesis, the targeted design further reduced the sample size compared to either of the individual subgroup analyses as shown in Table 11.5 (a 27% reduction

---

### TABLE 11.5
### No Improved Activity: Simple Subgroups or Targeted Method

| Stratum | Accrual | Rate | N(Simp) | Power(Simp) | N(SubT) | Power(SubT) | Cond. Prob. |
|---------|---------|------|---------|-------------|---------|-------------|-------------|
| 1 | 0.50 | 0.05 | 20.01 | 0.04 | 17.95 | 0.03 | 0.44 |
| 2 | 0.30 | 0.05 | 20.13 | 0.03 | 14.09 | 0.02 | 0.28 |
| 3 | 0.20 | 0.05 | 20.72 | 0.04 | 12.46 | 0.02 | 0.32 |

Min stratum = 15, max stratum = 25, min target = 20, max target = 50. Experiment-wise power (Simp) = 0.0988, experiment-wise power (Comb) = 0.0788. Target power = 0.0288.

**TABLE 11.6**

**Active within Subgroup: Simple Subgroups or Targeted Method**

| Stratum | Accrual | Rate | N(Simp) | Power(Simp) | N(SubT) | Power(SubT) | Cond. Prob. |
|---------|---------|------|---------|-------------|---------|-------------|-------------|
| 1 | 0.50 | 0.20 | 24.60 | 0.76 | 24.44 | 0.75 | 0.84 |
| 2 | 0.30 | 0.05 | 19.86 | 0.04 | 19.75 | 0.03 | 0.04 |
| 3 | 0.20 | 0.20 | 24.64 | 0.75 | 24.24 | 0.74 | 0.82 |

Min stratum=15, max stratum=25, min target=20, max target=50. Experiment-wise power (Simp)=0.9404, experiment-wise power (Comb)=0.9416. Target power=0.920.

in overall sample size). In addition, in Table 11.6, if the targeted strata had response probability of 0.20 and remaining strata had a response rate of 0.05, the simulation study showed that the targeted hypothesis significantly increased power (92%) (Type 1 error of 0.02) over individual subgroup analyses (approximately 77%) (Type 1 errors of 3% or 4%) for the two strata corresponding promising subgroups. The experiment-wise power of rejecting at least one of the strata was modestly higher than the experiment-wise power of the strategy including targeting. But this was, in part, due to the larger Type 1 error of the untargeted strategy compared to targeted 9.9% versus 2.9%. The reduction in Type 1 error for the targeted method is a result of the more directed futility testing that stops overall accrual if there is futility in the target subgroup, compared to considering each stratum separately in the untargeted strategy.

## 11.4   DISCUSSION

The Phase II strategies presented in this chapter fit into the class of recently developed methods for incorporating biologic subgroup variation into designed experiments. Our proposed Phase II method for unordered subgroups can be a useful alternative to either combining all groups to do a single Phase II study with a single endpoint evaluation or conducting multiple separate studies each with separate analyses. The former has the drawback of not acknowledging potential variation in activity in disease subtypes which are likely to occur, and the latter strategy may be logistically difficult if diseases are rare and the relative frequencies of subgroups cannot be well predicted before activating the study. We conduct individual subgroup tests and the overall combined tests all the while acknowledging the multiple testing properties of the design. The combination strategy yields smaller sample sizes when the drug is inactive across all strata and more power in cases when there is some activity across all strata compared to conducting individual Phase II studies in the subgroups. In addition, by retaining the stratum-specific tests, the design allows active subgroups to be identified.

While there are many variations for the Phase II design and implementation, we believe our results support the general proposal of appropriate "borrowing" of information in the Phase II setting where there are multiple biologic or histologic subgroups. For instance, for some diseases it may not be feasible to conduct as frequent futility testing (e.g., after every 5–10 patients are accrued). We believe the combined subgroup and overall analyses would still be useful even if only one interim analysis was possible. Furthermore, even in a single stage one-arm pilot study, the use of the either the unordered or targeted tests of the null hypotheses for efficacy testing could lead to improved overall power and insights into activity.

We have also chosen to use a method where futility stopping of a stratum only depends on stratum specific data. We only borrow information across strata for futility testing for the entire study. As noted earlier in the chapter, one could choose to borrow even for the stratum specific tests using the Bayesian proposals for multiple histology Phase II studies (Thall et al. 2003; Thall and Wathen 2008), but we prefer to evaluate the frequentist properties of any borrowing or shrinking method.

Another extension includes the use of time-to-event data. To evaluate progression-free survival and overall survival, one will typically need larger studies to achieve sufficient power and increase the promise that large sample results hold. Such studies may also be practically limited to a single interim or even no interim analysis. One could consider parametric survival estimates hazard ratio estimates or non-parametric estimates following work by Lin et al. (1996).

Software implementing this procedure is for response data available from the first author.

## ACKNOWLEDGMENT

This work was supported in part by grants NIH R01 CA90998 and CA038926.

## REFERENCES

Chugh R, Wathen JK, Maki RG, Benjamin RS, Patel RS, Myers PA, Priebat DA et al. 2009. Phase II multicenter trial of imatinib in 10 histologic subtypes of sarcoma using a Bayesian hierarchical statistical model, *Journal of Clinical Oncology*, 19:3148–3153.

Green SJ, Benedetti J, Crowley J. 2002. *Clinical Trials in Oncology*, 2nd edn. Chapman & Hall, Boca Raton, FL.

Green SJ, Dahlberg S. 1992. Planned versus attained design in phase II clinical trials, *Statistics in Medicine*, 11:853–862.

Hoering A, LeBlanc M, Crowley J. 2008. Randomized phase III clinical trial designs for targeted agents, *Clinical Cancer Research*, 14:4358–4367.

LeBlanc M, Rankin C, Crowley J. 2009. Multiple histology phase II trials, *Clinical Cancer Research*, 15(13):4256–4262.

Lin DY, Shen L, Ying Z, Breslow NE. 1996. Group sequential designs for monitoring survival probabilities, *Biometrics*, 52:1033–1042.

von Mehren M, Rankin C, Goldblum JR, Demetri GD, Bramwell V, Borden E. 2011. A phase II SWOG-directed intergroup trial (S0505) of sorafenib in advanced soft tissue sarcomas, July 12, 2011, Online, DOI: 10:1002/cncr.26334.

Simon R. 1989. Optimal two-stage designs for phase II clinical trials, *Controlled Clinical Trials*, 10:1–10.

Thall PF, Wathen JK. 2008. Bayesian designs to account for patient heterogeneity in phase II clinical trials, *Current Opinion in Oncology*, 20:407–411.

Thall PF, Wathen JK, Bekele BN, Champlin RE, Baker LO, Benjamin RS. 2003. Hierarchical Bayesian approaches to phase II trials in diseases with multiple subtypes, *Statistics in Medicine*, 22:763–780.

# 12 Phase II/III Designs

*Sally Hunsberger*

## CONTENTS

## 12.1 INTRODUCTION

Phase II/III, seamless phase II/III, and integrated II/III designs are terms that are used interchangeably and refer to study designs that combine aspects of phase II drug development and phase III drug development into one study. Phase II/III designs randomize patients in the phase II component and then include these patients in the phase III component of the study. An intermediate end point is evaluated in the phase II component.

Historically, phase II studies have been designed to have a single arm and are independent of a phase III. Phase II studies are used to screen agents for activity before launching a large phase III study. Since there are many agents to screen and many of the agents will provide no benefit, it is important to keep phase II studies as small as possible. Traditionally, the sample size for phase II studies has been 15–40 patients. As described in other chapters, phase III studies require large sample sizes since clinical benefit defined as overall survival (OS) or disease-free survival (DFS) is the endpoint of interest.

Although there has been more interest in using phase II/III designs recently (Goldman et al. 2008; Hunsberger et al. 2009; Parmar et al. 2008), the concept is not new. For example, Ellenberg and Eisenberger (1985) and Schaid et al. (1990) both proposed study designs that use the same patients to answer phase II and III questions, but the designs have rarely been used in practice in oncology. The renewed interest in phase II/III studies has occurred because of the need to perform more randomized phase II studies.

## 12.2 MOTIVATION FOR PHASE II/III DESIGNS

The need for randomized phase II studies is a result of significant changes in the drug development landscape in oncology. First, there are now agents known to extend survival in many types of cancer. Along with studying the single agent activity of a new agent, it is also of interest to study new agents in combination with agents that are known to be beneficial. Single-arm studies are less appropriate when studying combinations that include an established active agent. Due to heterogeneity of the population, some patients will respond to the active agent and some will not. An increase in an observed response rate over a value defined by the historical single agent response rate is difficult to interpret. The increase could be a result of accruing more patients to the study who respond to the active single agent or it could be due to the new agent. The only way to determine the population benefit of the addition of the new agent is through a randomized study.

Second, new molecularly targeted agents are being developed with different hypothesized mechanisms of action. Historically, antitumor activity has been evaluated by using an endpoint such as tumor shrinkage. Currently, many new agents are not expected to shrink tumors. It is thought that the molecularly targeted agents will inhibit tumor growth and stabilize disease. Therefore, progression-free survival (PFS) is often the endpoint of interest for phase II studies of molecularly targeted agents. This endpoint is preferred to OS for phase II studies, since it may occur significantly sooner than OS. Even when OS occurs early, it may not be a good endpoint for phase II studies, since often after progression patients are changed to a different therapy, thereby potentially diluting effects on OS and leading to the need for large sample sizes. Although PFS is a phase II endpoint of interest, it can be difficult to measure accurately and is more affected by population heterogeneity than tumor shrinkage. PFS can vary depending on individual patient characteristics; therefore, the median PFS for a study can be influenced greatly by patient selection. Consequently, studies involving molecularly targeted agents with PFS as the endpoint must be randomized in order to really learn if PFS has been increased with the new agent. Also, with molecularly targeted agents, patients may be selected based on having a positive or negative marker. If a population is selected based on a marker, there may be no historical data for the response rate or PFS rate in that population (McShane et al. 2009).

Third, molecularly targeted agents often have nonoverlapping toxicities with chemotherapeutic agents or very little toxicity, so it is of interest to study combinations of molecularly targeted agents along with combinations of molecularly targeted agents and cytotoxic chemotherapy. For all these reasons, an increasing number of phase II trials are needed, and many of them will require randomization.

Randomized phase II studies require at least two times more patients than single-arm phase II studies (Rubinstein et al. 2005). Given the increased number of regimens to study, efficient use of patients is required. For some experimental regimens, the same control arm would be used in a randomized phase II study and the phase III study. In this situation, an obvious efficient use of patients would be to include patients from the phase II study in the phase III study. A practical approach is to consider phase II/III designs, where patients in phase II can also be used in phase III.

## 12.3 SPECIFICS OF II/III DESIGNS

The elements of a phase II/III design are as follows: the overall sample size (total number of patients) is calculated based on the phase III endpoint. The phase II component of the study can be viewed as an interim futility analysis with an intermediate endpoint (Goldman et al. 2008). That is, patients are accrued to the study until a specified number of patients are on study. At that point, an analysis based on an intermediate endpoint (response or PFS) is performed. If a prespecified activity criterion is met, accrual is continued to the study until the overall sample size is met. All patients are then used in the phase III analysis (final analysis).

Challenges in designing phase II/III studies are the choice of the intermediate endpoint (or phase II endpoint), the decision criterion for stopping, and timing of the interim analysis. The intermediate endpoint should be related to the primary endpoint in such a way that at a minimum, lack of effect on the intermediate endpoint is a reliable indication of there being no effect on the primary endpoint. (This is the standard assumption that has historically been made when using PFS or response rate in single-arm phase II studies or randomized phase II studies.) The intermediate outcome should be observed earlier than the primary endpoint. If the intermediate endpoint is obtained late (or at a time that is not much different from the primary endpoint), then the benefit of the interim analysis (or the chance to stop the study early and save patients entering into the study) will be lost. The stopping criterion should be such that there is a high probability of stopping the study under the null hypothesis while having little impact on the overall power of the study to detect a true benefit on the primary endpoint. The timing of the interim analysis should be such that if the regimen is inactive, the study will stop as early as possible during accrual but late enough, so that a reliable decision can be made.

## 12.4   EXAMPLE

As a case study consider a Cancer and Leukemia Group B (CALGB) study of renal cell carcinoma (RCC). It is a placebo-controlled randomized study of bevacizumab in advanced RCC patients who have progressed after treatment with a tyrosine kinase inhibitor. The combination of everolimus (mTOR inhibitor) and bevacizumab (VEGFR inhibitor) is being compared to everolimus. Everolimus is approved for second line treatment of RCC based on a PFS endpoint (Motzer et al. 2008). Bevacizumab with interferon was shown to be an active combination in first line RCC (Escudier et al. 2007; Rini et al. 2008). Due to nonoverlapping toxicities of everolimus and bevacizumab, it was of interest to combine the two agents. A phase II/III design is of interest for the following reasons.

1. If the addition of bevacizumab to everolimus were shown to increase activity in a randomized phase II study, a phase III study with the same arms would definitely be designed.
2. Although both agents have been shown to increase PFS neither has demonstrated benefit on OS. Ultimately, the combination is only of interest if OS is shown to be increased.
3. The primary endpoint of interest is OS, but there is no data to indicate the addition of bevacizumab to everolimus increases activity. Obtaining the activity data before investing in a large phase III study is essential.

The actual phase II/III study design is as follows. The total study size is 676 patients with the primary endpoint being OS. With an accrual rate of 23 patients per month, the study will need to accrue for 30 months. The minimum follow-up will be 34 months. An interim analysis based on PFS will be performed after 100 patients have been followed for 4 months (since accrual will continue to the study while the patients are being followed for 4 months, approximately 191 patients will be on study). Patient accrual will continue if at the interim analysis, the estimate of 4 month PFS in the combination arm is at least 6% higher than the estimate in the everolimus alone arm.

The total sample size was chosen, so that $\beta_s$, the probability of incorrectly concluding no improvement in OS, would be less than 0.1 if the true median OS is improved from 12 to 15.6 months (hazard ratio, HR = 1.3). The calculation of the total sample size did not take into account the interim analysis on PFS. At the end of the study, a one-sided p-value less than 0.025 would be considered significant.

When the null hypothesis of no treatment effect on PFS is true, the study will stop with probability 0.76. If the combination truly improves median PFS from 4 to 8 months (hazard ratio of 2) and improves OS from 12 to 15.6 months, the overall probability of concluding a benefit of the combination is at least 0.855.

The choice of the phase II analysis time and criteria for continuing the study is critical to phase II/III studies and will be explored further for this example. The timing of the analysis will be determined by the type I and II error rates for the intermediate analysis, $\alpha_i$ and $\beta_i$, respectively. Here, $\alpha_i$ is the probability of continuing the study when the experimental agent is not active on the intermediate endpoint, and $\beta_i$ is the probability of not continuing the study when the experimental agent is active on the intermediate endpoint. Accrual to the study will continue if the p-value of the test comparing PFS in the two arms is less than $\alpha_i$. The selected $\alpha_i$ defines (and limits) the probability of continuing on to the phase III portion of the study when there is no benefit of the experimental agent on the intermediate endpoint. When there is no benefit on the intermediate endpoint, it is desirable to stop accrual to the study early to avoid continuing on to a foreseeable negative phase III study (assuming the predictive value of the intermediate endpoint). A measure of the impact of $\alpha_i$ is the expected sample size, E[S], or the average sample size if the study were repeated many times when the intermediate endpoint null hypothesis is true. It is given by $E[S] = n_i + \alpha_i(N - n_i)$ where $n_i$ is sample size at the interim analysis and N is the total sample size. Under the null hypothesis, we would like E[S] to be minimized; however, as $\alpha_i$ decreases, $n_i$ increases for fixed $\beta_i$ and N, so the relationship between $\alpha_i$ and E(S) is not monotonic. Figure 12.1 shows the relationship between E[S], $n_i$, and $\alpha_i$ for a specific example under the null hypothesis.

In Figure 12.1, N = 676, $\beta_i$ = 0.05 (the unusually small choice of $\beta_i$ will be described later), and $n_i$ is calculated assuming PFS is the intermediate endpoint and follows an exponential distribution with median of 4 months. The calculations use an accrual rate of 23 patients per month and target a hazard ratio of 1.5 or 2 (this is equivalent to an increase in median PFS to 6 or 8 months).

In Figure 12.1, the solid line is used to show E[S] and the dashed line to show $n_i$, as $\alpha_i$ varies. The figure shows that for small $\alpha_i$, $n_i$ is large and this increases E[S]. For the curves with HR = 1.5, $\alpha_i$ = 0.2 minimizes E[S]. For $\alpha_i$ = 0.2, E[S] = 365 and

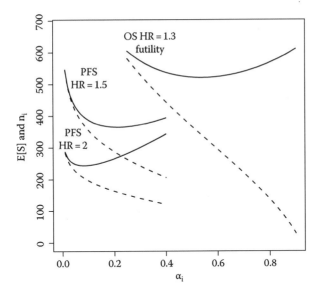

**FIGURE 12.1** Relationship between expected sample size, E[S], the sample size in phase II portion of study, $n_i$ (or before interim analysis), and $\alpha_i$ for the RCC study example. The solid line represents E[S] and the dashed line represents $n_i$. The lines labeled PFS HR are for stopping based on the PFS endpoint for different hazard ratios (HR). The lines labeled OS HR are for futility monitoring based on OS. The total sample size is fixed at 676 and $\beta_i = 0.05$.

$n_i = 287$. The E[S] curve is relatively flat for values of $\alpha_i$ between 0.2 and 0.3 but $n_i$ decreases rapidly. For example, for $\alpha_i = 0.3$, $E[S] = 372$ and $n_i = 241$, which means that $n_i$ has decreased by 46 patients while E[S] has only increased by 7. Therefore, $\alpha_i = 0.3$ is also a good choice for the interim analysis given the small increase in E[S] and large decrease in $n_i$. For the curves with HR = 2, $\alpha_i = 0.10$ minimizes E[S] with $E[S] = 244$ and $n_i = 196$. Again, the E[S] curve is relatively flat for an interval around $\alpha_i = 0.1$. For $\alpha_i = 0.15$, $E[S] = 252$ and $n_i = 177$. Here, $\alpha_i = 0.15$ is also an adequate choice for the stopping criteria.

The overall power is the probability of correctly concluding that the experimental treatment improves OS (given an interim analysis of PFS has occurred). In the phase II/III setting, this probability depends on $\beta_i$, the probability of incorrectly stopping a study when there is a true benefit on the intermediate endpoint and $\beta_s$ (the probability of concluding no benefit on OS if no interim analysis is performed). A simple calculation assuming the intermediate endpoint and the final endpoint are independent gives a lower bound on the overall power of the study. The overall power is the probability of rejecting the null hypothesis at the interim analysis multiplied by the probability of rejecting the null hypothesis at the end of the study given you rejected the null hypothesis at the interim analysis, that is $(1 - \beta_s)(1 - \beta_i)$, which, in our example, is $(1 - 0.1)(1 - 0.05) = 0.855$. By examining this equation, it can be seen that as $\beta_i$ decreases, the overall power increases. Typically, the intermediate endpoint and the final endpoint will be positively correlated (not independent), so the overall power will be between 0.9 and 0.855. We always assume that the treatment effects on the two variables are very highly correlated; otherwise, the intermediate endpoint is not a good surrogate for the primary endpoint.

Although there is a loss in power by using the phase II/III design rather than a phase III design with no interim analysis based on an intermediate endpoint, the power comparisons must be interpreted carefully. If a phase III design with no intermediate endpoint monitoring was performed, there would typically be an independent randomized phase II study based on the intermediate endpoint. Therefore, the correct comparison of power is to account for the phase II study before proceeding to the phase III study. If the phase II study was designed to have power of 0.95 and the phase III study to have power of 0.9, the overall probability of correctly concluding a benefit on OS would also be 0.855.

In the example, an overall power of 85% was specified, if instead, an overall power of 90% was desired, $\beta_s$ would need to be decreased from 0.10 to 0.05, since power would be $(1 - \beta_s)\ (1 - \beta_s) = (1 - 0.05)\ (1 - 0.05) = 0.90$. Now, $\beta_s$ is used in the calculation of the overall sample size and as $\beta_s$ decreases sample size increases. In this example, if we use the same type I error rate (0.025), hazard ratio (1.3), minimum follow-up (34 months), and accrual rate (23 patients per month), the overall sample size would be 826 (rather than 676). A figure similar to Figure 12.1 could be created for this new overall sample size. The $\alpha_i$'s that give the smallest E[S] are smaller (0.1–0.2). This is due to the larger overall sample size. If $\alpha_i$ is large, the study continues to the full size more often, which increases E[S] more dramatically. Thus, continuing to the full study size is more costly and should be done with a lower probability of erroneously moving forward.

A variant of the phase II/III design with an interim analysis based on an intermediate endpoint is to perform an aggressive futility analysis on the primary endpoint. This design does not work nearly as well for cases such as the one given, where the median time to the primary endpoint is much longer than that to the intermediate endpoint. In order to not impact power, the analysis must be performed late in the study, and due to the much later event times, the continuation criteria must be very low so that the study only stops in extreme cases. This is demonstrated in Figure 12.1, which shows the E[S] and $n_i$ as $\alpha_i$ varies for the futility design based on OS. In the Figure 12.1, the overall power is maintained at 0.855. Again, the solid line is E[S], and the dashed line is $n_i$. In this case, the null hypothesis involves OS. The figure indicates that $\alpha_i = 0.54$ minimizes E[S]. For this criteria E[S] = 520, $n_i = 330$. The study will continue with an observed hazard ratio of 0.979 (or 11.8 month median OS in the experimental arm), indicating that the placebo arm is performing slightly better than the experimental arm. The E[S] curve is relatively flat until about $\alpha_i = 0.6$, with this criteria E[S] = 523, $n_i = 294$, HR = 0.931, 11.18 median OS for the experimental arm. For both criteria, E[S] is 77% of the total sample size, whereas for the designs, using the intermediate endpoint, E[S] was 36% of the total sample size.

## 12.5 DISCUSSION

Phase II/III designs can be valuable designs in drug development, but they should not be used for all studies. Several issues should be evaluated when considering whether a phase II/III design is appropriate. A phase II/III study can be considered when there is an intermediate endpoint that is related to the phase III endpoint, and the intermediate endpoint can be obtained much earlier than the primary endpoint. If such an endpoint is not available, then there would be no savings in doing a II/III design.

A phase II/III design could be considered if a positive randomized phase II result (even using a relatively high $\alpha_i$, such as 0.2 or 0.3, as suggested in the example) would ensure moving to a phase III study. Typically, positive data from several single arm studies in a specific disease type are required before a phase III study is launched. For the phase II/III design, this may be the only phase II study in this disease type or stage. Therefore, there should be other types of data that would provide justification for a phase II/III study. For example, there may be evidence from other disease types, strong evidence from phase I studies, strong evidence from a different stage of disease, or a known molecular target that has shown activity in other settings with this regimen.

The key assumption in the phase II screening component of oncologic drug development for the past 50 years has been that a lack of effect on the intermediate endpoint is a reliable indication of there being no effect on the primary endpoint. This assumption is also crucial for phase II/III designs. If this assumption is not valid, the phase II component (either as an independent study or as part of a phase III study) will substantially reduce the probability of finding a treatment benefit on OS.

There is little savings in terms of the expected sample size, E[S], for the design with a futility analysis based on OS. However, the power does not depend on the experimental treatment affecting an intermediate endpoint. Therefore, this design could be considered when there is no intermediate endpoint that meets the previous assumption.

There are disadvantages of the phase II/III designs. Developing the protocol for a phase II/III design is complex and time consuming. It essentially requires developing a phase III protocol that requires more work than a phase II protocol. A phase III study often requires more sites to commit to the study since potentially more patients will be required. It may be possible to begin the study in a subset of sites for the phase II component and then expand to more sites for the phase III component but often this can lead to problems with sites not feeling invested in the study when they did not have much say in the development of the study. Thus, accrual to the phase III component may not increase as much as expected.

An unresolved issue is whether positive results from the phase II portion of the study should be published before the end of the phase III study (note accrual and treatment of patients would still be occurring). Typically, data from an interim analysis of an ongoing study are not published. This practice has been established so that doctors and patients will not base treatment decisions on unreliable information. For phase II/III studies, if $\alpha_i$ were chosen to be small, the phase II data may be the most reliable data available and one could argue that these should be published. Then again, publishing the data may negatively impact accrual to the study, since patients would want to be treated with the most promising regimen. A similar issue arises when an independent randomized phase II study is performed. Positive results from the study will be published potentially making it impossible to perform a phase III study. In a phase II/III study, if $\alpha_i$ were 0.2 or 0.3, publishing a positive phase II result early may result in treating patients with an experimental regimen when the probability of falsely concluding the regimen is active is high. The decision as to when positive phase II results could be published should be considered carefully for each study and clearly addressed in the protocol.

Although there are disadvantages and concerns to address, there are situations where phase II/III study designs should be considered.

## REFERENCES

Ellenberg, S. S. and Eisenberger, M. A. (1985). An efficient design for phase III studies of combination chemotherapies. *Cancer Treat Rep*, 69(10), 1147–1154.

Escudier, B., Pluzanska, A., Koralewski, P., Ravaud, A., Bracarda, S., Szczylik, C., Chevreau, C. et al. (2007). Bevacizumab plus interferon alfa-2a for treatment of metastatic renal cell carcinoma: A randomised, double-blind phase III trial. *Lancet*, 370(9605), 2103–2111.

Goldman, B., LeBlanc, M., and Crowley, J. (2008). Interim futility analysis with intermediate endpoints. *Clin Trials*, 5, 22.

Hunsberger, S., Zhao, Y., and Simon, R. (2009). A comparison of phase II study strategies. *Clin Cancer Res*, 15(19), 5950–5955.

McShane, L. M., Hunsberger, S., and Adjei, A. A. (2009). Effective incorporation of biomarkers into phase II trials. *Clin Cancer Res*, 15(6), 1898–1905.

Motzer, R. J., Escudier, B., Oudard, S., Hutson, T. E., Porta, C., Bracarda, S., Grunwald, V. et al. (2008). Efficacy of everolimus in advanced renal cell carcinoma: A double-blind, randomised, placebo-controlled phase III trial. *Lancet*, 372(9637), 449–456.

Parmar, M. K., Barthel, F. M., Sydes, M., Langley, R., Kaplan, R., Eisenhauer, E., Brady, M. et al. (2008). Speeding up the evaluation of new agents in cancer. *J Natl Cancer Inst*, 100(17), 1204–1214.

Rini, B. I., Halabi, S., Rosenberg, J. E., Stadler, W. M., Vaena, D. A., Ou, S. S., Archer, L. et al. (2008). Bevacizumab plus interferon alfa compared with interferon alfa monotherapy in patients with metastatic renal cell carcinoma: CALGB 90206. *J Clin Oncol*, 26(33), 5422–5428.

Rubinstein, L. V., Korn, E. L., Freidlin, B., Hunsberger, S., Ivy, S. P., and Smith, M. A. (2005). Design issues of randomized phase II trials and a proposal for phase II screening trials. *J Clin Oncol*, 23(28), 7199–7206.

Schaid, D. J., Wieand, S., and Therneau, T. M. (1990). Optimal 2-stage screening designs for survival comparisons. *Biometrika*, 77(3), 507–513.

# Part III

## Phase III Trials

# 13 Use of Covariates in Randomization and Analysis of Clinical Trials

*Garnet L. Anderson, Michael LeBlanc,*
*P.Y. Liu, and John J. Crowley*

## CONTENTS

## 13.1 INTRODUCTION

Randomization provides the basis for determining causality in scientific experiments. While there are settings in medicine and public health where convincing evidence may be obtained from nonrandomized studies, there is a clear shift toward requiring the higher quality evidence obtained from well-designed randomized trials. Rapidly changing diagnostic and disease assessment tools, the use of more subjective endpoints, requirements for diverse patient populations, and modest effect sizes all tend to weaken the inference from uncontrolled experiments. In oncology, where historically a single-arm phase II trial has often been adequately informative, randomized phase II trials are increasingly common.

Pure randomization, such as a simple coin flip, is almost never used in practice. Such a procedure assures balance between arms only in expectation. Given that clinical trials are almost never repeated, most researchers want to avoid the risk of a loss of power that would arise with a noteworthy imbalance in the number of patients on each arm by restricting the randomization to assure some degree of balance. Equal numbers in each arm are easily achieved but also considered insufficient, except in large trials, since imbalance on important prognostic factors may also diminish confidence in trial results. Hence the adage "block what you can and randomize what you cannot" (Box et al. 1978) is often invoked in trial design.

Multiple strategies exist to incorporate covariate information in randomization schemes. Kalish and Begg (1985) review a comprehensive list of treatment allocation strategies. These allocation rules generally fall into three categories based on their use of covariates: (1) rules that are independent of covariates, (2) rules that promote balance marginally for each covariate, and (3) rules that balance the treatment arms within each stratum. Another class of treatment allocation approaches, known as "response adaptive" randomization schemes (Hu and Rosenburg 2006), have been developed, which alter the probability of assignment to each arm over time based on interim results of the trial. We elected not to consider these here, because they are not well suited to the long-term and complex nature of randomized phase III trials in oncology (but see Chapter 18).

Any constrained randomization scheme can be applied overall, ignoring covariate information, or within strata defined by covariates (Hill 1951). Furthermore, a stratified randomization approach that does not constrain the treatment assignments to be approximately equal within strata does not introduce any true stratification. When the ratio of sample size to strata is small, however, stratified randomization may actually increase the potential for imbalance if balance is not adequately achieved in each cell of the design. For these settings, covariate-adaptive randomization schemes were developed to promote balance for each factor marginally (Taves 1974, Pocock and Simon 1975) or to optimize an objective function defined by a linear model (Begg and Iglewicz 1980).

The use of covariates in the analysis of randomized experiments is often guided by our understanding of linear models. In this setting, the model need not control for covariates to produce unbiased estimates of effect or a valid test (acceptable type I error), but may be used to improve power by reducing variance. In nonlinear models, however, omitting predictive covariates may reduce efficiency because the treatment effect estimators are biased toward zero (Gail et al. 1984, Lagakos and Schoenfeld 1984, Struthers and Kalbfleisch 1986, Anderson and Fleming 1995).

The choice of analytic approach in clinical trials is less clear when the randomization uses covariates (Peto et al. 1976, Friedman et al. 1981, Meinert 1986). Green and Byar (1978) demonstrated that an unstratified analysis of binary data generated from a trial using important prognostic covariates in a stratified treatment allocation rule yields a conservative test with noticeably reduced power. A stratified analysis in this setting preserves the nominal size of a test (Green and Byar 1978). For more complex randomization strategies, such as the adaptive designs, however, there is no direct link between the covariate structure in the design and the test statistic.

The Southwest Oncology Group (SWOG), an NCI-funded cooperative group, conducts numerous randomized trials of cancer therapeutics. These trials are designed to test the effects of specific treatment regimens on failure-time endpoints such as survival or progression-free survival. Baseline information on disease status and patient characteristics is often used in randomization. SWOG has adopted the biased-coin adaptive randomization rule proposed by Pocock and Simon (1975) to assure balance on the margins for key covariates. In reporting results, the majority of these studies use stratified logrank statistics or Cox proportional hazards regression to incorporate these covariates. It is of interest to know if there is a preferred analysis approach in this setting.

Here, we characterize the performance of the most commonly used survival analysis-based tests when applied to trials employing randomization strategies that differ in their use of covariates using simulations. Several factors come into play in these settings: the number of strata or covariates and their distribution in the sample, the magnitude of the covariate and treatment effects, and the degree of censoring. Though we cannot be comprehensive in examining these factors, we examined a variety of settings, some specifically chosen to violate model assumptions or create instability, with the hope that these would provide useful insight into the robustness of each approach.

## 13.2   RANDOMIZATION SCHEMES

We selected one allocation rule from each of the three categories defined earlier based on their use of covariate information to investigate.

### 13.2.1   RANDOMIZATION INDEPENDENT OF COVARIATES

Permuted blocks (PB) is the simplest and most commonly used randomization strategy (Rubin 1977, 1978). In this approach, a list or block of treatment assignments is generated in advance with each treatment arm appearing in random order in the predetermined proportion. The treatments are assigned sequentially to patients as they enter the trial. For the case of block size $N$, where $N$ is the total sample size for the study, a PB approach merely assures that the desired proportions on each treatment arm are reached. Typically multiple, smaller block are used (e.g., block sizes of 2, 4, 6, and 8 for two-armed trials). Table 13.1 gives an example of PB of size 4 and a simple method for their application. Since balance is attained at the completion of each block, smaller block sizes promote balance on the implicit covariate of time of entry, an important feature if there is a significant possibility of drift in patient characteristics over time or if interim analyses will be conducted. In unblinded trials, however, small block sizes increase the probability that the next treatment assignment can be accurately predicted, which may introduce selection bias. To reduce this problem, randomized PB algorithms have been proposed. Here, variable block sizes are used, with block size randomly selected from a few preselected sizes. More sophisticated algorithms, such as constrained block randomization (Berger et al. 2003) have been proposed to reduce the potential for selection bias while assuring reasonable balance over time. For this purpose, however, we examine a PB design with block size $N$, a method that imposes the fewest constraints on the randomization.

### 13.2.2   COVARIATE ADAPTIVE ALGORITHMS

The Pocock–Simon (PS; Pocock and Simon 1975) or minimization (Taves 1974) approach uses the covariate stream and a measure of covariate imbalance to determine

**TABLE 13.1**

**Permuted Blocks Example**

| Block | Randomization Assignments | | | |
|-------|---|---|---|---|
| 1 | A | A | B | B |
| 2 | A | B | A | B |
| 3 | A | B | B | A |
| 4 | B | A | B | A |
| 5 | B | A | A | B |
| 6 | B | B | A | A |

Assume 100 patients are to be randomized to two arms, designated A and B, using block size of 4. There are six potential blocks. One can generate a list of assignments by randomly sampling with replacement 25 times from these 6 blocks, and then assign patients to treatment in the order generated.

treatment assignment. Imbalance is defined as a function of the treatment imbalance for each covariate of interest, weighted by a measure of the importance of the covariate, if desired. If $A_{ij}$ and $B_{ij}$ represent the number of individuals currently assigned to arm $A$ and $B$, respectively, for the $j$th value of covariate $i$, then a typical measure of imbalance would be $\Delta = \Sigma$ abs$(A_{ij} - B_{ij})$, where the sum is over all $i$ and $j$ values. To emphasize balance for selected covariates, weights ($w_{ij}$) can be assigned to these covariates and incorporated into the measure of imbalance, as given by $\Delta = \Sigma w_{ij}$ abs$(A_{ij} - B_{ij})$. This function measure may be generalized to ensure balance within strata by summing the absolute differences between arms within combinations of covariates.

In adaptive randomizations, treatment arms are usually assigned at random with equal probability when there is perfect balance ($\Delta = 0$). When there is imbalance ($\Delta > 0$), minimization automatically assigns the next patient to the arm that minimizes $\Delta$. In many circumstances, then, minimization may not truly randomize. To introduce a stochastic component, Pocock and Simon (1975) proposed the biased coin design, where the next patient is randomized to the arm that minimizes $\Delta$ with probability greater than 0.5. Our simulations used the SWOG standard probability of 0.75. Figure 13.1 illustrates how the next assignment would be determined when balance on two covariates, in this case age and sex, is of interest. Here, the algorithm is designed to ensure approximately the same proportions of males and females on each arm and the same age distribution on each arm, but it does not assure balance between arms within each age by sex combination.

### 13.2.3 STRATIFIED RANDOMIZATION

For a stratified randomization, the intent is to assure balance in treatment arm assignments within each cell defined by the covariates. We evaluated the stratified

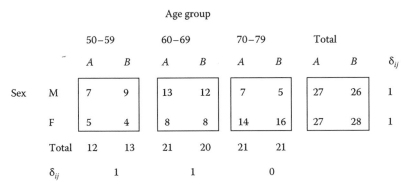

| | | Age group | | | | | | | | |
|---|---|---|---|---|---|---|---|---|---|---|
| | | 50–59 | | 60–69 | | 70–79 | | Total | | |
| | | A | B | A | B | A | B | A | B | $\delta_{ij}$ |
| Sex | M | 7 | 9 | 13 | 12 | 7 | 5 | 27 | 26 | 1 |
| | F | 5 | 4 | 8 | 8 | 14 | 16 | 27 | 28 | 1 |
| | Total | 12 | 13 | 21 | 20 | 21 | 21 | | | |
| | $\delta_{ij}$ | | 1 | | 1 | | 0 | | | |

**FIGURE 13.1**  Example of an adaptive randomization. Assume there are two treatment arms ($A,B$) and two stratification factors: Age (50–59, 60–69, 70–79) and Sex (M,F) of equal importance. For each possible value $j$ of covariate $i$, let $\delta_{ij}=abs(A_{ij} - B_{ij})$, the absolute value of the difference in the numbers currently assigned to $A$ and $B$ among patients with covariate $i$ value $j$. Then define the measure of total imbalance to be $\Delta=\Sigma\delta_{ij}$. If the current allocation by age and sex is given as shown, then the present value of $\Delta=4$. If the next patient is a male, age 60–69, the only $\delta$ values that would change are those for males and for 60–69 year olds. Assignment to $A$ would result in $\Delta=6$ whereas assignment to $B$ would result in $\Delta=2$. Under minimization, this patient would be assigned to arm $B$. Under a PS approach, this assignment would be made with probability 0.75. If the next patient is a female, age 50–59, assignment to $A$ or $B$ would result in $\Delta=2$ and $\Delta=6$, respectively. Again minimization would automatically assign this patient to arm $A$; PS would assign arm $A$ with probability 0.75.

block (SB) algorithm that applies PB within each stratum. This approach is easy to implement and common in multicenter studies where blocking within centers is recommended whenever sample size per center permits. Under well-controlled conditions, such as animal and agricultural studies, where the covariate distribution may be under the control of the researcher, this approach best assures balance on the design covariates. In clinical trials, where the distribution of covariates is unpredictable, balance within a block may not be achieved because the final block is incomplete.

## 13.3  BASIS FOR INFERENCE

Randomized experiments afford two options for interpreting results: randomization tests or population models. While randomization tests are free from assumptions about the sampling frame, they lack some appeal in that, strictly speaking, the conclusions have narrow applicability. If one were to use a randomization test as the basis for inference in a randomized clinical trial, there is a general agreement that the structure of the allocation scheme must be incorporated in the analysis to preserve power. The implementation of this is straightforward for PB and SB randomizations. The observed test statistic is compared to the distribution of test statistics obtained from a large number of simulations where each simulation merely generates a new sequence of PB under the original randomization structure. For nondeterministic adaptive designs, randomization tests can be similarly obtained through simulation by conditioning on the covariate stream and generating a new assignment with appropriate probability at each point of imbalance. We are not aware of anyone who has used this in published applications, however. For minimization designs, where a large fraction of the assignments are dictated by the preceding assignments and the cumulative covariate history, the proper specification of a randomization test is not clear.

Inference based on population models assumes that the sample under test is representative of a larger population to which the results apply. This assumption does not strictly hold for most clinical trials in the sense that the study population represents volunteers rather than a probability sample. Nevertheless, this approach is simpler to implement in that it allows us to rely on usual distribution theory for test statistics. Issues of generalizability are typically dealt with in the interpretation of results by considering eligibility and actual study subject characteristics. Because of its popularity, we evaluated this approach to inference.

## 13.4 ANALYTIC APPROACHES

Analyses of survival data from clinical trials are typically based on either unstratified or stratified logrank tests or on a test for the treatment assignment variable from a Cox proportional hazards regression model (Cox 1972). Each of these can be developed in the context of a Cox model given by $h(t;x,z) = h_0(t;z_2) \exp(\beta x + \alpha z_1)$, where $t$ is time from randomization, $x$ represents a binary treatment assignment variable, $z = (z_1, z_2)$ is a vector of covariates where $z_1$ corresponds to those covariates used in the regression function, $z_2$ covariates used for model stratification and $h_0(t;z_2)$ is the baseline hazard function for $z_2$.

The logrank test, a commonly employed test statistic for comparing survival curves, can be obtained from a Cox model as a maximum partial likelihood score test for $\beta = 0$ in a model were no other covariates are included (Kalbfleisch and Prentice 2002). The natural generalization to accommodate covariate information is the analogous score statistic in a Cox model where covariates are used as regressors in the model with a single baseline hazard function $h_0$. This model is of particular interest for the covariate adaptive randomization schemes because it uses the covariate information in the same manner—controlling for their main effects. A fully stratified logrank test or generalized score statistic can be computed in a similar fashion, where each stratum has a separate baseline hazard function.

## 13.5 DESIGN OF SIMULATION STUDIES

We evaluated the impact of randomization strategies on the size and power of these analytic strategies in simulated clinical trials using both purely hypothetical trial scenarios as well as several derived from completed SWOG trials.

For each hypothetical trial, the basic setting was a two-arm trial with 400 patients, 200 per arm. The underlying survival models were derived from Cox models assuming the existence of up to three binary covariates using the hazard models

$$h(t;x,z) = h_0(t) \exp(\beta x) \tag{A}$$

$$h(t; x, z) = h_0(t) \exp(\beta x + \alpha_1 z_1 + \alpha_2 z_2 + \alpha_3 z_3) \tag{B}$$

$$h(t; x, z) = h_0(t; z) \exp(\beta x_1) \tag{C}$$

where $h_0(t)$ is the hazard function from the exponential distribution for models $A$ and $B$. For all models, $x = 0$, 1 represents the randomization assignment and $z$ is the vector of binary covariates that jointly define membership into eight strata. For model $C$, with nonproportional covariate effects, the eight baseline hazard functions $h_0(t; z_1, z_2, z_3)$ were generated from Weibull $(\lambda_j, \kappa_j)$ distribution functions where $\lambda_j$ and $\kappa_j$ are the scale and shape parameters for stratum $j$, $j = 1, \ldots, 8$. The Weibull family of distributions was chosen because of the degree of flexibility it allows in describing nonproportional hazard functions. Values of $(\lambda_j, \kappa_j)$ used were (0.2, 0.7), (0.2, 0.8), (0.6, 1), (0.1, 1.2), (0.2, 1.5), (0.5, 2), and (0.2, 3). Note that for $\kappa_j = 1$, the Weibull model reduces to the exponential $(\lambda_j)$ distribution (constant hazard), and all covariate effects are proportional. When $\kappa > 1$ $(\kappa < 1)$, the baseline hazard functions are decreasing (increasing) with time. Hazard functions associated with a covariate will be nonproportional when values of $\kappa_j$ differ across levels of the covariates. Moderate covariate effects were defined as $\alpha_1 = \ln(0.33)$, $\alpha_2 = \ln(1.5)$, and $\alpha_3 = \ln(2.0)$. Larger covariate effects used hazard ratios of $\alpha_1 = \ln(0.2)$, $\alpha_2 = \ln(3)$, and $\alpha_3 = \ln(4)$. To examine the setting of highly stratified allocation, model $B$ was expanded to include five independent binary covariates (32 strata) with coefficients in the data generating model of $\ln(0.33)$, $\ln(1.5)$, $\ln(2)$, $\ln(0.67)$, and $\ln(1.5)$.

For each simulated trial, patient level covariates were generated with all combinations having equal probability. Two potential survival times were generated for each patient, one associated with each potential treatment assignment. Censoring times and the corresponding order of patient presentation were randomly generated from a uniform distribution to represent constant accrual over a designated interval. The two corresponding censored survival times and indicators were determined by comparing the survival times associated with each potential treatment assignment and the censoring time for each patient.

Three treatment allocation rules (PB, PS, and SB) were applied to this same patient dataset to simulate three trials in the same set of patients. As each patient in a trial was randomized, the appropriate censored survival time and indicator was selected from the source dataset to form the simulated trial data. All the test statistics (logrank, Cox regression, and stratified logrank) were then calculated for that trial. For each configuration, 5000 trials were simulated. Performance of each test statistic was assessed by calculating the proportion of test statistics exceeding 1.96, corresponding to a one-sided, 0.025-level test, to estimate size (under $\beta = 0$) and power (under the alternative $\beta = \beta_A$).

We conducted a similar set of simulations motivated by five completed SWOG trials known by protocol numbers SWOG-8516, SWOG-8501, SWOG-9210, SWOG-9308, and SWOG-8738 (Fisher et al. 1993, Gandara et al. 1993, Albert et al. 1996, Wozniak et al. 1998, Berenson et al. 2001). Key features of these trials extracted for the simulations are shown in Table 13.2. The number of design strata in these studies ranged from 4 to 38. For each stratum $j$ where sample size permitted, we estimated

**TABLE 13.2**

**Selected Parameters from Five SWOG Studies Used as the Basis for Simulation Studies**

| Protocol | Cancer Site | $N$ | No. of Covariates[a] | Strata | Weibull Parameter $(\lambda, \kappa)$ |
|---|---|---|---|---|---|
| 8516 | Non-Hodgkin's lymphoma | 435 | 5/3 | 38 | 27 cells with (0.185 and 0.845), 11 remaining cells have $\lambda = (0.205, 0.125, 0.097, 0.118, 0.070, 0.207, 0.570, 0.155, 0.096, 0.222,$ and $0.171)$ $\kappa = (1.46, 0.915, 0.865, 1.38, 0.796, 0.615, 0.840, 0.573, 0.566, 0.652,$ and $0.637)$ |
| 8501 | Ovary | 546 | 4/2 | 29 | 20 cells with (0.192 and 1.231), 9 remaining cells with $\lambda = (0.110, 0.182, 0.267, 0.191, 0.284, 0.168, 0.070, 0.208,$ and $0.255)$ $\kappa = (0.943, 1.239, 1.366, 1.218, 1.38, 1.256, 0.89, 1.506,$ and $1.283)$ |
| 9210 | Multiple myeloma | 247 | 2/0 | 6 | $\lambda = (0.309, 0.309, 0.286, 0.262, 0.343,$ and $0.344)$ $\kappa = (1.30, 1.30, 1.33, 1.148, 1.454,$ and $1.268)$ |
| 9308 | Non-small cell lung | 414 | 2/2 | 4 | $\lambda = (1.029, 0.605, 1.643,$ and $1.092)$ $\kappa = (1.213, 1.209, 1.031,$ and $1.151)$ |
| 8738 | Non-small cell lung | 356 | 2/2 | 6 | $\lambda = (1.079, 2.248, 0.914, 1.379, 1.737,$ and $1.471)$ $\kappa = (1.086, 1.55, 0.903, 0.922, 1.483,$ and $1.19)$ |

[a] Number of covariates used in the randomization scheme/number found to be significant $(p < 0.05)$ in a Cox proportional hazards model analysis.

the scale and shape parameters of a censored Weibull $(\lambda_j, \kappa_j)$ distribution. These Weibull hazard functions then formed the basis of the survival times for patients generated under model $C$.

SWOG trial-based simulations were conducted using the same general plan described for the hypothetical trials while preserving as much of the underlying data structures of the original trials as possible. The sample size $(N)$ was the same as the original trial and covariates for the $N$ patients were obtained by sampling with replacement from the observed covariate vectors. The simulated treatment effect $\beta_A$ was calculated separately for each trial to provide approximately 80% power for a one-sided 0.025-level test: $\ln(1.4)$ for SWOG-8516 and SWOG-8501; $\ln(1.65)$ for SWOG-9210; $\ln(1.4)$ for SWOG-9308; and $\ln(1.6)$ for SWOG-8738. Censoring was chosen to be uniform over an interval that varied between studies, yielding 15%–60% censoring, depending on the survival distributions. Results are summarized with estimated size and power, as described earlier.

## 13.6   RESULTS

In the hypothetical trials, all combinations of randomization schemes and test statistics provided statistically valid tests. The estimated size was never significantly above the nominal 0.025 level (Table 13.3), even in the settings where some of the underlying assumptions were violated (i.e., nonproportional covariate effects). Evidence of conservatism in the logrank statistics is seen under randomization schemes that use covariate information, however. In each scenario, where covariates were predictive of survival, the trials that used either covariate information in the design (PS or SB) show estimated type I error rates less than 0.025 and in some cases as low as 0.005.

**TABLE 13.3**

**Estimated Size and Power[a] for Three Randomization Strategies and Three Analytic Approaches Based on 5000 Simulated Trials Derived from Models *A–C***

| Model and Allocation Rule[b] | Analysis | | | | | |
|---|---|---|---|---|---|---|
| | Logrank | | Cox Model | | Stratified Logrank | |
| | Size | Power | Size | Power | Size | Power |
| **8 strata, no covariate effects** | | | | | | |
| PB | 0.023 | 0.923 | 0.026 | 0.923 | 0.026 | 0.902 |
| PS | 0.025 | 0.914 | 0.027 | 0.916 | 0.025 | 0.896 |
| SB | 0.025 | 0.920 | 0.025 | 0.918 | 0.025 | 0.912 |
| **8 strata, moderate PH covariate effects** | | | | | | |
| PB | 0.025 | 0.755 | 0.027 | 0.904 | 0.022 | 0.889 |
| PS | 0.012 | 0.790 | 0.023 | 0.908 | 0.024 | 0.890 |
| SB | 0.009 | 0.790 | 0.023 | 0.905 | 0.023 | 0.889 |
| **8 strata, large PH covariate effects** | | | | | | |
| PB | 0.025 | 0.579 | 0.025 | 0.930 | 0.026 | 0.915 |
| PS | 0.004 | 0.610 | 0.026 | 0.929 | 0.028 | 0.913 |
| SB | 0.005 | 0.584 | 0.029 | 0.926 | 0.026 | 0.926 |
| **8 strata, non-PH covariate effects** | | | | | | |
| PB | 0.027 | 0.654 | 0.026 | 0.820 | 0.024 | 0.857 |
| PS | 0.013 | 0.676 | 0.025 | 0.824 | 0.027 | 0.855 |
| SB | 0.013 | 0.697 | 0.027 | 0.841 | 0.027 | 0.874 |
| **32 strata, PH covariate effects** | | | | | | |
| PB | 0.027 | 0.764 | 0.027 | 0.905 | 0.026 | 0.825 |
| PS | 0.014 | 0.799 | 0.024 | 0.914 | 0.027 | 0.843 |
| SB | 0.015 | 0.792 | 0.027 | 0.908 | 0.026 | 0.853 |

Estimated type I error significantly less than 0.025

Estimated power significantly lower than the best performing approach

[a]   SE (estimated size) = 0.002; SE (estimated power) = 0.0055.

[b]   PB, permuted block; PS, Pocock–Simon adaptive allocation; SB, stratified permuted block.

Under the simple PB scheme, however, the size of the logrank statistic was unaffected by the presence of predictive covariates. The estimated type I error rates for the Cox model-based or stratified logrank tests appear unaffected by differences in randomization strategies.

Using covariates in the randomization appears to have a very modest effect on power throughout these simulations. Within any trial scenario and analytic approach, the differences in the estimated power between allocation strategies are less than 5% and are negligible for both the Cox model and stratified logrank tests.

The choice of analytic approach is more important. When covariates were not predictive of outcome, all tests were equally powerful. When there were predictive covariates, however, power for the Cox model and the stratified logrank test was higher than for the logrank test, regardless of whether these covariates were used in treatment allocation. With nonproportional covariate effects, the stratified logrank statistic improved power by 3% over the Cox model but in the setting of many covariates conforming to the proportional hazards assumption, the Cox model was more powerful. In all other cases examined, the Cox model and stratified logrank tests appear comparable.

Similar patterns are evident in the results simulated from the five SWOG trials (Table 13.4). The estimated size did not significantly exceed 0.025 in any of these simulated trials. In fact, the estimated type I errors observed in these simulations derived from actual trials more closely cluster around 0.025 than we observed in the hypothetical trials described earlier (Table 13.3). The estimate power for each combination of randomization scheme and test statistic yielded at most a 5% increment in power over the least favorable combination. For the majority of scenarios, the PH regression model performed slightly better than either the logrank or the stratified logrank, although the differences were generally quite small. In some settings, particularly, SWOG-8516 and SWOG-8501, there is a suggestion that the stratified logrank test does not provide as much power as the PH model based test, possibly related to the highly stratified nature of these trials.

In earlier work, we examined the effect of the number of covariates, their distribution in the study population, and the size of covariate effects on treatment effect inference (Anderson 1989). These simulations indicated that the number of covariates and their distribution have a smaller effect on the performance of these test statistics than the factors examined here. The magnitude of covariate effects was the key in determining the best analytic approach—the larger the effect, the more important it is to include that covariate in the analysis and to do so correctly.

## 13.7   DISCUSSION

The motivation behind this study was to examine the performance of various analytic strategies for clinical trials with failure time endpoints that employ randomization strategies that may or may not use important covariates. The approaches and scenarios examined via simulation were based on practical examples in which these very decisions are regularly made. Though not comprehensive in examining the many parameters that may influence the findings, these simulations provide a useful description of the magnitude of impact of the key aspects related to covariates in the design and analysis.

**TABLE 13.4**

**Estimated Size and Power[a] for Three Randomization Strategies and Three Analytic Approaches Based on 5000 Simulated Trials Derived from Five Swog Randomized Trials**

| Protocol and Allocation Rule[b] | Analysis | | | | | |
|---|---|---|---|---|---|---|
| | Logrank | | Cox Model | | Stratified Logrank | |
| | Size | Power | Size | Power | Size | Power |
| **SWOG-8516** | | | | | | |
| PB | 0.022 | 0.834 | 0.023 | 0.843 | 0.022 | 0.812 |
| PS | 0.024 | 0.835 | 0.027 | 0.850 | 0.026 | 0.816 |
| SB | 0.020 | 0.847 | 0.023 | 0.859 | 0.024 | 0.834 |
| **SWOG-8501** | | | | | | |
| PB | 0.025 | 0.836 | 0.026 | 0.841 | 0.026 | 0.821 |
| PS | 0.023 | 0.844 | 0.023 | 0.852 | 0.024 | 0.827 |
| SB | 0.027 | 0.831 | 0.027 | 0.832 | 0.027 | 0.819 |
| **SWOG-9210** | | | | | | |
| PB | 0.023 | 0.788 | 0.024 | 0.791 | 0.024 | 0.773 |
| PS | 0.021 | 0.793 | 0.021 | 0.799 | 0.022 | 0.780 |
| SB | 0.023 | 0.803 | 0.024 | 0.809 | 0.024 | 0.794 |
| **SWOG-9308** | | | | | | |
| PB | 0.019 | 0.836 | 0.024 | 0.884 | 0.022 | 0.871 |
| PS | 0.019 | 0.853 | 0.025 | 0.886 | 0.022 | 0.876 |
| SB | 0.023 | 0.843 | 0.028 | 0.886 | 0.027 | 0.875 |
| **SWOG-8738** | | | | | | |
| PB | 0.023 | 0.842 | 0.026 | 0.851 | 0.021 | 0.871 |
| PS | 0.019 | 0.843 | 0.025 | 0.860 | 0.026 | 0.878 |
| SB | 0.023 | 0.848 | 0.024 | 0.860 | 0.026 | 0.877 |

Estimated type I error significantly less than 0.025
Estimated power significantly lower than the best performing approach

[a] SE (estimated size) = 0.002; SE (estimated power) = 0.0055.

[b] PB, permuted block; PS, Pocock–Simon adaptive allocation; SB, stratified permuted block.

All combinations of randomization schemes and test statistics produced statistically valid tests but analyses that ignored predictive covariates, particularly if they were used in the design, produced smaller than expected type I error rates and significantly reduced power.

In realistic settings, the use of covariate information in treatment allocation may slightly improve power, but we found little evidence to suggest the superiority of one constrained allocation rule over another. With this knowledge, the choice of randomization scheme can be based primarily on other considerations including logistics and concern for selection bias associated with the predictability of the treatment assignment.

This work indicates that statistical power may be improved by including strongly predictive covariates in the analysis, regardless of their use in the randomization. Furthermore, there can be a substantial loss in power when highly predictive covariates were not accounted for in the analysis, consistent with previous work on omitted covariates, especially if they were used in the randomization. Where proportional hazards assumptions for the covariates are reasonable, a Cox model–based test is expected to provide better power than a stratified analysis. In most settings examined, however, there was little to distinguish these two approaches. Even when proportional hazards assumptions were known to be violated, the Cox model results were valid and nearly as powerful as the correct, stratified logrank tests.

In summary, the value of using of covariates in the randomization schemes is driven by their effect on the outcome variable. In most settings, covariate effects are relatively small, and their use in the treatment allocation or analysis will have a similarly modest effect. These simulations suggest that only when highly predictive covariates are used in the randomization but not in the analysis would we expect a marked degradation in performance (conservative type I error rates and a significant loss of power). In both the hypothetical trials and those derived from completed SWOG studies, we found that PS adaptive randomization and stratified PB schemes, paired with either tests from Cox regression models adjusting for important covariates or stratified logrank tests, provided similar operating characteristics.

## ACKNOWLEDGMENTS

This work was supported in part by grants #CA038926 and #CA90998 from the National Cancer Institute.

## REFERENCES

Alberts DS, Liu PY, Hannigan EV et al. 1996. Intraperitoneal cisplatin plus intravenous cyclophosphamide versus intravenous cisplatin plus intravenous cyclophosphamide for stage III ovarian cancer. *N Engl J Med* 335(26):1950–1955.

Anderson GL. 1989. Mismodelling covariates in Cox regression. Unpublished PhD thesis. University of Washington, Seattle, WA.

Anderson GL and Fleming TR. 1995. Model misspecification in proportional hazards regression. *Biometrika* 82(3):527–541.

Begg DB and Iglewicz B. 1980. A treatment allocation procedure for sequential clinical trials. *Biometrics* 36:81–90.

Berenson JR, Crowley JJ, Grogan TM et al. 2001. Maintenance therapy with alternate-day prednisone improves survival in multiple myeloma patients. *Blood* 99(9):3163–3168.

Berger VW, Ivanova A, and Knoll M. 2003. Minimizing predictability while retaining balance trough the use of less restrictive randomization procedures. *Stat Med* 22:3017–3028.

Box GEP, Hunter WG, and Hunter JS. 1978. *Statistics for Experimenters*. New York: Wiley.

Cox DR. 1972. Regression models and life-tables (with discussion). *J R Stat Soc B* 34:187–220.

Fisher RI, Gaynor ER, Dahlberg S et al. 1993. Comparison of a standard regimen (CHOP) with three intensive chemotherapy regimens for advanced non-Hodgkin's lymphoma. *N Engl J Med* 328:1002–1006.

Friedman LM, Furberg CD, and DeMets DL. 1981. *Fundamentals of Clinical Trials*. Boston, MA: John Wright PSG Inc., pp. 165–167.

Gail MH, Wieand S, and Piantadosi S. 1984. Biased estimates of treatment effect in randomized experiments with nonlinear regressions and omitted covariates. *Biometrika* 71:431–444.

Gandara DR, Crowley J, Livingston RB et al. 1993. Evaluation of cisplatin intensity in metastatic non-small-cell lung cancer: A phase III study of the Southwest Oncology Group. *J Clin Oncol* 11(5):873–878.

Green SB and Byar DB. 1978. The effect of stratified randomization on size and power of statistical tests in clinical trials. *J Chronic Dis* 31:445–454.

Hill AB. 1951. The clinical trial. *Br Med Bull* 7:278–282.

Hu F. and Rosenberg WF. 2006. *The Theory of Response-Adaptive Randomization in Clinical Trials*. New York: Wiley.

Kalbfleisch JD and Prentice R. 2002. *The Statistical Analysis of Failure Time Data*, 2nd edn. New York: Wiley, pp. 107–108.

Kalish LA and Begg CB. 1985. Treatment allocation methods in clinical trials: A review. *Stat Med* 4:129–144.

Lagakos SW and Schoenfeld DA. 1984. Properties of proportional-hazards score tests under misspecified regression models. *Biometrics* 40:1037–1048.

Meinert CL. 1986. *Clinical Trials: Design, Conduct and Analysis*. New York: Oxford University Press, pp. 193–195.

Peto R, Pike MC, Armitage P et al. 1976. Design and analysis of randomized clinical trials requiring prolonged observation of each patient (I). *Br J Cancer* 34:585–612.

Pocock SJ and Simon R. 1975. Sequential treatment assignment with balancing for prognostic factors in controlled clinical trials. *Biometrics* 31:103–115.

Rubin D. 1977. Estimating causal effects of treatments in randomized and nonrandomized studies. *J Educ Stat* 2:1–26.

Rubin D. 1978. Bayesian inference for causal effects: The role of randomization. *Ann Stat* 6:34–38.

Struthers CA and Kalbfleisch JD. 1986. Misspecified proportional hazards models. *Biometrika* 73:363–369.

Taves DR. 1974. Minimization: A new method of assigning patients to treatment and control groups. *Clin Pharmacol Ther* 15:443–453.

Wozniak AJ, Crowley JJ, Balcerzak SP et al. 1998. Randomized trial comparing cisplatin with cisplatin plus vinorelbine in the treatment of advanced non-small-cell lung cancer: A Southwest Oncology Group study. *J Clin Oncol* 16(7):2459–2465.

# 14 Factorial Designs with Time-to-Event Endpoints

*Stephanie Green*

## CONTENTS

## 14.1 INTRODUCTION

The frequent use of the standard two-arm randomized clinical trial is due in part to its relative simplicity of design and interpretation. Conclusions are straightforward: either the two arms are shown to be different or they are not. Complexities arise with more than two arms; with four arms, there are 6 possible pairwise comparisons, 19 ways of pooling and comparing two groups, 24 ways of ordering the arms, plus the global test of equality of all four arms. Some subset of these comparisons must be identified as of interest; each comparison has power, level, and magnitude considerations; the problems of multiple testing must be addressed; and conclusions can be difficult, particularly if the comparisons specified to be of interest turn out to be the wrong ones.

Factorial designs are sometimes considered when two or more treatments, each of which has two or more dose levels, possibly including level 0 or no treatment, are of interest alone or in combination. A factorial design assigns patients equally to each possible combination of levels of each treatment. If treatment $i$, $i = 1, \ldots K$, has $J_i$ levels, the result is a $J_1 \times J_2 \ldots \times J_K$ factorial. Generally, the aim is to study the effect of levels of each treatment separately by pooling across all other treatments. The assumption often is made that each treatment has the same effect regardless of assignment to the other treatments. Statistically, an assumption of no interaction is made.

The use of factorial designs in clinical trials has become more common, as noted in McAlister et al. (2003). Statistical papers on the topic include a theoretical discussion of factorials in the context of the proportional hazards model presented by Slud (1994). Other contributions to the topic include those by Byar (1990), who suggested potential benefit in the use of factorials for studies with low event rates such as screening studies; Simon and Freedman (1997), who discussed Bayesian design and analysis of $2 \times 2$ factorials, allowing for some uncertainty in the assumption of no interaction; Hung (1993), who discussed testing first for interaction when outcomes are normally distributed and interactions occur only if there are effects of both treatment arms; another by Hung (2000) concerning testing for unbalanced factorial clinical trials; and by Akritas and Brunner (1997), who proposed a nonparametric approach to the analysis of factorial designs with censored data making no assumptions about interaction. On the applied side, Green et al. (2002) discussed limitations of factorial designs and McAlister et al. (2003) discussed the quality of analysis and reporting in recently published factorial trials.

The multiple comparisons problem is one of the issues that must be considered in factorial designs. If tests of each treatment are performed at level $\alpha$, which is typical for factorial designs (Gail et al. 1998), then the experiment-wide level, defined as the probability that at least one comparison will be significant under the null hypothesis, is greater than $\alpha$. There is a disagreement on the issue of whether all primary questions should each be tested at level $\alpha$ or whether the experiment-wide level across all primary questions should be level $\alpha$, but clearly if the probability of at least one false-positive result is high, a single positive result from the experiment will be difficult to interpret and may well be dismissed by many as inconclusive. Starting with global testing followed by pairwise tests only if the global test is significant is a common approach to limit the probability of false-positive results. A Bonferroni approach where each of $T$ primary tests is performed at $\alpha/T$ is also an option. For comprehensive discussions of testing strategies in multiple testing settings, see Dmitrienko et al. (2010).

Power issues also must be considered. From the point of view of individual tests, power calculations are straightforward under the assumption of no interaction—calculate power according to the number of patients in the combined groups. A concern even in this ideal case may be the joint power. For instance, in a $2 \times 2$ trial of observation (O) versus treatment A versus treatment B versus the combination AB, if power to detect a specified effect of A is $1 - \beta$ and power to detect a specified effect of B is also $1 - \beta$, the joint power to detect the effects of both is closer to $1 - 2\beta$.

From the point of view of choosing the best arm, power considerations are considerably more complicated. The best arm must be specified for the possible true configurations; the procedures for designating the preferred arm at the end of the trial, which generally is the point of a clinical trial, must be specified; and the probabilities of choosing the best arm under alternatives of interest must be calculated. Various approaches can be considered in the context of a $2 \times 2$ trial. Three possibilities are considered in this chapter.

*Approach 1*

The first approach is to perform the analysis assuming there are no interactions, using two one-sided tests, A versus not-A and B versus not-B. For example, test $\alpha = 0$ and $\beta = 0$ in a two-parameter proportional hazards model $\lambda = \lambda_0 \exp(\alpha z_A + \beta z_B)$, where $\lambda$ is the survival hazard rate and $z_A$ and $z_B$ are treatment indicators. If neither test is significant, O is assumed to be the preferred arm. If A is better than not-A and B versus not-B is not significant, then A is assumed to be the preferred arm. B is assumed best if the reverse is true. If A is better than not-A and B is better than not-B, then AB is preferred.

## Approach 2

The second approach is to first perform a two-sided test for interaction using the model $\lambda = \lambda_0 \exp(\alpha z_A + \beta z_B + \gamma\, z_A z_B)$. If the interaction term $\gamma$ is not significant, then base conclusions on the tests of A versus not-A and B versus not-B as in Approach 1. If it is significant, then base conclusions on tests of the three terms in the model and on appropriate subset tests. The treatment of choice is as follows:

### Arm O if
1. $\gamma$ is not significant, A versus not-A is not significant, and B versus not-B is not significant
2. $\gamma$ is significant and negative (favorable interaction), $\alpha$ and $\beta$ are not significant in the three-parameter model, and the test of O versus AB is not significant
3. $\gamma$ is significant and positive (unfavorable interaction) and $\alpha$ and $\beta$ are not significant in the three-parameter model

### Arm AB if
1. $\gamma$ is not significant, and A versus not-A and B versus not-B are both significant
2. $\gamma$ is significant and favorable and $\alpha$ and $\beta$ are both significant in the three-parameter model
3. $\gamma$ is significant and favorable, $\alpha$ is significant and $\beta$ is not significant in the three-parameter model, and the test of A versus AB is significant
4. $\gamma$ is significant and favorable, $\beta$ is significant and $\alpha$ is not significant in the three-parameter model, and the test of B versus AB is significant
5. $\gamma$ is significant and favorable, $\alpha$ is not significant and $\beta$ is not significant in the three-parameter model, and the test of O versus AB is significant

### Arm A if
1. $\gamma$ is not significant, B versus not-B is not significant, and A versus not-A is significant
2. $\gamma$ is significant and favorable, $\alpha$ is significant and $\beta$ is not significant in the three-parameter model, and the test of A versus AB is not significant
3. $\gamma$ is significant and unfavorable, $\alpha$ is significant and $\beta$ is not significant in the three-parameter model
4. $\gamma$ is significant and unfavorable, $\alpha$ and $\beta$ are significant in the three-parameter model, and the test of A versus B is significant in favor of A

### Arm B if
1. Results are similar to A presented earlier but with the results for A and B reversed

*Arm A or Arm B if*

2. $\gamma$ is significant and unfavorable, $\alpha$ and $\beta$ are significant in the three parameter model, and the test of A versus B is not significant

*Approach 3*

The third approach is to control the overall level of the experiment by first doing an overall test of differences among the four arms, for example, the four-arm logrank test. Proceed with Approach 2 only if this test is significant. If the overall test is not significant, then arm O is concluded to be the treatment of choice.

## 14.2   SIMULATION STUDY

To illustrate the issues in factorial designs, a simulation of a $2\times2$ factorial trial will be used. The simulated trial had 125 patients per arm accrued over 3 years with 3 additional years of follow-up. Survival was exponentially distributed on each arm, and median survival was 1.5 years on the control arm. The sample size was sufficient for a one-sided 0.05 level test of A versus no-A to have power 0.9 with no effect of B, no interaction, and an A/O hazard ratio of 1/1.33. Various cases were considered using the model $\lambda = \lambda_0 \exp(\alpha z_A + \beta z_B + \gamma z_A z_B)$: neither A nor B effective ($\alpha$ and $\beta = 0$), A effective ($\alpha = -\ln(1.33)$) with no effect of B, A effective and B detrimental ($\beta = \ln(1.5)$), and both A and B effective ($\alpha$ and $\beta$ both $= -\ln(1.33)$). Each of these was considered with no interaction ($\gamma = 0$), favorable interaction (AB hazard improved compared to expected, $\gamma = -\ln(1.33)$), and unfavorable interaction (worse, $\gamma = \ln(1.33)$). For each case, 2500 realizations were used for estimating characteristics of the three approaches outlined previously. Table 14.1 summarizes the cases considered.

The possible outcomes of a trial of O versus A versus B versus AB are to recommend one of O, A, B, AB, or A or B, but not AB. Tables 14.2 through 14.4 show the simulated probabilities of making each of the conclusions in the 12 cases of

**TABLE 14.1**

**Median Survival Times from Arms** $\begin{pmatrix} 0 & A \\ B & AB \end{pmatrix}$ **Used in the Simulation**

| | | | Case | | | | | |
|---|---|---|---|---|---|---|---|---|
| | | | 2: Effect of A and No Effect of B | | 3: Effect of A and Effect of B | | 4: Effect of A and Detrimental Effect of B | |
| Interaction | 1: Null | | | | | | | |
| None | **1.5** | 1.5 | 1.5 | **2** | 1.5 | 2 | 1.5 | **2** |
| | 1.5 | 1.5 | 1.5 | 2 | 2 | **2.67** | 1 | 1.33 |
| Unfavorable | **1.5** | 1.5 | 1.5 | **2** | 1.5 | **2** | 1.5 | **2** |
| | 1.5 | 1.13 | 1.5 | 1.5 | **2** | 2 | 1 | 1 |
| Favorable | 1.5 | 1.5 | 1.5 | 1.5 | 1.5 | 2 | 1.5 | **2** |
| | 1.5 | **2** | 1.5 | **2.67** | 2 | **3.55** | 1 | 1.77 |

Each case has the median of the best arm in bold.

## TABLE 14.2
## Simulated Probability of Conclusion with
## Approach 1: No Test of Interaction

| | | | Conclusion | | |
|---|---|---|---|---|---|
| Case, Interaction | O | A | B | AB | A or B |
| 1, none | **0.890** | 0.055 | 0.053 | 0.002 | 0 |
| 1, unfavorable | **0.999** | 0.001 | 0 | 0 | 0 |
| 1, favorable | 0.311 | 0.243 | 0.259 | **0.187** | 0 |
| 2, none | 0.078 | **0.867** | 0.007 | 0.049 | 0 |
| 2, unfavorable | 0.562 | **0.437** | 0 | 0.001 | 0 |
| 2, favorable | 0.002 | 0.627 | 0.002 | **0.369** | 0 |
| 3, none | 0.010 | 0.104 | 0.095 | **0.791** | 0 |
| 3, unfavorable | 0.316 | 0.244 | 0.231 | 0.208 | **0** |
| 3, favorable | 0 | 0.009 | 0.006 | **0.985** | 0 |
| 4, none | 0.078 | **0.922** | 0 | 0 | 0 |
| 4, unfavorable | 0.578 | **0.422** | 0 | 0 | 0 |
| 4, favorable | 0.002 | **0.998** | 0 | 0 | 0 |

Each case has the median of the best arm in bold.

## TABLE 14.3
## Probability of Conclusion with Approach 2: Test of Interaction

| | | | Conclusion | | | Test for Interaction, |
|---|---|---|---|---|---|---|
| Case, Interaction | O | A | B | AB | A or B | Probability of Rejection |
| 1, none | **0.865** | 0.060 | 0.062 | 0.005 | 0.008 | 0.116 |
| 1, unfavorable | **0.914** | 0.036 | 0.033 | 0 | 0.017 | 0.467 |
| 1, favorable | 0.309 | 0.128 | 0.138 | **0.424** | 0 | 0.463 |
| 2, none | 0.086 | **0.810** | 0.006 | 0.078 | 0.019 | 0.114 |
| 2, unfavorable | 0.349 | **0.601** | 0.001 | 0.001 | 0.048 | 0.446 |
| 2, favorable | 0.003 | 0.384 | 0.002 | **0.612** | 0 | 0.426 |
| 3, none | 0.009 | 0.089 | 0.089 | **0.752** | 0.061 | 0.122 |
| 3, unfavorable | 0.185 | 0.172 | 0.167 | 0.123 | **0.353** | 0.434 |
| 3, favorable | 0 | 0.004 | 0.003 | **0.990** | 0.002 | 0.418 |
| 4, none | 0.117 | **0.883** | 0 | 0 | 0 | 0.110 |
| 4, unfavorable | 0.341 | **0.659** | 0 | 0 | 0 | 0.472 |
| 4, favorable | 0.198 | **0.756** | 0 | 0.046 | 0 | 0.441 |

Each case has the median of the best arm in bold.

TABLE 14.4

**Simulated Probability of Conclusion with Approach 3: Global Test Followed by Approach 2**

| Case, Interaction | Conclusion | | | | | Global Test, Probability of Rejection |
| | O | A | B | AB | A or B | |
|---|---|---|---|---|---|---|
| 1, none | **0.972** | 0.011 | 0.010 | 0.003 | 0.004 | 0.052 |
| 1, unfavorable | **0.926** | 0.032 | 0.026 | 0 | 0.015 | 0.578 |
| 1, favorable | 0.503 | 0.049 | 0.057 | **0.390** | 0 | 0.558 |
| 2, none | 0.329 | **0.578** | 0.001 | 0.074 | 0.018 | 0.684 |
| 2, unfavorable | 0.528 | **0.432** | 0 | 0 | 0.039 | 0.541 |
| 2, favorable | 0.014 | 0.374 | 0.001 | **0.611** | 0 | 0.987 |
| 3, none | 0.068 | 0.069 | 0.063 | **0.741** | 0.059 | 0.932 |
| 3, unfavorable | 0.466 | 0.067 | 0.072 | 0.109 | **0.286** | 0.535 |
| 3, favorable | 0 | 0.004 | 0.003 | **0.990** | 0.002 | 1.00 |
| 4, none | 0.117 | **0.882** | 0 | 0 | 0 | 0.997 |
| 4, unfavorable | 0.341 | **0.659** | 0 | 0 | 0 | 1.00 |
| 4, favorable | 0.198 | **0.756** | 0 | 0.046 | 0 | 0.999 |

Each case has the median of the best arm in bold.

Table 14.1, for the approach of ignoring interaction, for the approach of testing for interaction, and for the approach of doing a global test before testing for interaction. The global test was done at the two-sided 0.05 level. Other tests were done at the one-sided 0.05 level, with the exception of tests of A versus B and $\gamma = 0$, which were done at the two-sided 0.1 level. For each table the probability of drawing the correct conclusion is in bold.

Tables 14.2 through 14.4 illustrate several points. In the best case of using Approach 1, when in fact there is no interaction, the experiment level is 0.11, and the power when both A and B are effective is 0.79, about as anticipated and possibly insufficiently conservative. Apart from that, Approach 1 is best if there is no interaction. The probability of choosing the correct arm is reduced if Approach 2 testing first for interaction is used instead of Approach 1 in all four cases with no interaction.

If there is an interaction, Approach 2 may or may not be superior. If the interaction masks the effectiveness of the best regimen, it is better to test for interaction. See, for example, Case 4 with an unfavorable interaction, where the difference between A and not-A is diminished due to the interaction. If the interaction enhances the effectiveness of the best arm, testing is detrimental; see Case 4 with favorable interaction, where the difference between A and not-A is larger due to the interaction while B is still clearly ineffective. In all cases the power for detecting interactions is poor. Even using 0.1 level tests, the interactions were detected at most 47% of the time in these simulations.

Approach 3 does restrict the overall level, but this is at the expense of a reduced probability of choosing the correct arm when the four arms are not sufficiently different for the overall test to have high power.

Unfavorable interactions are particularly detrimental to a study. The probability of identifying the correct regimen is poor for all methods if the correct arm is not the control arm. Approach 1, assuming there is no interaction, is particularly poor.

## 14.3  EXAMPLES

### 14.3.1  Southwest Oncology Group Study 8300

As an illustration of how the use of a factorial design may compromise a study, consider Southwest Oncology Group Study 8300, which is similar to Case 4 with an unfavorable interaction, reported by Miller et al. (1998). In this study, in limited nonsmall cell lung cancer, the roles of both chemotherapy and prophylactic radiation to the brain were of interest. All 226 eligible patients received radiation to the chest and were randomized to receive prophylactic brain irradiation (PBI) versus chemotherapy versus both PBI and chemotherapy versus no additional treatment. PBI was to be tested by combining across the chemotherapy arms and chemotherapy was to be tested by combining across PBI arms. Investigators chose a Bonferroni approach to limit Type I error. The trial design specified level 0.025 for two tests, a test of whether PBI was superior to no PBI and a test of whether chemotherapy was superior to no chemotherapy. No other tests were specified. It was assumed that PBI and chemotherapy would not affect each other. Unfortunately, PBI was found to be detrimental to patient survival. Although the interaction term was not significant, the worst arm was PBI plus chemotherapy, followed by PBI, then no additional treatment, then chemotherapy alone. Using the design criteria, one would conclude that neither PBI nor chemotherapy should be used. With this outcome, however, it was clear that the comparison of no further treatment versus chemotherapy was critical, but the study had seriously inadequate power for this test, and no definitive conclusion could be made concerning chemotherapy.

### 14.3.2  North American Breast Cancer Intergroup Trial E1199

Another example is a $2 \times 2$ trial of docetaxel versus paclitaxel and weekly versus every 3 week administration as adjuvant treatment for breast cancer. Bria et al. (2006) in a letter to the editor in *Annals of Oncology* questioned whether it was reasonable to assume the effect of weekly versus every 3 week schedule would be the same for two different taxanes. They pointed to current evidence that weekly treatment might be beneficial for paclitaxel but not for docetaxel, expressed concern that ability to address each question within the trial might be compromised, and noted that preliminary results (Sparano et al. 2005) suggested the risk was real. They concluded "when planning such a trial, if a significant interaction is expected, it should be kept in mind that its occurrence could make the primary result of the trial practically useless, and the unique useful information could come from secondary, less powered analyses." In fact, as designed, the trial was negative for both of the primary comparisons, paclitaxel versus docetaxel and weekly versus every 3 weeks (Sparano et al. 2008). Unlike the previous example, however, this trial was designed to be large enough (4950 patients, 1038 events) to examine comparisons between control treatment (every 3 week paclitaxel) and the other three arms as secondary analyses. Both weekly paclitaxel and every 3 week docetaxel were observed to be beneficial with respect to disease-free survival, with weekly paclitaxel also showing a survival benefit. Significant interactions were also observed. The primary conclusion of the study was that weekly paclitaxel was beneficial. But as noted by Montgomery et al. (2003), "presentation of results should reflect the analytical strategy with an emphasis on the principal research questions." In the absence of difference in primary comparisons, secondary comparisons generally should be considered nondefinitive due to inflated Type I error. For this trial more emphasis on the planned primary comparisons might have been expected, with more cautionary interpretation of the secondary analyses. The results elicited a letter to the editor commenting that clinicians would have difficulty in drawing definitive conclusions due to the disparity of overall results with subset results (Tsubokura et al. 2008).

Once a $K \times J$ factorial study is recognized as not one $K$ arm study and one $J$ arm study that happen to be in the same patients but rather a $K \times J$ arm study with small numbers of patients per arm, the difficulties become evident. Perhaps in studies where A and B have unrelated mechanisms of action and are being used to affect different outcomes, assumptions of no biologic interaction may not be unreasonable. However, in general A cannot be assumed to behave the same way in the presence of B as in the absence of B. Potential drug interactions, overlapping toxicities, differences in compliance, and other confounding factors all make it more reasonable to assume there will be differences. Furthermore, interaction may occur simply as an artifact of the particular model chosen. In the simulation, *no interaction* meant the O/A and B/AB hazard ratios were equal. If instead, *equally effective* is defined as equal absolute increase in median, then two of the no interaction cases in Table 14.1 turn into interaction cases. There is no biologic reason that compels any particular mathematical formulation of *equally effective* to be correct. Thus, lack of biologic rationale does not necessarily provide reassurance with respect to interaction according to the model identified for analysis. Models are rarely completely correct, so statistical interactions of modest size are likely even if there is no evidence of biologic interactions.

## 14.4   OTHER APPROACHES TO MULTIARM STUDIES

Various approaches to multiarm studies are available. If the example study could be formulated as O versus A, B, and AB, as might be the case if lower doses of A and B are used for the combination, the problem of comparing control versus multiple experimental arms would apply. There is a long history of papers on this problem (e.g., Dunnet 1955, Marcus et al. 1976, Tang and Lin 1997) focusing on appropriate global tests or tests for subhypotheses. Liu and Dahlberg (1995) discussed design and provided sample size estimates based on the least favorable alternative for the global test for $K$-arm trials with time-to-event endpoints. Their procedure, a $K$-sample logrank test performed at level $\alpha$ followed by $\alpha$ level pairwise tests if the global test is significant, has good power for detecting the difference between a control arm and the best treatment. These authors emphasized the problems when power is considered in the broader sense of drawing the correct conclusions. Properties are good for this approach when each experimental arm is similar either to the control arm or the best arm, but not when survival times are more evenly spread out among the control arm and other arms.

Designs for ordered alternatives are another possibility. For example, suppose there are theoretical reasons to hypothesize superiority of A over B resulting in the alternative O<B<A<AB. Liu et al. (1998) proposed a modified logrank test for ordered alternatives,

$$T = \frac{\sum_{i=1}^{K-1} L(i)}{\left[ \sum_{i=1}^{K-1} L(i) + 2 \sum_{i<j} \left( \mathrm{cov}(L(i), L(j)) \right) \right]^{1/2}}$$

where $L(i)$ is the numerator of the one-sided logrank test between the pooled groups 1, ..., $i$ and pooled groups $i+1$, ..., $K$. This test is used as the global test before pairwise comparisons. Similar comments apply as to the more general case discussed earlier, with the additional problem that the test will not work well if the ordering is mis-specified. A related approach includes a preference ordering, say by expense of the regimens, which at least has a good chance of being specified correctly, and application of a bubble sort analysis. For example, the most costly treatment is preferred only if significantly better than the rest, the second most costly only if significantly better than the less costly arms and if the most costly is not significantly better, and so on. This approach is discussed by Chen and Simon (1994).

Any model assumption that is incorrect can result in problems. As with testing for interactions, testing any assumptions can either be beneficial or detrimental, with no way of ascertaining beforehand which is the case. If assumptions are tested, procedures must be specified for when the assumptions are shown not to be met, which changes the properties of the experiment and complicates sample size considerations. Southwest Oncology Group study S8738 (Gandara et al. 1993) provides an example of incorrect assumptions. This trial randomized patients to low-dose CDDP versus high-dose CDDP versus high-dose CDDP plus Mitomycin-C, with the obvious hypothesized ordering. The trial was closed approximately halfway through the planned accrual because survival on high-dose CDDP was convincingly shown *not* to be superior to standard dose CDDP by the hypothesized 25%. In fact, it appeared to be worse. A beneficial effect of adding Mitomycin-C to high-dose CDDP could not be ruled out at the time, but this comparison became meaningless in view of the standard-dose versus high-dose comparison.

## 14.5 CONCLUSION

The motivation for simplifying assumptions in multiarm trials is clear. The sample size required to have adequate power for multiple plausible alternatives, while at the same time limiting the overall level of the experiment, is large. If power for specific pairwise comparisons is important for any outcome, then the required sample size is larger. An even larger sample size is needed if detection of interaction is of interest.

To detect an interaction of the same magnitude as the main effects in a $2 \times 2$ trial, four times the sample size is required (Peterson and George 1993), thereby eliminating what most view as the primary advantage to factorial designs.

Likely not all simplifying assumptions are wrong, but disappointing experience tells us the risk is not negligible. Unfortunately, the reduced sample sizes resulting from oversimplification may lead to unacceptable chances of inconclusive results. The correct balance between conservative assumptions versus possible efficiencies is rarely clear. In the case of factorial designs, combining treatment arms seems to be a neat trick, yielding multiple answers for the price of one, until one starts to consider how to protect against the possibility that the assumptions underlying the trick are incorrect.

The conclusion of the Montgomery et al. (2003) paper is apt. "Difficulties in interpreting the results of factorial trials if an influential interaction is observed should be recognized as the cost of the potential for efficient, simultaneous consideration of two or more interventions ... factorial design does enable investigation of interactions in the analysis, albeit with limited power. Researchers should be aware of such issues."

## REFERENCES

Akritas, M. and Brunner, E. 1997. Nonparametric methods for factorial designs with censored data. *J. Am. Stat. Assoc.*, 92, 568–576.

Bria, E., De Maio, M., Nistico, C. et al. 2006. Factorial design for randomized clinical trials. Letter to the editor. *Ann. Oncol.*, 17, 1607–1608.

Byar, J. 1990. Factorial and reciprocal control design. *Stat. Med.*, 9, 55–64.

Chen, T. and Simon, R. 1994. Extension of one-sided test to multiple treatment trials. *Controlled Clin. Trials*, 15, 124–134.

Dmitrienko, A., Tamhane, A., and Bretz, F. eds. 2010. *Multiple Testing Problems in Pharmaceutical Statistics*. Boca Raton, FL: Chapman & Hall/CRC.

Dunnet, C. 1955. A multiple comparisons procedure for comparing several treatments with a control. *J. Am. Stat. Assoc.*, 60, 573–583.

Gail, M., You, W., Chang, Y. et al. 1998. Factorial trial of three interventions to reduce the progression of precancerous gastric lesions in Sandong, China: Design issues and initial data. *Controlled Clin. Trials*, 19, 352–369.

Gandara, D., Crowley, C., Livingston, R. et al. 1993. Evaluation of cisplatin intensity in metastatic non-small cell lung cancer: A Phase III study of the Southwest Oncology Group. *J. Clin. Oncol.*, 11, 873–887.

Green, S., Liu, P.Y., and O'Sullivan, J. 2002. Factorial design considerations. *J. Clin. Oncol.*, 20, 3424–3430.

Hung, H. 1993. Two-stage tests for studying monotherapy and combination therapy in two by two factorial trials. *Stat. Med.*, 12, 645–660.

Hung, H. 2000. Evaluation of a combination drug with multiple doses in unbalanced factorial design clinical trials. *Stat. Med.*, 19, 2079–2087.

Liu, P.Y. and Dahlberg, S. 1995. Design and analysis of multiarm clinical trials with survival endpoints. *Controlled Clin. Trials*, 16, 119–130.

Liu, P.Y., Tsai, W.Y., and Wolf, M. 1998. Design and analysis for survival data under order restrictions with a modified logrank test. *Stat. Med.*, 17, 1469–1479.

Marcus, R., Peritz, E., and Gabriel, K. 1976. On closed testing procedures with special reference to ordered analysis of variance. *Biometrika*, 63, 655–660.

McAlister, F., Straus, S., Sackett, D., and Altman, D. 2003. Analysis and reporting of factorial trials: A systematic review. *J. Am. Med. Assoc.*, 289, 2545–2553.

Miller, T., Crowley, J., Mira, J. et al. 1998. A randomized trial of chemotherapy and radiotherapy for stage III non-small cell lung cancer. *Cancer Therapeutics*, 1, 229–236.

Montgomery, A., Peters, T., and Little, P. 2003. Design, analysis and presentation of factorial randomized controlled trials. *BMC Med. Res. Methodol.*, 3, 26.

Peterson, B. and George, S. 1993. Sample size requirements and length of study for testing interaction in a $2 \times K$ factorial design when time to failure is the outcome. *Controlled Clin. Trials*, 14, 511–522.

Simon, R. and Freedman, L. 1997. Bayesian design and analysis of two $\times$ two factorial clinical trials. *Biometrics*, 53, 456–464.

Slud, E. 1994. Analysis of factorial survival experiments. *Biometrics*, 50, 25–38.

Sparano, J., Wang, M., Martino, S. et al. 2005. Phase III study of doxorubicin-cyclophosphamide followed by paclitaxel or docetaxel given every 3 weeks or weekly in patients with axillary node-positive or high-risk node-negative breast cancer: Results of North American Breast Cancer Intergroup Trial E1199. *Proceedings San Antonio Breast Cancer Symposium*, San Antonio, TX, 2005.

Sparano, J., Wang, M., Martino, S. et al. 2008. Weekly paclitaxel in the adjuvant treatment of breast cancer. *N. Engl. J. Med.*, 358: 1663–1671.

Tang, D.-I. and Lin, S. 1997. An approximate likelihood ratio test for comparing several treatments to a control. *J. Am. Stat. Assoc.*, 92, 1155–1162.

Tsubokura, M., Kami, M., and Kmatsu, T. 2008. Weekly paclitaxel in the adjuvant treatment of breast cancer. Letter to the editor. *N. Engl. J. Med.*, 359, 310.

# 15 Early Stopping of Clinical Trials

*Mary W. Redman*

## CONTENTS

## 15.1 INTRODUCTION

Monitoring of accumulating information on efficacy and toxicity data in a clinical trial is an important aspect of human subjects protection. The primary goal of monitoring a clinical trial is to protect patients while allowing sufficient information to be accumulated so that the study objectives can be addressed. Addressing study objectives may include stopping a trial as soon as there is sufficient evidence to demonstrate efficacy, harm, or even lack of benefit. The standards for these objectives may well depend on the disease setting, type of treatment, or other factors (Freidlin and Korn 2009). The objective of an interim monitoring plan is define pre-specified stopping rules that define when a study will be analyzed and under what conditions the trial will be stopped early, while controlling for the study design properties. A well-designed trial is the one in which the analyst has investigated and understands the properties of the trial design. In particular, it is important to have an understanding of when a trial may be stopped either for evidence of activity or for lack of benefit or harm.

Most treatments being developed in cancer are expected to work by acting on a biologic target: inhibiting some aspect of cell proliferation or some other mechanism within the host or tumor cell. In order for the drug to have some efficacy the patient must then have this target to inhibit, therefore this newer class of agents are called targeted agents. Patients who were once thought of as a homogenous group (e.g., a diagnosis with advanced non-small cell lung cancer with adenocarcinoma) are now being further stratified by more refined biologic markers. With the exception of a treatment with a known, validated, and reliably measured biomarker, an additional objective in drug development is to determine what patients may derive benefit or the most benefit from a drug. Therefore, it is generally expected that a clinical trial will answer a question about the experimental treatment and biomarker either as a primary objective or a secondary objective. Broadly speaking, there are four choices of clinical trial designs to address these objectives: (1) the all-comers design with secondary biomarker objectives, (2) a targeted design that restricts the patient population to "marker positive" patients, (3) a strategy design that randomizes patients to receive marker-based or non-marker-based treatments, and (4) a composite of the targeted and all-comers designs that address multiple hypotheses as co-primary objectives. As discussed by Hoering et al. (2008) and Mandrekar and Sargent (2009), the choice of a study design for evaluation of a targeted therapy with a potentially predictive biomarker depends on the specific scenario (see also Chapter 17). The objective of this chapter is to discuss considerations in the choice of an interim monitoring plan for different types of designs involving targeted therapies.

Throughout the chapter, the trial SWOG S0819 will be used to facilitate discussion of interim monitoring considerations for different trial designs. In 2009, SWOG (formally the Southwest Oncology Group) initiated a trial in first-line advanced non-small cell lung cancer to evaluate if the addition of cetuximab to chemoradiotherapy with or without bevacizumab improved progression-free survival (PFS). Support for the trial was based on two phase II trials, S0342 and S0536 (Gandara et al. 2009; Herbst et al. 2010). The first study evaluated the addition of cetuximab alone to chemoradiotherapy and the second evaluated cetuximab and bevacizumab added to chemoradiotherapy. Both of these studies met their pre-specified benchmarks indicating that cetuximab may improve PFS in this patient population. A retrospective analysis of tumor tissue in S0342 evaluated the predictive role of increased gene copy number of epidermal growth factor receptor (EGFR) measured by fluorescence in situ hybridization (FISH) (Hirsch et al. 2008). Tumors with four or more copies of the *EGFR* gene in $\geq 40\%$ of the cells (high polysomy) or tumors with *EGFR* gene amplification (gene-to-chromosome ratio $\geq 2$ or presence of gene cluster or $\geq 15$ gene copies in $\geq 10\%$ of the cells) were considered to be EGFR FISH positive, whereas all other tumors were considered to be EGFR FISH negative. This study found a near doubling of median PFS among EGFR FISH positive patients relative to EGFR FISH negative patients. Previous studies had found EGFR FISH to either be negatively prognostic or not prognostic (S0126). Therefore, in addition to evidence of improved PFS in the unselected population, based on these data, there was evidence that EGFR FISH could be a predictive biomarker for cetuximab.

While this chapter is not intended to be a comprehensive overview of group sequential designs, we now provide a brief overview of some relevant considerations.

For an extensive discussion of interim monitoring procedures and considerations, see, for example, Jennison and Turnbull (2000), Friedman et al. (1996), and Green et al. (2002).

## 15.2  INTERIM MONITORING CONSIDERATIONS

The typical goal in cancer clinical trials is to demonstrate that a regimen is either superior or equivalent (when the new regimen has other benefits such as being less toxic) to the standard of care. Therefore, the associated hypotheses are usually one-sided. Early stopping in this setting would then either be due to evidence of (1) benefit or (2) lack of benefit or harm. Throughout we will refer to the early closure of a study for evidence of benefit as stopping for efficacy and early closure due to lack of benefit or harm as stopping for futility.

### 15.2.1  INTERIM MONITORING

A test statistic commonly used to compare survival distributions is the log-rank test statistic. Under the proportional hazards assumption, the sequence of log-rank statistics is approximated by a multivariate normal and therefore group sequential procedures can be applied as developed for normally distributed data. Letting $T$ represent survival time with probability density function $f(t)$, then the survival function is defined as

$$S(t) = \Pr\{T > t\} = \int_t^\infty f(u)\,du, \quad t \geq 0,$$

and the hazard rate is

$$h(t) = \frac{f(t)}{S(t)}.$$

Letting $\lambda$ represent the hazard ratio between treatment the control arm $C$ and the experimental treatment arm $E$ and defining $\theta = \log(\lambda)$, then testing $\lambda = 1$ is equivalent to testing $\theta = \log(\lambda) = 0$. For $i$ indexing the discrete event times (assuming no ties), $k = 1, \ldots, K$ indexing the analyses and letting $d_k$ denote the number of uncensored events at analysis $k$, the log-rank statistic at analysis $k$ is

$$S_k = \sum_{i=1}^{d_k} \left( \delta_{Eki} - \frac{r_{Eki}}{r_{ki}} \right).$$

Here $\delta_{Eki} = 1$ if the $i$th event occurred on the experimental arm, $r_{Eki}$ is the number of participants on the experimental treatment arm at risk just before the $i$th event, and $r_{ki}$ is the total number of participants at risk. When $\theta$ is close to zero, the variance of $S_k$, which is equal to the observed information $I_k$ can be estimated by $d/4$ and further, it has been shown that $Z_k = S_k / \sqrt{I_k}$ follows a standard normal distribution.

Interim monitoring rules in the context of one-sided hypotheses for testing $H_0: \theta = 0$ against $H_A: \theta > 0$ define rules based on pairs of constants $(a_k, b_k)$, $a_k < b_k$ for $k = 1, \ldots, K - 1$ and $a_k = b_k$ such that if $Z_k \leq a_k$ the study is stopped for futility and if $Z_k \geq b_k$ the study is stopped for efficacy, otherwise the study is continued to the next stage. While originally proposed in the context of two-sided testing, two commonly used approaches to determine the critical values $(a_k, b_k)$ were proposed by Pocock (1977) and O'Brien and Fleming (1979).

### 15.2.1.1 Stopping for Efficacy

The approach of Pocock is to determine the critical value $b_k = C_p(K, \alpha)$ for all $k = 1, \ldots, K$ that preserves the overall type I error rate at $\alpha$, spending equal amounts of error across all analysis times, including the final analysis. The approach of O'Brien-Fleming (OBF) is to determine the critical value $b_k = C_B(K, \alpha)\sqrt{K/k}$ for all $k = 1, \ldots, K$, which also preserves type I error rates. Since the boundaries for OBF are a function of the percentage of information, relative to the Pocock boundaries, the OBF boundaries are quite conservative at earlier time points (less information) and become increasingly more aggressive with more information. There are numerous other approaches to determining the boundaries for group sequential testing. One other approach regularly used by SWOG is a modified Haybittle-Peto approach (Haybittle 1971). This approach is similar to the Pocock bounds in that for $k = 1, \ldots, K - 1$ the same critical value is used; however, the critical value at the final analysis is different. The bounds are specified on the fixed sample $p$-value scale by testing the null hypothesis at level $\alpha/10$ and then the final analysis is tested conservatively at $\alpha - K \times (\alpha/10)$. We note that the exact level can be determined exactly by simulation or in some software packages.

### 15.2.1.2 Stopping for Futility

As a result of the asymmetry of one-sided testing, formulation of the boundaries for futility testing can be specified in terms of testing the alternative hypothesis with boundaries determined to preserve the study type I and type II error rates. For testing the alternative hypothesis, the log-rank statistic is evaluated at $\theta = \delta$ and critical values are determined as for efficacy testing to spend a certain amount of error over the analysis times. The futility bound is a function of the alternative hypothesis $\delta$, the observed information $I_k$, and a critical value which now depends on both the type I error $\alpha$ and the type II error $\beta$ (Harrington et al. 1982). Specifically, the general form of the futility boundary $a_k$ is

$$a_k = \delta\sqrt{I_k} - C_k(K, \alpha, \beta), \quad k = 1, \ldots, K.$$

As before, the Pocock-style boundaries use a critical value that is constant across analysis times; the OBF-style boundaries are a function of the amount of information and are more aggressive as the study continues. The SWOG boundaries again are specified on the fixed sample $p$-value scale by testing the alternative hypothesis at level $\alpha/10$. The lower boundary is crossed in this set-up if $Z_k - \delta\sqrt{I_k}$ is less than the critical value.

An alternative to idea to specification of boundaries based on critical values as described earlier was proposed by Wieand et al. (1994). Their proposal is that once a study has reached at least 50% of the planned events, if the observed hazard ratio is greater than 1, then the study should be stopped for futility. This idea was further refined by Freidlin et al. (2010a) to provide boundaries that retain study design properties. While intuitively appealing, the simulations presented in their paper indicated that this approach was not that dissimilar from the SWOG approach, but is not as easily implemented and also results in a greater loss of power.

### 15.2.1.3  Other Considerations for Early Stopping

Emerson (2000) demonstrated that various approaches to error spending and stochastic curtailment approaches can all be mapped to each other one-to-one. Therefore, for this discussion of early stopping, the focus is on the use of error spending functions to determine the interim monitoring plan/boundaries. Clearly stopping early for evidence of benefit has an impact on the study-wide type I error rate and stopping early for evidence of no benefit or harm has an impact on the study-wide power.

Barber and Jennison (2002) demonstrated that minimizing the sample size under the null typically results in a larger sample size under the alternative (and vice versa) for asymmetric designs. It follows that designs with conservative stopping rules are closest to the fixed sample design; they spend less type I and II error at the interim analyses and therefore have smaller maximal sample sizes than designs with more aggressive stopping rules. Designs with more aggressive stopping rules are more likely to stop early for either efficacy or futility and therefore have smaller average sample sizes. However, these designs spend more type I and type II error at the interim analyses. It is possible that the associated increase in sample size to retain power may counteract the benefit to aggressive monitoring.

The timing of interim analyses in a clinical trial is usually based on the percentage of information accumulated. In cancer clinical trials, the number of events such as deaths or progression events is the typical measure of information. Protocol-specified stopping rules are defined in terms of the exact number of events. Deviations from the planned analysis schedule can have an impact on the operating characteristics of a trial. Even with careful and close monitoring of trial data, the interim analyses may not performed at precisely the protocol-specified number of events. This may be due to a variety of reasons. For example, in the cooperative group setting, cooperative groups typically have one DSMB for all studies within in the group that require monitoring. As such, these DSMBs usually have a set meeting schedule and meet for example on a biannual basis. The likelihood that accumulation of events in a study will follow the meeting schedule exactly is highly unlikely. Alternatively, an unplanned interim analysis may be called for given outside information. For example, due to safety concerns with the experimental drug arising from other studies, an unplanned interim analysis was performed in the SWOG trial S0023. This trial randomized stage III non-small cell lung cancer patients to receive either gefitinib or placebo for maintenance therapy following systemic chemotherapy. The unplanned analysis resulted in early closure of the trial (Kelly et al. 2008).

The Pocock and OBF boundaries were developed under the assumption of equal increments of information and analyses being performed exactly at the specified amounts of information. Lan and DeMets (1983) developed a method to adjust the testing thresholds to preserve the overall type I error. The SWOG boundaries do not determine the bounds based on the amount of information and use a conservatively adjusted *p*-value at the end of study and therefore does not need to be adjusted. Moreover, if the study investigators are willing to modify the maximal sample size, the design power can be maintained (Pampallona and Tsiatis 1994). These adjustments can be made to maintain the study properties accounting for both planned and unplanned analyses as long as the analyses do not depend on treatment effects at interim analyses.

Designs with multiple hypotheses have multiple groups on which to base the scheduling of interim analyses. Despite well-thought-out trial designs, it is almost a certainty that interim analyses will take place outside of the planned number of events for at least one of the groups. Therefore, the need to consider design properties resulting from analyses at non-pre-specified times may arise more often in designs with multiple hypotheses.

## 15.3 APPLICATIONS TO STUDY DESIGNS

Using the S0819 trial setting as a guide, we now evaluate and discuss the properties of different monitoring approaches for the all-comers, targeted, strategy, and multiple hypothesis designs. Design assumptions include an assumed prevalence of EGFR FISH positivity to be around 50% and the median PFS is estimated to be approximately 5–6 months. It is assumed that 80% of patients will have an EGFR FISH result and therefore 40% of the total population will be determined to be EGFR FISH positive. For designs that include the unselected population, it may be reasonable to include patients with unknown marker status. In this case, patients are classified as marker positive and marker non-positive. All designs will have 90% power for the primary hypothesis and 2.5% type I error based on one-sided testing. The target hazard ratio in the EGFR FISH positive group is a 33% improvement in median PFS. The target hazard ratio in the overall study population is a 20% improvement in median PFS. Further, accruals to the study are distributed uniformly over the accrual period, the accrual rate in the unselected population is 35 patients per month, and the follow-up time is 12 months. The interim monitoring plan considered for all designs will be interim analyses at 40%, 60%, and 80% of the expected PFS events.

### 15.3.1 Designs with a Single Hypothesis

The all-comers, targeted, and strategy designs evaluate one primary hypothesis. Referring to the motivating example S0819, the all-comers and targeted designs are based on the design assumptions stated earlier. The strategy design that would randomize patients to marker-based treatment or to receive the standard of care irrespective of marker value would then have a target hazard ratio equal to a 13% improvement in median PFS. The fixed-design sample sizes for these three designs are 1314 patients for the all-comers design, 1345 patients screened to achieve 538 marker-positive patients for the targeted design, and 2784 patients for the strategy design.

A comparison of properties of the all-comers, targeted, and strategy design for designs under the three monitoring approaches is presented in Table 15.1. While the

**TABLE 15.1**

**Properties of All-Comers, Targeted, and Strategy Designs under Pocock, OBF and SWOG Stopping Rules**

| | Study Time (If Continues to Full Accrual) | Events | Maximal Sample Size | Average Sample Size Under Null | Average Sample Size Under Alternative |
|---|---|---|---|---|---|
| | | | All-comers design: $H_a = 1.2$ | | |
| Pocock | 62 | 1678 | 1728 | 789 | 888 |
| OBF | 52 | 1333 | 1382 | 827 | 936 |
| SWOG | 51 | 1283 | 1334 | 950 | 963 |
| | | | Targeted design: $H_a = 1.33$ | | |
| Pocock | 63 | 686 | 706 | 323 | 363 |
| OBF | 53 | 545 | 566 | 338 | 382 |
| SWOG | 51 | 525 | 546 | 388 | 394 |
| | | | Strategy design: $H_a = 1.13$ | | |
| Pocock | 118 | 3627 | 3676 | 1707 | 1921 |
| OBF | 96 | 2881 | 2930 | 1787 | 2023 |
| SWOG | 93 | 2774 | 2824 | 2070 | 2083 |

sample size in the all-comers design is about 2.5 times that of the targeted design, accounting for the number needed to be screened, the two designs would take about the same amount of time to complete accrual. The ratio of the maximal and average sample sizes under the null and alternative hypotheses for the three monitoring approaches is constant across all scenarios. The strategy design requires approximately twice as many patients as the all-comers design and would take at least twice as long to complete. The strategy design requires about five times the number of patients needed for the targeted design and essentially performs the same comparison. The ratios of the average sample sizes under the null and alternative hypotheses are essentially the same for the different monitoring plans indicating that the fraction of times that the studies are stopped early is essentially the same, the strategy design just would take twice as long to get to the interim analyses.

The use of the all-comers design in this setting will likely include evaluation of a biomarker and a secondary objective. An important consideration in this setting is the power to look for subgroups deriving benefit when the overall null hypothesis is true. In this case, maximizing the sample size under the null is key indicating that a monitoring plan with conservative bounds is the most appropriate. Figure 15.1 demonstrates the properties of the boundaries for the all-comers design. The boundaries presented are based on OBF, Pocock, and the standard SWOG approach. The SWOG approach is the most conservative and the Pocock approach is the most aggressive.

## 15.3.2 Designs with Multiple Hypotheses

In the context of designs for targeted therapies, multiple hypothesis designs usually involve the specification of a hypothesis in the target population defined to be

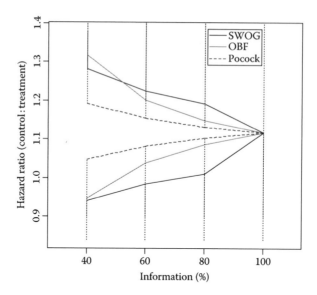

**FIGURE 15.1** A comparison of boundary shapes for the all-comers design.

biomarker-positive and in either the overall study population or in the biomarker-negative population (Chapter 17). These hypotheses are treated as "co-primary" and control the overall study false-positive rate; a fraction of the type I error is portioned to each of the hypotheses. Functionally, the study is designed around one of the hypotheses at the specified type I error rate and then the design associated with the other hypothesis is defined based on the sample size for the population associated with that hypothesis.

The specification of a design with multiple hypotheses not only has an impact on the design of the study itself, it has impact on the interim monitoring plan. No longer is there one hypothesis on which to base the monitoring plan. Decisions to stop a trial early for either efficacy or futility based on the evaluation of one hypothesis can have an impact on the ability to evaluate the other (or multiple other) hypotheses. Our primary driving framework for interim monitoring considerations for designs with multiple hypotheses is that the study design, study hypotheses, and the prioritization of the hypotheses should dictate the interim monitoring plan. Moreover, there has to be a trade-off between answering one question and answering multiple questions within the same study. Not only will the maximal sample size for these multiple hypothesis designs be larger than the standard phase III design, but the average sample size under the null and alternative hypotheses will be larger. Regular monitoring for safety and feasibility should not change significantly but the formal rules to guide under what conditions stopping the study should be considered.

We divide the scenarios for these multiple hypothesis designs into three categories: (1) subgroup-focused, (2) overall-population-focused, and (3) discrete-hypothesis designs. Subgroup-focused and overall-population-focused designs are trial designs where one of the hypotheses is nested within the other. Whereas discrete hypothesis designs are essentially parallel clinical trials with no overlap in hypotheses, subgroup-focused designs are designs where the subgroup drives the study design and is allotted the majority of the type I error. Design properties within the overall study population are based on the residual type I error to achieve the desired study type I error and the number of patients needed to be screened to achieve the number for the subgroup. Overall-population-focused designs are simply the opposite of the subgroup-focused design; the study design is based on the hypothesis within the overall study population and this hypothesis is allotted the majority of the type I error.

When deciding upon an interim monitoring plan in a study that has multiple primary objectives, all of the various scenarios should be taken into consideration. At each analysis time, one could decide to continue or stop the study in the overall study population or continue the study in one subgroup but not the other (e.g., continue in marker positive patients but stop in marker non-positive patients). Decisions regarding whether or not to continue the study in the marker non-positive group could be based on an evaluation within that subgroup or on the joint evaluation of the marker-positive group and the overall study population.

### 15.3.2.1  Subgroup-Focused Designs

In a subgroup-focused design, the hypothesis within the subgroup is the primary driver of the study design and this hypothesis is allotted the majority of the type I error. For example, Simon et al. (2005) recommend using 80% of the type I error for the subgroup hypothesis. An appropriate use of this design is when it is thought that the most likely group to benefit from the experimental regimen is the subgroup, but that it is also possible that the unselected population may also benefit from the experimental regimen, a likely scenario when the biomarker or biomarkers have not been validated.

The relationship between the subgroup-focused design versus a targeted design is depicted in Figure 15.2. In comparison to the targeted design, the subgroup-focused design requires more marker-positive patients and the analysis times are later, although these differences are very minor. The boundaries on the hazard ratio scale are essentially the same.

Therefore, in the scenario presented here, the relative cost of a subgroup-focused design to a targeted design is minimal, and the gains are that the treatment effect can be assessed in the entire study population.

The underlying implication of this study design is that the primary goal of the study is to monitor for efficacy in the subgroup. If the null hypothesis is rejected within the marker-positive group, then trial is a success and has demonstrated efficacy of the experimental regimen. However, the trade-off in this scenario is that by stopping a trial early for efficacy in the subgroup, the properties of the design in the overall study population are altered. The result of stopping a trial in the subgroup is that there is a loss of power to evaluate the hypothesis within the overall study population. Stopping the trial early can also reduce the false-positive rate within the overall study population because stopping the trial early could preempt studies that would have rejected the null hypothesis at full accrual. Additionally, if the study is stopped for efficacy in the marker positive group, a decision has to be made about whether or not to continue the trial in the marker non-positive group.

Determination of the rules for stopping a trial for futility is more complicated. In subgroup-focused designs, a clear component of futility monitoring is an evaluation

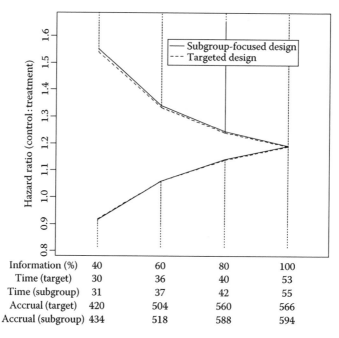

| Information (%) | 40 | 60 | 80 | 100 |
|---|---|---|---|---|
| Time (target) | 30 | 36 | 40 | 53 |
| Time (subgroup) | 31 | 37 | 42 | 55 |
| Accrual (target) | 420 | 504 | 560 | 566 |
| Accrual (subgroup) | 434 | 518 | 588 | 594 |

**FIGURE 15.2** The targeted design versus the subgroup-focused design with OBF boundaries.

within the target subgroup. However, if the biomarker or a set of biomarkers is not a predictive biomarker, then subgroup hypothesis is either not true or overly optimistic, but it is still possible that the overall study population hypothesis is true. In this scenario, one would not want the trial discontinued for lack of efficacy based on the target subgroup alone; the evaluation should also consider the overall study population. This scenario highlights that in these multiple hypothesis designs the trade-off for hedging your bets with multiple hypotheses is that more conservative stopping rules are needed to be able to address all of the trial objectives.

Futility monitoring could either occur separately within the marker positive and the marker negative groups or jointly within the marker positive group and in the overall study population. The subgroup-focused design specifies the target alternative hazard ratios for the subgroup and the overall study population. In order to define a monitoring plan for the marker negative group, the alternative hazard ratio for the negative subgroup needs to be determined based on the design hypotheses. If the data can be assumed to follow the exponential distribution, then the overall population hazard rate is simply a weighted average of the hazard rate in the marker-positive group and the marker-negative group. Moreover, if the marker is not prognostic, then the alternative hazard ratio is a weighted average of the hazard ratios for the marker positive and negative groups.

Referring to our example with EGFR FISH and cetuximab, if the objective within the EGFR FISH positive population was determined to be of greater importance than the objective within the unselected population, then a subgroup-focused design would be most appropriate. Based on the target hazard ratios for the EGFR FISH positive group and the overall study population, the associated alternative hypothesis within the EGFR FISH non-positive group is an 11% improvement in median PFS. Allocating 80% of the type I error to the subgroup results in a design with one-sided 0.02 type I error for the subgroup hypothesis. The residual type I error is conservatively 0.005; however, as the hypotheses are nested, the exact level can be determined to be greater than this level. Using simulations the exact residual type I error for this study was to use a one-sided $p$-value equal to 0.008 in the overall study population to achieve an overall study type I error rate of 2.5%. The sample size for this subgroup-focused design is a target accrual of 1440 patients needed to achieve 572 EGFR FISH positive patients. The power within the overall study population to detect a 20% improvement in median PFS is 83%.

Using the standard SWOG approach to interim monitoring, Figure 15.3 depicts stopping boundaries for the EGFR FISH positive group, the overall study population and the EGFR FISH non-positive group at 40%, 60% and 80% of PFS events. Futility boundaries for bounds based on monitoring the overall study (gray line) and the EGFR FISH non-positive group (dashed line) are presented. Boundaries in the EGFR FISH non-positive group are based on testing the alternative at the same level as the EGFR FISH positive group (overall level = 0.02).

This Figure 15.3 demonstrates that the underpowered aspect of the evaluation within the non-positive group is much more conservative than using an approach that uses an evaluation within the target subgroup and the overall population to determine if the study should be stopped for futility, even though the non-positive group is tested at a higher level than the overall study population. In fact, at the earlier interim

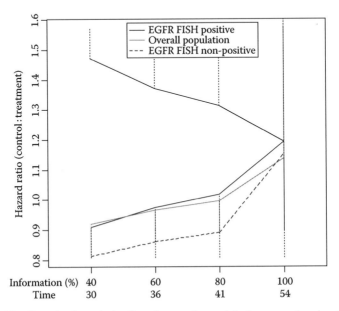

**FIGURE 15.3**  Stopping boundaries for subgroup-focused design example using the SWOG boundaries.

analyses, the futility boundary for the overall population is actually larger than that of the target subgroup due to the greater number of events in the entire study.

Given the complexity of a trial with multiple hypotheses, we recommend defining stopping rules for a limited set of conditions that are relatively conservative. In this example, the planned futility rules are to stop the trial for futility if both the alternative in the target subgroup and the overall study population are rejected. In addition, the plan includes stopping the trial for futility in the non-target subgroup if the alternative in the overall study population is rejected and the target subgroup is not rejected. This does result in a trial design with average sample size under the null that is not too dissimilar to the fixed design sample size. But again, the trade-off for complexity is conservatism, and conservatism results in a smaller maximal sample size but larger average sample size.

### 15.3.2.2  Overall-Population-Focused Designs

Designs that are overall-population-focused can be thought of as designs which add a safety net to the general all-comers design. Examples of designs which were overall population focused are the Sequential Tarceva in Unresectable NSCLC (SATURN) and INTEREST trials (Capuzzo et al. 2010; Kim et al. 2008). The INTEREST trial compared gefitinib, a tyrosine kinase inhibitor, which targets the EGFR receptor with docetaxel in previously treated non-small-cell lung cancer patients. The SATURN trial evaluated the role of erlotinib as maintenance therapy relative to no maintenance therapy (placebo) in advanced non-small-cell lung cancer patients. The biomarker used in the INTEREST trial was EGFR FISH and in the SATURN trial was EGFR measured by immunohistochemistry (IHC).

The interpretation of such a design is that the investigators believe that there is good evidence that an unselected population will benefit from the experimental regimen. However, it is possible that efficacy may be limited to a subset of the patients defined based on a biomarker or set of biomarker values. Given this set of suppositions, it makes sense that monitoring a study for early signs of efficacy would be based on the overall study population. If the null hypothesis is rejected within this population, then the trial is a success and has demonstrated the efficacy of the experimental regimen. The trade-off in this scenario is that by stopping a trial early for efficacy in the overall study population, there is a loss of power to evaluate the hypothesis within the subgroup. It is possible that the subgroup is the primary group that benefits and the rest of the patient population derives little or no benefit from the experimental drug. That said, if this is the case one hopes that the subgroup effect is so large that it is still well powered with the reduced sample size given that the trial is stopping early for large effect sizes.

Relative to the all-comers design, a consequence of smaller type I error is that the overall-population-focused design will stop less often under the null than the all-comers design. Futility monitoring in this setting is also more similar to the all-comers design except that it too is slightly more conservative than the all-comers design. A reasonable approach to futility monitoring may or may not include an evaluation of the subgroup. If the subgroup is known a priori and is evaluated, then stopping the trial for futility in the target subgroup would occur if both the overall-population and target subgroup futility boundary is crossed. If only the

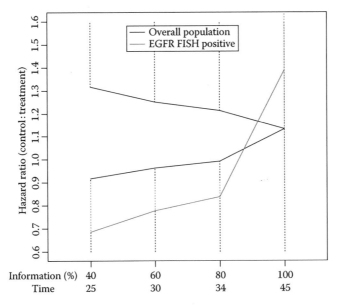

**FIGURE 15.4** Stopping boundaries for overall-population-focused design example using the SWOG boundaries.

overall-population hypothesis is rejected, it may still be of interest to continue the trial in the target subgroup alone.

Referring again to the example study S0819, an overall-population-focused design would be based on the target 20% improvement in median PFS and a type I error rate of 0.02. Under the design assumptions, the sample size is 1154 patients, 462 of them expected to be EGFR FISH positive. The split of type I error is the same for the overall-population-focused design as it was for the subgroup-focused design. Therefore, the power to detect a 33% improvement in median PFS in the EGFR FISH positive population is 38% using the 0.008 level. The stopping boundaries for this example are depicted in Figure 15.4.

As can be seen in Figure 15.4, the futility boundaries for both hypotheses are pretty conservative with stopping only for harm, and the boundaries for the EGFR FISH positive group will almost never be crossed. Any early closures for futility will almost certainly be based on the overall study population alone.

The overall-population-focused design can also be used in the situation where the biomarker or biomarker set is unknown, or where the exact threshold is unknown. For example, Freidlin and Simon (2005) proposed the adaptive signature design. This design can be used to both discover and validate a set of biomarker values that defines a subgroup most likely to benefit from treatment. Clearly, as the subgroup is not defined until the end of study, interim analyses will not include an evaluation of the subgroup.

### 15.3.2.3 Discrete Hypothesis Designs
Discrete hypothesis designs seem most appropriate when completely different hypotheses are to be evaluated within each subgroup. As the S0819 example is not appropriate

for this type of design, a different setting is used to motivate the discussion of this design. An example of a trial where the hypotheses are specified for discrete study populations is the MARVEL trial (Wakelee et al. 2008). The North Central Cancer Treatment Group initiated a trial in second-line advanced non-small cell lung cancer initiated a trial called MARVEL (marker validation for erlotinib in lung cancer). The study aimed to compare two drugs, both of which had been approved for treatment in the disease setting. This trial employed a biomarker-stratified design with separate hypotheses in each of the strata defined based on EGFR FISH status. The two hypotheses were that (1) erlotinib, an EGFR tyrosine kinase inhibitor was superior to pemetrexed, a multitargeted antifolate in patients who were EGFR FISH positive and (2) that pemetrexed was superior to erlotinib in EGFR FISH negative patients. The study was designed with 90% power to detect a 50% improvement with erlotinib in median PFS among EGFR FISH positive patients and to detect a 30% improvement with pemetrexed among EGFR FISH negative patients. They assumed that the proportion of patients determined to be EGFR FISH positive would be 30%. Interim analyses were specified to occur when 50% and 75% of the expected events had occurred within each stratum. For the purposes of this example, we assumed that the accrual rate was 15 patients per month and that the null median PFS was 3 months.

In contrast to the designs discussed earlier, the hypotheses for this trial were completely independent for the two strata; this trial design is one of two parallel phase III designs. Accordingly, the type I error levels were not split between the hypotheses. While a secondary objective was to test the interaction between EGFR FISH status and treatment effect, this objective was not the primary objective. Therefore, it makes sense that the interim analysis plan for this trial was specified separately for the two groups and any decision to stop early in one stratum would have no impact on the other stratum (Freidlin et al. 2010b). Part of this plan is an acceptance that the interim analyses may preclude the ability for the study to test the interaction (with much power). But in reality, if either group is stopped early either for efficacy or harm, the value of being able to definitely prove that the marker is prognostic is small relative to the overall benefit of determining one treatment is either more efficacious or more harmful within that subgroup.

The role of the biomarker in this trial is different from the other multiple hypothesis designs. In this setting, completely different questions are being asked of the subgroups defined by the biomarker and in fact, different monitoring approaches could be used for the studies within subgroups. In choosing the boundary shape parameters in this setting, on might want to take into consideration of the secondary objective to test the interaction and choose a more conservative monitoring plan. Table 15.2 details the trade-off between more or less aggressive monitoring and its impact on the maximal sample size and average sample sizes. As expected, the SWOG approach has the smallest maximal sample size and shortest time to study completion (if it goes to full accrual); the Pocock approach has the largest maximal sample size and longest time; and the OBF approach is in the middle. The average sample sizes for the OBF and Pocock boundaries are essentially the same under the null and the SWOG and OBF average sample sizes are essentially the same under the alternative hypothesis (Table 15.2).

**TABLE 15.2**

**Properties of the Discrete Hypothesis Design Example**

| | Study Time (If Continues to Full Accrual) | Events | Maximal Sample Size | Average Sample Size Under Null | Under Alternative |
|---|---|---|---|---|---|
| | | **FISH positive** | | | |
| Pocock | 78 | 321 | 324 | 176 | 191 |
| OBF | 67 | 267 | 272 | 174 | 195 |
| SWOG | 65 | 258 | 262 | 202 | 203 |
| | | **FISH negative** | | | |
| Pocock | 80 | 765 | 774 | 420 | 457 |
| OBF | 68 | 637 | 646 | 415 | 465 |
| SWOG | 66 | 616 | 624 | 482 | 485 |

## 15.4   DISCUSSION

In all the designs discussed in this chapter, a biomarker or set of biomarkers is evaluated either to establish eligibility to stratify for treatment assignment or to be evaluated during the course of the trial to determine subgroup membership (similar to stratify with prospective evaluation). Consideration of the operating characteristics of the interim monitoring plans is important to ensure that clinical trials, which are a huge undertaking, provide us with the necessary data to answer the pertinent scientific questions. Interim monitoring plans are best when they correspond to the setting. In particular, more complex trials designs may need less aggressive monitoring plans in order to address multiple objectives.

The evaluation of an interim monitoring plan includes the evaluation of all aspects. In settings where biomarker-driven hypothesis are primary, it is also important to monitor the study for the quality of biomarker data. Typically, the study design will specify the assumed marker prevalence, specimen submission rates, rates of adequate specimen submission, and assay failure rates. Therefore, in addition to evaluating clinical outcomes and adverse events, interim monitoring of the study should also include an evaluation of these assumptions. Incorrectly specified assumptions may require modification of screening and/or accrual targets or demonstrate a lack of feasibility to perform the biomarker-driven study. In any case, a carefully thought out plan should provide a good basis to evaluate accumulating information in a trial, with the goal to balance the risks and benefits for patients while addressing the scientific questions at hand.

## ACKNOWLEDGMENT

This work was supported in part by grants #CA038926 and #CA90998 from the National Cancer Institute.

## REFERENCES

Barber, S. and Jennison, C. 2002. Optimal asymmetric one-sided group sequential tests. *Biometrika* 89(1):1–18.

Cappuzzo, F., Ciuleanu, T., Stelmakh, L. et al. 2010. Erlotinib as maintenance treatment in advanced non-small cell lung cancer: A multicentre, randomized, placebo-controlled phase 3 study. *Lancet* 11(6):521–529.

Emerson, S.S. 2000. S+SeqTrial Technical Overview. Seattle: Insightful Corporation.

Freidlin, B. and Korn, E.L. 2009. Monitoring for lack of benefit: A critical component of a randomized clinical trial. *J. Clin. Oncol.* 27(4):629–633.

Freidlin, B., Korn, E.L., and Gray, R. 2010a. A general inefficacy interim monitoring rule for randomized clinical trials. *Clin. Trials* 7:197–208.

Freidlin, B., McShane, L.M., and Korn, E.L. 2010b. Randomized clinical trials with biomarkers: Design issues. *J. Natl Cancer Inst.* 102(3):152–160.

Freidlin, B. and Simon, R. 2005. Adaptive signature design: An adaptive clinical trial design for generating and prospectively testing a gene expression signature for sensitive patients. *Clin. Cancer Res.* 11(21):7872–7878.

Friedman, L.M., Furberg, C.D., and DeMets, D.L. 1996. *Fundamentals of Clinical Trials.* St. Louis, MO: Mosby.

Gandara, D.R., Kim, E.S., Herbst, R.S. et al. 2009. S0536: Carboplatin, paclitaxel, cetuximab, and bevacizumab followed by cetuximab and bevacizumab maintenance in advanced non-small cell lung cancer (NSCLC): A SWOG phase II study. *J. Clin. Oncol.* 27 (Suppl 15; abst 8015):A-11076.

Green, S., Benedetti, J., and Crowley, J. 2002. *Clinical Trials in Oncology*, 2nd edn. London, U.K.: Chapman & Hall.

Harrington, D., Fleming, T., and Green, S. 1982. Procedures for serial testing in censored survival data. In *Survival Analysis*, Eds. J. Crowley and R.A. Johnson, pp. 269–86. Hayward, CA: Institute of Mathematical Statistics.

Haybittle, J.L. 1971. Repeated assessments of results in clinical trials of cancer treatment. *Br. J. Radiol.* 44:793–797.

Herbst, R.S., Kelly, K., Chansky, K. et al. 2010. Phase II selection design of concurrent chemotherapy and cetuximab versus chemotherapy followed by cetuximab in advanced-stage non-small-cell lung cancer: Southwest Oncology Group study S0342. *J. Clin. Oncol.* 28(31):4747–4754.

Hirsch, F.R., Herbst, R.S., Olsen, C. et al. 2008. Increased EGFR gene copy number detected by fluorescent in situ hybridization predicts outcome in non-small cell lung cancer patients treated with cetuximab and chemotherapy. *J. Clin. Oncol.* 26(20):3351–3357.

Hoering, A., LeBlanc, M., and Crowley, J.J. 2008. Randomized phase III clinical trial designs for targeted agents. *Clin. Cancer Res.* 14:4358–4367.

Jennison, C. and Turnbull, B.W. 2000. *Group Sequential Methods with Applications to Clinical Trials.* Boca Raton, FL: Chapman & Hall/CRC.

Kelly, K., Chansky, K., and Gaspar, L.E. 2008. Phase III trial of maintenance gefitinib or placebo after concurrent chemoradiotherapy and docetaxel consolidation in inoperable stage III non-small-cell lung cancer: SWOG S0023. *J. Clin. Oncol.* 26(15):2450–2456.

Kim, E.S., Hirsch, V., Mok, T. et al. 2008. Gefitinib versus docetaxel in previously treated non-small-cell lung cancer (INTEREST): A randomized phase III trial. *Lancet* 372(9652):1809–1818.

Lan, K.K.G. and DeMets, D.L. 1983. Discrete sequential boundaries for clinical trials. *Biometrika* 70(3):659–663.

Mandrekar, S.J. and Sargent, D.J. 2009. Clinical trial designs for predictive biomarker validation: One size does not fit all. *J. Biopharm. Stat.* 19(3):530–542.

O'Brien, P.C. and Fleming, T.R. 1979. A multiple testing procedure for clinical trials. *Biometrics* 35:549–556.

Pampallona, S. and Tsiastis, A.A. 1994. Group sequential designs for one-sided and two-sided hypothesis testing with provision for early stopping in favor of the null hypothesis. *J. Stat. Plann. Infer.* 42:19–35.

Pocock, S.J. 1977. Group sequential methods in the design and analysis of clinical trials. *Biometrika* 64:191–199.

Wakelee, H., Kernstine, K., Vokes, E. et al. 2008. Cooperative group research efforts in lung cancer 2008: Focus on advanced-stage non-small-cell lung cancer. *Clin. Lung Cancer* 9(6):346–351.

Wieand, S., Schroeder, G., and O'Fallon, J.R. 1994. Stopping when the experimental regimen does not appear to help. *Stat. Med.* 13:1453–1458.

# 16 Noninferiority Trials

## Kenneth J. Kopecky and Stephanie Green

## CONTENTS

## 16.1 INTRODUCTION

Phase III therapeutic trials in oncology are conducted to compare the effectiveness of treatment regimens. In most settings, an accepted standard therapy exists and the motivation is the hope that a new treatment regimen ($E$) will prove to be superior to the standard therapy ($S$) in some respect, for example, survival or response rate. Such trials are called "superiority trials." Let $\rho(X,Y)$ denote a parameter that characterizes the difference between outcomes with treatments $X$ and $Y$. Without loss of generality, we assume that $\rho(E,S)$ is parameterized so that $\rho(E,S)=0$ if $E$ and $S$ are equally effective and $\rho(E,S)>0$ if $E$ is superior to $S$. For example, for comparisons of response rates, $\rho(E,S)$ might be rate difference $P_E-P_S$ or the log odds ratio $\ln\{P_E(1-P_S)/[P_S(1-P_E)]\}$, where $P_X$ denotes the response rate for arm $X=S$ or $E$. Similarly $\rho(E,S)$ might be the log hazard ratio for $S$ relative to $E$ in comparing censored outcomes such as overall or progression-free survival, or $\rho(E,S)$ might be the difference in mean values of a continuous outcome variable measured without censoring, such as a quantitative measure of molecular response. In the hypothesis testing context, a superiority trial tests the null hypothesis $H_0:\rho(E,S)\leq0$ against the one-sided alternative $H_A:\rho(E,S)>0$.

In some circumstances, however, a trial is motivated by the hope that $E$ is nearly as effective as $S$ in some respect. In cancer trials, such studies can be of particular interest since many treatment regimens have significant detrimental consequences, for example, severe and even life-threatening toxicity, high cost, or inconvenience or difficulty of administration that reduces adherence to the regimen. A new regimen that is less toxic, expensive, or difficult but nearly as effective as the standard regimen may therefore be the preferred treatment approach. Trials in this setting can be classified as either equivalence trials or noninferiority trials.

The term "equivalence trial" has generally come to refer to trials for which the hypothesis of interest is that results with $E$ are similar to $S$, that is, neither better nor worse beyond reasonable limits. In general, such trials are of little value for studies of the effectiveness of new treatments, since there would be little reason to reject $E$ if it proved significantly more effective than $S$. Equivalence trials will not be discussed in this chapter.

Noninferiority trials, in contrast, are inherently one-sided. The hypothesis of interest is that $E$ is, at worst, inferior to $S$ by a defined margin. In the hypothesis testing context, the null hypothesis for a noninferiority trial is therefore $H_0:\rho(E,S)\leq M$ against the one-sided alternative $H_A:\rho(E,S)>M$ where $M<0$ is the allowable margin of inferiority, that is, the maximum loss of effectiveness that is considered acceptable. $M$, referred to herein as the noninferiority margin, is sometimes called the equivalence limit or irrelevant difference (Wiens 2002, Lange and Freitag 2005).

Recent years have seen a great deal of research into the methods for designing, analyzing, and interpreting noninferiority trials; see, for example, the January 30, 2003 issue of *Statistics in Medicine* (volume 22, number 2), the December, 2004 issue of the *Journal of Biopharmaceutical Statistics* (volume 14, number 2), and the February 15, 2005 issue of *Biometric Journal* (volume 47, number 1). Standards for reporting results of noninferiority trials have been established (Piaggio et al. 2006). In this chapter, we address some practical issues regarding noninferiority trials in the setting of cancer therapy research.

## 16.2 HYPOTHESIS TESTS AND CONFIDENCE INTERVALS

There are two general approaches to analyzing the results of noninferiority trials: significance testing and confidence interval (CI) estimation. The distinction between the two approaches is to some extent artificial. Although these are sometimes viewed as alternative approaches to statistical analysis, they provide complementary information and are indeed often used together. Nevertheless the design and analysis of noninferiority trials is generally presented in terms of one or the other approach.

In the hypothesis testing approach, the aim is to perform a significance test of the null hypothesis of unacceptable inferiority, $H_0:\rho(E,S)\leq M$ (recall $M<0$ is the largest allowable margin of inferiority), against the one-sided alternative $H_A:\rho(E,S)>M$. If the null hypothesis is rejected, then noninferiority is concluded. The study's statistical power is the probability of correctly rejecting the null hypothesis of unacceptable inferiority. Ordinarily the study's sample size is determined to ensure that this test has a high level of power, typically 90% or 80%, if $E$ and $S$ are indeed equally effective, that is, under the specific alternative hypothesis $H_A:\rho(E,S)=0$.

The aim of the CI approach is to calculate a lower confidence limit $\hat{\rho}^L(E, S)$ for $\rho(E,S)$. In this chapter, we assume $\hat{\rho}^L(E, S)$ is the lower limit of a two-sided

$100(1-\alpha)\%$ CI. If $M < \hat{\rho}^L(E, S)$, then the study's results are inconsistent with unacceptable inferiority, and noninferiority within the margin $M$ is concluded. If, on the other hand, $\hat{\rho}^L(E, S) \leq M$, then the possibility of unacceptable inferiority cannot be ruled out. The sample size is determined to ensure a high level of power, in other words, a high probability that $\hat{\rho}^L(E, S)$ will exceed $M$ if in fact $E$ is not inferior to $S$. As in the hypothesis testing approach, it is usually reasonable to calculate sample size under the assumption that $\rho(E,S)=0$, that is, that $E$ and $S$ are equally effective.

As is generally the case, the two approaches are closely related, for example, one can define significance tests on the basis of CIs including or excluding hypothesized values. Nevertheless the CI approach provides more information than the simple result of the hypothesis test, since it gives a range of plausible values for the treatment difference parameter $\rho(E,S)$. Therefore, the following development is based on the CI approach.

In some circumstances, it may be appropriate to test both superiority and noninferiority hypotheses in a single trial, since this allows three possibilities: rejecting the superiority null hypothesis $H_0 : \rho(E,S) \leq 0$ might suggest that $E$ should replace $S$ as the standard therapy; otherwise rejecting the noninferiority null hypothesis $H_0 : \rho(E,S) \leq M$ might support a recommendation that $E$ may be used as an alternative to $S$, while failing to reject the latter hypothesis would support a conclusion that $E$ is unacceptably inferior to $S$ and should not be used (Dunnett and Tamhane 1997, Friedlin et al. 2007). As in simple noninferiority trials without superiority testing, the general approach based on CIs can be applied to both hypotheses in this setting (Tsong and Zhang 2005).

In the following sections, sample size formulas are presented for simple noninferiority trials, without superiority testing, in which the treatments are compared with respect to a binary outcome such as response to therapy, a time-to-event outcome subject to censoring such as overall or disease-free survival, or a continuous outcome variable not subject to censoring such as a quantitative measure of response. These relatively simple models may be appropriate for noninferiority trials of cancer therapies in many if not most settings. Indeed models of such simplicity have been used to design a number of published cancer trials although, as described in the following examples, they have not always been used with sufficient attention to the selection of appropriate design specifications.

## 16.3   SAMPLE SIZE DETERMINATION

### 16.3.1   Noninferiority Trial with Binary Outcome

For a binary outcome variable such as complete response (CR), a noninferiority trial can be based on the difference in outcome probabilities: $\rho(E,S)=P_E-P_S$. The $100(1-\alpha)\%$ two-sided confidence limits for $P_E-P_S$ are given by

$$\hat{P}_E - \hat{P}_S \pm z_{\alpha/2} \sqrt{\frac{\hat{P}_E\left(1-\hat{P}_E\right)}{N_E} + \frac{\hat{P}_S\left(1-\hat{P}_S\right)}{N_S}}$$

where

$N_x$ and $\hat{P}_x$ are the number of patients and proportion of patients with the outcome, respectively, in arm $x = E$ or $S$

$z_p$ denotes the $100p$th percentile of the standard normal distribution

For a noninferiority trial comparing $E$ and $S$, one wants a high probability (power) that the lower confidence limit will be greater than the noninferiority margin $M$ if $E$ is indeed not inferior. The sample size required to ensure statistical power of $100(1 - \beta)\%$ if the true event probabilities are $P_E$ and $P_S$ may therefore be calculated using the formula

$$N = \left[ \frac{z_{\alpha/2} + z_\beta}{M + (P_E - P_S)} \right]^2 \times \left[ \frac{P_E(1 - P_E)}{K_E} + \frac{P_S(1 - P_S)}{1 - K_E} \right] \tag{16.1}$$

where

$N$ is the total number of patients
$K_E$ is the proportion randomized to $E$

Ordinarily trials are designed to have adequate power to reject inferiority if the regimens are equally effective, that is if $P_E = P_S = P$ for a value of $P$ specified by the investigators. Also for any fixed $P$, $M$, $\alpha$, and $\beta$, $N$ is minimized when $K_E = 0.5$. With these assumptions, Equation 16.1 simplifies to

$$N = 4 \times \left[ \frac{z_{\alpha/2} + z_\beta}{M} \right]^2 \times \left[ P(1 - P) \right] \tag{16.2}$$

Table 16.1 displays the numbers of patients required for various combinations of $P$, $M$, $\alpha$, and $\beta$, calculated using Equation 16.2.

Alternatively, the difference in event rates can be expressed as the log odds ratio: $\rho(E,S) = \ln\{P_E(1 - P_S)/[P_S(1 - P_E)]\}$ (Wang et al. 2002a). The estimated log odds ratio is

$$\hat{\rho}(E, S) = \ln\left( \frac{\hat{P}_E}{1 - \hat{P}_E} \right) - \ln\left( \frac{\hat{P}_S}{1 - \hat{P}_S} \right)$$

which has estimated standard error

$$\sqrt{\frac{1}{N_E \hat{P}_E \left(1 - \hat{P}_E\right)} + \frac{1}{N_S \hat{P}_S \left(1 - \hat{P}_S\right)}}$$

For inferiority margin $M$, now expressed as the log odds ratio, the sample size formula analogous to Equation 16.1 is

## TABLE 16.1

### Study Sizes Required for Noninferiority Comparison of Binary Outcome, Based on Arithmetic Difference in Outcome Probabilities

| Probability of Outcome with Standard Therapy | Noninferiority Margin M, Expressed as Additive Change in Outcome Probability | Confidence Level[a] | | | |
|---|---|---|---|---|---|
| | | 95% | | 90% | |
| | | Statistical Power | | | |
| | | 90% | 80% | 90% | 80% |
| 0.50 | −0.05 | 4204 | 3140 | 3426 | 2474 |
| | −0.10 | 1052 | 786 | 858 | 620 |
| 0.75 | −0.05 | 3154 | 2356 | 2570 | 1856 |
| | −0.10 | 790 | 590 | 644 | 464 |
| 0.90 | −0.05 | 1514 | 1132 | 1234 | 892 |
| | −0.10 | 380 | 284 | 310 | 224 |

[a] Confidence level for two-sided confidence interval.

$$N = \left[ \frac{z_{\alpha/2} + z_\beta}{M - \ln(OR)} \right]^2 \times \left[ \frac{1}{K_E P_E (1 - P_E)} + \frac{1}{(1 - K_E) P_S (1 - P_S)} \right] \qquad (16.3)$$

where $\ln(OR) = \ln[P_E/(1 - P_E)] - \ln[P_S/(1 - P_S)]$ is defined by the values of $P_E$ and $P_S$ under the alternative hypothesis. If this is chosen as the hypothesis of equivalence $(P_E = P_S = P)$ and $K_E = 0.5$, then Equation 16.3 simplifies to

$$N = 4 \times \left( \frac{z_{\alpha/2} + z_\beta}{M} \right)^2 \times \left[ \frac{1}{P(1 - P)} \right] \qquad (16.4)$$

Table 16.2 displays the numbers of patients required for selected values of $P$, $M$, $\alpha$, and $\beta$, calculated using Equation 16.4. If $P_S > 0.5$, and therefore $P > 0.5$, then for any fixed values of $M$, $\alpha$, and $\beta$, the sample size increases with increasing $P$. This occurs because the absolute difference between $P_E$ and $P_S$ corresponding to the log odds ratio $M$ decreases.

### 16.3.2 NONINFERIORITY TRIAL WITH TIME-TO-EVENT OUTCOME

For cancer clinical trials in which the outcome of interest is time until some event such as death or disease progression, it is often reasonable for sample size calculations to assume that times to events are exponentially distributed. Assume $N$ patients will accrue at a uniform rate from time 0 until $A$, and that follow-up will continue for an additional period of duration $F$, at which point observation will be censored for all patients remaining alive (censoring at time $A + F$). Assuming $E$ and $S$ are

**TABLE 16.2**

**Study Sizes Required for Noninferiority Comparison of Binary Outcome, Based on Odds Ratio**

| Probability of Outcome with Standard Therapy ($P_S$) | Noninferiority Margin, Expressed as Odds Ratio [$M$=Log Odds Ratio] ($P_E$[a]) | Confidence Level[b] | | | |
|---|---|---|---|---|---|
| | | 95% | | 90% | |
| | | Statistical Power | | | |
| | | 90% | 80% | 90% | 80% |
| 0.50 | 0.80 [−0.22] (0.44) | 3377 | 2523 | 2752 | 1987 |
| | 0.70 [−0.36] (0.41) | 1322 | 988 | 1078 | 778 |
| 0.75 | 0.80 [−0.22] (0.71) | 4502 | 3363 | 3670 | 2649 |
| | 0.70 [−0.36] (0.68) | 1763 | 1317 | 1437 | 1037 |
| 0.90 | 0.80 [−0.22] (0.88) | 9379 | 7006 | 7644 | 5519 |
| | 0.70 [−0.36] (0.86) | 3671 | 2743 | 2992 | 2160 |

[a] Event probability for arm $E$ assuming probability $P_S$ for arm $S$ and the indicated $E$:$S$ odds ratio.

[b] Confidence level for two-sided confidence interval.

exponentially distributed, the hazard rates can be parameterized as $\lambda_E = e^{\alpha}$ and $\lambda_S = e^{\alpha + \rho(E,S)}$, respectively, so that the log hazard ratio for $S$ relative to $E$, $\rho(E,S)$ is greater than 0 if $E$ is superior to $S$, and the noninferiority hypothesis is $H_0 : \rho(E,S) \leq M$ for a specified $M < 0$. For example, in Southwest Oncology Group study SWOG-8412, which compared carboplatin plus cyclophosphamide to the standard therapy of cisplatin plus cyclophosphamide with respect to overall survival of patients with stage III or IV ovarian cancer, the margin was chosen to correspond to a mortality hazard ratio ($E$ relative to $S$) of 1.3, corresponding to a noninferiority margin $M = -\ln(1.3) = -0.262$ (Alberts et al. 1992).

Letting $\rho = \rho(E,S)$, the maximum likelihood estimator of the log hazard ratio is

$$\hat{\rho} = \ln\left(\frac{d_E}{T_E}\right) - \ln\left(\frac{d_S}{T_S}\right)$$

with estimated standard error

$$SE(\hat{\rho}) = \sqrt{\frac{(d_E + d_S)}{d_E d_S}}$$

where $d_x$ and $T_x$ are the number of events and total observation time (sum of all times from study entry until observation of the event or censoring), respectively observed on arm $x = E$ or $S$. Thus the $100(1 - \alpha)\%$ confidence limits are given by

$$\hat{\rho} \pm z_{\alpha/2} \times SE(\hat{\rho})$$

The total number of patients required to ensure at least $100(1-\beta)\%$ probability that the lower limit of the two-sided $100(1-\alpha)\%$ CI will exceed $M$ when the true value of the log hazard ratio is $\rho(E,S)$ can be calculated as

$$N = \left(\frac{z_{\alpha/2} + z_{\beta}}{M - \rho(E,S)}\right)^2 \times \left[\frac{1}{K_E Q_E} + \frac{1}{(1-K_E)Q_S}\right] \qquad (16.5)$$

where
  $K_E$ is the proportion of patients randomized to $E$ and $Q_E$
  $Q_S$ are the expected proportions of patients whose deaths will be observed in the two arms

For exponentially distributed times to events,

$$Q_x = 1 - \frac{\exp(-\lambda_x F) \times \left[1 - \exp(-\lambda_x A)\right]}{\lambda_x A} \qquad (16.6)$$

for $x=E$ or $S$. Typically the study requires adequate power under the alternative hypothesis $\rho(E,S)=0$, in which case $\lambda_E=\lambda_S$, $N$ is again minimized if $K_E=0.5$ and Equation 16.5 simplifies to

$$N = \left(\frac{4}{Q_S}\right)\left(\frac{z_{\alpha/2} + z_{\beta}}{M}\right)^2 \qquad (16.7)$$

The value of $\lambda_S$, and of $\lambda_E$, if needed, can be determined from parameters of the anticipated true exponential distributions. For example, if the median event time is predicted to be $T_{0.5}$, then $\lambda_x = \ln(2)/T_{0.5}$. Note from Equation 16.6 that the required number of patients depends on the accrual and follow-up times through their ratios to the median event time, $A/T_{0.5}$ and $F/T_{0.5}$. A JavaScript program that calculates $N$ using Equation 16.5 for the alternative hypothesis that the true value of $\rho(E,S)$ is 0 and for arbitrary $Q_E$ and $Q_S$ is available at http://www.swogstat.org/stat/public/equivsurv.htm.

Table 16.3 displays examples of the sample size required for various combinations of $M$, $\alpha$, and $\beta$, calculated using Equations 16.6 and 16.7, assuming $A/T_{0.5}=4$ and $F/T_{0.5}=1$. Whether an accrual goal can be met within an accrual period depends, of course, on the accrual rate. For example, if the noninferiority margin is set at 1.10, and the study uses the two-sided 95% confidence level and requires 90% power if the true hazard ratio is 1.0, the study must accrue 5569 patients in a period that is four times the median survival time with standard therapy. If the median is 1.5 years, then an accrual rate of about 929 per year is required for 6 years. Having specified the noninferiority margin, confidence level, and power, a combination of $A$, $F$, and accrual rate, if any is indeed feasible, can be found by trial and error.

In general, increasing the duration of follow-up will not reduce the study size greatly. For example, with margin 1.10, confidence level 95%, and power 90% for true hazard ratio 1.0, increasing the follow-up from one to four times the median

**TABLE 16.3**

**Study Sizes Required for Noninferiority Comparison of Exponentially Distributed Time-To-Event Outcome, Based on Hazard Ratio**

| Noninferiority Margin, Expressed as E:S Hazard Ratio (Corresponding M) | Duration of Study Periods, Expressed as Ratios to Median Event Time with S | | Confidence Level[a] | | | |
|---|---|---|---|---|---|---|
| | | | 95% | | 90% | |
| | | | Statistical Power | | | |
| | Accrual | Follow-Up | 90% | 80% | 90% | 80% |
| 1.05 (−0.049) | 4 | 1 | 21249 | 15873 | 17319 | 12503 |
| 1.10 (−0.095) | 4 | 1 | 5569 | 4160 | 4539 | 3277 |
| 1.30 (−0.262) | 4 | 1 | 735 | 549 | 599 | 433 |

[a] Confidence level for two-sided confidence interval.

survival with standard therapy decreases the required number of patients to from 5569 to 4727. This is because the power depends heavily on $NQ_S$, the expected number of patients whose events will be observed. For the specifications in Table 16.3, $Q_S$ increases from 0.83 if $F = 1$ to 0.98 if $F = 4$, a modest increase. Note that increasing $F$ further above four would clearly yield little additional power. Shortening the accrual interval increases the necessary number of patients and consequently the required accrual rate. For example, under the same specifications that were discussed earlier, total accrual of 6343 would be required for the study to complete accrual in a period twice, rather than four times, as long as the median event time. Note that this more than doubles the required accrual rate.

The results in Table 16.3 show that the sample sizes required to demonstrate noninferiority within reasonable margins may be very large. For outcomes such as death or, for highly lethal diseases, disease progression, it may be difficult to justify a 30% or even 10% increase in mortality as an acceptable trade-off for some other benefit such as decreased toxicity or cost. Moreover, allowing a large noninferiority margin increases the risk that an apparently noninferior $E$ will not be significantly superior to no treatment. However, it may not be possible to conduct an adequately powered noninferiority trial targeting a smaller margin. The likelihood that the accrual period will need to extend for several multiples of the median time to event may render a noninferiority trial impractical. This is especially true for studies of patients with good prognosis for long median event times, a circumstance in which noninferiority questions may be most likely to arise. Shorter accrual periods may be appropriate for studies in patients with poor prognosis, however in such settings superiority trials aimed at improving treatment outcomes are likely to have much higher research priority than noninferiority trials.

## 16.3.3 Noninferiority Trial with Uncensored Continuous Outcome

In cancer trials, the primary endpoints have commonly been either binary outcomes such as CR to remission induction therapy, or time-to-event outcomes that are subject to censoring such as overall or progression-free survival. However, continuous variables that are not subject to censoring can also serve as outcomes of interest. For example, assays that produce quantitative results such as real-time polymerase chain reaction (RT-PCR) or flow cytometry might be used to measure an impact of treatment. A noninferiority trial for such an outcome might be based on the difference in mean values of a continuous outcome variable. Let $Y$ denote the outcome variable, with larger values of $Y$ corresponding to better results, and let $\mu_E = E_E Y$ and $\mu_S = E_S Y$ be the mean values of $Y$ for the experimental and standard regimens, respectively. Then a noninferiority trial might be based on the difference $\rho(E,S) = \mu_E - \mu_S$, with noninferiority margin $M < 0$ representing the absolute decrease in the mean value of $Y$ that is considered acceptable. If the variance of $Y$, $\sigma^2$, is the same for both $E$ and $S$, then under suitable regularity conditions, the asymptotic $100(1-\alpha)\%$ CI for the true difference $\mu_E - \mu_S$ is

$$\hat{\mu}_E - \hat{\mu}_S \pm s \times z_{\alpha/2} \sqrt{\frac{1}{N_E} + \frac{1}{N_S}} \qquad (16.8)$$

where
  $N_E$ and $N_S$ are the numbers of patients
  $s^2$ is the pooled estimate of the common variance $\sigma^2$

The total sample size $N = N_E + N_S$ required to ensure statistical power of $100(1-\beta)\%$ if the true event means are $\mu_E$ and $\mu_S$ may therefore be calculated using the formula

$$N = \frac{\left\{ (z_{\alpha/2} + z_\beta)\sigma/M - (\mu_E - \mu_S) \right\}^2}{\left[ K_E(1 - K_E) \right]} \qquad (16.9)$$

where $K_E$ is the proportion of patients randomized to $E$. If the goal is to ensure adequate power when $E$ and $S$ are in fact equivalent, that is, under the alternative hypothesis $\rho(E,S) = \mu_E - \mu_S = 0$, and if $K_E = 0.5$, Equation 16.9 simplifies to

$$N = 4 \times \left[ \frac{(z_{\alpha/2} + z_\beta)\sigma}{M} \right]^2 \qquad (16.10)$$

Note that $N$ is a function of $[M - (\mu_E - \mu_S)]/\sigma$ in (16.9) and simply $M/\sigma$ in (16.10). Thus $N$ depends only on $M$ measured in units of the standard deviation. For example, if $\sigma = 12$, then a noninferiority margin $M = -3$ corresponds to a decrease of 0.25 standard deviations: $M = -0.25\sigma$. Table 16.4 shows the numbers of patients required for various combinations of $M$ (expressed as a multiple of $\sigma$), $\alpha$, and $\beta$ based on Equation 16.10. Expressing the noninferiority margin as a multiple of the true standard deviation $\sigma$ may be a useful approach to defining $M$ for a given study, since it represents the loss of benefit in relation to the variability of the response variable.

  If $Y$ is positive, that is, cannot have values $\leq 0$, an alternative approach is to define a noninferiority margin for the ratio of the means, that is, $E$ is unacceptable

**TABLE 16.4**

**Study Sizes Required for Noninferiority Comparison of Uncensored Continuous Outcome, Based on Arithmetic Difference in Means**

| Noninferiority Margin, $M$, Expressed as a Multiple of the Standard Deviation $\sigma$ | Confidence Level[a] | | | |
|---|---|---|---|---|
| | 95% | | 90% | |
| | Statistical Power | | | |
| | 90% | 80% | 90% | 80% |
| $-0.10\sigma$ | 4203 | 3140 | 3426 | 2474 |
| $-0.25\sigma$ | 673 | 503 | 549 | 396 |
| $-0.50\sigma$ | 169 | 126 | 138 | 99 |

[a] Confidence level for two-sided confidence interval.

if $\mu_E/\mu_S \leq R_M < 1$ where $R_M$ is close to 1.0. Note that $100(1-R_M)\%$ corresponds to a proportional decrease in the mean of $Y$. For example, if $R_M = 0.95$, then the noninferiority margin corresponds to a 5% decrease in the mean. This may be a useful way to express the magnitude of the noninferiority margin. Laster and Johnson, noting that $\mu_E/\mu_S \leq R_M$ is equivalent to $\mu_E - R_M\mu_S \leq 0$, described testing for noninferiority by, in effect, calculating the asymptotic $100(1-\alpha)\%$ CI for $\mu_E - R_M\mu_S$:

$$\hat{\mu}_E - R_M\hat{\mu}_S \pm s \times z_{\alpha/2}\sqrt{\frac{1}{N_E} + \frac{R_M^2}{N_S}} \qquad (16.11)$$

where $s$ is the pooled estimate of the common variance as in Equation 16.8 (Laster and Johnson 2003).

If the lower confidence limit for $\mu_E - R_M\mu_S$ is greater than 0, then the null hypothesis of unacceptable inferiority can be rejected. In this approach, sometimes called "ratio-based" noninferiority testing, the total sample size to ensure $100(1-\beta)\%$ power under the alternative hypothesis of equivalence, $\mu_E/\mu_S = 1$ for a study with $N_E = N_S = N/2$ is

$$N_{RB} = 2 \times \left(1 + R_M^2\right) \times \left[\frac{(z_{\alpha/2} + z_\beta)\sigma}{\mu_S\left(1 - R_M\right)}\right]^2 \qquad (16.12)$$

Note that this ratio-based approach differs from the general formulation described earlier, in which $\rho(E,S)$ does not involve the noninferiority margin $M$, but the null hypothesis does: $\rho(E,S) \leq M$. In the ratio-based approach the measure of difference between $E$ and $S$, $\mu_E - R_M\mu_S$, includes $R_M$, a defined constant analogous to the noninferiority margin, while its value under null hypothesis does not: $\mu_E - R_M\mu_S = 0$. As a result, the power of the ratio-based test using (16.12) depends not only on $R_M$ but also on $\mu_S/\sigma$. This occurs because, under the noninferiority alternative hypothesis $\mu_E = \mu_S$, the expected value of $\hat{\mu}_E - R_M \hat{\mu}_S$ in (16.11) is $\mu_S(1 - R_M)$, while the expected value of $\hat{\mu}_E - \hat{\mu}_S$ in (16.8) is 0 for any value of $\mu_S$. However, as Laster and Johnson pointed out, for a given value of the noninferiority ratio $R_M$, the corresponding absolute noninferiority margin in (16.10) is simply $M = \mu_E - \mu_S = -\mu_S(1 - R_M)$. Substituting this expression for $M$ in (16.10), it follows that for any given $M$ and corresponding $R_M$, the ratio-based test requires fewer patients (Laster and Johnson 2003). Specifically, comparing (16.12) and (16.10), $N_{RB}/N = (1 + R_M^2)/2$. Since $R_M < 1$, $N_{RB}$ will always be less than $N$ for any $\alpha$ and $\beta$. For example, if $R_M = 0.95$, which corresponds to an absolute noninferiority margin of $M = -0.05\,\mu_S$, the ratio-based noninferiority comparison using (16.11) will require only 95.1% as many patients as the comparison based on absolute differences as in (16.8).

In general, the decision to base a trial on an absolute specification of the noninferiority margin (Equations 16.8 through 16.10), as opposed to a ratio-based specification (Equations 16.11 and 16.12) cannot be based solely on the greater efficiency (smaller sample size) of the ratio-based design. The ratio-based approach is appropriate for positive outcome variables (after reparameterization if necessary). If $\mu_E$ and $\mu_S$ have different signs, the ratio is no longer a useful characterization of noninferiority. Also the sample size formulas (16.10) and (16.12) assume that the variance of $Y$ is the same for both $E$ and $S$, which may be untrue for a positive outcome variable. Often, the variance of a positive outcome variable $Y$ is positively related to its mean. Generalizations of (16.10) allowing for the variance of $Y$ to differ between $E$ and $S$ are possible, but applying a variance-stabilizing transformation to $Y$, for example, logarithmic transformation, may be more appropriate. The transformed variable in such cases may also be more nearly symmetrically distributed than $Y$, thereby improving the accuracy of the large-sample approximations in Equations 16.8 through 16.12.

## 16.4 EXAMPLE

Two recent papers provide interesting examples of noninferiority trials (Major et al. 2001, Rosen et al. 2001). Each study compared the experimental treatment zoledronic acid ($E = Zol$) to the standard therapy, pamidronate ($S = Pam$), with respect to skeletal-related events (SREs, i.e., skeletal metastases or osteolytic lesions) in cancer patients, or hypercalcemia related to malignancy (HCM). The primary endpoints for the noninferiority comparisons were binary outcomes: avoidance of SRE (excluding HCM) during treatment and follow-up in the first trial (the "SRE trial"), and complete response (CR) of HCM in the second trial (the "HCM trial"). Since these two trials did not address the same endpoint, they cannot be compared directly. Nevertheless, they present an interesting contrast.

Both studies were designed to test noninferiority of $Zol$ by comparing the upper limit of a two-sided $100(1-\alpha)\%$ CI for the difference in event rates $(P_{Zol} - P_{Pam})$ to a specified margin $M$. For the SRE trial, the upper limit of the 90% CI for $P_{Zol} - P_{Pam}$ was required to exceed $-0.08$ in order to conclude noninferiority of $Zol$, that is, $\alpha = 0.1$ and $M = -0.08$. The trial was designed to ensure 80% power ($\beta = 0.2$) if the true probabilities were $P_{Zol}=P_{Pam}=0.5$ and therefore from Equation 16.2 required $N=968$ patients. The HCM trial was designed with very different specifications that led to a much smaller study size: the criterion for noninferiority of *Zol* required that the upper limit of the 95% CI exceed a margin of $M=-0.10$ and the trial was designed to ensure 80% power if the true event probabilities were $P_{Zol}=0.92$ and $P_{Pam}=0.90$. Consequently from Equation 16.1 the HCM trial had a goal of only $N=180$ patients.

Ordinarily noninferiority trials are designed to have adequate power to reject inferiority if the two regimens are equivalent. However, the HCM trial was designed to have adequate power if *Zol* was in fact slightly superior to *Pam*. Had the power been targeted to the conventional alternative hypothesis that *Zol* is equivalent to *Pam*, that is, $P_{Zol}=P_{Pam}=0.90$, the study would have required $N=284$ patients (Table 16.1) rather than 180. Therefore, the HCM trial was seriously underpowered and had an unacceptably high probability of failing to reject the hypothesis of *Zol*'s inferiority if it was in fact equivalent to *Pam*.

## 16.5  DETERMINING THE NONINFERIORITY MARGIN

Determining an appropriate value for the noninferiority margin $M$ requires careful clinical and statistical consideration. Wiens (2002) described general approaches for selecting noninferiority margins. One is to choose a margin small enough to ensure that if $E$ is nearly as effective as $S$, then it is reasonable to conclude that $E$ is superior to no treatment or placebo ($P$). To do this, one might try to choose a specific value of $M$, which is "close enough" to 0 to provide assurance of $E$'s benefit; this appears to be the approach taken in the two *Zol* vs. *Pam* trials described earlier. Alternatively, one may choose to define $M$ as a fraction of the benefit of $S$ compared to $P$: $M=-\varphi\rho(S,P)$ where $0<\varphi<1$. This way of defining $M$ has an appealingly intuitive interpretation: the noninferiority margin corresponds to preserving $100(1-\varphi)\%$ of the benefit of $S$ relative to $P$. Note that the latter approach corresponds to the formulation of ratio-based testing described earlier. The general problem of assessing benefits of $S$ and/ or $E$ relative to $P$ is discussed further below. In either case, this may be a useful approach when there is very strong evidence that $S$ is very effective. However, if the statistical significance or the magnitude of the benefit of $S$ is modest, then a noninfe-riority margin chosen solely by this approach may not provide the desired assurance that $E$ has some benefit.

A second approach described by Wiens is to choose a margin based solely on clinical importance, that is, a difference that is judged to be clinically unimportant. Choosing a margin in this way is clearly fraught with subjectivity and uncertainty. Nevertheless, it may be a reasonable approach when there is little information avail-able from which to predict the likely benefit of $S$ compared to $P$ in the planned trial. For example, Michallet et al. designed a noninferiority comparison of $E=$ pegylated interferon alpha-2b (rIFN-$\alpha$2b) compared to $S=$ rIFN-$\alpha$2b as therapy for chronic myelogenous leukemia (CML) in chronic phase (Michallet et al. 2004). They speci-fied a 20% decrease in the odds of major cytogenetic response (MCR) as the non-inferiority margin. Although the authors did not describe their rationale for this specification, it was perhaps justified by a combination of the two approaches mentioned earlier. In particular, regarding Wiens' first approach, it is plausible to assume that spontaneous MCR is a very unlikely event, so if $S$ is clearly beneficial relative to $P$ and the trial showed that $E$ preserved a large proportion of the benefit of $S$, then it might be reasonable to conclude that $E$ is sufficiently beneficial to replace $S$. However, the trial was unlikely to reach such a conclusion for two reasons. First, the rate of MCR with $S$ was not very high: 20% in the investigators' assumption for design purposes. Thus even if $E$ could be shown to preserve a large proportion of the benefit of $S$, it would probably remain unclear whether $E$ had sufficient benefit compared to no treatment to warrant its use. Moreover, the study as designed was badly underpowered. The sample size was calculated to ensure that the lower limit of a two-sided 95% CI for the log odds ratio had 80% probability of exceeding a noninferiority margin corresponding to an odds ratio of 0.8 if the true MCR rates were 20% with $S$ and 30% with $E$, that is, if under an alternative hypothesis that $E$ was substantially superior to $S$. Using Equation 16.3 or a similar formula, the study was designed to include 300 patients, although 344 were actually included. The trial was therefore badly underpowered: a total of 3941 patients would be required to have 80% power if $E$ and $S$ are in fact equivalent with MCR rates of 20%. As it turned out, the study failed to reject the hypothesis of inferiority. However, due to the study's low power, this result is in fact inconclusive.

The third approach described by Wiens is to select a margin that ensures the distributions of outcomes for patients on the $E$ and $S$ arms are similar in some respect other than the parameter for which they are being compared (Wiens 2002). A simple example of this is the use of the difference in rates to determine the noninferiority margin for the odds ratio in trials with binary outcome variables: the difference in rates may be more readily understood by clinicians than the odds ratio. For example, in the CML trial described earlier, the noninferiority margin corresponded to a 20% decrease in the odds of MCR, and the MCR rate was assumed to be 20% with $S$ (Michallet et al. 2004). The noninferiority margin therefore corresponds to a decrease in the MCR rate from 20% with $S$ to 17% with $E$, which is easy to interpret clinically.

## 16.6   BENEFIT OF $E$ COMPARED TO NO TREATMENT

In order for $E$ to be a suitable replacement for $S$ on the basis of noninferiority, it is important to consider not only (1) whether $E$ is nearly as effective as $S$, but also (2) whether $E$ is superior to no treatment or placebo ($P$), that is, whether $\rho(E,P) > 0$. The ideal equivalence trial would randomize to all three approaches, $P$, $S$, and $E$, provided it is ethical to randomize to $P$. This might be the case if evidence supporting $S$ is weak, such as the lower bound of CI being close to 0, uncertainty due to poorly conducted previous trials, changes over time, short-term effects, or highly variable differences in treatment effect across previous studies. Koch and Röhmel describe conduct of "gold standard" non-inferiority trials (Koch and Röhmel 2004). The experimental regimen $E$ is accepted if $E$ is significantly better than $P$ and if it is non-inferior to $S$. $S$ itself need not be significantly better than $P$. Hypotheses are ordered hierarchically. $H_{01}$:$\rho(E,P)= 0$ vs. $\rho(E,P)>0$ is tested in step one and, if rejected, $H_{02}$: $\rho(E,S)=M$ vs. $\rho(E,S)>M$ is tested in step two, each typically at the 0.025 level. If both hypotheses are rejected, the trial is concluded successful. If the trial is successful, further tests can be done to address questions about superiority of $S$ compared to $P$ and of $E$ compared to $S$ without compromising family-wise type-one error.

If a treatment of established effectiveness exists (i.e., $S$), it would be unethical to randomize patients to the nontreatment arm $P$. In this circumstance, only historical experience may be available to address (2). Therefore, the benefit of $E$ relative to $P$ must be inferred from the current trial comparing $E$ to $S$ and from whatever information is available regarding the benefit of $S$ relative to $P$. The latter inference typically relies on the assumption of some kind of "constancy condition," that is, that the benefit of $S$ compared to $P$ observed in prior studies carries over to the current noninferiority trial (Jones et al. 1996, D'Agostino et al. 2003). If the noninferiority margin is defined as a fraction of the benefit of $S$ compared to $P$, $M=-\varphi\rho(S,P)$ for a specified value of $\varphi$, then the need to infer $\rho(S,P)$ from historical experience also affects the inference regarding (1).

Some approaches to estimating or testing $\rho(E,P)$ are described briefly in the following. First, however, it is important to recognize that the validity of inferences concerning the benefit of $E$ relative to $P$ in a trial with no $P$ arm can be very sensitive to the validity of the constancy condition (Wang et al. 2002b, Hung et al. 2003, Rothman et al. 2003, Fleming 2008). Therefore, the constancy condition requires careful, critical consideration. Any number of effects may operate to violate the constancy condition: patterns of referral of patients to study centers may change, diagnostic criteria may change, or supportive care may become more effective. Moreover, variations in the design and conduct of the current and prior trials may invalidate the constancy condition: differences in eligibility criteria, response criteria, adherence to treatment regimens and follow-up requirements, subsequent "rescue" therapy for treatment failures, and many other factors may reduce the actual effect of $S$ compared to $P$ (Rothman et al. 2003). These are basically the same pitfalls that arise in any comparison of current to historical data. The potential for error in this extrapolation is of particular concern in studies of cancer therapies, since there may be few or even no historical studies that can provide a solid basis for estimating the benefit of $S$ compared to no treatment.

To reduce the bias that can arise from imputing the standard regimen's effectiveness using historical placebo-controlled studies, the current study should be as similar as possible to the prior successful trials (Jones et al. 1996). However, a high degree of similarity may be difficult to achieve. For example, in adult AML (excluding AML-M3), the most widely used remission induction regimens, including ara-C and an anthracycline such as daunorubicin or idarubicin, have been arguably standard therapy for two decades or more. During that time there have been no placebo-controlled trials of AML remission induction chemotherapy. Moreover, it has recently been proposed to revise the diagnostic criteria for AML to include a condition, RAEB-T, which was previously classified as one of the myelodysplastic syndromes. This reclassification was based on evidence that RAEB-T and AML patients under age 60 have similar prognoses for overall survival (Bennett 2000).

Such a revision makes it even more difficult for future noninferiority trials of chemotherapy for AML, if any are attempted, to infer reliably the benefits of $S$ and $E$ relative to $P$.

Simon has argued that noninferiority trials cannot produce reliable results unless there is very strong evidence that the benefit of $S$ compared to $P$ is large (Simon 2001). This would not be the case if, for example, the benefit of $S$ was established in placebo-controlled trials with marginal levels of statistical significance or, equivalently, CIs for the magnitude of the benefit barely excluded zero. Similarly, suppose $S$ is the latest in a series of two or more standard therapies that have been adopted sequentially based on trials, without placebo controls, that have each demonstrated marginally significant incremental superiority over the previous standard regimen. In such situations, it may be extremely difficult to infer the benefit of $S$ relative to no treatment. In particular, if the current $S$ was adopted on the basis of a noninferiority trial, or perhaps a series of noninferiority trials, then its benefit relative to $P$ may be diminished, a phenomenon that has been called "biocreep" (D'Agostino et al. 2003). D'Agostino et al. suggest dealing with biocreep by always using the "best" regimen as the active control arm, however this may not be practical: selection of the best arm may need to rely on nonrandomized historical comparisons and a new trial in which standard care is a therapy that is no longer widely used may fail to accrue patients. Moreover, biocreep in the opposite direction might also occur in a series of superiority trials as a result of publication bias: if superiority trials with statistically significant results are more likely to be published than those with significant results, then the benefit of $S$ may be overestimated. This kind of biocreep would be less likely if positive results of superiority trials were routinely investigated in confirmatory trials.

Several approaches have been proposed for what is sometimes called "putative placebo analysis," used for inferring the comparison of $E$ to $P$ from the current noninferiority trial of $E$ vs. $S$ and historical data regarding the benefit of $S$ relative to $P$.

Fisher (1998) and Hasselblad and Kong (2001) exploited the fact that if treatment differences can be represented on an additive scale, then

$$\rho(E,P) = \rho(E,S) + \rho(S,P) \tag{16.13}$$

Note that this may require transformation to an additive scale, for example, to log odds ratios or log hazard ratios. If the two terms on the right side of Equation 16.13 are estimated from independent studies, we also have

$$\mathrm{var}\left[\hat{\rho}(E,P)\right] = \mathrm{var}\left[\hat{\rho}(E,S)\right] + \mathrm{var}\left[\hat{\rho}(S,P)\right] \tag{16.14}$$

The terms on the right sides of Equations 16.13 and 16.14 can be estimated from the current noninferiority trial [$\rho(E,S)$] and the historical data [$\rho(S,P)$]. For example, $\rho(S,P)$ and var[$\hat{\rho}(S,P)$] might be estimated from a meta-analysis of prior trials of $S$ vs. $P$. Thus, $\rho(E,P)$ and its variance can be estimated, and the hypothesis $H_0:\rho(E,P) \leq 0$ can be tested against the one-sided alternative $H_A:\rho(E,P) > 0$, or a CI for $\rho(E,P)$ can be calculated to support inference regarding the benefit of $E$ compared to $P$.

Rothman described a "two confidence interval" approach in which a lower confidence limit for the effect of $E$ relative to $S$, $\hat{\rho}^L(E,S)$, is compared to a multiple of an upper confidence limit for the benefit of $S$ relative to $P$, $\delta\hat{\rho}^U(S,P)$, based on historical data. The confidence level of the latter interval must be chosen to ensure the desired probability of type I error (Rothman et al. 2003).

Simon described a Bayesian approach to analysis after a trial of $E$ vs. $S$ in which the expected responses for $P$, $S$, and $E$ are $\mu$, $\mu+\eta$, and $\mu+\theta$, respectively. In terms of Equation 16.13, $\theta=\rho(E,P)$ and $\eta=\rho(S,P)$ (Simon 1999, 2001). Thus, since positive values of $\eta$ and $\theta$ indicate benefit, $E$ would be of interest if $\eta>0$ ($S$ has benefit) and $\theta>(1-\varphi)\eta$ for a specified value of $\varphi$ between 0 and 1 ($E$ preserves at least $100(1-\varphi)\%$ of $S$'s benefit). Note that the latter condition corresponds to $\theta-\eta>-\varphi\eta$, and the noninferiority margin for $\rho(E,S)=\theta-\eta$ is therefore $M=-\varphi\eta$, which is proportional to $\eta=\rho(S,P)$. Through straightforward Bayesian analysis, the posterior joint distribution of $(\mu, \eta, \theta)$ is estimated, allowing in turn estimation of the posterior probabilities of the events $\{\eta>0\}$ and $\{\theta>(1-\varphi)\eta\}$, and perhaps more usefully of the event $\{\eta>0$ and $\theta>(1-\varphi)\eta\}$. Simon also describes a variation of this model for the proportional hazards regression model assuming the hazard ratios for $S$ and $E$ relative to $P$ are $\exp(\eta)$ and $\exp(\theta)$, respectively (Simon 1999, 2001).

Note that in Simon's approach, there is no attempt to compare $E$ to $P$ directly as in the approach of Hasselblad and Kong. Instead the benefit of $E$ compared to $P$ is inferred from the findings that (1) $S$ is superior to $P$, and (2) $E$ retains at least $100(1-\varphi)\%$ of the benefit of $S$. If the results do not favor (1), that is if the posterior probability of $\{\eta>0\}$ is small, then inference regarding (2) is of little interest and the validity of the constancy condition is in doubt, however the posterior probability of $\{\theta>0\}$ may still provide useful information about the benefit of $E$. Allowing for uncertainty in $\mu$ and $\eta$ is appealing, but as always with Bayesian approaches, care must be taken that choice of priors does not unduly influence the conclusion concerning $E$.

## 16.7 EXAMPLE, CONTINUED

For neither the SRE trial nor the HCM trial did the study's reported design or implementation provide for testing or estimating the benefit of *Zol* compared to a putative untreated control. No rationale for this omission was provided. The investigators may have assumed that the benefits of *Pam* are sufficiently large and precisely estimated that showing *Zol* is almost as effective as *Pam* would ensure that it must have benefit compared to no treatment. The risk in this assumption was clearly shown by the results of the HCM trial, in which the CR rate with *Pam* (69.7%) was markedly lower than had been expected based on earlier HCM trials (Major et al. 2001). Had the trial been designed to have 80% power if $P_{Zol}=P_{Pam}=0.7$, it would have required $N=660$ patients, rather than the 180 required by targeting the power to $P_{Zol}=0.92$ and $P_{Pam}=0.90$.

In further analysis of the SRE results, an estimate of *Pam*'s benefit was derived from three prior placebo-controlled studies (Ibrahim et al. 2003). It was estimated that *Pam* increased the rate of SRE avoidance from the placebo's 48.0% to 61.1%, an improvement of 13.1% with 95% CI (7.3%, 18.9%). In the SRE trial, the estimated event rates were 56% with *Zol* and 54% with *Pam*, for a difference of 2% with 95% CI (−3.7%, 7.9%). Comparing these confidence intervals, it was concluded that *Zol* retained at least (7.3 − 3.7)/7.3 = 49.3% of *Pam*'s benefit relative to placebo. Had the lower confidence limit for *Zol*'s inferiority been less than −7.3%, the study could not have ruled out the possibility that *Zol* had no benefit compared to placebo. Again it was noteworthy that *Pam* was less effective in the SRE trial (54%) than might have been predicted from the earlier placebo-controlled trials (61.1%), raising doubt about the validity the constancy condition.

As it turned out, the proportions of patients with favorable outcomes were higher with *Zol* than with *Pam* in both of the SRE and HCM trials. While this may obviate some of the concerns about these trials' limitations as noninferiority studies, it must be emphasized that these trials were at risk of producing inconclusive or even misleading results concerning their stated noninferiority objectives.

## 16.8  INTENTION-TO-TREAT VS. PER-PROTOCOL

The principle of making treatment comparisons on the basis of intention to treat (ITT) is widely accepted for superiority trials, since the inclusion of ineligible or untreated patients, lack of adherence to treatment regimens, and other inevitable "flaws" in study conduct are generally expected to increase the noise in the study and may reduce the apparent benefit, if any, of the experimental treatment. That is, comparisons of treatment groups based on ITT are expected to be conservative in superiority trials. In contrast, "per-protocol" (PP) analysis is limited to eligible patients who received treatment according to protocol. PP analysis, which may be unbiased with regard to treatment differences, may have severely limited generalizability. For noninferiority trials, however, the situation regarding ITT analysis may be reversed: the "flaws" in study conduct, by increasing the noise and reducing the apparent difference between $E$ and $S$, may bias the study toward a conclusion of noninferiority (Jones et al. 1996, CDER/CBER 1998). Thus ITT may be anticonservative for noninferiority trials. Jones et al. recommend carrying out both ITT and PP analyses and careful examination of the patients who are excluded from PP analysis, in order to investigate the impact on the anticonservatism of ITT analysis (Jones et al. 1996).

## 16.9  DISCUSSION

It is widely understood that failure to reject the null hypothesis that two regimens have equivalent effectiveness does not constitute proof that they are equivalent. However, this understanding is not universal. One still hears, for example, estimated survival curves that are quite close together (described sometimes as "superimposable") interpreted as evidence of equivalence, with no mention of the variability inherent in the estimates. In a similar vein, a large $p$-value for a test of the hypothesis of equality may also be taken inappropriately to imply equivalence, for example, $p = 0.9$ may be misinterpreted to mean that there is a 90% chance the null hypothesis is true. Krysan and Kemper reviewed 25 randomized controlled trials that claimed equivalence of case mortality between treatments for bacterial meningitis in children, and found that the claim was based on absence of significant superiority in 23 trials, and that only 3 of the 25 trials had adequate power to rule out a 10% difference in mortality (Krysan and Kemper 2002). Others have reported similar results (Greene et al. 2000). While noninferiority questions may frequently arise in cancer therapy research, the questions of whether and how such questions should be addressed require careful consideration.

The conduct, analysis, and interpretation of noninferiority trials have been the subject of extensive methodological research in recent years, and a number of valuable insights and methods have resulted. However, in the context of cancer therapy trials, relatively simple methods may be adequate and even preferred. Much of the recent methodological research has addressed the problem of inferring whether $E$ is superior to $P$, and the validity of this inference is heavily dependent on the validity of a constancy condition that permits extrapolation from prior studies comparing $S$ to $P$. In the setting of cancer therapy trials, it may be very difficult to justify this extrapolation. In that setting, if a noninferiority trial is necessary and appropriate, a practical approach may be the following: define a fixed noninferiority margin $M$ that preserves a sufficient fraction of the benefit of $S$ relative to $P$, based on the best judgment of the magnitude of that benefit and the best clinical opinion as to the fraction of that benefit that must be preserved; and then perform an adequately powered trial to produce a hypothesis test or CI to support an inference about whether $E$ is or is not inferior to $S$. See the commentaries by Hung et al. (2005) and Fleming (2008) for further discussion of issues regarding the selection of $M$.

The requirement that noninferiority trials be adequately powered would seem to be self-evident. And yet, as the previous examples illustrate, even published studies have failed to meet this minimal quality requirement. Adequate power may require extraordinarily large study sizes, especially for studies of highly significant outcomes such as survival or, for some diseases, response to therapy. Reducing these sample sizes can be achieved in either of two ways. First the margin of noninferiority, $M$ (or $R_M$ for a ratio-based comparison), can be chosen to have a comparatively large magnitude. However, such a value of $M$ may represent an unacceptable trade-off for the benefits that the experimental treatment offers. The other way to reduce study size is to require that the study only have adequate power to reject inferiority if $E$ is in fact superior to $S$, as was done in the HCM and CML trials described earlier. However, this requires one to accept less than adequate power to conclude noninferiority if the two treatments are in fact equivalent. In other words, it has too large a probability of missing the benefits that accrue from using $E$ in place of $S$ if $E$ and $S$ are in fact equivalent.

In studies of cancer therapy, most superiority trials include interim analyses to permit early stopping if sufficiently conclusive results are obtained before the trial is completed. Several approaches have been developed to ensure that the study maintains the intended probabilities of Type I and II error when interim analyses are performed. These approaches generally carry over to the setting of simple noninferiority trials, that is, to trials that do not also include tests for superiority. However as mentioned earlier, some trials may be designed to test both noninferiority and superiority of $E$ compared to $S$. In such trials, the superiority comparison may only require sufficient statistical power to detect an improvement that is substantially larger in magnitude than the noninferiority margin $M$. In other words, the superiority comparison may require many fewer patients than the noninferiority comparison. A number ways to conduct interim analyses for studies with both noninferiority and superiority comparisons have been proposed in recent years, and research in this area is ongoing (see, e.g., Dunnett and Tamhane 1997, Wang et al. 2001, Lai et al. 2006, Öhrn and Jennison 2010).

It should also be noted that the requirements for reporting results of noninferiority trials differ somewhat from requirements for superiority trials. A version of the CONSORT (Consolidated Standards of Reporting Trials) statement for noninferiority trials, published in 2006, provides a useful guide to the information that should be reported, including the predefined noninferiority margin "with the rationale for its choice" (Piaggio et al. 2006). Notably, in a 2005 review, Lange and Freitag found that the rationale for choice of the noninferiority margin was reported for only 43% of 314 published noninferiority trials not limited to cancer trials (Lange and Freitag 2005). A review of 162 reports (116 noninferiority trials and 46 equivalence trials) found frequent and serious deficiencies in the descriptions of study design and results (Le Hananff et al. 2006).

Noninferiority trials requiring large numbers of patients may be difficult to complete; however, smaller trials having insufficient statistical power should be avoided since, as is true of any statistical study, they are too likely to produce inconclusive results. It remains true, as Simon pointed out in the first edition of this handbook (Simon 2001), that superiority trials remain the preferred means to improve cancer therapy whenever possible.

## ACKNOWLEDGMENT

This work was supported in part by grant #CA038926 from the National Cancer Institute.

## REFERENCES

Alberts, D. S., Green, S., Hannigan, E. V. et al. 1992. Improved therapeutic index of carboplatin plus cyclophosphamide versus cisplatin plus cyclophosphamide: Final report by the Southwest Oncology Group of a phase III randomized trial in stages III and IV ovarian cancer. *J. Clin. Oncol.* 10: 706–717.

Bennett, J. M. 2000. World Health Organization classification of the acute leukemias and myelodysplastic syndrome. *Int. J. Hemat.* 72: 131–133.

CDER/CBER, Food and Drug Administration. 1998. Guidance for Industry. E9 Statistical Principles for Clinical Trials. Rockville, MD: Center for Biologics Evaluation and Research (CBER).

D'Agostino, R. B., Massaro, J. M., and Sullivan, L. M. 2003. Non-inferiority trials: Concepts and issues—The encounters of academic consultants in statistics. *Stat. Med.* 22: 169–186.

Dunnett, C. W. and Tamhane, A. C. 1997. Multiple testing to establish superiority/equivalence of a new treatment compared with $k$ standard treatments. *Stat. Med.* 16: 2489–2506.

Fisher, L. 1998. Active control trials: What about a placebo? A method illustrated with clopidogrel, aspirin and placebo. *J. Am. Coll. Cardiol.* 31: 49A.

Fleming, T. R. 2008. Current issues in non-inferiority trials. *Stat. Med.* 27: 317–332.

Friedlin, B., Korn, E. L., George, S. L., and Gray, R. 2007. Randomized clinical trial design for assessing noninferiority when superiority is expected. *J. Clin. Oncol.* 25: 5019–5023.

Greene, W. L., Concato, J., and Feinstein, A. R. 2000. Claims of equivalence in medical research: Are they supported by the evidence? *Ann. Intern. Med.* 132: 715–722.

Hasselblad, V. and Kong, D. F. 2001. Statistical methods for comparison of placebo in active-control trials. *Drug Inf. J.* 35: 435–449.

Hung, H. M. J., Wang, S., and O'Neill, R. O. 2005. A regulatory perspective on choice of margin and statistical inference issue in non-inferiority trials. *Biom. J.* 47: 28–36.

Hung, H. M. J., Wang, S., Tsong, Y., Lawrence, J., and O'Neil, R. T. 2003. Some fundamental issues with noninferiority testing in active controlled trials. *Stat. Med.* 22: 213–225.

Ibrahim, A., Scher, N., Williams, G. et al. 2003. Approval summary for zoledronic acid for treatment of multiple myeloma and cancer bone metastases. *Clin. Cancer Res.* 9: 2394–2399.

Jones, B., Jarvis, P., Lewis, J. A., and Ebbutt, A. F. 1996. Trials to assess equivalence: The importance of rigorous methods. *BMJ* 313: 36–39.

Koch, A. and Röhmel, J. 2004. Hypothesis testing in the "gold standard" design for proving the efficacy of an experimental treatment relative to placebo and a reference. *J. Biopharm. Stat.* 14: 315–325.

Krysan, D. J. and Kemper, A. R. 2002. Claims of equivalence in randomized controlled trials of the treatment of bacterial meningitis in children. *Pediatr. Infect. Dis. J.* 21: 753–757.

Lai, T. L., Shih, M. C., and Zhu, G. 2006. Modified Haybittle-Peto group sequential designs for testing superiority and non-inferiority hypotheses in clinical trials. *Stat. Med.* 25: 1149–1167.

Lange, S. and Freitag, G. 2005. Choice of delta: Requirements and reality—Results of a systematic review. *Biom. J.* 47: 12–27.

Laster, L. L. and Johnson, M. F. 2003. Non-inferiority trials: The "at least as good as" criterion. *Stat. Med.* 22: 187–200.

Le Hananff, A., Giraudeau, B., Baron, G., and Ravaud, P. 2006. Quality of reporting of noninferiority and equivalence randomized trials. *JAMA* 295: 1147–1151.

Major, P., Lortholary, A., Hon, J. et al. 2001. Zoledronic acid is superior to pamidronate in the treatment of hypercalcemia of malignancy: A pooled analysis of two randomized, controlled clinical trials. *J. Clin. Oncol.* 19: 558–567.

Michallet, M., Maloisel, F., Delain, M. et al. 2004. Pegylated recombinant interferon alpha-2b vs recombinant interferon alpha-2b for the initial treatment of chronic-phase chronic myelogenous leukemia: A phase III study. *Leukemia* 18: 309–315.

Öhrn, F. and Jennison, C. 2010. Optimal group-sequential designs for simultaneous testing of superiority and non-inferiority. *Stat. in Med.* 29: 743–749.

Piaggio, G., Elbourne, D. R., Altman, D. G. et al. 2006. Reporting of noninferiority and equivalence trials. An extension of the CONSORT statement. *JAMA* 295: 1152–1160.

Rosen, L. S., Gordon, D., Kaminski, M. et al. 2001. Zoledronic acid versus pamidronate in the treatment of skeletal metastases in patients with breast cancer or osteolytic lesions of multiple myeloma: A phase III, double-blind, comparative trial. *Cancer J.* 7: 377–387.

Rothman, M., Li, N., Chen, G., Chi, G. Y. H., Temple, R., and Tsou, H. 2003. Design and analysis of non-inferiority mortality trials in oncology. *Stat. Med.* 22: 239–264.

Simon, R. 1999. Bayesian design and analysis of active control clinical trials. *Biometrics* 55: 484–487.

Simon, R. 2001. Therapeutic equivalence trials. In *Handbook of Statistics in Clinical Oncology*, ed. J. Crowley, pp. 173–87. New York: Marcel Dekker, Inc.

Tsong, Y. and Zhang, J. 2005. Testing superiority and non-inferiority hypotheses in active controlled clinical trials. *Biom. J.* 47: 62–74.

Wang, H., Chow, S., and Li, G. 2002a. On sample size calculation based on odds ratio in clinical trials. *J. Biopharm. Stat.* 12: 471–483.

Wang, S. J., Hung, H. M. J., and Tsong, Y. 2002b. Utility and pitfalls of some statistical methods in active controlled clinical trials. *Control. Clin. Trials* 23: 15–28.

Wang, S. J., Hung, H. M. J., Tsong, Y., and Cui, L. 2001. Group sequential test strategies for superiority and non-inferiority hypotheses in active controlled trials. *Stat. Med.* 20: 1903–1912.

Wiens, B. L. 2002. Choosing an equivalence limit for noninferiority or equivalence trials. *Control. Clin. Trials* 23: 2–14.

# 17 Phase III Trials for Targeted Agents

*Antje Hoering, Michael LeBlanc,*
*and John J. Crowley*

## CONTENTS

## 17.1  INTRODUCTION

The paradigm of cancer research has been changing and cancer therapies with new mechanisms of action from conventional chemotherapies are being developed. Conventional chemotherapies are also often known as cytotoxic agents and utilize various mechanisms important in mitosis to kill dividing cells, such as tumor cells. Cytostatic agents, on the other hand, exploit alternate mechanisms, such as inhibiting the formation of new blood vessels (antiangiogenic agents), initiating tumor cell death (proapoptotic agents), or inhibiting tumor cell division (epidermal growth factor inhibitors). Many newer therapies (including both cytostatic and cytotoxic agents) are also often referred to as targeted, as they target specific molecules or pathways important to cancer cells. It is expected that by focusing treatment on important molecules or mechanisms, the therapies will be more effective and result in less toxicity than many traditional treatments. While many of these compounds are at a preclinical stage or in early clinical testing, there are already some well-known targeted therapies.

Gleevec (imatinib mesylate) is a small-molecule drug approved by the FDA to treat CML. Gleevec interferes with the protein produced by the bcr/abl oncogene. Velcade (bortezomib) is a proteasome directed drug approved by the FDA to treat multiple myeloma and is being tested in other cancers. Another approved targeted agent is Herceptin (trastuzumab), which blocks the effects of the growth factor protein Her-2, which transmits growth signals to breast cancer cells. Iressa (gefitinib) and Tarceva (erlotinib) both target the epidermal growth factor receptor (EGFR). Recent phase III studies do not support the use of Iressa but a phase III trial of Tarceva showed a significant improvement in survival in non-small cell lung cancer (NSCLC) [12].

The story for EGFR inhibitors is complicated because there may be benefits in the subgroup of patients who are nonsmokers due to genetic differences in the tumors. It is not clear if the survival benefit may be due to mutations, gene copy number, or protein expression [5]. The results for these EGFR inhibitors motivate several more general targeted therapy questions: Is there a genetic subgroup where such treatments are effective (or more effective) and how should study designs be modified where feasible? Should all patients of a particular tumor type be treated with a targeted agent or should only those patients who are positive for the target (or marker) be so treated? As mentioned earlier, traditional cytotoxic agents "target" dividing cells, thus killing tumor cells but at the cost of collateral damage (toxicity), especially for other organs with a high proliferative fraction. Also, targeted agents can have collateral benefit, in that they can be effective in patients classified as negative for the target, either because there is a weak signal for the target in such patients, or because the agent hits a different target. For example, there is now evidence that trastuzumab has some effect on Her-2 neu negative breast cancer patients [9]. Another example is imatinib, which was developed to target the CML defining bcr-abl translocation but also destroys tumor cells that are c-kit positive (which virtually defines GI stromal tumors) [4].

Technological and scientific advances in fields such as gene expression profiling and proteomics have made it possible to detect possible tumor markers very efficiently. Research laboratories at universities and pharmaceutical companies have been very productive in developing targeted agents specifically for those tumor markers. The next challenge then is to validate such biomarkers in the clinical trial setting and to determine the subgroup of patients with good prognosis and the subgroup of patients most likely to benefit from a new therapy as a function of these biomarkers. Hoering and Crowley [6] recently discussed some general issues with respect to targeted therapies and cytostatic agents in the context of clinical trials for multiple myeloma.

Two classes of biomarkers can be distinguished. Prognostic markers give information about a likely disease outcome independent of a treatment, and can be used for risk stratification. For example, high-risk patients, who do poorly with conventional approaches, may be treated more aggressively, or may be reserved for highly experimental regimens. Other markers, on the other hand, give information on a likely disease outcome based on a specific treatment. These therefore represent treatment by marker interactions, and are now known in some clinical literature as "predictive" markers [11]. Predictive markers can be used to indicate which patients should be treated with a particular targeted agent, developed to attack that marker. In general, a prognostic marker is not necessarily a predictive marker, but the hope is that some of the prognostic markers may be predictive as well.

Such markers are often based on levels of a specific chemical in the blood or in other tissue compartments, on the abundance of certain proteins or peptides, or on a combination of gene expression levels. Thus, in practice, the underlying marker distribution, and the response probability as a function of the marker value, is often continuous. The actual cut-point to distinguish marker-positive from marker-negative patients may not be able to be determined precisely, or the best cut-point among various possibilities may be unknown. In that scenario it is advantageous to take the actual marker distribution into account when designing the trial. In this chapter we investigate the performance of several phase III clinical trial designs, both for testing the overall efficacy of a new regimen and for testing its efficacy in a subgroup of patients with a tumor marker. We recently studied the impact of designs assuming continuous markers to assess the trade-off between the number of patients on study and the effectiveness of treatment in the subgroup [7]. This formulation also allows us to explore the effect of marker prevalence in the patient population, and the effect of marker misclassification if the actual cut-point that distinguishes the group of patients associated with the greatest potential treatment effect is not known. Here we evaluate possible trial designs for predictive markers, but we also consider scenarios with an underlying prognostic marker, as it is often unknown whether or not a novel marker is prognostic or predictive. The results of this investigation can serve as a guide in the decision as to which trial design to use in a specific situation. While we present the results for binary outcome data, the same strategy can be easily implemented for other outcomes including survival data.

## 17.2   PHASE III TRIAL DESIGNS FOR TARGETED AGENTS

A variety of designs for assessing targeted treatments using biomarkers have been proposed. Figure 17.1 illustrates three such phase III trial designs for predictive markers. For illustration purposes, we restrict our discussion to two treatments: T1 and T2, where T1 could be the standard of care and T2 the new therapy of interest. These do not have to be limited to single agents but can include entire treatment strategies, as is common for many cancers. We also assume that the marker distinguishes between two groups—marker-positive patients (M+) and marker-negative

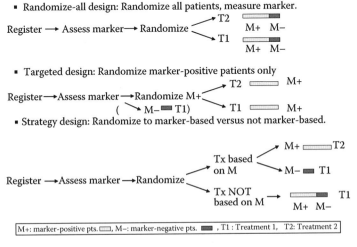

**FIGURE 17.1**   Possible clinical trial designs for targeted therapy: *randomize-all* design, *targeted* design, and *strategy* design.

patients (M–). It is conjectured that the new therapy to be studied, T2, benefits M+ patients. For this illustration we also assume that for continuous markers, a cut-point has been determined to distinguish these two groups.

In the *randomize-all* design, the marker status of the patient is assessed and all patients are randomized to one of two treatments. The treatment assignment for patients can also be stratified by observed marker status. If stratification is deemed not necessary, assessing the marker status of the patient can occur after randomization, which may speed up the start of treatment. If we hypothesize that the treatment is mostly efficacious in marker-positive patients, but it is unclear whether the therapy is beneficial (possibly to a lesser extent) for marker-negative patients as well, this is a good design to test for overall benefit, regardless of marker status, and to explore the M– and M+ subsets. One possibility is to use this design and power it for the subgroup of marker positive patients. This will then allow us to determine, with appropriate power, whether or not the treatment is effective overall and in the subgroup of M+ patients. A similar procedure in the context of hazard ratios was recently discussed by Jiang et al. [8]. SWOG has recently adopted this trial design for an NSCLC trial (S0819). In this trial, patients with advanced NSCLC are randomized to carboplatin and pacitaxel plus or minus cetuximab. Two hypotheses are being tested. The overall hypothesis tests whether cetuximab increases the efficacy of concurrent chemotherapy (carboplatin and pacitaxel) in patients with advanced NSCLC. The targeted hypothesis tests whether EGFR FISH+ patients benefit to a larger degree. More specifically, the hazard ratio to be tested in the EGFR FISH+ group was chosen to be larger than that of the hazard ratio to be tested in the entire study population.

Simon and Manitournam [13] evaluated the efficiency of a *targeted* trial design. In this design, patients are first assessed for their marker value and only marker-positive patients are enrolled in the trial and randomized to the two treatment options. They evaluated the effectiveness of the *targeted* design versus the *randomize-all* design with respect to the number of patients required for screening and the number of patients needed for randomization. A *targeted* design proves to be a good design if the underlying pathways and biology are well enough understood, so that it is clear that the therapy under investigation only works for a specific subset of patients, namely marker-positive patients. Such a *targeted* design generally requires a smaller number of patients to be randomized than the *randomize-all* design to determine the efficaciousness of a new treatment in M+ patients; however, no insight is gained on the efficaciousness of the new treatment in M– patients, and a large number of patients still needs to be assessed for their marker status. Freidlin and Simon [2] also proposed an adaptive two-stage trial design specifically for developing and assessing markers using gene expression profiling. We do not evaluate this trial design here as we focus our discussion on one-stage designs.

Hayes et al. [3] suggested a trial design for predictive markers, where patients are randomized between marker-based treatment (M+ patients getting new therapy, M– patients getting standard of care) and every patient, independent of their marker status, getting standard of care. Such a trial is designed to test whether marker-based treatment strategy is superior to standard therapy. We refer to this trial design as the *strategy* design. Sargent [10] suggested an *augmented strategy* design, extending this strategy design to the case where patients are randomized between marker-based treatment (as in the strategy design) and treatment independent of marker, where in the latter arm a second randomization to new versus standard therapy is added. We evaluate the *strategy* design rather than the *augmented strategy* design since the former is more frequently used. As an example, the *strategy* design was recently used in an NSCLC trial to test individualized cisplatin-based chemotherapy dependent on the patients ERCC1 mRNA [1].

These various trial designs test different hypotheses. The *randomize-all* design addresses the question whether the treatment is beneficial for all patients, with the possibility of testing whether or not the new treatment is beneficial in the subset of marker-positive patients. We also investigate testing both the *targeted* and the *overall* hypothesis in the *randomize-all* design with appropriate adjustment for multiple comparisons. The *targeted* design tests whether or not the treatment is beneficial for marker-positive patients. The *strategy* design addresses the question of whether the marker-based treatment strategy is better than everyone receiving standard of care (T1) regardless of marker status. The *strategy* design does not directly address the question of whether treatment T2 is more efficacious than treatment T1; however, it is frequently used in that context and we thus felt it important to assess its properties.

In this chapter we evaluate the effectiveness of the *randomize-all*, the *targeted* and the *strategy* phase III trial designs under several scenarios. These scenarios include the presence of a prognostic marker, several possible scenarios for the presence of a predictive marker, and no valid marker. We assume that the underlying distribution of the biomarker is continuous in nature. We further assume that a cut-point is used to distinguish patients with marker values above (below) such a threshold, who are then referred to as marker-positive (negative) patients. We recently investigated the performance of several test statistics for the different trial designs discussed in this section as a function of the marker distribution and the marker cut-off [7]. The performance was evaluated as a function of the cut-point, the number of patients screened, and the number of patients randomized to obtain a certain power and significance for the various test statistics. We studied these designs under some simple marker and effect assumptions.

## 17.3   UNDERLYING MODEL ASSUMPTIONS AND SIMULATIONS

In practice, the underlying marker distribution, and the response probability as a function of the marker value, are often continuous. Assume that the log-transformed marker value $X$ is normally distributed, $X \sim N(\mu, \sigma^2)$ and its density function is denoted by $f(X)$. Other distributional assumptions may be used instead. If multiple markers are of interest, a combined distribution of a linear combination of the markers can be used. We assume that two treatments T1 and T2 are being investigated and that the treatment assignment has been determined using one of the various trial designs discussed in Section 17.2. The treatment assignment is indexed by $j = 1, 2$ and we focus our analysis on binary outcomes. However, this approach can be easily extended to a survival outcome. The expected outcome for the subgroup M+ patients, $M+ = \{X : X > c\}$, can be written, assuming a logit link, as

$$g_j(c, M+) = \int\limits_{x>c} \frac{e^{a_{0j}+a_{1j}x}}{1+e^{a_{0j}+a_{1j}x}} f(x)\,dx / v_{M+}(c),$$

where $c$ is the cut-point that distinguishes M+ from M− subjects and where the fraction of marker-positive patients is given by $v_{M+}(c) = \int\limits_{x>c} f(x)dx$ and the marker-negative fraction by $v_{M-}(c) = 1 - v_{M+}(c)$. Analogous calculations for the M− patients give the summary measures, $g_j(c, M−)$ for those groups. We study design properties indexed by the cut-point $c$. Therefore, important parameters in the design assessments are $(g_j(c, M+), g_j(c, M−), v_{M+}(c))$, which constitute the outcome and the fractions of patients in the M+ group.

Figure 17.2 presents several scenarios based on this simple marker treatment model. Scenario 1 is the scenario where the marker under investigation is a false marker, that is, it has no effect on the outcome. Scenarios 2 through 4 are different scenarios for a predictive marker. In Scenario 2 the new treatment (T2) does not help M− patients more than the standard treatment (T1), but has additional benefit for marker positive patients, increasing with the marker value. In Scenario 3 the two treatment curves are diverging with increasing marker value. The marker does not have any effect on Treatment 1, but the effect of Treatment 2 is increasing with increasing marker value. In scenario 4 the new therapy benefits M+ patients, but has a negative impact on M− patients. Finally, for a prognostic marker, where T2 is overall better than T1, both are increasing with increasing marker value (scenario 5). All these graphs are on a logit scale.

We investigated the overall performance of the different designs in the various scenarios presented in Figure 17.2 [7]. We simulate the underlying log-marker distribution from a normal distribution $X \sim N(\mu, \sigma^2)$. We then evaluated the response probability to the marker using the distribution functions discussed previously for the various scenarios. The actual parameters used to evaluate the response probabilities for the five different scenarios can be found in [7]. We performed 5000 simulations to calculate $g_j(c, M−)$ and $g_j(c, M+)$. These derived quantities were then used to evaluate power or sample size for the different scenarios assuming an underlying binomial distribution. For the power calculations we used a one-sided significance level $\alpha$ of 0.05.

## 17.4   RESULTS

Figure 17.3 shows the power of the three designs as a function of the sample size of patients randomized for each of the five scenarios discussed earlier. In Scenario 1, which is the scenario with no valid marker, the *randomize-all* and the *targeted* design achieve the same power for all sample sizes, as response to treatment is independent of the marker status. The lowest power is achieved with the *strategy design* as this design assigns subsets of patients in both of the randomized arms to the identical treatment, and is thus inefficient if there is no true underlying marker. For Scenario 2, in which the new treatment T2 only helps patients with the marker, the *targeted* design outperforms both the *randomize-all* and the *strategy* design, as this is the

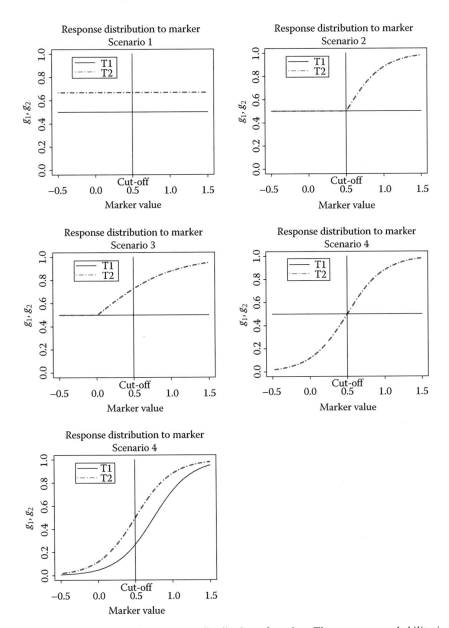

**FIGURE 17.2** Scenarios for response distribution of marker. The response probability is plotted versus the log-transformed marker value *x*.

scenario of a true marker for which this trial has been designed. The *randomize-all* design and the *strategy* design achieve the same power. This is due to the fact that in the experimental arm the same fraction of marker-positive patients are treated with the effective treatment T2 and the same fraction of marker-negative patients are treated with T1 (in the *strategy* design) or T2 (in the *randomize-all* design), and

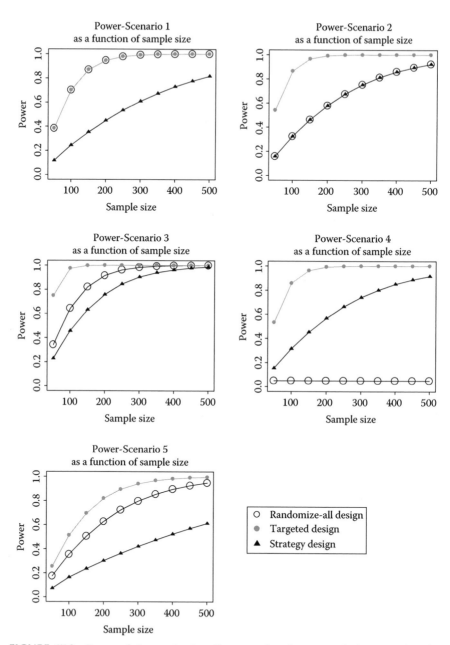

**FIGURE 17.3** Power of the *randomize-all, targeted,* and *strategy* designs as a function of sample size (number of randomized patients) for different scenarios. In Scenario 1 the power of *the randomize-all* and *targeted* designs are identical. In Scenario 2 the power of the *randomize-all* and *strategy* designs are identical.

the effect of both treatments is the same for marker-negative patients. Scenario 3 is the scenario in which M− patients benefit less than M+ patients. In that scenario the *targeted* design performs the best, followed by the *randomize-all* design, and then the *strategy* design. In this case the efficacy is the largest in the M+ patients and thus best picked up by the *targeted* design. However, the new therapy also helps M− patients. This fact is missed by the *targeted* design, since no information is obtained on M− patients. In the strategy design the M− patients in the experimental arm are treated with the less effective treatment T1 and the power of that design is thus lower than that of the other two designs. In Scenario 4, where the new therapy is beneficial for M+ patients, but is actually harmful for M− patients, the *targeted* design outperforms the others. The *randomize-all* design does the worst, as the two effects in this example cancel each other out. Lastly, in Scenario 5, the example for a purely prognostic marker, the *targeted* design performs the best, followed by the *randomize-all* design and lastly the *strategy* design.

For a new marker or a new assay that has not been thoroughly tested yet, the cut-point corresponding to the strongest therapeutic effect is often not known precisely. Using an underlying continuous marker model makes it possible to investigate this effect on power and sample size for the various scenarios. We thus performed simulation studies in which we vary the cut-point $c$, which distinguishes M+ from M− patients. Shifting the cut-point results in some patients being incorrectly (or inappropriately) classified as M+, when treatment T2 is not more effective for this patient and vice versa. We investigated the effect on the power for a fixed sample size in the three designs. Moving the cut-point does not affect power in the *randomize-all* design, as all patients are being randomized independent of their marker status and the underlying marker distribution is not affected by moving the cut-point. Moving the cut-point has an effect on whether a subject is *classified* as being marker positive or being marker negative and thus has a large effect on power for the *targeted* and the *strategy* design.

We found that overall the improvements in power for the *targeted* design are impressive for most scenarios. Only in the case in which there is a constant odds ratio between treatment arms is there a decrease in power for the *targeted* design, and then only for the most extreme marker group. The worst case for the *randomize-all* design is the hypothetical total interaction model of Scenario 4, where the overall treatment effect is null. This is also the only case in which the *strategy* design performs slightly better than the *randomize-all* design.

We also explored the effect of maker prevalence in the patient population on power for the different designs and scenarios. In our simulations we achieve this by shifting the marker distribution, but leaving the cut-point at $X = 0.5$. Shifting the marker distribution increases or decreases the fraction of M+ and M− patients. We evaluated the effect of marker prevalence on power and sample size. The *targeted* design performs the best in all scenarios with an underlying true predictive marker (Scenarios 2–4). In those scenarios the treatment benefit for M+ patients is diluted in the *randomize-all* and the *strategy* design and many more patients are needed to test the respective hypothesis. However, the *targeted* design misses the benefit of the T2 for marker-negative patients in Scenario 3. In the case of a prognostic marker (Scenario 5) with a constant odds ratio between treatment arms the *targeted* design has smaller power than the *randomize-all* design but only for the extreme marker values when the cut-point is shifted such that most patients are marker negative. The *randomize-all* design performs as well or in most cases better than the *strategy* design except for the hypothetical total interaction model of Scenario 4, where the overall treatment effect is null.

We also studied the feasibility and performance of testing both the overall and the targeted hypothesis in the *randomize-all* design with appropriate adjustment for multiple comparisons. We split the significance level $\alpha$ and test the overall hypothesis at $\alpha = 0.04$ and the targeted hypothesis at $\alpha = 0.01$. Other splits of the significance level can be considered, but the outcome would qualitatively stay the same. In general, there is little change in power for the overall hypothesis for $\alpha = 0.04$ versus $\alpha = 0.05$ [7]. The change in power for the targeted hypothesis for $\alpha = 0.01$ versus $\alpha = 0.05$ is slightly larger since there is a larger difference in alpha. The main question, however, is whether it is feasible to test both the targeted and the overall hypothesis in the scenarios with a predictive marker using this trial design. In the scenarios with a predictive marker (Scenarios 2–4), with exception of the scenario of total interaction (Scenario 4), the power for the two hypotheses (with Bonferroni adjusted alpha-levels) is comparable and only a modest increase of sample size (compared to the *randomize-all* design with just the overall hypothesis and $\alpha = 0.05$) is needed to test both hypotheses. We note that in the context of a given real study, one can simulate from the large sample joint normal distribution of the two test statistics to less conservatively control for the overall type-1 error. For instance, if the overall hypothesis is fixed at $\alpha = 0.04$, then by using this calculation one could increase alpha for subgroup test to greater than 0.01, yet have overall $\alpha = 0.05$.

This approach was recently used in the SWOG trial S0819, a randomized, phase III study comparing carboplatin/paclitaxel or carboplatin/paclitaxel/bevacizumab with or without concurrent cetuximab in patients with advanced NSCLC. This study was designed to have two primary objectives. The primary objective for the entire study population is to compare overall survival in advanced NSCLC patients treated with chemotherapy plus bevacizumab (if appropriate) versus chemotherapy and bevacizumab (if appropriate) and cetuximab. The addition of cetuximab will be judged to be superior if the true increase in median OS is 20% (overall hypothesis). The second primary objective is to compare progression-free survival (PFS) by institutional review in EGFR FISH–positive patients with advanced NSCLC treated with chemotherapy plus bevacizumab (if appropriate) versus chemotherapy and bevacizumab (if appropriate) and cetuximab. The addition of cetuximab will be judged to be superior in this subset of patients if the true increase in median PFS is 33% (targeted hypothesis). The overall sample size for this study is 1546 patients, which includes approximately 618 EGFR FISH+ patients. The overall one-sided significance level, $\alpha$, was chosen to be 0.025. The overall hypothesis was tested at $\alpha = 0.015$ and the targeted hypothesis at $\alpha = 0.020$; the split of $\alpha$ was determined using simulation studies. The power for the overall hypothesis is 86% and the power for the targeted hypothesis is 92%. These calculations are based on 4 year accrual and 1 year follow-up. The estimate for the overall survival in the EGFR FISH+ subgroup and the entire patient population for the control arm were determined by estimating the proportion of patients deemed to be in the bevacizumab-appropriate versus the bevacizumab-inappropriate. A targeted design, testing the targeted hypothesis only with the same statistical properties as used in S0819 (except for using a one-sided $\alpha = 0.025$) would take 582 patients. The strategy design testing the marker-based treatment (only EGFR FISH+ patients receiving the addition of cetuximab) versus treatment not based on marker (none of the patients receiving cetuximab independent of marker status) results in testing a hazard ratio of 1.14 and would require approximately 2580 patients. These calculations are based on using the preceding parameters and statistical assumption for the overall hypothesis and a one-sided $\alpha = 0.025$.

We investigated the effect of the marker prevalence on the ratio of the number of patients randomized in the *randomize-all* design and the number of patients screened in the *targeted* design [7]. The number of patients required to be screened in the *targeted* design is given by the ratio of the number of patients randomized in the *targeted* design divided by the fraction of M+ patients. If the fraction of M+ patients is equal to one, the *targeted* and the *randomize-all* design are equivalent. For a small fraction of M+ patients the mass of the marker distribution is centered at very low marker values. Scenarios 1 and 5 are similar. In the case of no marker (Scenario 1) and a constant difference in treatment efficacy independent of the marker value, this ratio increases linearly with the fraction of M+ patients. In Scenario 5 this ratio increases too, but is not linear as the difference in response is not constant. Scenarios 2, 3, and 4, the scenarios with an underlying predictive marker, are also similar. The ratio of the number of patients randomized in the *randomize-all* design and the number of patients screened in the *targeted* design gets larger with smaller M+ prevalence. If the marker prevalence is small in those scenarios we have to screen more patients in the targeted design. However, we have to randomize even more patients in the randomize-all design than screen in the targeted design, as the treatment effect gets diluted.

## 17.5   DISCUSSION

We evaluated three different trial designs commonly considered for situations when an underlying predictive marker is hypothesized. We consider the *randomize-all* design, the *targeted* design and the *strategy* design. We also evaluate testing both, the overall and the targeted hypothesis in the *randomize-all* design. Even if a promising marker is found in the laboratory, it is not clear that this marker is an actual predictive marker for the treatment of patients or that the new treatment under investigation only helps marker-positive patients. We investigated five realistic scenarios, considering several different types of predictive markers, a prognostic marker, and no marker. Since many biologic markers are continuous in nature, we assume an underlying continuous marker distribution rather than a discrete distribution as has been used in the current literature. This is more realistic for most markers and thus allows for a more precise design and analysis of clinical trial data. It also allows us to determine the effect of range of cut-points on the performance of the various designs. For a newly developed marker or assay the cut-point has often not been determined precisely. This formulation also allows us to take into account marker prevalence in the patient population by shifting the underlying marker distribution. Finally, while the results are stated for a single continuous marker, the same strategy holds for a linear combination potentially based on two or more biologic markers. For instance, the continuous marker could be a linear combination of gene expression measurements.

The large impact on power we have observed due to differences in treatment efficacy as a function of marker values and fraction of selected marker positive patients highlights the need for a thorough investigation of properties prior to committing to a specific design and initiating a phase III study with targeted agents. If the actual underlying scenario (marker response distribution) is known, it is easy to decide on the most appropriate trial design using our results. In reality, however, the true underlying marker response distribution is often unknown and we have to consider several possibilities.

The SWOG trial S1007 provides a recent example when using a continuous marker is essential. S1007 is a phase III randomized clinical trial of standard adjuvant endocrine therapy ± chemotherapy in patients with 1–3 positive nodes, hormone receptor positive and HER2-negative breast cancer with recurrence score (RS) of 25 or less. Women who have been diagnosed with node-positive (1–3 positive nodes), HER2-negative, endocrine-responsive breast cancer who meet the eligibility criteria will undergo testing by the 21-gene RS assay (OncotypeDX®). Enough patients will initially be tested to obtain a total of 4000 eligible women with RS of 25 or less accepting to be randomized. The primary question is to test whether chemotherapy benefit (if it exists) depends on the RS. Thus, the underlying hypothesis is that there is an interaction of chemotherapy and RS. This trial tests Scenario 4 (interaction) versus Scenario 5 (prognostic marker). The interaction is tested in a Cox regression model of disease-free survival. If the interaction of chemotherapy and the linear RS term is statistically significant (two-sided $\alpha$) and there is a point of equivalence between the two randomized treatments for some RS value in the range 0–25, then additional steps are undertaken. Based on simulation studies, power to find a significant interaction with an equivalence point is 81%. Assuming there is a significant predictive effect of RS on chemotherapy benefit, a clinical cut-point for recommending chemotherapy will be estimated. This estimated cut-point is the upper bound of the 95% confidence interval on the point of equivalence. If there is no statistical interaction between linear RS and chemotherapy, then chemotherapy will be tested in a Cox model adjusting for RS, but without an interaction term. This test will be conducted at a one-sided $\alpha = 0.025$ since chemotherapy would be expected to improve outcomes. Chapter 19 in this handbook describes this trial in greater detail.

We suggest some general guidelines to help with the decision on which trial design is most appropriate. In general, the *targeted* design performs the best in all scenarios with an underlying true predictive marker. There is only one exception which is in the case of a prognostic marker with constant odds ratio between treatment arms (Scenario 5) when the *targeted* design has less power than the *randomize-all* design, but only for the extreme marker values when the cut-point is shifted such that most patients are marker negative. In addition, more patients still need to be assessed for their marker status compared to the *randomize-all* and the *strategy* designs. If the new treatment may also help marker-negative patients there is the question whether the targeted design is appropriate. The *strategy* design tends to be inefficient to compare the efficacy difference of two treatments as patients in different randomized arms are treated with the same therapy. The *randomize-all* design performs as well or in most cases better than the *strategy* design except for the hypothetical total interaction model on Scenario 4, where the overall treatment effect is null. We thus recommend using the *randomize-all* design over the *strategy* design except for cases where the actual strategy hypothesis is of greater interest than the efficacy hypothesis or if almost all patients in the marker-based treatment arm receive the experimental treatment T2.

We recommend using the *targeted* design if it is known with little uncertainty that the new treatment does not help all patients to some degree, if the marker prevalence (indicating patients helped by the new therapy) is small, and if the cut-point of marker-positive and marker-negative patients is relatively well established. If the cut-point is not well established yet, the power of the study can be severely compromised. Likewise, if only the most extreme marker values are classified as marker positive, but if the treatment is more broadly effective, then some patients who are classified as marker-negative will not get randomized even though they would have benefited from the new treatment.

Scenario 3 is a very likely scenario. In this scenario the treatment works better for M+ subjects but also benefits M− subjects, for instance to a lesser extent. Even if one pathway of action is well understood for M+ patients, there is always the possibility that the new agent works via a different pathway for the M− patient. This has recently been observed in the case of Her-2 over-expression in breast cancer, there is still the possibility that the new therapy under investigation works through other pathways not yet investigated [9]. If there is the possibility that the new treatment helps marker-negative patients, that the cut-point determining marker status has not yet been well established, and if the marker prevalence is large enough to make the study effective, we recommend using the *randomize-all* design with the power adjusted for multiple comparison such that both the overall and the targeted hypothesis can be tested. Our results show that if there is an underlying predictive marker and if the cut-point determining marker status is not too far off the correct cut-point, the targeted hypothesis and the overall hypotheses (with split alpha-level) achieve similar power as the overall hypothesis tested at $\alpha = 0.05$ and thus both hypotheses can be tested with only a modest increase in sample size compared to testing the overall hypothesis alone in the *randomize-all* design. In addition, we found that even in the case of extreme (large or small) marker prevalence both the targeted and the overall hypotheses (with split alpha-level) achieve comparable power as the overall hypothesis tested at $\alpha = 0.05$ and again both hypotheses can be tested with only a modest increase in sample size compared to testing the overall hypothesis only in the *randomize-all* design.

## REFERENCES

1. Cobo M, Isla D, Massuti B et al., Customizing cisplatin based on quantitative excision repair cross-complementing 1 mRNA expression: A phase III trial in non–small-cell lung cancer. *Journal of Clinical Oncology* 25:2747–2754, 2007.

2. Freidlin B, Simon R. Adaptive signature design: And adaptive clinical trial design for generating and prospectively testing a gene expression signature for sensitive patients. *Clinical Cancer Research* 11:7872–7878, 2005.
3. Hayes DF, Trock B, Harris AL. Assessing the clinical impact of prognostic factors: When is statistically significant clinically useful? *Breast Cancer Research Treatment* 52:305–319, 1998.
4. Heinrich MC, Corless CL, Demetri GD et al., Kinase mutations and imatinib response in patients with metastatic gastrointestinal stromal tumor. *Journal of Clinical Oncology* 21:4342–4349, 2003.
5. Hirsch FR, Varella-Garcia M, Bunn PA et al., Epidermal growth factor receptor in non-small-cell lung carcinomas: Correlation between gene copy number and protein expression and impact on prognosis. *Journal of Clinical Oncology* 21(20):3798–3807, 2003.
6. Hoering A, Crowley J. Clinical trial designs for multiple myeloma. *Clinical Advances in Hematology* 5:309–316, 2007.
7. Hoering A, LeBlanc M, Crowley J. Randomized phase III clinical trial designs for targeted agents. *Clinical Cancer Research* 14:4358–4367, 2008.
8. Jiang W, Freidlin B, Simon R. Biomarker-adaptive threshold design: A procedure for evaluating treatment with possible biomarker-defined subset effect. *Journal of the National Cancer Institute* 99:1036–1043, 2007.
9. Menendez JA, Mehmi I, Lupu R. Trastuzumab in combination with heregulin-activated Her-2 (erbB-2) triggers a receptor-enhanced chemosensitivity effect in the absence of Her-2 overexpression. *Journal of Clinical Oncology* 24(23):3735–3746, 2006.
10. Sargent D, Allegra C. Issues in clinical trial design for tumor marker studies. *Seminars in Oncology* 29:222–230, 2002.
11. Sargent DJ, Conley BA, Allegra C, Collette L. Clinical trial designs for predictive marker validation in cancer treatment trials. *Journal of Clinical Oncology* 9:2020–2027, 2005.
12. Shepherd FA, Pereira J, Ciuleanu TE et al., Erlotinib in previously treated non-small-cell lung cancer. *New England Journal of Medicine* 353:123–132, 2005.
13. Simon R, Maitournam A. Evaluating the efficiency of targeted designs for randomized clinical trials. *Clinical Cancer Research* 10:6759–6763, 2004.

# 18 Adaptive Trial Designs

*Brian P. Hobbs and J. Jack Lee*

## CONTENTS

## 18.1 INTRODUCTION

Adaptive designs can be broadly defined as all designs that allow mid-trial modifications based on *interim information* from sources both *internal* and *external* to the trial. Methodology has been proposed to facilitate adaptivity for prospective modification to many features of clinic trial design.[1–3] For example, eligibility criteria can be modified to enrich the study population and enhance the chance of success. Adaptive randomization (AR) methods have been proposed based upon baseline covariates,[4–6] outcomes,[7–12] and biomarkers.[13–16] Several authors have proposed designs for phase I trials that use methods for adaptively allocating patients to dose levels.[17–23] Methods have been proposed for adding or dropping study arms (or doses) or sequential stopping,[24–33] for adaptive sample size reestimation,[34–40] adaptively modifying study endpoints or hypotheses,[41–43] and "seamless" designs that even adaptively alter the trial's phase.[44–49]

The use of adaptive designs has gained much attention lately thanks to its potential for improving study efficiency by reducing sample size, facilitating higher statistical power for identifying efficacious drugs or important biomarkers associated with the drug efficacy, and treating more patients with more effective treatments during the trial. As the data accrue, these designs allow learning about the efficacy and safety profiles of the experimental treatment under study to guide the ongoing trial, which reflects actual clinical practice. Both the Center for Biologics Evaluation and Research (CBER) and the Center for Drug Evaluation and Research (CDER) at the U.S. FDA have issued guidance documents for the use of adaptive methods in clinical trials.[3] In addition, the Center for Devices and Radiological Health (CDRH) also issued guidance for applying Bayesian methods to the design and analysis of clinical trials,[50] which is closely related to the use of adaptive designs.

The main part of this chapter is divided into three sections. In Section 18.2 we discuss frequentist methods for sequential analysis and sample size reestimation. Then in Section 18.3 we consider Bayesian approaches for interim monitoring, AR, seamless phase II/III designs, and hypothesis testing. In addition, we describe two recent high profile large scale clinical trials that highlight the potential impact of new innovative adaptive clinical trial designs that use Bayesian methods. Finally, Section 18.4 briefly discusses practical issues that arise when implementing adaptive design methods in clinical trials.

## 18.2   FREQUENTIST PERSPECTIVE

Classical analysis of outcomes observed in a randomized controlled trial is based upon the frequentist perspective of probability as long-run frequency behavior. To ensure a high probability of making correct inference, a clinical trial must enroll sufficient number of patients to satisfy the prespecified Type I and Type II error constraints. The frequentist approach regards parameters as fixed and not subject to probability distributions. Probability is assigned on the space of the observed data through a model (or likelihood) by assuming fixed values of the unknown parameters. In the frequentist hypothesis-testing framework, the $P$-value is defined as the probability of observing events as extreme as or more extreme than the observed data, given that the null hypothesis ($H_0$) is true. The $P$-value is not the probability that the null hypothesis is true, but rather a measure of evidence against the null hypothesis, with smaller $P$-values corresponding to stronger evidence. Conventionally, $P \leq 0.05$, has been used to indicate that the data provide a statistically significant result. However, if analyses of two distinct designs (e.g., different sample sizes) testing the same null hypothesis result in identical $P$-values, the amount of "evidence" against the null hypothesis supplied by the two studies need not be equivalent.[51] Since $P$-values are computed conditionally with respect to possible, yet unobserved, values of the experimental data, they depend upon the experimental design. Consequently, frequentist designs lack flexibility. This lack of design flexibility exposes a fundamental limitation of frequentist-based methods, because statistical inferences are made by computing the probability of observing data conditioned on a particular design and sampling plan. When there is a disparity between the proposed design and the actual trial conduct (more the norm than an exception in clinical trials), adjustments must be made to all statistical inferences.

In Section 18.2.1 we consider sequential approaches that enable stopping at interim analyses while maintaining Type I error at the preplanned rate. Frequentist sample size calculations depend upon the accurate assessment of uncertain parameters, but potential inaccuracies in these assessments are not formally acknowledged with prior distributions as in the Bayesian framework. Section 18.2.2 considers methods for reassessing these parameters at interim stages of the trial in order to achieve the preplanned operating characteristics. Many authors have compared Bayesian and frequentist approaches to clinical trial design.[52-58]

### 18.2.1 SEQUENTIAL ANALYSIS

Most clinical trials are designed with a fixed sample size (or expected number of events for time-to-event studies). This is in contrast to sequential designs in which the sample size is not fixed by design but depends on the accumulating results of the study. Sequential designs are used to minimize the number of patients enrolled into the trial by stopping early if interim analysis of the primary outcome suggests unequivocal evidence of treatment benefit or harm, or clear absence of treatment differences (i.e., equivalence). Often these designs assume that the outcomes can be assessed quickly relative to patient accrual and the duration of the trial. Trials may also be stopped early by data safety monitoring board for reasons unrelated to interim analysis of the primary outcome, such as unexpected toxicities that prevent the treatment from being used, poor enrollment, insufficient follow-up, or poor compliance to one or more of the treatments.

The simplest sequential trial designs[24] involve patients enrolling into the trial in pairs and randomly allocated to each of two treatments (A or B). The pairs need not necessarily be matched. After the outcomes are observed for each pair of patients, a decision is made to continue randomizing or stop the study. This is referred to as an "open" sequential plan since, in theory, randomization continues indefinitely. A subsequent variation or "closed" plan[59] restricts the maximum enrollment. A consequences of repeated interim analyses of accumulating trial data is Type I error inflation. Both the "open" and "closed" plans involve the determination of boundary lines based on the Type I and Type II error rates and the proportion of untied pairs with preference for one of the treatments.

Given the limitations of the simple sequential designs, several alternative group sequential approaches to interim monitoring that control for the Type I error rate have been proposed. These designs require that interim analyses occur at predetermined sample sizes. Consider a trial designed to test the null hypothesis $H_0: \delta = 0$, and let $\alpha$ denote the desired overall Type I error rate. Suppose the trial is designed to conduct $J$ interim analyses after outcomes for $n_j$ patients have been observed and denote the associated critical value for the $j$th analysis by $Z_j, j = 1, \ldots, J$. The frequentist approach to group sequential trial design in essence involves methods for bounding the critical values at each interim analysis by scalars $c_1, \ldots, c_J$, such that

$$f(|Z_1| < c_1, |Z_2| < c_2, \ldots, |Z_J| < c_J \mid \delta = 0) = 1 - \alpha. \tag{18.1}$$

That is $H_0$ is rejected and the trial is terminated at the $j$th interim analysis if $|Z_j| \geq c_j$.

Haybittle[25] and Peto et al.[26] propose requiring very large critical value, such as $c_j = 3.3$ for stopping the trial at interim, $j < J$, then using the conventional $c_J = 1.96$

at the final analysis. Pocock[27] proposed dividing the sample size into $J$ equal-sized groups and testing the null hypothesis using the same critical value at each interim analysis, $c_j = c^*(\alpha, j)$, where $c^*(\alpha, j)$, a function of the number of interim analyses and $\alpha$, preserves the overall Type I error rate at $\alpha$. O'Brien and Fleming[28] propose using a declining critical value, $c_j = b^* \sqrt{J/j}$, where $b^*$ is a scalar that preserves the overall Type I error rate at $\alpha$. Stopping the trial at an earlier interim analysis requires stronger evidence against the null hypothesis since $c_{j'} > c_j$ for all $j' < j$. For the final analysis, after outcomes are observed for all planned $n_J$ patients, $c_J$ is very close to 1.96.

To provide flexibility in monitoring, Lan and DeMets[60] proposed the "alpha spending function" approach to interim analyses which does not require that the number of interim analysis be prespecified nor that an equal number of outcomes are observed between each analysis; also see DeMets and Lan.[29] The spending function defines the rate at which the overall Type I error is used up at repeated interim analyses. To use this approach, one has to define the scale on which information is accumulated. In trials with morbidity/mortality outcomes in which time-to-event methods will be used for analysis, the information accumulated corresponds to the number of events observed, not the number of patients under follow-up. For further discussion of group sequential methods see Friedman et al.[5] A number of authors have recently proposed modifications to the conventional approach to group sequential analysis.[61-63]

## 18.2.2 ADAPTIVE SAMPLE SIZE REESTIMATION

Traditional methods for clinical trial design fix the sample size (or target number of events) to deliver a prespecified power to detect a clinically meaningfully treatment effect size for fixed values of "nuisance" parameters. The nuisance parameters are usually estimates of the variability of the outcome or the underlying event rate. These are assessed using available pretrial information in the design stage. Sample size formulation in the frequentist paradigm is based upon the convergence of various test statistics to standard (typically normal) probability distributions for large sample sizes. For example, for continuous, approximately normally distributed responses and a test of $H_0: \mu_1 = \mu_2$ versus $H_1: \mu_1 \neq \mu_2$, the sample size per group required by a standard frequentist design to deliver power $1 - \beta$ and Type I error rate $\alpha$ satisfies

$$\frac{N}{2} = \frac{2(Z_{\alpha/2} + Z_\beta)^2 \sigma^2}{\Delta^2}, \tag{18.2}$$

where
   $\Delta = \mu_1 - \mu_2$, the true change in mean response between the treatment and control groups
   $\sigma^2$ is the common variance of the assumed distributions of responses to which observations from both groups belong
   $Z_\gamma$ denotes the $1 - \gamma$-quantile of the standard normal probability distribution function

Since we do not know $\sigma^2$, it must be assumed or estimated in some capacity from prior data. Similarly, since $\Delta$ is also unknown, one typically chooses a value that is pragmatically attainable, yet small enough to distinguish between groups with truly disparate conditions. A frequentist design would fix $\Delta$ at the minimally clinically significant difference (i.e., the smallest improvement the clinician would consider meaningful), and "powers" the trial to detect a true effect difference of $\Delta$ or greater.

At interim stages of the trial, investigators would have gained additional information to assess these parameters. To avoid sample size under- or overestimation several proposals for sample size reestimation based on interim estimates of the variability have been offered.[35,37–39] The general intention of these methods is to preserve the prespecified power/Type I error in case of a priori misspecification of the "nuisance" parameters. The final analysis must account for the reassessment procedure in order to avoid inflating the Type I error rate.

Posch and Bauer[38] propose an adaptive procedure for sample size reassessment that incorporates sequential stopping rules for early rejection and acceptance of the null hypothesis in a two-stage design. Consider a two-stage test of the one-sided hypothesis $H_0:\Delta=\mu_1-\mu_2=0$ versus $H_1:\Delta>0$ for the difference of means from two independent normal populations assuming a common unknown variance $\sigma^2$. Denote the sample sizes in each treatment arm for the first and second stages by $n_1$, $n_2$ (balanced over treatment arms). Denote the one-sided $P$-values calculated before and after the adaptive interim analysis by $p_1$ and $p_2$. Suppose that the trial proceeds to the second stage, only if $\alpha_1 \leq p_1 < \alpha_0$, where the null hypothesis is rejected at the first stage if $p_1 < \alpha_1$, and accepted if $p_1 \geq \alpha_0$. At the second stage, the null hypothesis is rejected only if $p_2 < c_{\alpha_2}/p_1$, where $c_{\alpha_2}$ is based on Fisher's product criterion. To obtain an $\alpha$ level test, $\alpha_0$, $\alpha_1$, and $\alpha_2$ must satisfy

$$\alpha_1 + c_{\alpha_2}\{\log(\alpha_0) - \log(\alpha_1)\} = \alpha, \qquad (18.3)$$

where $c_{\alpha_2} = \exp(-0.5\chi^2_{4,1-\alpha})$ and $\chi^2_{4,1-\alpha}$ denote the $1-\alpha$ quantile of the $\chi^2$ distribution with 4 degrees of freedom. For fixed $\alpha_2$, $\alpha_0$ can be expressed as a monotonically decreasing function of $\alpha_1$,

$$\alpha_0(\alpha_1) = \alpha_1 \exp\left(\frac{\alpha - \alpha_1}{c_{\alpha_2}}\right), \qquad (18.4)$$

where $\alpha_0(c_{\alpha_2}) = 1$ and $\alpha_0(\alpha) = \alpha$

The product test may reject the null hypothesis after the second stage even if a fixed sample test of the pooled data at the same $\alpha$-level does not. Posch and Bauer[38] suggest aiming at a prespecified conditional power, (power of the remainder of the trial given the observed information in the first stage), $1-\beta$, at the final analysis by choosing the sample size for the second stage using fixed sample size calculations with modified significance level equal to $c_{\alpha_2}/p_1$. Therefore, if $\alpha_1 < p_1 < \alpha_0$ after the first stage, then $n_2$ can be chosen to satisfy

$$n_2(p_1, \hat{\sigma}_1, \alpha_2) = \frac{2\hat{\sigma}_1^2 \ (Z_\beta + Z_{c_{\alpha_2}/p_1})}{\Delta^2}, \tag{18.5}$$

where $\hat{\sigma}_1^2$ is the estimated variance from the first stage. Therefore, the sample size in the second stage depends on the prespecified treatment effect size under the alternative hypothesis $\Delta$, the observed variance in the first stage $\hat{\sigma}_1^2$, and the $P$-value from the first stage such that the power conditional on the event that the second stage is necessary is near $1-\beta$. For $n_1 \to \infty$ such that $\hat{\sigma}_1$ converges to $\sigma$ almost surely, the conditional power for the second stage converges almost surely to $1-\beta$.

In order to obtain an overall power of $1-\beta$, the power conditional on stopping at the first stage has to be equivalent to the conditional power for the second stage analysis, $1-\beta$. Therefore, under the alternative hypothesis $\beta$ must satisfy

$$\beta = \frac{p(p_1 > \alpha_0)}{p(p_1 > \alpha_0) + p(p_1 < \alpha_1)}. \tag{18.6}$$

For given $\alpha_0$ and $\alpha_1$, the sample size for stage 1 follows from (18.6). Denote the difference between the sample means in the two groups at the first stage by $\hat{\Delta}$. For large $n_1$, (18.6) is approximated by

$$\beta = \frac{p\left( \left( \hat{\Delta}\sqrt{n_1}/\sigma\sqrt{2} \right) < Z_1 - \alpha_0 \right)}{p\left( \left( \hat{\Delta}\sqrt{n_1}/\sigma\sqrt{2} \right) < Z_{\alpha_0} \right) + p\left( \left( \hat{\Delta}\sqrt{n_1}/\sigma\sqrt{2} \right) > Z_{\alpha_1} \right)}. \tag{18.7}$$

Let $\xi = \Delta(n_1)^{1/2}/(2^{1/2}\sigma)$. Then $\xi$ satisfies

$$\frac{1-\beta}{\beta} \Phi_{(\xi,1)}(Z_{\alpha_0}) = 1 - \Phi_{(\xi,1)}(Z_{\alpha_1}), \tag{18.8}$$

where $\Phi_{(\mu,\sigma)}()$ denotes the cumulative distribution function of the normal distribution with mean $\mu$ and standard deviation $\sigma$. Posch and Bauer[38] denote the unique solution of (18.8) (solved numerically) by function $\xi(\alpha_0,\alpha_1)$, defined for all $\alpha_1 \in \{c_{\alpha_2(\alpha_0,\alpha_1)}, \alpha\}$, $\alpha_0 \in \{\alpha_1, 1-\alpha_1\}$, and fixed $\beta < 1/2$, such that if the sample size for the first stage is chosen by

$$n_1(\alpha_0, \alpha_1) = \frac{2\hat{\sigma}_0^2 \ \xi(\alpha_0,\alpha_1)^2}{\Delta^2}, \tag{18.9}$$

where $\hat{\sigma}_0$ denotes the fixed prestudy estimate of $\sigma$. The power conditional on stopping in at the first stage is $1-\beta$, given that the variance estimate is indeed correct. If early stopping after the first stage is not allowed ($\alpha_0 = 1$), applying the sample size reestimation procedure based on the conditional power of $1-\beta$ leads to an expected overall power that is greater than $1-\beta$.

Fisher[34] and Shen and Fisher[36] propose so-called self-designing clinical trials based on a sequential monitoring method that uses the trial's accumulating data to assign a "weight" to the next patient. The method uses the interim results to expand or contract the implicit sample size in stages while maintaining the Type I error rate. The approach does not require that the maximum sample size is specified in the design stage. Yin and Shen[40] expand the approach to correlated data using the general estimating equations framework.

## 18.3   BAYESIAN METHODS

The general Bayesian approach involves combining prior knowledge about the distributions of the unknown model parameters with the observed data to provide direct estimation of "evidence" for the parameter of interest using posterior probabilities. In contrast, frequentist hypothesis tests based on $P$-values offer indirect evidence for the parameters of interest that is based on conditional probabilities of the *observed data* given a fixed values of the parameters. The Bayesian approach to inference enables relevant existing information to be formally incorporated into the statistical analysis. This is done through the specification of prior distributions, which summarize our preexisting understanding or beliefs regarding any unknown model parameters $\boldsymbol{\theta}=(\theta_1,\ldots,\theta_K)'$. Inference is conducted on the posterior distribution of $\boldsymbol{\theta}$ given the observed data $\mathbf{y}=(y_1,\ldots,y_N)'$, via the Bayes rule as

$$p(\boldsymbol{\theta}\,|\,\mathbf{y}) = \frac{p(\boldsymbol{\theta},\mathbf{y})}{p(\mathbf{y})} = \frac{f(\mathbf{y}\,|\,\boldsymbol{\theta})p(\boldsymbol{\theta})}{\int f(\mathbf{y}\,|\,\boldsymbol{\theta})p(\boldsymbol{\theta})d\boldsymbol{\theta}}.$$

This simple formulation assumes the prior $p(\boldsymbol{\theta})$ is fully specified. However, when we are less certain about $p(\boldsymbol{\theta})$, or when model variability must be allocated to multiple sources (say, centers and patients within centers), a hierarchical model may be more appropriate. One of the greatest contributions of Bayesian statistics to biomedical research is the use of hierarchical models to borrow strength across related subpopulations. This approach places prior distributions on the unknown parameters of previously specified priors in stages. Posterior distributions are again derived by Bayes theorem, where the integral in the denominator is more difficult to compute, but remains feasible using modern Markov chain Monte Carlo (MCMC) methods.[54,57,64]

Another advantage of the Bayesian approach is the ability to find probability distributions of as yet unobserved results. Often the goal of a statistical analysis is to predict how the system under study will behave in the future. Let $y_{N+1}$ denote a future observation that is conditionally independent of $\mathbf{y}$ given the model parameters $\boldsymbol{\theta}$. The posterior predictive distribution for $y_{N+1}$ follows as

$$p(y_{N+1}\,|\,\mathbf{y}) = \int f(y_{N+1}\,|\,\boldsymbol{\theta})p(\boldsymbol{\theta}\,|\,\mathbf{y})\,d\boldsymbol{\theta}.$$

The posterior predictive distribution synthesizes information concerning the likely value of a new observation, given the likelihood, prior, and the data observed so far.

Generally speaking, the goal for conducting clinical trials is to provide evidence for estimating or making inference on the unknown parameter of interest, for example, the treatment efficacy. Bayesian methods assume that all unknown parameters follow certain statistical distributions. Before the trial begins, available information on the parameter can be incorporated into the prior distribution. By conducting a clinical trial, new data are collected to refine the estimate of the parameter by computing the posterior distribution which can be used for the updated estimator or inference making. Clinical trials can be considered as an iterative learning process. The Bayesian framework is adaptive in nature and ideal for learning. Recently there have been several articles [51,55,65,66] discussing fundamental concepts of applying Bayesian methods in the design and analysis of clinical trials. Specific examples are given hereafter.

Over the past two decades many authors have proposed various Bayesian clinical trial designs that incorporate adaptive features. The *continual reassessment method* (CRM)[18] seems to have been the first Bayesian model-based phase I design introduced in the literature. Details of the CRM[23] and other seminal works in this area have been thoroughly investigated in the literature.[7,8,30,31,67,68] The proposed methodologies differ widely by complexity, attention to practical details, use of predictive probabilities, inclusion of decision theoretic arguments, sequential decisions, and more. Bayesian methods offer a different approach for designing and monitoring clinical trials by permitting calculation of the posterior probability of various events given the data. Bayesian design conforms to the likelihood principle,[69] which states that all information pertinent to the parameters is contained in the data and is not constrained by the design. Bayesian methods are particularly appealing in clinical trial design because they inherently allow for flexibility in trial conduct and impart the ability to examine interim data, update the posterior probability of parameters, and accordingly make relevant predictions and sensible decisions.[66] Furthermore, the pioneers of Bayesian methods in medical research argue that in addition providing more efficient designs of trials and of drug development programs, the Bayesian approach is more ethical for physicians who participate in randomized clinical trials.[52,53] Given the aforementioned advantages, the Bayesian approach has become a standard in designing clinical trials at the University of Texas MD Anderson Cancer Center[70] and have generated considerable interest elsewhere.

Many Bayesian clinical trial designs can be described as follows. The parameter of interest is defined based on the primary objective of the clinical trial. Relevant prior distributions of the parameters should be elicited before the trial. Data are collected during the trial. Posterior probabilities of clinically meaningful events are computed. Thresholds on these posterior probabilities are constructed to define decision rules. The thresholds are calibrated to attain certain desired frequentist properties, such as the control of Type I and Type II error rates, mean sample size, etc. In the context of clinical trial design such frequentist summaries, that is, probabilities and means under repeat experimentation of the design quantities of interest, are also known as frequentist operating characteristics. Berry et al.[58] discuss the frequentist operating characteristics of many Bayesian designs. In summary, posterior probabilities can be used to construct a valid inference with desirable frequentist properties. Such approaches are sometimes referred to as "proper Bayes" methods and are widely used. The proper Bayes approach uses informative prior distributions based on available evidence and summaries of the posterior distributions to reach conclusions without explicit incorporation of utility functions, as in the decision-theoretic framework.[54] A typical example is sequential stopping for futility and efficacy[30,31] which is discussed in Section 18.3.1. Bayesian methods are also used to assign patients to better performing treatments, as discussed in Section 18.3.2. Seamless phase II/III designs are discussed in Section 18.3.3. Bayesian hypothesis testing methodology is introduced in Section 18.3.4. In Section 18.3.5 we discuss two recent high profile large-scale clinical trials that highlight the potential impact of new innovative adaptive clinical trial designs that use Bayesian methods.

## 18.3.1 INTERIM MONITORING

One of the advantages of the Bayesian approach to inference is its flexibility to include sequential stopping compared to the more restrictive requirements under a frequentist approach. Stopping rules do not affect a Bayesian inference given that they are a priori independent of the parameters. In this case posterior inference remains unchanged regardless of the reason why a trial is stopped.

### 18.3.1.1 Posterior Inference

Thall and Simon[30] and Thall et al.[31] introduce a class of phase II Bayesian clinical trial designs that include stopping rules based on decision boundaries for clinically meaningful events. To illustrate, let $y_i \in \{0,1\}$ denote an indicator for response for the $i$th patient. Let $\theta_E$ and $\theta_S$ denote the probability of response for the experimental therapy ($E$) and standard of care ($S$), respectively. Many phase IIA studies do not include randomization to control. In such cases we assume that either $\theta_S$ is known, or at least that an informative prior distribution $p(\theta_S)$ is available. Let $\mathbf{y} = (y_1, \ldots, y_n)$ denote all data up to patient $n$. Bayes rule allows for the direct evaluation of the posterior probability that the response probability under the experimental therapy exceeds that under the standard of care by at least $\delta$, which follows as

$$\pi_n = p(\theta_E > \theta_S + \delta \mid \mathbf{y}). \tag{18.10}$$

The offset $\delta$ is fixed by the investigator, and should reflect the minimum clinically meaningful improvement. It also depends on the nature of the response, the disease, and the range of $\theta_S$. The probability $\pi_n$ is updated after each patient (or patient cohort), and is subsequently used to define sequential stopping rules reminiscent of the form

$$\text{decision} = \begin{cases} \text{stop and declare } E \text{ promising} & \text{if } \pi_n \geq U_n \\ \text{continue enrolling patients} & \text{if } L_n < \pi_n < U_n . \\ \text{stop and declare } E \text{ not promising} & \text{if } \pi_n \leq L_n \end{cases} \tag{18.11}$$

The decision boundaries $\{(L_n, U_n), n = 1, 2, \ldots\}$ are parameters of the design. They determine the design's frequentist operating characteristics. For example, a "symmetric" rule could use $L_n \equiv 0.05$ and $U_n \equiv 0.95$ for all $n$.

The considerations for choosing stopping boundaries in the frequentist group sequential designs discussed in Section 18.2.1 apply when designing a clinical trial from the Bayesian perspective. In practice, one starts with a reasonable first choice, evaluates frequentist operating characteristics, and iteratively adjusts the decision boundaries until desired operating characteristics are achieved. For example, we might start with $L_n = 0.1$ and $U_n = 0.8$. Next we compute operating characteristics. We might consider two scenarios: a null scenario $S0$ with $\theta_E = \theta_S$ and an alternative scenario $S1$ with $\theta_E > \theta_S + \delta$ as the simulation truth. Type I error is then the probability with respect to repeat experimentation under $S0$ of ending the trial with the conclusion that $E$ is promising, while power is the probability, with respect to repeated simulation of possible trial histories under $S1$, that the trial ends with the conclusion that $E$ is promising. Suppose that the Type I error implied by rule (18.11) is 0.08, thus larger than the desired. The upper bound $U_n$ needs to be increased (e.g., to $U_n = 0.85$) to reduce the Type I error. Now we might find an acceptable Type I error under $S0$, but a power of only 0.7 under $S1$. To increase power we might now try to reduce the upper bound, say to $U_n = 0.825$ for example. A sequence of such iterative corrections on $L_n$, $U_n$, and $N$ will eventually lead to a set of bounds that achieve desirable operating characteristics.

Thall et al.[31] extend the design from a single outcome to multiple outcomes, including, for example, an efficacy and a toxicity outcome. This allows us to consider the phase II analog of phase I–II dose-finding trials that trade off efficacy and toxicity following the approach of Thall and Simon.[21] In our present context, let $CR$ denote an efficacy event (e.g., complete response) and $TOX$ a toxicity event. Thall and Simon[30] describe an example with $K = 4$ elementary events $\{A_1 = (CR, TOX)$, $A_2 = (noCR, TOX)$, $A_3 = (CR, noTOX)$, $A_4 (noCR, noTOX)\}$. Efficacy is $CR = A_1 \cup A_3$, while toxicity is $TOX = A_1 \cup A_2$, etc. The design again involves stopping boundaries as in (18.11), but now using posterior probabilities of $CR$ and $TOX$.

Let $\{p_T(A_1), p_T(A_2), p_T(A_3), p_T(A_4)\}$ denote the (unknown) probabilities of the four elementary events $A_1$, $A_2$, $A_3$, and $A_4$ under treatment $T$, where $T \in \{E, S\}$ (experimental or standard therapy). Suppose we assume a Dirichlet prior for these probabilities. Under standard therapy, we assume a priori that $(p_{s1}, \ldots, p_{s4}) \sim \mathrm{Dir}(\theta_{s1}, \ldots, \theta_{s4})$. Similarly, under experimental therapy we assume $(p_{E1}, \ldots, p_{E4}) \sim \mathrm{Dir}(\theta_{E1}, \ldots, \theta_{E4})$, where $\theta_s$ and $\theta_E$ are fixed hyperparameters. Let $y_i^n$ denote the number of patients among the first $n$ who report event $A_i$ and let $y^n = (y_1^n, \ldots, y_4^n)$. The conjugate Dirichlet prior allows for easy posterior updating, since

$$p_E(p_1, \ldots, p_4 | y^n) = \mathrm{Dir}(\theta_{E1}^n, \ldots, \theta_{E4}^n),$$

where $\theta_{Ei}^n = \theta_{Ei} + y_i^n$. Let $\eta_S(CR) = \sum_{A_i \in CR} p_{Si}$ denote the probability of complete remission under standard therapy, and similarly for $\eta_E(CR), \eta_S(TOX)$, and $\eta_E(TOX)$. The posterior $p_E\{n_E(CR)/y^n\}$ then emerges as a beta distribution, $\mathrm{Beta}(\theta_{E1}^n + \theta_{E3}^n, \theta_{E2}^n + \theta_{E4}^n)$. Here we used the fact that the beta is the special case of a Dirichlet distribution having just two probabilities. Similarly, $p\{\eta_E(TOX)|y^n\} = \text{Beta}(\theta_{E1}^n + \theta_{E2}^n, \theta_{E3}^n + \theta_{E4}^n)$. The distributions for $\eta_S(.)$ remain unchanged throughout as $p\{\eta_S(TOX)\} = \text{Beta}(\theta_{S1} + \theta_{S2}, \theta_{S3} + \theta_{S4})$, and similarly for $p\{\eta_S(CR)\}$.

As before, thresholds on posterior probabilities determine sequential stopping. We track the two posterior probabilities

$$\pi_n(CR) = p\{\eta_E(CR) > \eta_S(CR) + \delta_{CR}|y^n\} \quad \text{and}$$

$$\pi_n(TOX) = p\{\eta_E(TOX) > \eta_S(TOX) + \delta_{TOX}|y^n\}. \tag{18.12}$$

After each patient cohort, the posterior probabilities $\pi_n(\cdot)$ are updated and compared against thresholds (in this sequence):

decision

$$= \begin{cases} \text{stop, declare } E \text{ not promising} & \text{if } \pi_n(CR) < L_n(CR) \\ \text{stop, declare } E \text{ too toxic} & \text{if } \pi_n(TOX) > U_n(TOX) \\ \text{stop, declare } E \text{ promising} & \text{if } \pi_n(CR) > U_n(CR), \pi_n(TOX) < L_n(TOX) \\ \text{continue enrolling patients} & \text{otherwise} \end{cases}$$

$$\tag{18.13}$$

The evaluation of $\pi_n(CR)$ requires integration with respect to the two independent beta-distributed random variables $\eta_E(CR)$ and $\eta_S(CR)$, and similarly for $\pi_n(TOX)$.

The stopping rules discussed previously are based on a binary response variable. The nature of a response of this sort varies across studies. For example, a typical response might be an indicator for patient survival beyond 6 months. Response variables based on a dichotomized continuous outcome involve a loss of information compared to the original data. Their main advantage is increased robustness; it is easy to be very general about a probability model for a binary outcome. By contrast, inference is often very sensitive with respect to the choice of a specific parametric form for the distribution of a continuous outcome and the corresponding cutoff values. On the other hand, the likelihood function for the continuous outcome is more informative (i.e., more peaked) and allows more decisive inference with fewer observations. In other words, we achieve faster learning with the same number of patients. Also, in some studies it is scientifically inappropriate to reduce the outcome to a dichotomized binary variable, for example, a quadratic dose–response curve. Another limitation of binary outcomes is their inherent delays. For example, we might have to wait up to 100 days after treatment to record a response when the binary outcome is defined as transplant rejection within 100 days.

Thall et al.[32] propose study designs that allow early stopping for futility and/or efficacy based on a time-to-event outcome. Assume that an event time $T_i$ is recorded for each patient, say, time to disease progression (*TTP*). We assume a parametric model for the sampling distribution, say, an exponential distribution. Let $\mu_S$ denote the mean event time under the standard of care, and let $\mu_E$ denote the unknown mean event time under the experimental therapy. Rather than reducing $T_i$ to a binary outcome (such as $TTP > 6$), the authors replace the posterior probabilities $\pi_n$ in (18.10) with corresponding probabilities on the $\mu$ scale, for example,

$$\pi_n = p(\mu_E > \mu_S + \delta | \mathbf{y}).$$

On the basis of $\pi_n$ they define stopping rules similar to (18.11): for example, stop for futility when $\pi_n < L_n$, stop for efficacy when $\pi_n > U_n$, and continue enrollment otherwise. As before, the tuning parameters $\delta$ and $\{(L_n, U_n), n = 1, 2, \ldots\}$ are chosen to achieve desired operating characteristics. A public domain software implementation of this approach is available from http://biostatistics.mdanderson.org/SoftwareDownload/. Thall et al.[32] also discuss extensions to multiple event times, such as $TTP$, severe adverse event, and death.

### 18.3.1.2  Predictive Probability*

Given the observed data and assuming that the current trend continues, the predictive probability of concluding superiority/inferiority at the end of the trial can be computed should the trial continue to enroll patients until it reaches the planned sample size. Computing predictive probability can be a useful tool for interim monitoring during the trial such that an informative decision can be made based on the observed data. The concept of predictive probability can also be applied to clinical trial design, for example, consider a phase IIA trial designed to evaluate the response rate $p$ for a new drug by testing the hypothesis $H_0: p \leq p_0$ versus $H_1: p \geq p_1$. Suppose we assume that the prior distribution of the response rate, $\pi(p)$, follows a Beta$(a_0, b_0)$ distribution. The beta family of densities has mean equal to $a_0/(a_0 + b_0)$. The quantity $a_0 + b_0$ characterizes "informativeness." Since the quantities $a_0$ and $b_0$ can be considered as the numbers of effective prior responses and nonresponses, respectively, $a_0 + b_0$ can be thought of as a measure of prior precision, a larger sum results in a more informative the prior.

Suppose we set a maximum number of accrued patients $N_{max}$ and assume that the number of responses $X$ among the current $n$ patients $(n < N_{max})$ follows a binomial$(n, p)$ distribution. By the conjugacy of the beta prior and binomial likelihood, the posterior distribution of the response rate follows another a beta distribution, $p|x \sim$ Beta$(a_0 + x, b_0 + n - x)$. The predictive probability approach is based upon interim assessment of the future probability of a positive conclusion at the end of study given the current observed data. Let $Y$ be the number of responses in the potential $m = N_{max} - n$ future patients. Suppose our design is to declare superiority (efficacy) if the posterior probability of $p$ exceeding some prespecified level $p_0$ is greater than some threshold $\theta_T$. Marginalizing $p$ out of the binomial likelihood, it is well known that $Y$ follows a *beta-binomial* distribution, $Y \sim$ Beta-Binomial$(m, a_0 + x, b_0 + n - x)$. When $Y = i$, the posterior distribution of $p|(X = x, Y = i)$ is Beta$(a_0 + x + i, b_0 + N_{max} - x - i)$.

* J. J. Lee and D. D. Liu, A predictive probability design for phase II cancer clinical trials, Clinical Trials, 5(2):93–106, 2008. SAGE Publications pp. 96 and 97 (section titled: Predictive probability approach in a Bayesian setting), 2008.

The predictive probability ($PP$) of trial success can then be calculated as follows.[56] Letting $B_i = Pr(p > p_0 | x, Y = i)$ and $I_i = (B_i > \theta_T)$, we have

$$PP = E\{I[p(p > p_0 | x, Y) > \theta_T] | x\}$$

$$= \int I[p(p > p_0 | x, Y) > \theta_T] dP(Y | x)$$

$$= \sum_{i=0}^{m} p(Y = i | x) \times I(p(p > p_0 | x, Y = i) > \theta_T)$$

$$= \sum_{i=0}^{m} p(Y = i | x) \times I(B_i > \theta_T)$$

$$= \sum_{i=0}^{m} p(Y = i | x) \times I_i.$$

The quantity $B_i$ is the probability that the response rate is larger than $p_0$ given $x$ responses in $n$ patients in the current data and $i$ responses in $m$ future patients. Comparing $B_i$ to a threshold value $\theta_T$ yields an indicator $I_i$ for considering if the treatment is efficacious at the end of the trial given the current data and the potential outcome of $Y = i$. The weighted sum of indicators $I_i$ yields the predictive probability of concluding a positive result by the end of the trial based on the cumulative information in the current stage. A high $PP$ means that the treatment is likely to be efficacious by the end of the study, given the current data, whereas a low $PP$ suggests that the treatment may not be efficacious. Therefore, $PP$ can be used to determine whether the trial should be stopped early due to efficacy/futility or continued because the current data are not yet conclusive.

Lee and Liu[56] define a decision rule by introducing two thresholds on $PP$ as follows: if $PP < \theta_L$, stop the trial and reject the alternative hypothesis; if $PP > \theta_U$, stop the trial and reject the null hypothesis; otherwise continue to the next stage until reaching $N_{max}$ patients.

Typically, $\theta_L$ is chosen as a small positive number and $\theta_U$ as a large positive number, both between 0 and 1 (inclusive). $PP < \theta_L$ indicates that it is unlikely the response rate will be larger than $p_0$ at the end of the trial given the current information. When this happens, we may as well stop the trial and reject the alternative hypothesis at that point. On the other hand, when $PP > \theta_U$, the current data suggest that, if the same trend continues, we will have a high probability of concluding that the treatment is efficacious at the end of the study. This result, then, provides evidence to stop the trial early due to efficacy. By choosing $\theta_L > 0$ and $\theta_U < 1.0$, the trial can terminate early due to either futility or efficacy. For phase IIA trials, we often allow for early stopping due to futility ($\theta_L > 0$), but not due to efficacy ($\theta_U = 1.0$).[56]

Following Lee and Liu,[56] suppose an investigator plans to enroll a maximum of $N_{max} = 40$ patients into a phase II study. At a given time, $x = 16$ responses are observed

**TABLE 18.1**

**Bayesian Predictive Probability Calculation for $p_0 = 0.60$, $\theta_T = 0.90$, $N_{max} = 40$, $x = 16$, $n = 23$, and a Beta(0.6,0.4) Prior Distribution on $p$**

| $Y = i$ | $Pr(Y = i \mid x)$ | $Bi = Pr(p > 0.60 \mid x, Y = i)$ | $I(Bi > 0.90)$ |
|---|---|---|---|
| 0 | 0.0000 | 0.0059 | 0 |
| 1 | 0.0000 | 0.0138 | 0 |
| 2 | 0.0001 | 0.0296 | 0 |
| 3 | 0.0006 | 0.0581 | 0 |
| 4 | 0.0021 | 0.1049 | 0 |
| 5 | 0.0058 | 0.1743 | 0 |
| 6 | 0.0135 | 0.2679 | 0 |
| 7 | 0.0276 | 0.3822 | 0 |
| 8 | 0.0497 | 0.5085 | 0 |
| 9 | 0.0794 | 0.6349 | 0 |
| 10 | 0.1129 | 0.7489 | 0 |
| 11 | 0.1426 | 0.8415 | 0 |
| 12 | 0.1587 | 0.9089 | 1 |
| 13 | 0.1532 | 0.9528 | 1 |
| 14 | 0.1246 | 0.9781 | 1 |
| 15 | 0.0811 | 0.9910 | 1 |
| 16 | 0.0381 | 0.9968 | 1 |
| 17 | 0.0099 | 0.9990 | 1 |

*Source:*   Lee, J.J. and Liu, D.D., *Clin. Trials*, 5(2), 97, 2008. With permission.

in $n = 23$ patients. What is *P(response rate > 60%)*? Assuming a vague Beta(0.6,0.4) prior distribution on the response rate $p$ and letting $Y$ be the number of responses in a future $m = 17$ patients, $Y$'s marginal distribution is beta-binomial(17,16.6,7.4). At each possible value of $Y = i$, the conditional posterior of $p$ follows a beta distribution, $p|x$, $Y = i \sim \text{Beta}(16.6 + i, 24.4 - i)$. In this example we can set $\theta_T = 0.90$.

Table 18.1 shows that when $Y$ lies in [0,11], the resulting *P(response rate > 0.60)* ranges from 0.0059 to 0.8415. Therefore, one would conclude $H_0$ for $Y \leq 11$. On the other hand, when $Y$ lies in [12,17], the resulting *P(response rate > 0.60)* ranges from 0.9089 to 0.9990. In these cases we would instead decide in favor of $H_1$. The predictive probability is then the weighted average (weighted by the probability of the realization of each $Y$) of the indicator of a positive trial should the current trend continue and the trial be conducted until the end of the study. The calculation yields $PP = 0.5656$. If we were to choose $\theta_L = 0.10$, the trial would not be stopped due to futility because $PP$ is greater than $\theta_L$. Similarly, if we were to choose $\theta_U = 0.95$, the trial would not be stopped due to efficacy either. Therefore, based on the interim data, the trial should continue because the evidence is not yet sufficient to draw a definitive conclusion.

## 18.3.2 ADAPTIVE RANDOMIZATION

Randomization ensures that on average, the effects of the unknown dependent variables will be balanced among all treatment arms, thus providing unbiased comparisons. Many authors have written on the advantages and disadvantages of randomization.[7,8,11,58,71] Friedman et al.[5] broadly refer to randomization procedures that adjust the allocation ratio as the study progresses as *adaptive*. Two types of the AR designs are commonly used in clinical trials. Baseline AR designs are used to balance prognostic factors available at baseline among the treatment arms.[4,6] Response adaptive or outcome-adaptive designs were developed for the purpose of assigning more patients to the better treatments based on the interim data.

One of the goals of the outcome AR designs is to minimize the expected number of treatment failures for patients enrolled in the trial. Such designs have been proposed to mitigate the ethical dilemma of equally allocating patients to treatments when the evidence available during the trial with respect to the comparative treatment efficacy violates the requirement of equipoise. In this section we consider applying outcome response adaptive randomization to phase IIB multiarm clinical trials. The multiple arms could be different treatments (possibly including a control arm), different doses or schedules of the same agent, or any combination of such comparisons.

Thall and Wathen[11] propose Bayesian adaptive randomization (BAR) in the context of a multicenter trial comparing two chemotherapy regimens in patients with advanced/metastatic unresectable soft tissue sarcoma. Let $A_1$ and $A_2$ denote the two treatment arms. Let $p_{1<2}$ denote the posterior probability that arm $A_2$ is better than arm $A_1$. For example, assume that the outcome is a binary efficacy response, and let $\theta_1$ and $\theta_2$ denote the probability of response under each treatment arm. Let $y$ generically denote the currently available data. Then $p_{1<2} = p(\theta_1 < \theta_2|y)$. One proposal is to allocate patients to treatments $A_2$ and $A_1$ with probability proportional to $r_2(y) = \{p_{1<2}(y)\}^c / [\{p_{1<2}(y)\}^c + \{1 - p_{1<2}(y)\}^c]$ and $r_1(y) = \{1 - p_{1<2}(y)\}^c / [\{p_{1<2}(y)\}^c + \{1 - p_{1<2}(y)\}^c]$, where $c > 0$ is a tuning parameter. In general, for K arms (K>=2),

$$r_j(\mathbf{y}) \propto \frac{\{p(\theta_i = \max_k \theta_k |\mathbf{y})\}^c}{\sum_{i=1\,\text{to}\,K} \{p(\theta_i = \max_k \theta_k |\mathbf{y})\}^c}. \qquad (18.14)$$

Notice that when $c = 0$, (18.14) corresponds to equal randomization (ER). When $c = \infty$, (18.14) yields the "play-the-winner" design. That is, the process is deterministic since the next patient is assigned to the current winning treatment. The randomization ratio becomes more "imbalanced" as $c$ increases.

Thall and Wathen[11] propose using $c = n/(2N)$, where $N$ is the maximum number of patients and $n$ is the number of currently enrolled patients. This recommendation is based on empirical evidence under typical scenarios. The results of extensive simulations studies and specific recommendations for the implementation of BAR can be found in Wathen and Cook.[72] Thall and Wathen[9] apply the approach to a study where the probability model for an ordinal outcome includes a covariate. The outcome is ternary (response, stable, failure), while the covariates are two binary patient-specific baseline values. The definition of (18.14) remains unchanged; only the relevant probability model with respect to which the posterior probabilities are evaluated changes. Cheung et al.[10] apply the method with $r_j$ based on posterior probabilities of survival beyond day 50 under three competing treatment regimens.

Lee et al.[16] propose response adaptive randomization (RAR) using a ratio that is based upon the posterior mean probability of success of the $j$th treatment, denoted $\hat{\theta}_j$, in each group. In the simple case of testing the response rates of only two treatments the authors propose randomization ratios of the form, $r_2(\mathbf{y}) = \hat{\theta}_2^c/[\hat{\theta}_1^c + \hat{\theta}_2^c]$ and $r_1(\mathbf{y}) = \hat{\theta}_1^c/[\hat{\theta}_1^c + \hat{\theta}_2^c]$ .

Figure 18.1 compares the randomization probabilities and the observed response rates (plotted by assignment) of the RAR and ER designs for five simulated trials of $n = 80$ patients, where $\theta_1 = 0.1$ and $\theta_2 = 0.3$. It is assumed that patients are enrolled sequentially and that the patient outcomes are observed instantaneously.

For ER, the plots show that the randomization probabilities converge to 0.5 as the trial progresses (upper left). Furthermore, the observed response rates converge to their corresponding true values, 0.1 and 0.3, for treatments 1 and 2, respectively (bottom left). The right panels show the performance of RAR. This procedure randomizes the first 20 patients equally, then adaptively assigns the last 60. After 20 patients, the randomization ratio decreases for treatment 1 and increases for treatment 2, and therefore more patients are randomized into the better treatment. The plots show that resulting observed response rates also converge to their corresponding true values as the trial continues.

Adaptive designs enable the investigators to learn about the clinical activities of novel treatments during the trial. We can apply this knowledge to better treat patients in real time by implementing an AR design that randomizes more patients to the more effective treatments. AR designs preserve Type I and Type II error rates at the cost of a slight increase in sample size when compared to ER.[16] However, decision rules can be implemented to stop the trial at interim when sufficient evidence for futility and/or efficacy has accumulated. Lee et al.[16] also consider AR designs that facilitate simultaneous evaluation of the effects of treatment and biomarkers for the purpose of treating more patients with more effective treatments according to their biomarker profiles.

Strategies for accruing patients into clinical trials are integral parts of adaptive trial design. This is especially important because adaptive rules based on the outcomes of patients who have been treated previously are used to assign patients to treatments. But there often is a time lag between treatment and evaluation of outcome. Efficient patient accrual is especially vital in oncology, where the full effects of radiation therapy or toxicities from chemotherapy are often observed months after treatment.[73]

For this reason it is customary in cancer phase II studies to use a proxy early outcome in place of the ultimate outcome. The ultimate outcome is overall survival, or at least progression-free survival. To avoid the long delay involved in recording these event times, many phase II studies use instead tumor response as an intermediate endpoint. For solid tumors, response might be defined in terms of tumor size after a fixed number of days after treatment. Thall et al.[31] provide another example of a phase II trial of a post transplant prophylaxis for graft versus host disease (GVHD) in which patients were monitored for 100 days post transplant before outcome was determined.

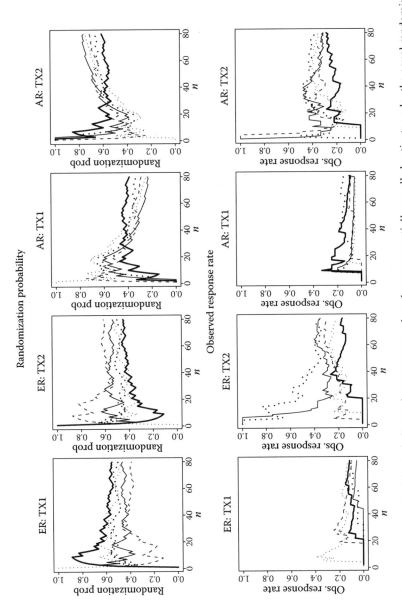

**FIGURE 18.1** Randomization probability and observed response rate plotted over sequentially enrolled patients under the equal randomization (ER) and response adaptive randomization (RAR) designs for 5 simulated trials in each design, respectively. The probabilities of response in treatment 1 (TX1) and treatment 2 (TX2) are 0.1 and 0.3, respectively. For RAR design, RAR starts after the first 20 patients are equally randomized. (From Lee, J.J. et al., *Clin. Trials*, 7(5), 586, 2010. With permission.)

In a recent publication Korn and Freidlin[74] argue that for two-arm trials response AR is inferior to 1:1 randomization in terms of acquiring information for the general clinical community, and that the benefits to the patients on the trial are modest at best and do not justify the added complexity required for implementing designs that incorporate AR schemes in practice. The authors recommend a fixed 1:1 randomization given no differential rates in patient accrual because of the trial design, and 2:1 randomization if assigning more patients to the experimental arm can increase the study's accrual rate. In the corresponding editorial, Berry[44] acknowledges the added complexities involving implementation of designs that incorporate response AR, but argues that the disadvantages should be considered along with the potential advantages. Berry contends that while the benefits of AR are limited but real in two-arm trials, they can be more evident in trials with more than two arms. Furthermore, Berry suggests that AR can shorten the time of cancer drug development and better identify responding patient populations. Further discussions on this issue can be found in Yuan and Yin[87] and Lee et al.[88]

### 18.3.3 SEAMLESS PHASE II/III DESIGNS

In traditional cancer drug development, phase II addresses tumor response. Sufficient success in phase II leads to phase III, which is designed to determine if the drug provides an improvement in survival. Seamless phase II/III designs refer to multi-stage clinical trials that begin with multiple doses of one or more experimental agents. In the first stage a pre-specified dose arm is graduated to a second stage wherin the experimental agent undergoes a more traditional comparision to a control arm at the graduated close.

Seamless phase II/III trials combine phase II and phase III into a single trial consisting of a phase II stage and a phase III stage. Phase II trials generally require more than 18 months, after which phase III generally requires at least another 2 years.[58] In contrast, seamless phase II/III trials allow for moving from phase II to phase III without stopping patient accrual, which accelerates the drug development process. Inoue et al.[45] compared the seamless design with more conventional designs having the same frequentist operating characteristics and found reductions in average sample size ranging from 30% to 50%, in both the null and alternative hypothesis cases. In addition, the total time of the trial was similarly reduced. Several phase II/III clinical designs have been proposed more recently. Kimani et al.[47] propose a dose-selection procedure in an adaptive phase II/III trial that incorporates the dose–response relationship when the experimental treatments are different dose levels of the same drug for binary outcomes. Stallard[49] considers strong control of the family wise Type I error rate when short-term endpoint data are used for the treatment selection at the phase II stage. Bischoff and Miller[48] compare an adaptive two-stage test procedure to a seamless phase II/III trial design and provide formulae for the expected sample size of the design.

One of the major challenges of drug development is the high failure rate of phase III confirmatory studies. More than 50% of phase III studies in cancer are reported to fail,[75] despite the promising results in the preceding phase II studies. Huang et al.[12] speculate that one of the reasons for this disconnect is that often, an improvement in response rate does not necessarily translate into an improvement in survival. The main reason why investigators nevertheless continue to use tumor shrinkage are the practical considerations arising from the substantial lag between treatment assignment and reporting of a delayed survival response. To mitigate the problem they propose a novel clinical trial design that explicitly includes the delayed survival response, in addition to tumor response for adaptive treatment allocation. They consider a phase IIB trial with two treatment arms, $A$ and $B$.

The key feature of the design is a joint probability model for tumor response ($S$) and survival ($T$). Let $x_i \in \{A,B\}$ denote the treatment assignment for the $i$th patient, and let $(S_i, T_i, \delta_i)$ denote the outcome for the $i$th patient, with $S_i$ denoting tumor response (i.e., tumor shrinkage), $T_i$ denoting the survival time, and $\delta_i \in \{0,1\}$ a binary indicator with $\delta_i = 1$ when $T_i$ is observed and $\delta_i = 0$ when only a censored time $t_i \leq T_i$ is recorded. In other words, at calendar time $t$ the recorded response for a patient who was recruited at (calendar) time $t_i^0$ is $t_i = \min(T_i, t - t_i^0)$, with $\delta_i$ indicating whether $t_i$ is an observed survival time. The authors assume that tumor response is reported as a categorical outcome with four possibilities, $S_i \in \{1,2,3,4\}$, referring to resistance to treatment or death ($S_i = 1$), stable disease ($S_i = 2$), partial remission ($S_i = 3$), and complete remission ($CR$; $S_i = 4$). The joint probability model for $(S_i, T_i)$ is

$$P(S_i = j \mid x_i = x) = p_{xj} \quad \text{and} \quad P(T_i \mid S_i = j, x_i = x) = \text{Exp}(\lambda_{xj}), \qquad (18.15)$$

where $\text{Exp}(\lambda)$ indicates an exponential distribution with mean $\mu = 1/\lambda$. The model is completed with a prior

$$(p_{x1}, \ldots, p_{x4}) \sim \text{Dir}(\gamma_{x1}, \ldots, \gamma_{x4}), \quad \text{and} \quad \mu_{xj} \equiv \frac{1}{\lambda_{xj}} \sim IG(\alpha_{xj}, \beta_{xj}) \qquad (18.16)$$

independently for $x \in \{A,B\}$. Here $\text{Dir}(a_1, \ldots, a_4)$ denotes a Dirichlet distribution with parameters $(a_1, \ldots, a_4)$ and $IG(a,b)$ is an inverse gamma distribution with mean $b/(a-1)$. The model is chosen to allow closed-form posterior inference. Let $n_{xj} = \sum_{i=1}^{n} I(S_i = j \text{ and } x_i = x)$ denote the number of patients with response $j$ under treatment $x$, let $t$ denote the current calendar time, let $\gamma'_{xj} = \gamma_{xj} + n_{xj}$, and let

$$\alpha'_{xj} = \alpha_{xj} + \sum_{i:S_i=j,x_i=x} \delta_i \quad \text{and} \quad \beta'_{xj} = \beta_{xj} + \sum_{i:S_i=j,x_i=x} t_i \qquad (18.17)$$

with $t_i = \min\{T_i, t - t_i^0\}$ denoting the observed survival time $T_i$ if $\delta_i = 1$, and the censoring time $t - t_i^0$ if $\delta_i = 0$. Letting $Y$ generically denote the observed data, we have

$$p(p_{x1}, \ldots, p_{x4} \mid Y) = \text{Dir}(\gamma'_{x1}, \ldots, \gamma'_{x4}) \quad \text{and} \quad p(\mu_{xj} \mid Y) = IG(\alpha'_{xj}, \beta'_{xj}). \qquad (18.18)$$

Huang et al.[12] propose a trial design that includes continuous updating of the posterior distributions (18.18), adaptive allocation based on current posterior inference and early stopping for futility and for superiority. For adaptive allocation they consider the posterior probability

$$p = P(\mu_A > \mu_B | Y),$$

with $\mu_x = \sum p_{xj}\mu_{xj}$ for $x \in \{A,B\}$ indicating the mean progression-free survival on treatment arm $x$. By allocating patients to arm $A$ with probability $p$, the design increases the probability that patients receive the best treatment. The same posterior probability is used to define early stopping for futility when $p < p_L$ and for superiority when $p > p_U$, using, for example, $p_L = 0.025$ and $p_U = 1 - p_L$. The authors discuss an application of the proposed design to a phase II trial for acute myelogenous leukemia.

### 18.3.4 BAYESIAN HYPOTHESIS TESTING

Johnson and Cook[33] argue that Bayesian clinical trial designs should use decision rules based upon formal Bayesian hypothesis tests instead of posterior credible intervals, which result in a loss of efficiency and involve unnecessary subjectivity. Consider two competing models and let $\theta \in \Theta$ denote the parameter of interest. Let $H_0$ and $H_1$ denote the null and alternative hypotheses, respectively, and $\mathbf{x}$ denote the current observable trial data. Classical tests of two hypotheses typically involve partitioning the parameter space into two disjoint subspaces, $H_0: \theta \in \Theta_0$ and $H_1: \theta \in \Theta_1$, such that $\Theta_0 \cup \Theta_1 = \Theta$. Hypothesis testing in the Bayesian paradigm involves computing the posterior odds in favor of the alternative hypothesis. This requires that prior distributions are specified on $\theta$ under the alternative and null hypotheses $\pi_1(\theta)$, $\pi_0(\theta)$, respectively, and that the prior probabilities are assigned to the hypotheses themselves. Let $\gamma$ denote the prior probability assigned to the alternative hypothesis, and $f_1(x|\theta)$ and $f_0(x|\theta)$ denote the sampling distributions of the data under the alternative and null models. The posterior odds in favor of the alternative hypothesis is equal to the product of the *Bayes factor* (BF)[76] and the prior odds in favor of the alternative hypothesis. The BF is defined as the ratio of the marginal densities of the data defined under the alternative and null hypotheses

$$\mathrm{BF} = \frac{m_1(\mathbf{x})}{m_0(\mathbf{x})} = \frac{\int_\theta f_1(\mathbf{x}|\theta)\pi_1(\theta)d\theta}{\int_\theta f_0(\mathbf{x}|\theta)\pi_0(\theta)d\theta}. \qquad (18.19)$$

Thus, the posterior odds follow as

$$\frac{p(H_1|\mathbf{x})}{p(H_0|\mathbf{x})} = \frac{m_1(\mathbf{x})}{m_0(\mathbf{x})} \frac{\gamma}{1-\gamma}. \qquad (18.20)$$

Bayesians use the logarithm of the BF, or "weight of evidence," to summarize the result of a hypothesis test.[33]

In an effort to be "objective," there is a temptation to specify improper vague prior densities on model parameters under the alternative hypothesis. Yet, BFs for two competing hypotheses are only defined for proper prior distributions, $\pi_1(\theta)$ and $\pi_0(\theta)$. This fact has precluded widespread use of Bayesian testing methodology in clinical trial design.[77] However, Johnson and Cook[33] show that these concerns about objectivity are in fact misguided since misspecification of the prior density under the alternative model in single-arm clinical trials can only decrease the expected weight of evidence in favor of the alternative model. In other words, there is no danger that proponents of an experimental treatment can bias the results of a Bayesian test-based trial in favor of the alternative model by specifying an overly optimistic alternative model. In fact, they show that prior distributions on the parameters for the alternative model, $\pi_1(\theta)$, that assign positive probability to regions of the parameter space that are consistent with the null hypothesis, referred to as "local alternative" prior densities, dramatically decreases the rate at which a trial can accumulate evidence in favor of a true null hypothesis because parameter values under the alternative model are then also consistent with the observed data. Instead, they propose formal test-based designs that use a class of "nonlocal" prior densities for specifying alternative hypotheses, referred to as inverse moment densities and argue that these designs provide better operating characteristics, use fewer patients per correct decision, and provide more directly interpretable results than other commonly used Bayesian and frequentist designs of phase II single-arm trials.

### 18.3.5  EXAMPLES

In this section we briefly describe two recent high profile large-scale clinical trials that highlight the potential impact of new innovative adaptive clinical trial designs that use Bayesian methods. Both trials use AR schemes that account for heterogeneity with respect to treatment response relative to biomarker profiles and decision rules for interim monitoring of treatment arms.

### 18.3.5.1  BATTLE

The BATTLE trial[14,78] is a phase II trial for patients with advanced non-small cell lung cancer (NSCLC) that considers five subpopulations defined by biomarker profiles. BATTLE stands for "biomarker-integrated approaches of targeted therapy for lung cancer elimination." Biomarker profiles include EGFR mutation/amplification, K-ras and B-raf mutation, VEGF and VEGFR expression and Cyclin D1/RXR expressions. Four targeted therapies are evaluated with one therapy targeting each one of the four biomarker profiles. The primary outcome is the disease control rate at 8 weeks. The outcome is reported as a binary response. We refer to the binary outcome as "disease control." The design calls for adaptive treatment allocation based on a patient's biomarker profile. Let $\gamma_{jk}$ denote the current posterior mean probability of disease control for a patient in biomarker group $k$ under treatment $j$. The next patient in biomarker group $k$ is assigned to treatment $j$ with probability

$$r_j \equiv \frac{\gamma_{jk}}{\sum_i \gamma_{jk}}. \tag{18.21}$$

Posterior probabilities are with respect to a hierarchical probit model. The probit model is written in terms of latent probit scores $z_{jki}$ for patient $i$ under treatment $j$ in biomarker group $k$. The model assumes a hierarchical normal/normal model for $z_{jki}$. The model includes mean effects $\mu_{jk}$ of treatment $j$ in biomarker group $k$, and mean effects for treatment $j$.

The hierarchical probit model[79] is used to borrow strength across related subpopulations. The model is also used to define early stopping of a treatment arm $j$ for the $k$th disease group. An arm is dropped for futility when the posterior probability for disease control being beyond $\theta_1$ is less than $\delta_L$. Here, $\theta_1$ would naturally be chosen to be the probability of disease control under the experimental treatment. Similarly, treatment $j$ is recommended for biomarker group $k$ if the posterior probability of mean probability for disease control being greater than $\theta_0$ is greater than $\delta_U$. Here $\theta_0 > \theta_1$ and the difference would indicate a clinically meaningful improvement from the standard therapy. The BATTLE trial enrolled 341 patients and randomized 255 of them under the proposed AR scheme. The trial confirmed several prespecified hypotheses and identified interesting subgroups of patients for further study.[78]

### 18.3.5.2  I-SPY-2

ISPY-2[15] is an adaptive phase II clinical trial of neoadjuvant treatments for women with locally advanced breast cancer. The trial title is an acronym for "investigation of serial studies to predict *your* therapeutic response with imaging and molecular analysis." The little word "your" in the name signifies revolution. The trial evaluates a large number of potential treatments but considers up to five different experimental therapies at any given time. All are given in combination with standard chemotherapy, before surgery (thus "neoadjuvant"). In the case of I-SPY-2 the adaptation includes changing probabilities of assigning patients to the treatment arms, the possibility of dropping arms early for futility or graduating an arm for efficacy. In the latter case, the protocol recommends a following small phase III study. These decisions are based on posterior predictive probabilities of being successful in a (future) phase III study. These probabilities can only be meaningfully accurately reported under a Bayesian framework with a complete description of all underlying uncertainties.

In contrast to common practice the trial is designed to allocate patients to the therapy that is best for them. To achieve this goal the trial explicitly allows for population heterogeneity, considering up to 256 different subpopulations (although only about 14 remain as practically interesting, due to prevalence and biologic constraints). For each patient the investigators record presence or absence of a list of biomarkers, including presence of hormone receptors (estrogen and progesterone), human epidermal growth factor receptor 2 (HER2), and MammaPrint risk score. These biomarkers are recorded from core biopsies taken during screening. Patients are allocated to the competing treatment arms using AR. Let $\pi(z,t)$ denote the probability of pCR for a patient characterized by biomarkers $z$ under treatment $t$. I-SPY 2 uses adaptive allocation probabilities proportional to

$$P(\pi(z,t) > \pi(z,t'), t' \neq t | \text{data}),$$

that is, the posterior probability of treatment $t$ being optimal for subgroup $z$. As usual the randomization is restricted to some minimum allocation probability for all active treatment arms. In addition, to increase the study efficiency, the results of a series of MRI scans are used to inform the probability of pCR. The trial is a collaboration of the U.S. National Cancer Institute, the U.S. Food and Drug Administration, pharmaceutical companies and academic investigators. See http://www.ispy2.org for more details.

## 18.4 PRACTICAL CONSIDERATIONS

Success of clinical investigation requires that trials are properly designed and meticulously implemented. There are many available computer software tools to facilitate the trial design and conduct.[80] Compared to the standard, fixed designs, adaptive designs demand more attention in both the study design and trial conduct phases. The operating characteristics of the trial design need to be thoroughly examined under a spectrum of plausible conditions. Special tools need to be developed to implement adaptive designs such that data can be timely updated to allow interim statistical monitoring.

Requesting interim data frequently from the trial creates additional pressure on data collection. Response AR requires that responses are assessed accurately in a relatively short time period. This requires that robust infrastructure be put into place to allow timely and more frequent monitoring of interim results. Adaptive designs also require more frequent involvement of statisticians since they will be asked to provide calculations to assess the strength of the available data for interim decision making. Another consideration for the adaptive design is that because changes in patient characteristics over the course of the trial can lead to biased treatment comparisons, all clinical trial designs should adhere to strict eligibility criteria to ensure homogeneity in the patient population as patients enroll over time. Designs that incorporate outcome AR are more sensitive to population drifts[74] than standard designs that utilize 1:1 randomization among the study arms. However, regression analysis can be used to adjust for an imbalance of prognostic factors between the treatment groups. There are several recent articles[81-86] that discuss many practical issues that arise when implementing adaptive design methods in clinical trials.

## REFERENCES

1. S.-J. Wang, Biomarker as a classifier in pharmacogenomics clinical trials: A tribute to 30th anniversary of PSI, *Pharmaceutical Statistics*, 6: 283–296, 2007.
2. F. Bretz, F. Koenig, W. Brannath, E. Glimm, and M. Posch, Adaptive designs for confirmatory clinical trials, *Statistics in Medicine*, 28: 1181–1217, 2009.
3. FDA, Guidance for industry: Adaptive design clinical trials for drugs and biologics, Technical report, U.S. Department of Heath and Human Services, Food and Drug Administration (CDER/CBER), 2010. http://www.fda.gov/downloads/DrugsGuidance ComplianceRegulatoryInformation /Guidances/UCM201790.pdf
4. S. J. Pocock and R. Simon, Sequential treatment assignment with balancing for prognostic factors in the controlled clinical trial, *Biometrics*, 31: 103–115, 1975.
5. L. Friedman, C. Furberg, and D. L. DeMets, *Fundamentals of Clinical Trials*. New York: Springer-Verlag, 3rd edn., 1998.

6. G. Anderson, M. LeBlanc, P. Y. Liu, and J. Crowley, On use of covariates in randomization and analysis of clinical trials, in *Handbook of Statistics in Clinical Oncology* (J. Crowley and A. Hoering, eds.), 3rd edn., ch. 13, Boca Raton, FL: Chapman & Hall/ CRC Press, 2011.

7. D. A. Berry and C.-H. Ho, One-sided sequential stopping boundaries for clinical trials: A decision-theoretic approach, *Biometrics*, 44: 219–227, 1988.

8. D. A. Berry and S. Eick, Adaptive assignment versus balanced randomization in clinical trials: A decision analysis, *Statistics in Medicine*, 14: 231–246, 1995.

9. P. F. Thall and J. K. Wathen, Covariate-adjusted adaptive randomization in a sarcoma trial with multi-stage treatments, *Statistical in Medicine*, 24: 1947–1964, 2005.

10. Y. K. Cheung, L. Y. T. Inoue, J. K. Wathen, and P. F. Thall, Continuous Bayesian adaptive randomization based on event times with covariates, *Statistics in Medicine*, 25: 55–70, 2006.

11. P. F. Thall and J. K. Wathen, Practical Bayesian adaptive randomization in clinical trials, *European Journal of Cancer*, 43: 859–866, 2007.

12. X. Huang, J. Ning, Y. Li, E. Estey, J.-P. Issa, and D. A. Berry, Using short-term response information to facilitate adaptive randomization for survival clinical trials, *Statistics in Medicine*, 28: 1680–1689, 2009.

13. B. N. Bekele and Y. Shen, A Bayesian approach to jointly modeling toxicity and biomarker expression in a phase I/II dose-finding trial, *Biometrics*, 61: 344–354, 2005.

14. X. Zhou, S. Liu, E. S. Kim, R. S. Herbst, and J. J. Lee, Bayesian adaptive design for targeted therapy development in lung cancer—A step toward personalized medicine, *Clinical Trials*, 5: 181–193, 2008.

15. A. D. Barker, C. C. Sigman, G. J. Kelloff, N. M. Hylton, D. A. Berry, and L. J. Esserman, I-SPY 2: An adaptive breast cancer trial design in the setting of neoadjuvant chemotherapy, *Clinical Pharmacology and Therapeutics*, 86: 97–100, 2009.

16. J. J. Lee, X. Gu, and S. Liu, Bayesian adaptive randomization designs for targeted agent development, *Clinical Trials*, 7: 584–597, 2010.

17. B. E. Storer, Design and analysis of phase I clinical trials, *Biometrics*, 45: 925–937, 1989.

18. J. O'Quigley, M. Pepe, and L. Fisher, Continual reassessment method: A practical design for phase I clinical trials in cancer, *Biometrics*, 46: 33–48, 1990.

19. P. F. Thall and K. T. Russell, A strategy for dose finding and safety monitoring based on efficacy and adverse outcomes in phase I/II clinical trials, *Biometrics*, 54: 251–264, 1998.

20. P. F. Thall, J. J. Lee, C.-H. Tseng, and E. H. Estey, Accrual strategies for phase I trials with delayed patient outcome, *Statistical in Medicine*, 18: 1155–1169, 1999.

21. P. F. Thall and J. D. Cook, Dose-finding based on efficacy-toxicity trade-offs, *Biometrics*, 60: 684–693, 2004.

22. P. Müller, D. Berry, A. Grieve, and M. Krams, A Bayesian decision-theoretic dose finding trial, *Decision Analysis*, 3: 197–207, 2006.

23. J. O'Quigley, Dose-finding using continual re-assessment method, in *Handbook of Statistics in Clinical Oncology* (J. Crowley and A. Hoering, eds.), 3rd edn., ch. 2, Boca Raton, FL: Chapman & Hall/CRC Press, 2011.

24. P. Armitage, Restricted sequential procedures, *Biometrika*, 44: 9–26, 1957.

25. J. L. Haybittle, Repeated assessment of results in clinical trials of cancer treatment, *British Journal of Radiology*, 44: 793–797, 1971.

26. R. Peto, M. C. Pike, P. Armitgae, N. E. Breslow, D. R. Cox, S. V. Howard, N. Mantel, K. McPherson, J. Peto, and P. G. Smith, Design and analysis of randomized clinical trials requiring prolonged observations of each patient. I. Introduction and design, *British Journal of Radiology*, 34: 585–612, 1976.

27. S. J. Pocock, Group sequential methods in the design and analysis of clinical trials, *Biometrika*, 64: 191–199, 1977.

28. P. C. O'Brien and T. R. Fleming, A multiple testing procedure for clinical trials, *Biometrics*, 35: 549–556, 1979.

29. D. L. DeMets and K. K. G. Lan, Interim analyses: The alpha spending function approach, *Statistics in Medicine*, 13: 1341–1352, 1994.

30. P. F. Thall and R. Simon, Practical Bayesian guidelines for phase IIB clinical trials, *Biometrics*, 50: 337–349, 1994.

31. P. F. Thall, R. M. Simon, and E. H. Estey, Bayesian sequential monitoring designs for single-arm clinical trials with multiple outcomes, *Statistics in Medicine*, 14: 357–379, 1995.

32. P. F. Thall, L. Wooten, and N. Tannir, Monitoring event times in early phase clinical trials: Some practical issues, *Clinical Trials*, 2: 467–478, 2005.

33. V. E. Johnson and J. D. Cook, Bayesian design of single-arm phase II clinical trials with continuous monitoring, *Clinical Trials*, 6: 217–226, 2009.

34. L. Fisher, Self-designing clinical trials, *Statistics in Medicine*, 17: 1551–1562, 1998.

35. A. L. Gould and W. Shi, Modifying the design of ongoing trials without unblinding, *Statistics in Medicine*, 17: 89–100, 1998.

36. Y. Shen and L. Fisher, Statistical inference for self-designing clinical trials with a one-sided hypothesis, *Biometrics*, 55: 190–197, 1999.

37. C. S. Coffey and K. E. Muller, Exact test size and power of a Gaussian error linear model for an internal pilot study, *Statistics and Medicine*, 18: 1199–1214, 1999.

38. M. Posch and P. Bauer, Interim analysis and sample size reassessment, *Biometrics*, 56: 1170–1176, 2000.

39. L. Gould, Sample size re-estimation: Recent developments and practical considerations, *Statistics in Medicine*, 20: 2625–2643, 2001.

40. G. Yin and Y. Shen, Adaptive design and estimation in randomized clinical trials with correlated observations, *Biometrics*, 61: 362–369, 2005.

41. T. Lang, A. Auterith, and P. Bauer, Trend tests with adaptive scoring, *Biometrical Journal*, 42: 1007–1020, 2000.

42. M. Neuhäuser, An adaptive location-scale test, *Biometrical Journal*, 43: 809–819, 2001.

43. M. Kieser, B. Schneider, and T. Friede, A bootstrap procedure for adaptive selection of the test statistics in flexible two-stage designs, *Biometrical Journal*, 44: 641–652, 2002.

44. D. A. Berry, Adaptive clinical trials: The promise and the caution, *Journal of Clinical Oncology,* 21: 606–609, 2010.

45. L. Y. T. Inoue, P. Thall, and D. A. Berry, Seamlessly expanding a randomized phase II trial to phase III, *Biometrics*, 58: 823–831, 2002.

46. M. Krams, K. R. Lees, and D. A. Berry, The past is the future: Innovative designs in acute stroke therapy trials, *Stroke*, 36: 1341–1347, 2005.

47. P. K. Kimani, N. Stallard, and J. L. Hutton, Dose selection in seamless phase II/III clinical trials based on efficacy and safety, *Statistics in Medicine*, 28: 917–936, 2009.

48. W. Bischoff and F. Miller, A seamless phase II/III design with sample-size re-estimation, *Journal of Biopharmaceutical Statistics*, 19: 595–609, 2009.

49. N. Stallard, A confirmatory seamless phase II/III clinical trial design incorporating short-term endpoint information, *Statistics in Medicine*, 29: 959–971, 2010.

50. FDA, Guidance for the use of Bayesian statistics, Technical report, U.S. Department of Heath and Human Services, Food and Drug Administration (CDRH) http://www.fda.gov/MedicalDevices/DeviceRegulationandGuidance/ GuidanceDocuments/ucm071072.htm

51. S. N. Goodman, Introduction to Bayesian methods I: Measuring the strength of evidence, *Clinical Trials*, 2: 282–290, 2005.

52. P. F. Thall, Ethical issues in oncology biostatistics, *Statistical Methods in Medical Research*, 11: 429–448, 2002.

53. D. A. Berry, Bayesian statistics and the efficiency and ethics of clinical trials, *Statistical Science*, 1: 175–187, 2004.
54. D. J. Spiegelhalter, K. R. Abrams, and J. P. Myles, *Bayesian Approaches to Clinical Trials and Health-Care Evaluation*. London, U.K.: Wiley, 2004.
55. D. A. Berry, Bayesian clinical trials, *Nature Reviews Drug Discovery*, 5: 27–36, 2006.
56. J. J. Lee and D. D. Liu, A predictive probability design for phase II cancer clinical trials, *Clinical Trials*, 5: 93–106, 2008.
57. B. P. Carlin and T. A. Louis, *Bayesian Methods for Data Analysis*. Boca Raton, FL: Chapman & Hall/CRC Press, 3rd edn., 2009.
58. S. M. Berry, B. P. Carlin, J. J. Lee, and P. Müller, *Bayesian Adaptive Methods for Clinical Trials*. Boca Raton, FL: Chapman & Hall/CRC Press, 2010.
59. P. Armitage, *Sequential Medical Trials*. New York: John Wiley & Sons, 2nd edn., 1975.
60. K. K. G. Lan and D. L. DeMets, Discrete sequential boundaries for clinical trials, *Biometrika*, 70: 659–663, 1983.
61. A. A. Tsiatis and C. Mehta, On the inefficiency of the adaptive design for monitoring clinical trials, *Biometrika*, 90: 367–378, 2003.
62. W. Brannath, P. Bauer, and M. Posch, On the efficiency of adaptive designs for flexible interim decisions in clinical trials, *Journal of Statistical Planning and Inference*, 136: 1956–1961, 2006.
63. C. Jennison and B. W. Turnbull, Adaptive and nonadaptive group sequential tests, *Biometrika*, 93: 1–21, 2006.
64. A. Gelman, J. B. Carlin, H. S. Stern, and D. B. Rubin, *Bayesian Data Analysis*. Boca Raton, FL: Chapman & Hall/CRC Press, 2nd edn., 2004.
65. T. A. Louis, Introduction to Bayesian methods II: Fundamental concepts, *Clinical Trials*, 2: 291–294, 2005.
66. D. A. Berry, Introduction to Bayesian methods III: Use and interpretation of Bayesian tools in design and analysis, *Clinical Trials*, 2: 295–300, 2005.
67. D. A. Berry, A case for Bayesianism in clinical trials (with discussion), *Statistics in Medicine*, 12: 1377–1404, 1993.
68. D. J. Spiegelhalter, L. S. Freedman, and M. K. B. Parmar, Bayesian approaches to randomized trials (with discussion), *Royal Statistical Society: Series A*, 157: 357–416, 1994.
69. A. Birnbaum, On the foundations of statistical inference (with discussion), *Journal of the American Statistical Association*, 57: 269–326, 1962.
70. S. Biswas, D. D. Liu, J. Lee, and D. A. Berry, Bayesian clinical trials at the University of Texas MD Anderson Cancer Center, *Clinical Trials*, 6: 205–216, 2009.
71. W. F. Rosenberger, N. Stallard, A. Ivanova, C. N. Harper, and M. L. Ricks, Optimal adaptive designs for binary response trials, *Biometrics*, 57: 909–913, 2001.
72. J. Wathen and J. Cook, Power and bias in adaptively randomized clinical trials, Technical report, Department of Biostatistics, MD Anderson Cancer Center, 2006.
73. Y. K. Cheung and R. Chappell, Sequential designs for phase I clinical trials with late-onset toxicities, *Biometrics*, 56: 1177–1182, 2000.
74. E. L. Korn and B. Freidlin, Outcome-adaptive randomization: Is it useful? *Journal of Clinical Oncology*, 29: 771–776, 2011.
75. I. Kola and J. Landis, Can the pharmaceutical industry reduce attrition rates? *Nature Reviews Drug Discovery*, 3: 711–715, 2004.
76. V. E. Johnson, Bayes factors based on test statistics, *Journal of the Royal Statistical Society: Series B*, 67: 689–701, 2005.
77. V. E. Johnson and D. Rossell, On the use of non-local prior densities in Bayesian hypothesis tests, *Journal of the Royal Statistical Society: Series B*, 72: 143–170, 2010.

78. E. S. Kim, R. S. Herbst, I. I. Wistuba, J. J. Lee, G. R. Blumenschein, A. Tsao, D. J. Stewart et al., The BATTLE trial: Personalizing therapy for lung cancer, *Cancer Discovery*, 1: 44–53, 2011.

79. J. H. Albert and S. Chib, Bayesian analysis of binary and polychotomous response data, *Journal of the American Statistical Association*, 88: 669–679, 1993.

80. J. J. Lee and N. Chen, Software for design of clinical trials, in *Handbook of Statistics in Clinical Oncology* (J. Crowley and A. Hoering, eds.), 3rd edn., ch. 21, Boca Raton, FL: Chapman & Hall/CRC Press, 2011.

81. P. Bauer and W. Brannath, The advantages and disadvantages of adaptive designs for clinical trials, *Drug Discovery Today*, 9: 351–357, 2004.

82. P. Gallo, C. Chuang-Stein, V. Dragalin, B. Gaydos, M. Krams, and J. Pinheiro, Adaptive designs in clinical drug development–An executive summary of the PhRMA working group, *Journal of Biopharmaceutical Statistics*, 16: 275–283, 2006.

83. M. Chang, S.-C. Chow, and A. Pong, Adaptive design in clinical research: Issues, opportunities, and recommendations, *Journal of Biopharmaceutical Statistics*, 16: 299–309, 2006.

84. M. Krams, C.-F. Burman, V. Dragalin, B. Gaydos, A. P. Grieve, J. Pinheiro, and W. Maurer, Adaptive designs in clinical drug development: Opportunities, challenges, and scope reflections following PhRMA's November 2006 workshop, *Journal of Bio-Pharmaceutical Statistics*, 17: 957–964, 2007.

85. S.-C. Chow and M. Chang, Adaptive design methods in clinical trials—A review, *Orphanet Journal of Rare Diseases*, 3: 1–13, 2008.

86. F. Bretz, M. Branson, C.-F. Burman, C. Chuang-Stein, and C. S. Coffey, Adaptivity in drug discovery and development, *Drug Development Research*, 70: 169–190, 2009.

87. Y. Yuan and G. Yin, On the usefulness of outcome-adaptive randomization, *Journal of Clinical Oncology*, 29: 3390–3392, 2011.

88. J. J. Lee, N. Chen, and G. Yin, Worth adapting? Revisit the usefulness of outcome-adaptive randomization, Submitted, 2011.

# 19 Design of a Clinical Trial for Testing the Ability of a Continuous Marker to Predict Therapy Benefit

*William E. Barlow*

## CONTENTS

## 19.1 INTRODUCTION

### 19.1.1 BACKGROUND

Biologic markers are commonly used as prognostic indicators of outcome following a diagnosis of disease and subsequent treatment. In oncology, tumor-based markers are used to suggest the potential for cancer to recur or to cause death. These markers are regarded as "prognostic" in that they provide information to patients about what they might expect in the future, but the markers may not help choose appropriate treatment (Schumacher et al., 2006). On the other hand, "predictive" markers do suggest that a particular therapy is optimal and may reflect that the prognostic effect of the marker differs by treatment or that the efficacy of a particular treatment depends on the marker. The distinction between prognostic and predictive factors is usually attributed to the late William McGuire (McGuire et al., 1992). Marker discovery begins by noting the important prognostic effect of a marker, which may in turn be found to be predictive upon greater examination of the prognostic effect conditional on different treatment choices. Ideally, treatment has been randomized, thus providing an unbiased assessment of predictive ability of a marker with regard to treatment choice.

### 19.1.2 STATISTICAL MODELING OF PROGNOSIS AND PREDICTION

Prognostic effects are typically coded as a main effect in statistical models, since their effect is present for all patients regardless of treatment choice. On occasion, prognostic effects will be considered only within patients treated in a uniform fashion or even in untreated patients to determine the natural course of disease. In contrast, predictive effects are often represented as interactions of the marker with treatment. Suppose we have treatment (trt) and a marker Z. A simple Cox regression model of survival at time $t$ on the log hazard rate scale would be the following:

$$\log \lambda(t; trt, z) = \log \lambda_0(t) + trt \, \beta_1 + z \, \beta_2 + trt * z \, \beta_3 \qquad (19.1)$$

The treatment is considered to be dichotomous for simplicity, and the marker $Z$ could be either dichotomous or continuous. A typical approach is to test whether the interaction term adds significantly to a statistical model, which has only the two main effects of treatment and the marker. A significant interaction may imply that the effect of treatment differs by the value of the marker. It can also imply that the prognostic effect of the marker $Z$ is conditional on the choice of treatment.

### 19.1.3 QUALITATIVE VERSUS QUANTITATIVE INTERACTIONS

Interaction terms can be described as quantitative or qualitative. A "quantitative" interaction describes an interaction that is in a consistent direction even though the magnitude may vary. Thus, even though the magnitude of the treatment effect may depend on the covariate $z$, one treatment is always superior to the other treatment for all choices of $z$. For example, in Model (19.1), $\beta_1 + z\beta_3 < 0$ for all $z$ implies that treatment is always effective in increasing survival even though the magnitude of benefit may depend on the marker $z$. In this case, the marker may not guide the choice of treatment, since a particular treatment is always dominant. Thus, an interaction of treatment and the marker may be necessary for a predictive effect, but it is not sufficient. The work by Janes et al. (2011) gives other examples within this context. On the other hand, a qualitative interaction implies that the benefit of treatment may differ for different values of the marker such that the treatment is beneficial in some situations, but not others. In terms of the model, it implies that that there is a cutoff $z_0$, such that $\beta_1 + z\beta_3 \leq 0$ for $z \geq z_0$ and that $\beta_1 + z\beta_3 \geq 0$ for $z < z_0$. Thus, treatment may be valuable for high values of the marker, but may not be effective (or even harmful) for low values of the marker. In this situation, we would term the marker as "predictive" since it may suggest treatment strategy depends on the value of the marker.

### 19.1.4   RETROSPECTIVE EVALUATION OF MARKERS AS PREDICTIVE

Often, predictive markers are tested in the context of a more general comparative trial of two treatments or the addition of an experimental treatment compared to standard treatment. In most cases, the trial was powered to find an overall difference between two treatments despite the possible presence of subgroups who may not have benefitted from treatment. Consequently, analyses of interaction terms will often be inadequately powered to find a statistically significant difference unless the interaction is large. Even in the presence of a statistically nonsignificant interaction, separate analyses of treatment by a marker may demonstrate an effect of treatment in one group, but not another. These apparent effects can then lead to a new trial with sufficient power or to similar analyses in other trials to validate the original findings. On the other hand, separate analyses of treatment by marker values may be convincing that there is little predictive effect of the marker. For example, forest plots of treatment by marker values may show strong concordance of the treatment difference across subgroups suggesting little predictive effect of the markers.

## 19.2   CONTINUOUS MARKERS

### 19.2.1   CUTPOINTS FOR CONTINUOUS MARKERS

In many cases, marker values are dichotomous or cutpoints are designated to divide the marker into positive or negative values. Well-known examples of predictive markers in breast cancer include hormone-receptor status as a guide to using endocrine therapy and HER2-status as a determinant of trastuzumab efficacy. Both markers are viewed as positive or negative for decision making, but in fact often arise from continuous or ordinal values. Testing of dichotomous markers and associated trial designs are discussed by Hoering et al. (2008) and Sargent et al. (2005). It is well known that categorization of continuous markers may lose power (Royston et al., 2006). In this work, we will focus on continuous markers and attempts to categorize the marker when needed for final clinical decision making.

### 19.2.2   STATISTICAL MODEL FOR CONTINUOUS MARKERS

We assume that we have a continuous marker $Z \geq 0$ and use a standard Cox regression model that included an interaction term

$$\log \lambda(t; trt, z) = \log \lambda_0(t) + trt\,\beta_1 + z\,\beta_2 + trt * z\,\beta_3$$

For the purpose of illustration, we define treatment as being a comparison of chemotherapy to no chemotherapy, and the continuous marker is labeled as recurrence

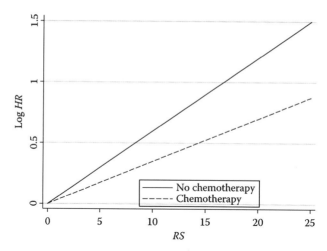

**FIGURE 19.1**   Modeled relationship of the Cox regression log hazard ratio (HR) relating survival to Recurrence Score (RS) and therapy. In this model chemotheraphy has a lower failure rate than no chemotheraphy for all values of RS.

score (*RS*) for recurrence score. Figure 19.1 illustrates a quantitative interaction between *RS*, a continuous marker, and treatment with chemotherapy. The log hazard ratio (HR) for no chemotherapy is always higher than that for chemotherapy at all *RS* values, so chemotherapy is always the preferred therapy. Within each therapy, higher *RS* is a predictor of worse prognosis with slope $\beta_2$ and $(\beta_2 + \beta_3)$ per unit increase in *RS* for no chemotherapy and chemotherapy, respectively. Clinically, chemotherapy is always more efficacious, though some patients may still feel that the gain is too small to outweigh the adverse effects of treatment.

For a qualitative interaction, the appropriate illustration may be more like that in Figure 19.2. There is a point at approximately $RS = 12.5$ for which the benefit of treatment would change. Below this value, no chemotherapy is the preferred choice, but above this point, chemotherapy would have a lower failure rate. In both cases, *RS* appears to be prognostic within its treatment group though the slope for chemotherapy is much less pronounced. Note that if one started with a simple model with only main effects in this scenario $\log \lambda(t;trt, z) = \log \lambda_0(t) + trt\,\beta_1 + z\,\beta_2$, then the treatment parameter estimate $\hat{\beta}_1$ would be close to zero due to the interaction masking the impact of treatment. Thus, a significant treatment effect is not a precondition to investigate a predictive effect, particularly when there is an a priori hypothesis that the interaction exists. Finally, we note that we describe the crossover point in the model as a fixed point, but it is of course subject to sampling error as we consider later.

### 19.2.3 EXAMPLE FROM SWOG TRIAL S8814

To illustrate this approach, we use SWOG study S8814, which compared no chemotherapy to chemotherapy for node-positive hormone-receptor positive breast cancer (Albain et al., 2009). The overall trial showed a significant benefit of chemotherapy particularly if delivered before tamoxifen therapy commenced (Albain et al., 2009).

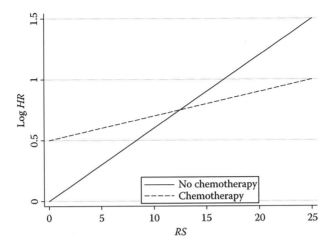

**FIGURE 19.2**    Modeled relationship of the Cox regression log HR relating survival to RS and therapy. In this model chemotherapy has a lower failure rate than no chemotherapy only for higher values of RS.

For available tumor samples, the 21-gene assay (OncotypeDX) was evaluated (Albain et al., 2010). This assay yields *RS* on a scale of 0–100 indicating likelihood of a recurrence. It had previously been shown to be predictive in node-negative disease (Paik et al., 2006), but not yet in node-positive disease. For disease-free survival up to 5 years, there was a significant interaction of chemotherapy and continuous *RS* ($p=0.029$) with adjustment for the main effects of chemotherapy, *RS*, and number of positive nodes (1–3 versus 4+). The estimated model leads to a crossing of the log HRs at an approximate *RS* value of 19. Above this value, the model suggests that chemotherapy has better outcomes than no chemotherapy, though the sampling variability around this point is large. The model also indicates that below this value, chemotherapy may not be beneficial despite the results of the overall trial. We did assume that the impact of *RS* on the log hazard rate was linear. The assumption of linearity was supported by testing with fractional polynomials as described by Royston and Sauerbrei (2004). This retrospective study has limitations including the small sample size, evolution of chemotherapy since the original trial was conducted, and addition of new endocrine therapies. Therefore, a prospective trial is necessary to confirm that chemotherapy may not be beneficial for some values of *RS* and to establish the correct cutoff.

## 19.3    TRIAL DESIGN FOR TESTING A PREDICTIVE MARKER

### 19.3.1    STATISTICAL MODEL

Designing a trial to test prediction of treatment benefit using a continuous marker requires categorizing the marker (e.g., as positive or negative based on the cutoff) or using the marker as a continuous value. Preservation of the marker as continuous will increase power compared to using cutpoints (Royston et al., 2006). A continuous marker can be used directly in the model or the marker can be converted into percentile values based on a known distribution of the marker values in a population and modeled directly on the percentile scale (Huang et al., 2007). In the absence of a known distribution, one may have to model the marker directly. Again, we assume an underlying model using the interaction term

$$\log \lambda(t; trt, z) = \log \lambda_0(t) + trt\ \beta_1 + z\ \beta_2 + trt * z\ \beta_3$$

The first requirement is that power be sufficient so that testing of the estimate of $\beta_3$ has high probability of rejecting the null hypothesis that $\beta_3 = 0$. A significant interaction will suggest that the value of the marker may determine the efficacy of treatment for patient with that marker value. The second requirement is that the log HRs for the two treatment groups cross for some value of the marker internal to the range of values for the marker (Figure 19.2). This point of equivalence is designated as $\theta$. If the model is correct, then equivalence between treatments is achieved at marker value $\theta = -\beta_1/\beta_3$ estimated by $\hat{\theta} = -\hat{\beta}_1/\hat{\beta}_3$ from the fitted Cox model. However, the crossover point has estimated variance based on the delta method of $\text{Var}(\hat{\theta}) = 1/\hat{\beta}_3^2 \left[ V_{11} + 2\hat{\theta}V_{13} + \hat{\theta}^2 V_{33} \right]$ using the appropriate covariance terms from the fitted model. Before a treatment is designated as beneficial, it must be convincingly superior to no treatment, not just equivalent. For that reason, we take the upper limit of the 95% CI on $\hat{\theta}$ as the point for which there is convincing evidence of benefit. This cutpoint can be based on the upper limit of a 1-sided Wald confidence interval for the point of equivalence:

$$c = \left( \hat{\theta} + 1.645 * \sqrt{\text{Var}(\hat{\theta})} \right)$$

This is illustrated in Figure 19.3. The actual value of the HR at the upper limit of the confidence interval will vary, but may provide a reasonable estimate of a clinically meaningful difference. One can see that the variance depends on the strength of the interaction term and the individual variances of the treatment effect, interaction effect, and their covariance. The Wald confidence interval assumes asymptotic normality of the estimate of the point of equivalence, $\hat{\theta}$. Alternatively, one can determine the upper bound of the interval using profile likelihood methods. Let $ll(\beta)$ be the partial log-likelihood at $\beta$. We would search for the upper bound $\tilde{\theta}$ that satisfies the following $2[ll(\hat{\beta}) - ll(\beta)] = \chi_\alpha^2(1df)$, where

$$\log \lambda(t; trt, z) = \log \lambda_0(t) + trt\ \beta_1 + z\ \beta_2 + trt * z\ \beta_3$$

is maximized subject to the constraint that $\beta_1 = -\theta\beta_3$ defining an upper bound on the range of equivalency.

## 19.3.2 SAMPLE SIZE, POWER, AND HYPOTHESIS TESTING

Sample sizes for testing interaction terms are often larger than sample sizes for testing constant treatment effects. However, testing a continuous interaction may not require the huge sample sizes that a dichotomized marker would require. Simulation

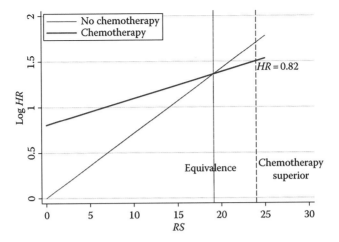

**FIGURE 19.3**   Modeled relationship of the Cox regression log HR relating survival to RS and therapy. The short dashed line indicates the RS value where treatments are equivalent. The long dash line indicates the upper bound of the 95% confidence interval on the point of equivalence.

is probably required in most complex situations. The goal is to choose a sample size that gives 80%–90% power to reject the null hypothesis of no interaction when comparing the model with an interaction of marker and treatment to a reduced model without the interaction term. If the interaction is statistically significant, then one would determine if the point of equivalency is interior to the range of marker values. This would then be followed by construction of a one-sided confidence limit on the point of equivalence that will allow estimation of the cutoff point for recommending therapy. Should the interaction term not be statistically significant, then step-down testing would suggest that the interaction term be dropped and that the treatment effect be tested using the marker as a prognostic term only (main effect). We assume that there is already sufficient evidence that the marker is prognostic, so testing the marker per se may not be of interest. To summarize the steps:

1. Test the interaction term in the model

$$\log \lambda(t; trt, z) = \log \lambda_0(t) + trt\, \beta_1 + z\, \beta_2 + trt * z\, \beta_3$$

   versus

$$\log \lambda(t; trt, z) = \log \lambda_0(t) + trt\, \beta_1 + z\, \beta_2$$

2.
   a.  If the interaction term is significant, establish the cutoff point based on

$$\hat{\theta} = -\frac{\hat{\beta}_1}{\hat{\beta}_3} \quad \mathrm{Var}\left(\hat{\theta}\right) = \frac{1}{\hat{\beta}_3^2}\left[V_{11} + 2\hat{\theta}V_{13} + \hat{\theta}^2 V_{33}\right]$$

$$c = \left( \hat{\theta} + 1.645 * \sqrt{\mathrm{Var}\left(\hat{\theta}\right)} \right)$$

    b.  If the interaction term is not significant, test the treatment effect overall using

$$\log \lambda(t; trt, z) = \log \lambda_0(t) + trt\,\beta_1 + z\,\beta_2$$

versus

$$\log \lambda(t; trt, z) = \log \lambda_0(t) + z\,\beta_2$$

In the presence of a significant interaction with crossing HRs, a cutpoint for use of therapy can be derived, and one can give predicted benefit from either treatment at each value of the marker. In the absence of a significant interaction, the effect of treatment can be estimated as a single HR over the entire range of marker values tested.

### 19.3.3   MODEL DIAGNOSTICS

The assertion that the marker acts linearly on the log HR may be a strong assumption. After testing the primary hypotheses, secondary analyses can consider model form. There are several methods available for checking this assumption. The first method would be a fractional polynomial model of degree 2 that would allow departure from linearity and provide a direct likelihood-based test of the linearity assumption (Royston and Sauerbrei, 2004). A second method would be the subpopulation treatment effect pattern plot (STEPP)—a nonparametric approach described by Bonetti and Gelber (2000). A third method would be derived from a model fit based on $\log \lambda(t; trt, z) = \log \lambda_0(t) + trt\,\beta_1$ without inclusion of the marker at all. After fitting the model, delta beta diagnostics for treatment would be computed assessing each individual's effect on the treatment coefficient. A plot of these delta betas against the marker $z$ can indicate the nature of the functional association of the marker and log hazard rate separately by treatment group (Barlow and Prentice, 1988). Finally, one may wish to use the ranks of the marker values, rather than the actual marker values, to test the model $\log \lambda(t; trt, z) = \log \lambda_0(t) + trt\,\beta_1 + \mathrm{rank}(z)\,\beta_2 + trt*\mathrm{rank}(z)\,\beta_3$. This approach is very similar to that described by Janes et al. (2011) who use the marker percentile as the predictor where the percentiles are known from external data, but could be generated from internal data using the ranked data.

## 19.4   APPLICATION TO TRIAL DESIGN

### 19.4.1   SWOG TRIAL S1007

The earlier results of SWOG trial S8814 suggested that chemotherapy was beneficial, but only for higher values of the *RS*. Giving chemotherapy to women with node-positive breast cancer has become standard of care, but clearly some women may not benefit if they have a low risk for recurrence. The recently launched S1007 RxPONDER trial will test the efficacy of chemotherapy in women with low *RS*s (0–25) who have only one to three positive nodes and who have endocrine-responsive disease. This group is at low risk for recurrence and did not seem to benefit from chemotherapy in the retrospective evaluation of S8114. The sample size is constructed on finding a significant interaction of *RS* and randomized treatment (chemotherapy or no chemotherapy; two-sided $\alpha = 0.05$) with 80% power followed by the identification of the cutoff using the aforementioned procedure. Note that this is not a test of the 21-gene assay directly, which might be directly tested by randomization to its use or not. Instead, we assume that women with $RS > 25$ need chemotherapy and only examine the relationship of *RS* to the efficacy of chemotherapy for women with *RS* in the range 0–25.

### 19.4.2 POWER CALCULATIONS

While there may be closed form sample size estimation procedures for estimation of interaction terms (Schmoor et al., 2000), we believed that this situation was complex enough to use simulation. Parameter estimates were derived from the S8814 study restricting consideration to women with 1–3 positive nodes and *RS* in the range 0–25. A Weibull model provided a better fit than the exponential model, so this model was used to simulate 10,000 replications of the trial. For each replication, we used a Cox model to test the interaction term. Empirical power was determined by the probability of rejection of the null hypothesis for the interaction term. If it was significant and the point of equivalence was interior to the range 0–25, then the upper bound of the 95% Wald CI was computed to determine the cutpoint. In some cases, the upper cutpoint would exceed 25, and therefore the clinical interpretation is that chemotherapy is not needed for the entire range 0–25. If the interaction was not significant, then a main effect of chemotherapy was tested over the entire range.

Other parameter configurations were tested beyond using the direct estimates from the S8814 trial. For example, under the null hypothesis of no interaction, the correct test size of 5% was obtained. If the model is further simplified and thus there is no treatment effect, again the correct test size is obtained. Examination of the 95% confidence interval for the point of equivalence showed 95% of the obtained intervals included the true equivalence point. Other simulations showed remarkable robustness to some violations of the linearity assumption. There was a concern that the linearity assumption may lead to an optimistic sample size estimate if the relationship was monotonic in *RS*, but not linear. Simulations showed that these concerns were not warranted. Departures from linearity tend to depress the magnitude of the interaction term thus resulting in more conservative estimates. Furthermore, while estimates at the extremes are affected, estimation of the point of equivalence and its confidence interval is less affected, thus making the calculations somewhat robust to misspecification.

It was also expected that there will be treatment crossovers from patients who do not want to comply with their treatment assignment and get the opposite treatment from that randomized with a probability depending on the *RS*. This inflates the sample size since the analysis is intent-to-treat and patients are analyzed by randomization assignment. The actual simulated population was 3800 (including 5% treatment crossovers), but the sample size goal was increased to 4000 to allow for dropouts and ineligibility. The final sample size of 4000 will require screening approximately 9000 women to determine if their *RS* value is ≤25 since the 21-gene assay is not routinely done.

### 19.4.3 PLANNED ANALYSES

The protocol includes interim analyses of the interaction as well as safety analyses that could indicate the no chemotherapy group has lower survival than expected compared to the chemotherapy group early on. The primary analysis of the interaction is consistent with how the simulations were performed. Nonetheless, the underlying model assumes that the effect of *RS* on the log hazards ratio is linear with different slopes for each treatment group. This assumption will be tested in the analysis using alternative models such as fractional polynomials. A successful trial would include (1) a statistically significant linear interaction, (2) an estimated cutpoint below the upper bound of 25, (3) Kaplan–Meier displays showing no benefit of chemotherapy below the cutpoint, but benefit above the cutpoint, and (4) estimated benefit of treatment at each value on the range 0–25 with 95% confidence intervals. The last goal may require a departure from the linearity assumption if the diagnostic tools indicate that the linear model does not provide a sufficient description.

## 19.5 CONCLUSIONS

While methods to test prediction of treatment benefit for dichotomous markers are available, there has been less development using continuous markers. We are unaware of any clinical trials that have been designed to primarily test prediction using linear markers. Testing the ability of a continuous marker to optimize treatment assignment can be done by a sequence of steps. The first is to demonstrate a significant interaction of the marker value with treatment assignment, followed by a determination of a point of equivalence and its associated confidence interval. The upper bound of that confidence interval can mark a cutoff for choosing a treatment. The same logic can be applied to designing a trial to test marker prediction. While sample sizes can be large, the sample size is moderated by using a continuous marker in a linear prediction model. Use of cutpoints to design the trial will require larger sample sizes and thus imperil the likelihood of the trial going forward.

## ACKNOWLEDGMENT

This work was supported in part by grant #CA038926 from the National Cancer Institute.

# REFERENCES

Albain KS, Barlow WE, Ravdin PM, Farrar WB, Burton GV, Ketchel SJ et al. 2009. Adjuvant chemotherapy and timing of tamoxifen in postmenopausal patients with endocrine-responsive, node-positive breast cancer: A phase 3, open-label, randomised controlled trial. *Lancet*, 374: 2055–2063.

Albain KS, Barlow WE, Shak S, Hortobagyi GN, Livingston RB, Yeh IT et al. 2010. Prognostic and predictive value of the 21-gene recurrence score assay in postmenopausal women with node-positive, oestrogen-receptor-positive breast cancer on chemotherapy: A retrospective analysis of a randomised trial. *Lancet Oncology*, 11: 55–65.

Barlow WE, Prentice RL. 1988. Residuals for relative risk regression models. *Biometrika*, 75: 65–74.

Bonetti M, Gelber RD. 2000. A graphical method to assess treatment–covariate interactions using the Cox model on subsets of the data. *Statistics in Medicine*, 19: 2595–2609.

Hoering A, Leblanc M, Crowley JJ. 2008. Randomized phase III clinical trial designs for targeted agents. *Clinical Cancer Research*, 14: 4358–4367.

Huang Y, Sullivan Pepe M, Feng Z. 2007. Evaluating the predictiveness of a continuous marker. *Biometrics*, 63: 1181–1188.

Janes H, Pepe MS, Bossuyt PM, Barlow WE. 2011. Measuring the performance of markers for guiding treatment decisions. *Annals of Internal Medicine*, 154: 253–259.

McGuire WL, Tandon AK, Allred DC, Chamness GC, Ravdin PM, Clark GM. 1992. Prognosis and treatment decisions in patients with breast cancer without axillary node involvement. *Cancer*, 70: 1775–1781.

Paik S, Tang G, Shak S, Kim C, Baker J, Kim W et al. 2006. Gene expression and benefit of chemotherapy in women with node-negative, estrogen receptor-positive breast cancer. *Journal of Clinical Oncology*, 24: 3726–3734.

Royston P, Altman DG, Sauerbrei W. 2006. Dichotomizing continuous predictors in multiple regression: A bad idea. *Statistics in Medicine*, 25: 127–141.

Royston P, Sauerbrei W. 2004. A new approach to modelling interactions between treatment and continuous covariates in clinical trials by using fractional polynomials. *Statistics in Medicine*, 23: 2509–2525.

Sargent DJ, Conley BA, Allegra C, Collette L. 2005. Clinical trial designs for predictive marker validation in cancer treatment trials. *Journal of Clinical Oncology*, 23: 2020–2027.

Schmoor C, Sauerbrei W, Schumacher M. 2000. Sample size considerations for the evaluation of prognostic factors in survival analysis. *Statistics in Medicine*, 19: 441–452.

Schumacher M, Hollander N, Schwarzer G, Sauerbrei W. 2006. Prognostic factor studies. In *Handbook of Statistics in Clinical Oncology*, 2nd edn., J. Crowley and D.P. Ankerst (eds.), pp. 289–333. Boca Raton, FL: Chapman & Hall/CRC.

# 20 Software for Design and Analysis of Clinical Trials

*J. Jack Lee and Nan Chen*

## CONTENTS

## 20.1  INTRODUCTION

Recent advances in molecular biology, genomics, and targeted agent development have fueled the rapid progress in clinical oncology. In parallel, developments in statistical theory and computation have continued to provide better methods and tools for dealing with complex problems. All these efforts lead to more advanced, yet complicated study design, conduct, and analysis, which depend more and more heavily on computing resources from both the software and hardware points of view. Because a wide range of complex calculation methods are involved, it is difficult and complicated for statisticians to develop their own codes from scratch every time when a new design is implemented or an analysis is performed. Moreover, the emerging Bayesian methods and adaptive trial designs (Berry 2006, Biswas et al. 2009, Berry et al. 2010, Lee et al. 2010), which introduced many new concepts and calculation methods, pose new challenges for software development. Developing and debugging codes could take a huge amount of time, and, without thoroughly being tested, the best effort from any individual is also subject to errors. Fortunately, many useful and valuable computer software and resources are now available from both research and commercial entities. Instead of developing their own codes from scratch every time, statisticians and clinical trial researchers will benefit much from using available design and analysis software that has been developed and tested. In this chapter, we will give a broad overview on selected software resources relevant to cancer clinical trials. It is impossible to do a comprehensive review in this knowledge explosion era. The choice of the software is limited by the authors' knowledge and experience. Undoubtedly, many valuable tools could be omitted and not covered. However, we hope the information provided in this chapter can be used as a starting point for the quest of identifying and developing more and better software for cancer clinical trials.

In the recent literature, there are some reviews on software packages relevant to clinical trials. Tai and Seldrup (2000) reviewed software packages on data management, design, and analysis of clinical trials. Some clinical trial packages (nQuery, PEST, and POWER) and analysis tools (SAS, SPSS, and STATA) were discussed in the review. Arena and Rockette (2005) provided an overview of software that is related to the design, management, and analysis of clinical trials. Wassmer and Vandemeulebroecke (2006) reviewed many popular group sequential and adaptive design software packages for clinical trials. They evaluated packages such as ADDPLAN, EAST, PASS, and PEST and some source code for SAS, Fortran, and R. A comprehensive review on nQuery and PASS is given by Lane (2002). This review listed the features for each software package and provided a detailed comparison between them. However, this review was published in 2002, and many new features have been developed in nQuery and PASS since then.

Most reviews discussed earlier focused on a specific field (i.e., group sequential designs) and included much calculation details. In this review, our intent is to give readers a brief introduction of popular software packages for clinical trial designs. However, due to the space limit, we are not able to discuss the calculation in detail in this review, which can be easily found in the related literature.

Most previous reviews are based on frequentist methods, and almost no Bayesian method–based software is discussed. In the past decade, at the MD Anderson Cancer Center, many Bayesian clinical trial designs have been developed and applied due to their unique strength and flexibility of handling complex designs (Biswas et al. 2009). Many software packages for implementing such designs have been developed, and users can download them for free from the software downloading website (https://biostatistics.mdanderson.org/SoftwareDownload/). In this review, we will also introduce some Bayesian clinical trial design software to the readers who are interested. The source of all the software described below can be found in Table 20.1.

## 20.2 SOFTWARE PACKAGES FOR POWER/SAMPLE SIZE CALCULATION

### 20.2.1 POWER ANALYSIS AND SAMPLE SIZE

Power analysis and sample size (PASS) is a commercial software package for power analysis and sample size calculation based on frequentist methods. Its power and sample size calculation procedure library includes analysis of mean and proportion of one or two groups, correlated or paired, cross-over design, ANOVA, regression/correlation, survival analysis, noninferiority, group sequential analysis, equivalence tools, and many other procedures. The package comes with a detailed manual containing tutorials, examples, references, and instructions; users can easily become familiar with its usage. Each procedure in PASS is validated using published document examples, and the validation examples are attached with the manual. It has a very good graphic user interface (GUI) on the Windows platform (Figure 20.1) and a detailed help system, making its usage convenient and straightforward.

### 20.2.2 NQUERY

nQuery is a commercial software package for sample size and power calculation for a wide range of frequentist analysis. It calculates the sample size and power for means, proportions, agreements, regression, survival analysis, and nonparametric test and offers analysis for more than 90 different tests. It has a function for generating randomization lists for patient treatment allocation, and one can use this tool for patient treatment assignment in a randomized trial. It has a user-friendly GUI

**TABLE 20.1**

**Software Packages for Clinical Trial Design and Analysis**

| Name | URL | Free or Commercial[a] |
|---|---|---|
| | **Power and Sample Size** | |
| nQuery | http://www.statistical-solutions-software.com/products-page/nquery-advisor-sample-size-software/ | C |
| PASS | http://www.ncss.com/pass.html | C |
| STPLAN | https://biostatistics.mdanderson.org/SoftwareDownload/ | F |
| StudySize | http://www.studysize.com/ | F |
| | **Phase I** | |
| CRM simulator | https://biostatistics.mdanderson.org/softwaredownload | F |
| EffTox | https://biostatistics.mdanderson.org/softwaredownload/ | F |
| BMA-CRM | https://biostatistics.mdanderson.org/softwaredownload/ | F |
| TITE-CRM | http://roadrunner.cancer.med.umich.edu/wiki/index.php/TITE-CRM | F |
| ATDPH1 | http://linus.nci.nih.gov/~brb/Methodologic.htm | F |
| Modified CRM v2.0 | http://www.cancerbiostats.onc.jhmi.edu/software.cfm | F |
| JLB design | http://odin.mdacc.tmc.edu/~yuanj/software.htm | F |
| EWOC | https://apps.winship.emory.edu/biostatistics/software_ewoc.php | F |
| | **Phase II** | |
| Simon two-stage design | http://linus.nci.nih.gov/~brb/Opt.htm | F |
| Green-Benedetti-Crowely | http://www.swogstat.org/stat/public/TwoStage/2stage1.htm | F |
| Bryant-Day design | http://www.upci.upmc.edu/bf/ClinicalStudyDesign/Phase 2 BryantDay.cfm | F |
| Predictive probability design | https://biostatistics.mdanderson.org/softwaredownload | F |
| BFDesigner | https://biostatistics.mdanderson.org/softwaredownload | F |
| Multc99 | https://biostatistics.mdanderson.org/softwaredownload | F |
| CTD system | http://www.cancer.duke.edu/modules/CTDSystems54/index.php?id = 3 | F |
| One-arm binomial | http://www.swogstat.org/stat/public/one_binomial.htm | F |
| One-arm survival | http://www.swogstat.org/stat/public/one_survival.htm | F |
| Two-arm survival | http://www.swogstat.org/stat/public/survival_twoarm.htm | F |
| Biomarker-targeted randomized design | http://linus.nci.nih.gov/brb/samplesize/td.html | F |
| Biomarker-stratified randomized design | http://linus.nci.nih.gov/brb/samplesize/sdpap.html | F |
| Optimal Two-stage designs for phase II clinical trials | http://linus.nci.nih.gov/brb/samplesize/otsd.html | F |
| Sample size for integrated phase II/III trial | http://linus.nci.nih.gov/brb/samplesize/ip23study1.html | F |

## TABLE 20.1 (continued)
## Software Packages for Clinical Trial Design and Analysis

| Name | URL | Free or Commercial[a] |
|---|---|---|
| **Phase III** | | |
| EAST | http://www.cytel.com/software/east.aspx | C |
| PEST | http://www.maths.lancs.ac.uk/department/research/ statistics/mps/pest | C |
| gsDesign | R package | F |
| ADDPLAN | http://www.addplan.com/ | C |
| S + SeqTrial | http://spotfire.tibco.com/products/splus-seqtrial.aspx | C |
| Expected death on a study | http://www.swogstat.org/stat/public/expdeath.htm | F |
| **Tools and Others** | | |
| Adaptive randomization | https://biostatistics.mdanderson.org/softwaredownload | F |
| Parameter solver | https://biostatistics.mdanderson.org/softwaredownload | F |
| Predictive probability calculation | https://biostatistics.mdanderson.org/softwaredownload | F |
| TTEDesigner | https://biostatistics.mdanderson.org/softwaredownload | F |
| Interaction survival | http://www.swogstat.org/stat/public/int_survival.htm | F |
| **Web-based Calculators and Resources** | | |
| Biometric research of NCI | http://linus.nci.nih.gov/~brb/ | F |
| Power and sample size | http://www.epibiostat.ucsf.edu/biostat/sampsize.html | F |
| Sample size | http://www.swogstat.org/statoolsout.html | F |
| Simon's two-stage design | http://www.upci.upmc.edu/bf/resources.cfm | F |
| MD Anderson | https://biostatistics.mdanderson.org/ SoftwareDownload/ | F |
| Sidney Kimmel Comprehensive Cancer Center in Johns Hopkins | http://www.cancerbiostats.onc.jhmi.edu/software.cfm | F |
| MGH biostatistics center at Harvard University | http://hedwig.mgh.harvard.edu/biostatistics/ software?tid_1 = All | F |
| SAS | http://www.sas.com/ | C |
| R | http://www.r-project.org/ | F |
| SPlus | http://spotfire.tibco.com/products/s-plus/statistical- analysis-software.aspx | F |
| SPSS | http://www.spss.com/ | C |
| Stata | http://www.stata.com/ | C |
| GraphPad Prism | http://www.graphpad.com/prism/prism.htm | C |
| BUGS, WinBUGS, and JAGS | http://www.mrc-bsu.com.ac.uk/bugs/ | F |

[a] F, Free; C, Commercial.

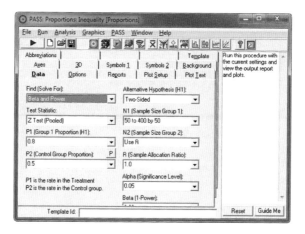

**FIGURE 20.1**    Screenshot of software PASS.

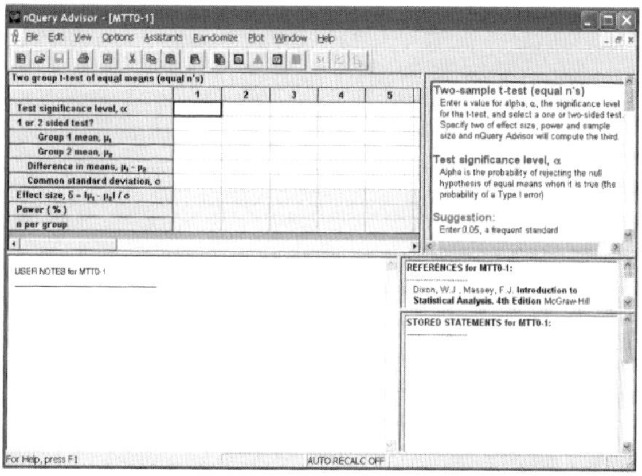

**FIGURE 20.2**    Screenshot of software nQuery.

(Figure 20.2) and detailed help documents, making sample size and power calculation straightforward. A new module nTerim is shipped with the nQuery Advisor 7 for group sequential trial designs, and it includes the spending functions of Pocock (1977), O'Brien and Fleming (1979), Hwang et al. (1990), and other functions.

## 20.2.3 STPLAN

STPLAN is a software package for designing frequentist clinical trial. It covers a wide range of frequentist tests and performs power, sample size, and significance calculation for different types of analysis. It offers tests for binomial distribution, Poisson distribution, normal distribution, exponential distribution, and survival time analysis. Most common frequentist one-sample and two-sample tests are included in the package. For a practical test, users need to set an unknown variable from distribution parameters, significance level, power, and sample size, and the package then calculates the value of the unknown variable from other specified parameters. The program is useful and free for downloading. It is easy to use and has a simple command line tool, running on DOS/Windows operating systems, but lacks a more sophisticated user interface.

### 20.2.4 StudySize

StudySize is a commercial software package for performing most standard hypothesis testing, point estimation, and confidence interval calculation. It includes equivalence and noninferiority tests. It also can perform nonparametric tests (Wilcoxon test and Sign test). It can run group sequential interim analyses for most tests and confidence interval calculation. It has a user-friendly Windows GUI.

## 20.3 PHASE I CLINICAL TRIAL SOFTWARE

### 20.3.1 CRM Simulator

Continual reassessment method (CRM) simulator is a useful tool for phase I clinical trial based on the CRM (O'Quigley et al. 1990). It can be used for trial planning and implementation. Using this software package, one can simulate trials with different parameter values, observing the operating characteristics for different scenarios. Input parameters include the prior mean probability of toxicity at each dose level, target probability of toxicity, different scenarios (true probability of toxicity at each dose level), and simulation setting parameters (e.g., repeat numbers of the simulations). The software package simulates each trial with a different random number sequence and at the end collects all data to produce the output. The output includes the selection probability at each dose level, average number of patients treated at each dose level, average toxicities for each simulated trial, and other information. It has a user-friendly graphical GUI on Windows platforms (Figure 20.3), and users can easily adjust each parameter and analyze output data.

### 20.3.2 BMA-CRM

This software package implements the Bayesian model average continual reassessment method (Yin and Yuan 2009) for dose finding in the phase I clinical trial, and it can be used for clinical trial design and trial conduct. The difference between the BMA-CRM and the CRM is that the BMA-CRM utilizes the Bayesian model average method for dose level selection based on multiple sets of probability of prior mean of toxicity and the traditional CRM uses only one set of prior mean of toxicity for the dose level selection. Usually, the BMA-CRM gives more robust results than the traditional CRM. Parameters for the BMA-CRM are similar to that of the CRM except that multisets of prior are needed. This package has a user-friendly GUI and runs on Windows platforms (Figure 20.4).

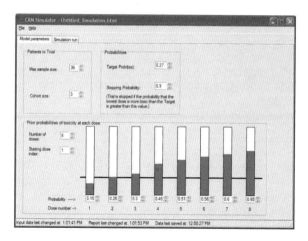

**FIGURE 20.3**    Screenshot of software CRM simulator.

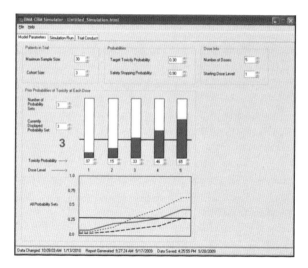

**FIGURE 20.4**    Screenshot of software BMA-CRM.

## 20.3.3   TITE-CRM

The TITE-CRM (Cheung and Chappell 2000) software is used for dose finding in
the situation that patient outcomes are not instantaneous and late-onset effects play
an important role. It is based on the time-to-event continual reassessment method
and a weighted dose model to extend the CRM method. For ongoing trials, it has the
functions of estimating the probability of toxicities, selecting dose level for the successive patient based on current data. With this software package, one can perform
trial simulations with different scenarios and calculate the operating characteristics
for phase I trial design planning. This package is an SAS program but does not have
a GUI. It has a detailed user guide for users to run the program.

## 20.3.4   EWOC

EWOC (escalation with overdose control) is a software tool for conducting cancer phase I clinical trial based on such design (Babb et al. 1998). It calculates the maximum tolerated dose level by utilizing an adaptive escalation scheme with all information available at the time of dose assignment. The design reaches the maximum tolerated dose level at a fast rate, while still subject to the constraints of the prespecified overdose proportion. Compared with the CRM, this method demonstrates lower overdose rates, fewer toxicities, and comparable accuracy. This software tool is based on windows platforms. It has a user-friendly GUI and well-organized introduction documents.

## 20.3.5   JLB DESIGN

The software package for the JLB design (Ji et al. 2007) is distributed in the form of an Excel macro, and one can easily use it to carry out the phase I trial if he/she has some basic knowledge of the Excel macro. The calculation method has two important components: a beta/binomial model and a dose-assignment rule based on posterior toxicity probability. Two parameters are required for running the macro: target toxicity probability and the maximum sample size. Once the parameters are specified, the macro will generate a spreadsheet to guide users for trial monitoring and dose assignment for each patient enrolled. This software is not compatible with Mac OS, Unix, or Linux; it works only on the Excel Windows version.

## 20.3.6   EffTox

Software package EffTox is a dose-finding tool for phase I/II trial designs based on trade-offs between treatment efficacy and toxicity (Thall and Cook 2004, 2006). It can handle trinary or bivariate binary patient outcomes for both efficacy and toxicity. One can adjust different parameter combinations to balance the drug efficacy and toxicity for patient dose level assignment. The dose level for the successive patients is determined by the current outcome and the efficacy-toxicity contour. One can use this package to design trials by performing trial simulations or to conduct real trial by enrolling patients, recording their outcomes, and determining the dose for treating subsequent patients. The package has a user-friendly GUI and runs on Windows platforms (Figure 20.5).

## 20.4   PHASE II TRIAL DESIGN SOFTWARE

### 20.4.1   Simon Two-Stage Design

Simon two-stage design (Simon 1989) is a small program for the popular two-stage optimal and minimax designs. The optimal design minimizes the expected sample size under the null hypothesis, and the minimax design attains the smallest total sample size that satisfies the error constraints. The usage of the program is very simple, and only several parameters (null and alternative response rates, maximum

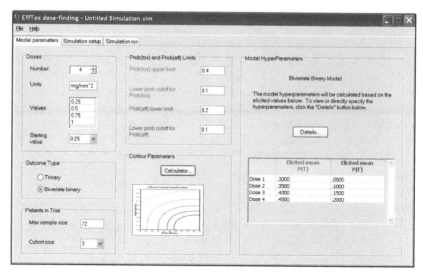

**FIGURE 20.5**   Screenshot of software EffTox.

sample size, and Type I and II error constraints) are required. It calculates the total sample size, the interim sample size, and the stopping boundary. It runs very fast on a DOS platform (or using a command line console on Windows). However, in the latest Windows 7 OS, it has a compatibility problem, but running the program in a DOS simulator (i.e., DOSBox) can easily solve the problem.

## 20.4.2   WEB-BASED TWO-STAGE DESIGN

A very useful two-stage phase II trial design tool is based on a web-application at SWOG (http://www.swogstat.org/stat/public/TwoStage/2stage1.htm). The calculator can estimate the sample size, interim analysis points, stopping boundaries, and power values for a two-stage Green–Benedetti–Crowely design (Green et al. 1997). It allows both futility and efficacy stopping after the first stage of the trial. It has two versions: The JavaScript version can be saved as a web-page, and one can run it in a web-browser without internet connection. The server version is provided in case the user's web-browser does not support JavaScript.

CTD system (clinical trial design system), developed at Duke Cancer Institute, is a user-friendly web-based two-stage design tool. It plots the expected sample size versus total sample size curve and indicates the points corresponding to the optimal and minimax designs. It supports two types of two-stage designs: allowing only futility stopping (Simon's two-stage design) or allowing both futility and efficacy stopping.

Another free web-based two-stage phase II calculator is for Bryant-Day design (Bryant and Day 1995) calculation. The toxicity is incorporated into the Simon's two-stage design, and a trial will be stopped either by unacceptable clinical response or toxicity. Probabilities of accepting poor responses, accepting toxic drug, rejecting good drug, and other parameters are required for the calculation. The application calculates the stopping boundaries based on patients' response and toxicity. It is web-based and users can easily run the application from their web-browser.

### 20.4.3    PREDICTIVE PROBABILITY DESIGN

Predictive probability design (Lee and Liu 2008) is a useful tool for designing single-arm phase II trial based on the predictive probability calculation. Stopping boundaries at each interim look are calculated based on the predictive probability of the final inference decision. The software package helps users find the cut-off values of the predictive probability and the corresponding stopping boundary calculation. Users need to specify the type I and type II error constraints, interim look points, the search domain of the cut-off values and priors, the program will search the parameter domain to find whether a solution exists to satisfy both type I and type II error constraints. If a solution is found, the cut-off value, stopping boundaries, and the corresponding operating characteristics will be calculated and displayed. The software has a user-friendly GUI on Windows platforms, and one can easily use it with the assistance from the embedded user guide (Figure 20.6).

### 20.4.4    MULTC99

Multc99 (Thall et al. 1995) is a program for designing single-arm phase I/II trial with multiple outcomes, typically, efficacy and toxicity. A Dirichlet-multinomial model is applied to describe discrete multivariate outcomes, and Bayesian stopping rules are set for high rates of adverse outcomes or low rates of desirable outcomes. Users can use this software to calculate the operating characteristics of different scenarios and stopping boundaries. The software is a command line DOS program and a simplified Windows version covers only the basic features.

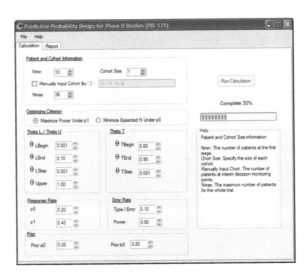

**FIGURE 20.6**    Screenshot of software predictive probability designer.

### 20.4.5 BFDESIGNER

BFDesigner is a useful tool for single-arm phase II clinical trial design. The software package is based on the method of Bayesian hypothesis tests via Bayes factor and nonlocal alternative prior density proposed by Johnson and Cook (2009). This method provides more efficient stopping rules than the commonly used Bayesian posterior credible interval and frequentist methods. The software package is a command line tool, but a detailed manual is attached with the package, making the usage of this tool straightforward.

## 20.5 PHASE III CLINICAL TRIAL SOFTWARE

### 20.5.1 EAST

EAST is a widely used commercial package for group sequential trial planning and analysis. It supports normal, binomial, survival, and other type of end points and can be applied for superiority, noninferiority, and equivalence trial designs. Its spending function family includes Pocock, O'Brien–Fleming, Wang–Tsiatis, and other functions. Calculation results include stopping boundaries, power, expected number of events, and sample size with different scenarios. The software (Figure 20.7) comes with a user-friendly wizard system to help one design a group sequential trial in a very convenient way. A detailed manual includes many software usage tutorials and examples.

### 20.5.2 PEST

The PEST ("planning and evaluation of sequential trials") is a commercial software package for sequential trial design and analysis. PEST offers a wide range of response types including binary, normal, survival, and interval censored survival

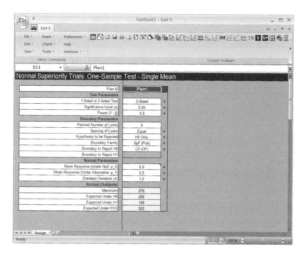

**FIGURE 20.7** Screenshot of software EAST.

times. It includes five modules: design, simulator, monitor, analyze, and view for different purposes of usage. Using this package, one can calculate stopping boundary and sample size in the design stage and perform analysis such as significance level and interval estimation at the end of the trial. The package is developed using C and SAS and runs within an SAS session on Windows platforms, making communicating with other SAS codes easy.

### 20.5.3 GSDESIGN (R PACKAGE)

gsDesign is an R package for group sequential design, and it can be installed using the R installation function. It supports common spending functions including Pocock, O'Brien–Fleming, and Hwang–Shih–DeCani types. For a standard group sequential design, it is not as convenient as the commercial packages such as the EAST package, but it is free and offers flexibility for accommodating nonstandard designs in the R environment.

### 20.5.4 ADDPLAN

The ADDPLAN (adaptive designs-plan and analysis) is a commercial software package for adaptive clinical trial designs. It offers a comprehensive design planning tools for means, proportions and survivals, one-sided and two-sided, noninferiority, and equivalence tests. At interim monitoring points, it can recalculate the sample size for the ongoing trial based on the current data and adaptively adjust the trial based on the patient outcomes.

### 20.5.5 S + SEQTRIAL

S + SeqTrial is a S-Plus software library for designing, monitoring, and analyzing the group sequential trials. It is integrated into the S-Plus software and allows users to directly use or extend the package functions for their designs. It includes many spending functions such as Pocock, O'Brien–Fleming, Whiteheard triangular and double triangular, Wang–Tsiatis, and others. It can evaluate design operating characteristics including power curve, average sample size calculation, sample size distribution, stopping probabilities, and maximum sample size.

### 20.5.6 EXPECTED DEATH ON A STUDY

Expected death on a study is a useful web-based tool to estimate the expected number of death at specific time point in a time-to-event trial design. The program can be used to plan various types of phase III trials. The program assumes the uniform accrual and the time to death follows an exponential distribution. Users need to specify the accrual time, follow-up time, hazard rate, and sample size, and the program calculates the expected number of deaths at a specific time point. The program can also calculate the time at which a given potion of deaths has occurred. The program is developed using JavaScript, and one can run it from a web-browser.

## 20.6 TOOLS AND OTHERS

### 20.6.1 ADAPTIVE RANDOMIZATION

Adaptive randomization is a software package for helping statisticians design adaptive randomization-based Bayesian clinical trials. Users can study operating characteristics of different scenarios and randomization rates by running trial simulations in this software. For binary outcome cases, treatment response rates are described with a Beta distribution. For time-to-event cases, survival times are described with an inverse Gamma distribution. Users can easily adjust parameters including trial sample size, tuning parameters for adaptive randomizations, early stopping rules, threshold values, and final decision rules. Users can also input multiple scenarios simultaneously, and the software carries out all scenario simulations as a batch job. The output includes expected sample size, rejection rates, allocation rates, early stopping rates, and other useful operating characteristics. Users can modify and improve trial designs based on software output. The software runs on Window platforms with a user-friendly GUI (Figure 20.8).

### 20.6.2 PARAMETER SOLVER

Parameter solver (Figure 20.9) is a useful tool for understanding properties of common distributions and for studying Bayesian statistics and inference. This application calculates properties of a given distribution determined by mean and variance or other combinations of two parameters. It supports beta, gamma, inverse gamma, log normal, normal, and Weibull distributions. It is a very useful tool for studying the properties of the distributions of random variables.

### 20.6.3 PREDICTIVE PROBABILITY CALCULATION

The predictive probability calculation (Figure 20.10) program is a useful tool for calculating the predictive probability based on the current patient outcomes and future

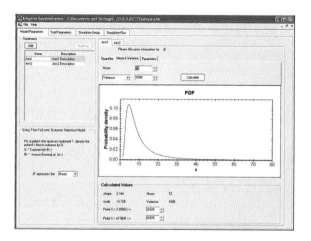

**FIGURE 20.8**  Screenshot of software adaptive randomization.

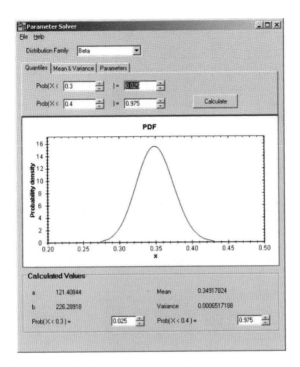

**FIGURE 20.9**    Screenshot of software parameter solver.

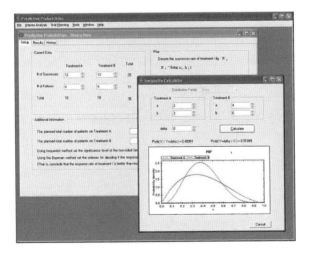

**FIGURE 20.10**    Screenshot of software predictive probability calculation.

sample size. This software includes the parameter solver and the inequality calculator to help users adjust distribution parameters and compare distributions. The program runs on Windows platforms and has a user-friendly GUI.

The difference between this program and the predictive probability design software is that this one calculates predictive probability for both binary and survival endpoints. Users can use this tool as a tutorial to understand how the predictive probability works. Predictive probability calculation can also be used by the Data Safety and Monitoring Board for monitoring the study based on the interim outcomes and making decision on whether to stop or continue the trial.

On the other hand, the predictive probability design calculates the stopping boundaries and sample sizes for designing trials based on a binary endpoint. One can use the predictive probability design tool for planning a single-arm phase II trial design.

### 20.6.4　OTHER TOOLS FOR BAYESIAN AND NON-BAYESIAN ADAPTIVE DESIGNS

Traditional frequentist clinical trial methodology is known to be more rigid and less adaptive. On the other hand, Bayesian framework naturally incorporates prior knowledge to current data to make proper inference. Bayesian methods are adaptive in nature and are ideal for learning. Methods and software tools for Bayesian adaptive designs can be found in a recent book by Berry et al. (2010). Discussions on non-Bayesian adaptive designs are covered by books by Chow and Chang (2006,2007).

### 20.6.5　OTHER PROGRAMS

There are many other well-known programs that are frequently used in clinical trial design, conduct, and analysis. Many statisticians rely heavily on those packages such as SAS, R, SPlus, SPSS, Stata, and others in their daily work. There are also many user-developed add-on's such as SAS macros, R libraries, and Stata ado files that are helpful for clinical trial design and analysis. In addition, Graphpad Prism is a very useful tool for curve fitting, statistical comparison, column statistics, linear regression and correlation, clinical lab statistics, and other functions. It also provides a lot of scientific graphing functions to draw and edit scientific plots. Lastly, the developments of BUGS, WINBUGS, and JAGS have greatly enhanced the implementation of computations using Bayesian approaches.

## 20.7　WEB-BASED CALCULATORS AND RESOURCES

### 20.7.1　HTTP://WWW.SWOGSTAT.ORG/STATOOLSOUT.HTML

Online calculators for sample size calculation of one-arm, two-arm, normal, binomial, and survival clinical trials. It also includes the Fisher's exact test and some probability calculations for common distributions.

### 20.7.2　HTTP://WWW.UPCI.UPMC.EDU/BF/RESOURCES.CFM

University of Pittsburgh Cancer Institute website includes online calculators for Simon's and Bryant-Day two-stage designs.

### 20.7.3　HTTPS://BIOSTATISTICS.MDANDERSON.ORG/SOFTWAREDOWNLOAD/

MD Anderson statistical software download site offers many software packages for a wide variety of statistical calculations and clinical trial designs. It has many packages for Bayesian clinical trial design including adaptive randomization, CRM packages, predictive probability designs, Multc design, EffTox design, and some frequentist packages as well, such as STPLAN.

### 20.7.4   HTTP://CALCULATORS.STAT.UCLA.EDU/

This website, developed by UCLA, offers online calculation for distribution, graphic chart, and statistical analysis.

### 20.7.5   HTTP://WWW.CANCERBIOSTATS.ONC.JHMI.EDU/SOFTWARE.CFM

This website, developed by Sidney Kimmel Comprehensive Cancer Center in Johns Hopkins, offers some statistical software packages for clinical trials, including randomization, CRM, optimization, and power/sample size calculation.

### 20.7.6   HTTP://HEDWIG.MGH.HARVARD.EDU/BIOSTATISTICS/SOFTWARE?TID _ 1 = ALL

This website, developed by MGH biostatistics center at Harvard University, provides some software packages for clinical trials including sample size, model fitting, sequential boundaries, failure time analysis, power/sample size for logistic, and Cox models and others.

### 20.7.7   HTTP://WWW.BETTYCJUNG.NET/STATPGMS.HTM

This website, developed by Berry C. Jung, covers a large variety of online statistical resources. It includes statistical software sites, online calculator sites, specific data management software sites, and general software (R, SAS, SPSS, and STATA).

### 20.7.8   HTTP://STATPAGES.ORG/#COMPARISONS

This page includes many useful links for performing statistical analyses and tests. Users can find most common statistical test software packages and many useful statistical analysis resources.

## 20.8   SUMMARY

In the last few decades, significant progress in clinical trial design software has been made, thanks to the efforts of statisticians and software developers. Statisticians and end users have many software options (Table 20.1) for implementing their designs: commercial packages, free software, online tools, and R-packages, etc. Finding and learning clinical trial software usages has become an important component of statisticians' routine responsibilities, which can save them a large amount of time rather than developing their own codes for trial design and conduct.

With the development of statistical methods and information technology, clinical trial software will become more convenient and powerful for users to design sophisticated trials and perform complex analyses. For instance, high-speed computers make the MCMC sampling much faster than before, resulting in rapid progress in Bayesian clinical trial methods. Cloud computing technology provides a very convenient environment for users to run calculation from a web-browser, without installing any software on their computers. We can expect continual advance in clinical trial software design in future with the development of computation and computer technologies. More powerful and user-friendly software will be available and used to facilitate clinical trial design, conduct, and analysis.

## REFERENCES

Arena, V.C. and Rockette, H.E. 2005. Software for clinical trials. In *Encyclopedia of Biostatistics*, pp. 5019–5040, 2nd edn., P. Armitage and T. Colton, eds., John Wiley & Sons, New York.

Babb, J., Rogatko, A., and Zacks, S. 1998. Cancer phase I clinical trials: Efficient dose escalation with overdose control. *Stat Med* 17:1103–1120.

Berry, D.A. 2006. A guide to drug discovery: Bayesian clinical trials. *Nat Rev Drug Discov* 5(1):27–36.

Berry, S.M., Carlin, B.P., Lee, J.J., and Müller P. 2010. *Bayesian Adaptive Methods for Clinical Trials*. Boca Raton, FL: Chapman & Hall.

Biswas, S., Liu, D.D., Lee, J.J., and Berry, D.A. 2009. Bayesian clinical trials at the University of Texas M.D. Anderson Cancer Center. *Clin Trials* 6(3):205–216.

Bryant, J. and Day, R. 1995. Incorporating toxicity considerations into the design of two-stage phase II clinical trials. *Biometrics* 51(4):1372–1383.

Chang, M. 2007. *Adaptive Design Theory and Implementation Using SAS and R*. (Chapman & Hall/CRC Biostatistics Series). Boca Raton, FL: Chapman & Hall.

Cheung, Y.K. and Chappell, R. 2000. Sequential designs for phase I clinical trials with late-onset toxicities. *Biometrics* 56:1177–1182.

Chow, S. and Chang, M. 2006. *Adaptive Design Methods in Clinical Trials* (Chapman & Hall/CRC Biostatistics Series). Boca Raton, FL: Chapman & Hall.

Green, S.J., Benedetti, J., and Crowely J. 1997.*Clinical Trials in Oncology*, 1st edn., Boca Raton, FL: Chapman & Hall.

Hwang, I.K., Shih, W.J., and De Cani, J.S. 1990. Group sequential designs using a family of Type I error probability spending functions. *Stat Med* 9:1439–1445.

Ji, Y., Li, Y., and Bekele B.N. 2007. Dose-finding in phase I clinical trials based on toxicity probability intervals. *Clin Trials* 4:235.

Johnson, V.E. and Cook, J.D. 2009. Bayesian design of single-arm phase ii clinical trials with continuous monitoring. *Clin Trials* 6:217–226.

Lane, P. 2002. Review of nQuery and pass for power and sample-size calculations. *Pharm Stat* 1:135–140.

Lee, J.J., Gu, X., and Liu, S. 2010. Bayesian adaptive randomization designs for targeted agent development. *Clin Trials* 7(5):584–596.

Lee, J.J. and Liu, D.D. 2008. A predictive probability design for phase II cancer clinical trials. *Clin. Trials* 5(2):93–106.

O'Brien, P.C. and Fleming, T.R. 1979. A multiple testing procedure for clinical trials. *Biometrics* 35:549–556.

O'Quigley, J., Pepe, M., and Fisher, L. 1990. Continual reassessment method: A practical design for phase I clinical trials in cancer. *Biometrics* 46:33–48.

Pocock, S.J. 1977. Group sequential methods in the design and analysis of clinical trials. *Biometrika* 64(2):191–199.

Simon, R. 1989. Optimal two stage designs for phase II clinical trials. *Control Clin. Trials* 10:1–10.

Tai, B.C and Seldrup, J. 2000. A review of software for data management, design and analysis of clinical trials. *Ann Acad Med Singapore* 5:576–581.

Thall, P.F. and Cook, J.D. 2004. Dose-finding based on efficacy-toxicity trade-offs. *Biometrics* 60:684–693.

Thall, P.F. and Cook, J.D. 2006. Adaptive dose-finding based on efficacy-toxicity trade-offs. In *Encyclopedia of Biopharmaceutical Statistics*, 2nd edn., S.-C. Chow, ed., New York: Marcel Dekker.

Thall, P., Simon, R., and Estey, E. 1995. Bayesian sequential monitoring designs for single-arm clinical trials with multiple outcomes. *Stat Med* 14:357–379.

Wassmer, G. and Vandemeulebroecke, M. 2006. A brief review on software developments for group sequential and adaptive designs. *Biom J* 48:732–737.

Yin, G. and Yuan, Y. 2009. Bayesian model averaging continual reassessment method in phase I clinical trials. *J Am Stat Assoc* 104:954.

# 21 Cure-Rate Survival Models in Clinical Trials

*Megan Othus, John J. Crowley, and Bart Barlogie*

## CONTENTS

## 21.1 INTRODUCTION

Advances in therapy have made cure a possibility for some cancers. For example, multiple myeloma (MM) is generally considered an incurable disease [14], but recent research suggests that some MM patients could be cured. Investigators at the University of Arkansas for Medical Sciences (UAMS) have developed an approach called total therapy (TT) that has recently been shown to cure up to 30% of MM patients [13].

The most common regression model for survival data, the proportional hazards (PH) model [12], is often not appropriate for heterogeneous patient populations including both cured and uncured patients because the PH assumptions fails [37]. In this situation, alternative models are needed, and a number of cure regression models have been proposed for this type of data.

Cure models can be useful for applications where patients are not technically "cured," but rather there is a proportion of patients who will not fail during the follow-up of the study. These patients can be referred to as long-term survivors rather than cured. Cure models often can more adequately describe survival trends when there is a non-negligible proportion of patients alive at the end of follow-up with a plateau at the end of the survival curve. In this case, the "cured" proportion from cure models provides an estimate of the proportion of patients who will not fail during follow-up, which may be a clinically relevant value.

This chapter is organized as follows: Section 21.2 reviews cure models proposed in the statistical literature; Section 21.3 summarizes important assumptions common to cure models; Section 21.4 outlines cure modeling options available in R, SAS, and Stata; Section 21.5 outlines design considerations for clinical trials where some patients may be cured; and Section 21.6 summarizes an analysis of the UMAS MM data by several cure models to highlight differences, common features, and interpretations of models.

## 21.2 MODEL OPTIONS

Cure models can be classified into two groups: mixture and non-mixture. Each group will be reviewed in the following.

### 21.2.1 MIXTURE CURE MODELS

Mixture cure models assume that the underlying population includes both cured and uncured patients. The first cure models were motivated by cancer survival trends and assumed that survival for cured patients was different and better than survival for uncured patients [7]. The authors assumed a simple parametric model:

$$S(t) = pS_0(t) + (1-p)S_0(t)\exp(-\lambda t),  \tag{21.1}$$

where

$p$ denotes the proportion of cured patients
$S_0(t)$ denotes the survival of the "general" or "normal" population
$\lambda$ denotes the death rate due to cancer [7]

The authors were "surprised as well as gratified" to find that such a simple formulation with only two parameters fit observed data quite well.

Further research on mixture cure models has focused on developing more general and flexible formulations of Equation 21.1. Most mixture cure models can be written as

$$S(t|X) = p(X) + (1-p(X))S_0(t|X),  \tag{21.2}$$

where

$X$ is a set of covariates
$p(X)$ is a model for the probability that an individual is cured
$S_0(t|X)$ is the survival function for patients who are not cured

Most mixture cure models use a logistic model for $p(X)$. Proposed models for $S_0(t|X)$ include the exponential and Weibull distributions [16], the PH model [20,34,38], a semiparametric accelerated failure time model [24], and a semiparametric transformation model that includes both the PH and proportional odds [6] models as special cases [28].

Recent research on mixture cure models has focused on more complicated survival data including interval censoring [27], dependent censoring [26,32], longitudinal data [23,36,44], current status data [29], and grouped survival data [45].

## 21.2.2 NON-MIXTURE CURE MODELS

Most non-mixture cure models parametrize the survival function as

$$S(t) = \exp(-\theta F(t)). \tag{21.3}$$

where $F(t)$ is the distribution function for a non-negative random variable. In this model, the cumulative hazard function $\theta F(t)$ is bounded, and so the survival function is an improper survival function in the sense that $\lim_{t \to \infty} S(t) > 0$. In Equation 21.3, the proportion of cured patients is equal to $\exp(-\theta)$. When $F(t)$ does not depend on covariates, Model (21.3) has a PH structure. Covariates are incorporated into this model through both $\theta$ and $F(t)$. Often $\theta$ is modeled with the relationship $\theta(X) = \exp(\beta'X)$. Common parametric forms for $F(t)$ include the Weibull, lognormal, logistic, and gamma distributions.

Parametric forms for $F(t)$ can incorporate covariates and have been considered by a number of authors [8,37,40]. Models with semiparametric $F(t)$ have also been proposed [41]. Some work has been done for non-mixture cure models with alternative transformations of $\theta F(t)$ [39,46].

Non-mixture cure models are a popular framework for Bayesian cure models because mixture cure models yield improper posterior distributions for many non-informative priors, and the PH structure is computationally convenient [8,18,41]. Proposals for Bayesian extensions to Equation 21.3 include models for multivariate survival data [9], models for spatial data with interval censoring [1], and general transformations of $\theta F(t)$ into survival functions [42,43].

## 21.2.3 DIFFERENCES BETWEEN MIXTURE AND NON-MIXTURE CURE MODELS

Choosing between mixture and non-mixture models is a matter of preference. Frequentist results are available for both mixture and non-mixture models, but Bayesian work has focused on non-mixture models due to computational ease. Because in mixture models the probability of being cured is modeled separately from the survival for those who are not cured, mixture models allow for separate covariate relationships for cured and uncured patients.

## 21.3 ASSUMPTIONS AND IDENTIFIABILITY

All cure models, parametric, semiparametric, mixture, and non-mixture, assume that that a cured fraction exists. This assumption ensures that there is enough data to estimate parameters related the cure proportion. This assumption can be checked in a dataset by looking at empirical survival curves. Survival functions for populations with cured patients exhibit a plateau at the end of the curve beyond which there are no more failures and the survival curve is flat. Given this feature of cure survival curves, Kaplan–Meier plots that exhibit plateaus at the end of the curve are often interpreted to describe cured populations and that shape of curve is often taken as evidence that a cure model may be appropriate. For mixture cure models, a test of the existence of a cure fraction based on the tail of the Kaplan–Meier curve has been proposed [30], though it is not straightforward to implement the test.

Additionally, care needs to be taken to ensure that semiparametric models are identifiable. Proofs of identifiability or nonidentifiability exist for some general classes of semiparametric mixture and non-mixture cure models. For example, the logistic-PH model and Equation 21.3 with $\log(\theta)$ linear in covariates without an intercept and $F(t)$ unspecified are both identifiable [25]. The mixture cure model (Equation 21.2) with survival for those not cured modeled nonparametrically and assuming a constant probability of cure [$p(x) = p$ for all $x$] is not identifiable [25].

Although common semiparametric mixture models have been proved to be identifiable, in finite samples, the models can exhibit "near-nonidentifiability" in which the likelihood for cure parameters can be flat. To address this issue in mixture cure models, authors have proposed setting the survival function for patients who are not cured $S_0(t)$ in Equation 21.2 equal to zero after the last observed failure time [28,34,38]. The justification for this computational adjustment is that cure models are only appropriate when some patients are cured and that long follow-up is required to identify the plateau of the tail of a survival curve. If there is sufficient follow-up to support the assumption of a cured proportion, authors argue that it is reasonable to set the survival function to zero after the last failure. If there is not sufficient follow-up or there is no rational for why a cure might exist, the model should not be used. Similarly, semiparametric non-mixture survival models usually assume that $F(t)$ from Equation 21.3 is equal to zero at the last failure. Many Bayesian models can control the degree to which a model is semiparametric. Bayesian semiparametric non-mixture models often model $F(t)$ as having a piecewise constant hazard. The number of pieces controls the "nonparametricity" of the model, and so small-to-moderate numbers of pieces are required to have the models behave well [9].

## 21.4  COMPUTATIONAL IMPLEMENTATION

One barrier to implementation of cure models is that there are limited computational resources available. Cure models are not standard functions in most statistical packages. Some authors have made personal code available for their methods, but for the most part interested parties would need to hand code complicated formulae. Some methods only require a straightforward implementation of built-in optimization routines, but many methods propose EM algorithms that require more work on the part of the user. Later, we review the limited R packages, SAS macros, and Stata modules available for cure analyses.

## 21.4.1   R

There is one package for cure modeling in R. The package nltm provides frequentist estimates for non-mixture PH and proportional odds models based on [39]. Additionally, some authors have made R code available on personal websites. There is S-PLUS and R code available for an implementation of the logistic-PH mixture cure model [20,33,34,38] using an EM algorithm. The website for the code is http://www.math.mun.ca/~ypeng/research/semicure/, and details of the method are provided in [33]. S-PLUS code for evaluating a generalized F mixture cure model using a simulated annealing algorithm [35] is available at http://www.math.mun.ca/~ypeng/research/.

WinBUGS code is available for a Bayesian hierarchical model that includes models of the form (21.2) and (21.3) as special cases. The method proposed in [10] has code available at http://www.biostat.umn.edu/~sudiptob/Software.html. The book [19] has a chapter on Bayesian cure survival models. Code for the book can be found on the website http://www.stat.uconn.edu/~mhchen/survbook/.

## 21.4.2   SAS

A SAS macro was published that fits some frequentist parametric and semiparametric mixture cure survival models [11].

## 21.4.3   STATA

There is a Stata module available to fit a frequentist parametric non-mixture cure model as detailed in ref. [37]. The module can be downloaded from http://ideas.repec.org/c/boc/bocode/s446901.html. Details on Stata commands to fit cure models that incorporate expected background mortality and that can estimate relative morality have been published [21].

## 21.5   DESIGN CONSIDERATIONS

Limited work has been done for power and sample size calculations assuming a proportion of patients have been cured. All of the work as focused on mixture cure survival models and most of that work has focused on power of tests of the cure proportion. Gray and Tsiatis [17] proposed a linear rank test derived to focus power at the alternative that cure proportions are different but that survival among those not cured is the same between the two groups. This test has improved power over the log-rank test when less than 50% of the population is cured. Laska and Meisner [22] proposed a test of cure proportions based on the tails of the Kaplan–Meier curves. Ewell and Ibrahim extended the results of [17] to cases in which the survival distributions for non-cured populations may differ [15]. There currently do not exist calculators to determine power and sample size for clinical trials assuming a cure proportion, and so simulations are the most straightforward way to determine sample size.

## 21.6   ANALYSIS OF MULTIPLE MYELOMA DATA

In an effort to distinguish between the available models, we will evaluate several models on the MM dataset mentioned in the introduction of this chapter. The UAMS has developed three TT protocols since 1989 with the intent of curing some MM patients. The first protocol, TT1, used a tandem autotransplant approach [3,5]. The second protocol intensified induction, added posttransplant consolidation, and randomized between the addition of thalidomide, TT2+, or no thalidomide, TT2– [4]. The most recent protocol, TT3, incorporated thalidomide and bortezomib for induction [2,31]. Patient outcomes have improved over the protocols, so we will investigate the trends in progression-free survival (PFS) over the protocols using several cure models. PFS is defined from the time of registration to the first of death or progression, with patients last known to be alive without progression censored at the date of last contact.

First, we look at the survival curves for the four groups to evaluate whether cure models are appropriate for this data. Figure 21.1 shows Kaplan–Meier plots of PFS stratified by TT protocol. PFS has improved over time, and each PFS curve has a plateau at the tail indicating the potential that some patients may be cured.

Table 21.1 summarizes estimates and standard errors (SEs) for a mixture cure model (Equation 21.2) with a constant probability of cure, $p(X)=p$, and exponential survival, $S_0(t|X)=\exp(-\lambda t)$ fit to each protocol. The estimated cure proportions increase over the protocols, as Figure 21.1 indicated. The proportion of cured patients more than doubled between TT1 and TT2+/TT3. Survival for patients who are not cured has also improved over the TT protocols. Based on the exponential

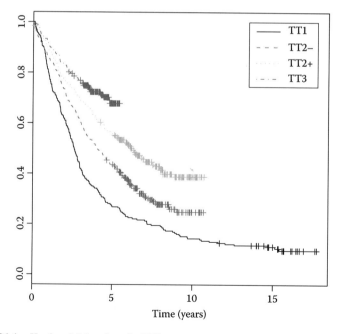

**FIGURE 21.1**   Kaplan–Meier plots for PFS.

**TABLE 21.1**
**Exponential Cure Model Regression Results**

|        | Cure Proportion (%) | SE | Survival Parameter λ | SE |
|--------|:---:|:---:|:---:|:---:|
| TT1    | 9.4  | 2.1  | 0.30 | 0.02 |
| TT2−   | 10.3 | 6.1  | 0.20 | 0.03 |
| TT2+   | 23.2 | 7.8  | 0.17 | 0.03 |
| TT3    | 52.7 | 11.5 | 0.22 | 0.08 |

assumption, median survival for patients who were not cured was 2.3 years in TT1 and 3.2 years in TT3. Survival among those not cured in TT2−, TT2+, and TT3 was relatively stable.

We can incorporate covariates into a parametric mixture cure model though a logistic-Weibull cure model. In this model, the probability of being cured, $p(X)$, follows a logistic distribution, and the survival for those who are not cured, $S(t|X)$, follows a Weibull distribution. We incorporate covariates into the Weibull survival function by $S(t|X) = \exp(-\exp(\beta'X)\lambda t^{\gamma})$, where $\beta$ is a vector of parameters corresponding to the covariate matrix $X$, $\lambda$ is the Weibull shape parameter, and $\gamma$ is the Weibull scale parameter. Table 21.2 summarizes results (odds ratios [ORs], hazard ratios [HRs], and 95% confidence intervals [CIs]) from a model with covariates for protocol, age at diagnosis, and an indicator of presence of metaphase cytogenetic abnormalities (CA) at diagnosis. The conclusions from the logistic-Weibull models are similar to the conclusions from the simple cure model summarized in Table 21.1; the probability of cure increased over the protocols. Survival among those not cured in TT2+ was significantly improved over TT1, though survival among those not cured in TT2−, and TT3 was not significantly improved over TT1. Additionally, we have information on age and CA. Both increased age and presence of CAs were associated with a decreased probability of being cured and an increased hazard of

**TABLE 21.2**
**Logistic-Weibull Regression Results**

|              | Cure Model | | Weibull Model | |
|--------------|:---:|:---:|:---:|:---:|
|              | OR | 95% CI | HR | 95% CI |
| TT1 (ref)    |       |                |      |                |
| TT2−         | 1.51  | (1.06, 5.26)   | 0.65 | (0.57, 1.00)   |
| TT2+         | 4.75  | (2.22, 10.18)  | 0.64 | (0.44, 0.91)   |
| TT3          | 20.23 | (9.11, 44.90)  | 0.91 | (0.48, 1.73)   |
| Age          | 1.03  | (1.00, 1.05)   | 1.01 | (1.00, 1.02)   |
| CA           | 2.38  | (1.43, 4.00)   | 1.46 | (1.17, 1.83)   |
| λ (shape)    |       |                | 0.16 | (0.09, 0.30)   |
| γ (scale)    |       |                | 1.11 | (1.02, 1.19)   |

failure. The exponential distribution is a special case of the Weibull distribution when $\gamma = 1$. In this model, the 95% CI for $\gamma$ excludes 1 implying the model does not simplify to the exponential case.

The PH model can be more flexible than the Weibull model because it does not assume a parametric form for the hazard function. Table 21.3 summarizes results from a logistic-PH model, where $S(t|X) = \exp(-\exp(\beta'X) \Delta(t))$ and $\Delta(t)$ is an unspecified cumulative hazard function. The point estimates for the ORs and HRs from the logistic-PH model are fairly similar to the estimates from the logistic-Weibull model. In contrast to the logistic-Weibull model, the survival among those not cured with TT2− was significantly improved over TT1, and the HR for CA is not significantly different from 1.

An alternative semiparametric model is a non-mixture model (Equation 21.3) with an unspecified $F(t)$ and $\theta = \exp(\beta'X)$. Results for this model were summarized in Table 21.4. The results for the PH non-mixture model indicate that there was continued improvement in survival for all patients, on average, from TT1 through TT3. Older age and presence of CAs are associated with decreased survival.

**TABLE 21.3**
**Logistic-Proportional Hazards Regression Results**

|           | Cure Model | | PH Model | |
|-----------|------|--------------|------|--------------|
|           | OR   | 95% CI       | HR   | 95% CI       |
| TT1 (ref) |      |              |      |              |
| TT2−      | 1.90 | (1.08, 3.34) | 0.69 | (0.57, 0.84) |
| TT2+      | 3.97 | (2.31, 6.82) | 0.57 | (0.46, 0.70) |
| TT3       | 21.35| (12.32, 37.03) | 0.87 | (0.67, 1.24) |
| Age       | 1.031| (1.05, 1.02) | 1.01 | (1.00, 1.01) |
| CA        | 2.48 | (1.86, 3.69) | 1.44 | (0.89, 1.21) |

**TABLE 21.4**
**PH Non-Mixture Model Regression Results**

|           | HR   | 95% CI       |
|-----------|------|--------------|
| TT1 (ref) |      |              |
| TT2−      | 0.64 | (0.53, 0.78) |
| TT2+      | 0.45 | (0.36, 0.55) |
| TT3       | 0.29 | (0.22, 0.37) |
| Age       | 1.03 | (1.01, 1.05) |
| CA        | 1.72 | (1.47, 2.01) |

**TABLE 21.5**

**Weibull Non-Mixture**

**Model Regression Results**

|  | HR | 95% CI |
|---|---|---|
| **TT1 (ref)** | | |
| TT2− | 0.64 | (0.53, 0.78) |
| TT2+ | 0.45 | (0.36, 0.55) |
| TT3 | 0.29 | (0.22, 0.37) |
| Age | 1.03 | (1.01, 1.05) |
| CA | 1.72 | (1.47, 2.01) |
| **Scale** | | |
| Intercept | −7.03 | (−8.24, −5.83) |
| Age | −0.02 | (−0.04, 0.01) |
| **Shape** | | |
| Intercept | 0.56 | (0.18, 0.94) |
| Age | −0.01 | (−0.01, −0.001) |

The non-mixture model can also take use parametric forms for $F(t)$. Table 21.5 summarizes results for $F(t)$ following the Weibull distribution with the covariate age and letting $\theta = \exp(\beta'X)$. The results for this model are virtually identical to the results form the semiparametric model.

As a final comparison, the standard survival model, the PH model, is summarized in Table 21.6. The PH model has very similar estimates as the non-mixture cure models.

Given the number of different models applied to the data, we were interested in how the estimates of cured fractions differed between the models. Table 21.7 summarizes estimates of cure fractions for each of the protocols from the five cure models summarized earlier. Each model was fit with only covariates for the protocols. Estimates were fairly stables between the models even though each model had

**TABLE 21.6**

**Proportional Hazards**

**Model Regression Results**

|  | HR | 95% CI |
|---|---|---|
| TT1 (ref) | | |
| TT2− | 0.65 | (0.53, 0.79) |
| TT2+ | 0.45 | (0.36, 0.55) |
| TT3 | 0.29 | (0.22, 0.37) |
| Age | 1.02 | (1.01, 1.02) |
| CA | 1.72 | (1.48, 2.01) |

**TABLE 21.7**

**Estimates of Cure Proportions for Mixture and Non-Mixture Models**

|      | Exponential Mixture | Weibull Mixture | PH Mixture | Weibull Non-Mixture | PH Non-Mixture |
|------|---------------------|-----------------|------------|---------------------|----------------|
| TT1  | 9.4                 | 9.4             | 9.6        | 6.0                 | 8.9            |
| TT2– | 10.3                | 15.7            | 10.2       | 15.5                | 18.7           |
| TT2+ | 23.2                | 28.8            | 22.8       | 27.3                | 31.0           |
| TT3  | 52.7                | 59.0            | 58.7       | 42.9                | 45.5           |

different modeling assumptions. TT1 had the smallest range in estimates, and TT3 had the largest range of estimates, reflecting that there is more follow-up for TT1 than TT3 and so more information for estimating the cure proportion.

As highlighted in the interpretation of the results, one main difference between mixture and non-mixture models is that the mixture models explicitly model separately the probability of being cured and the survival for those not cured. This allows for covariates to have distinct relationships for cured and uncured patients. In contrast, the interpretation of covariates within the non-mixture model is for survival averaged across patients, while functionally allowing some patients to be cured. In this application, the mixture model picked out different trends in the cure and survival functions. The proportion of cured patients has increased continuously from TT1 to TT3, while survival in TT2+/– and TT3 for those not cured was fairly similar (and better than TT1).

As a final note, the exponential cure model and the logistic-Weibull models were fit using personal code. The logistic-PH model was fit in SAS using the macro described in Section 21.4. The Weibull non-mixture was fit in Stata using the module cureregr. The semiparametric non-mixture model was fit using the R package ntlm, and the PH model was fit using the R package survival.

## 21.7  CONCLUDING THOUGHTS

While cure survival models have been a popular topic of methodologic work, straightforward implementation of the models is constrained by the limited software available. Currently, someone interested in using a cure survival model will likely need to put some effort into writing new code or adapting available code to their application. Incorporating cure models into standard survival packages will be important to encourage more widespread use of such models in applications. Additionally, more work on design considerations for cure models would be useful.

## ACKNOWLEDGMENTS

This work was supported in part by grants #CA038926, #CA90998, and #CA055819 from the National Cancer Institute.

# REFERENCES

1. S. Banerjee and B.P. Carlin. Parametric spatial cure rate models for interval-censored time-to-relapse data. *Biometrics*, 60(1):268–275, 2004.
2. B. Barlogie, E. Anaissie, F. Van Rhee, J. Haessler, K. Hollmig, M. Pineda-Roman, M. Cottler-Fox et al. Incorporating bortezomib into upfront treatment for multiple myeloma: Early results of total therapy 3. *British Journal of Haematology*, 138(2):176–185, 2007.
3. B. Barlogie, S. Jagannath, D.H. Vesole, S. Naucke, B. Cheson, S. Mattox, D. Bracy et al. Superiority of tandem autologous transplantation over standard therapy for previously untreated multiple myeloma. *Blood*, 89(3):789, 1997.
4. B. Barlogie, G. Tricot, E. Anaissie, J. Shaughnessy, E. Rasmussen, F. van Rhee, A. Fassas et al. Thalidomide and hematopoietic-cell transplantation for multiple myeloma. *New England Journal of Medicine*, 354(10):1021–1030, 2006.
5. B. Barlogie, G.J. Tricot, F. Van Rhee, E. Angtuaco, R. Walker, J. Epstein, J.D. Shaughnessy et al. Long-term outcome results of the first tandem autotransplant trial for multiple myeloma. *British Journal of Haematology*, 135(2):158–164, 2006.
6. S. Bennett. Analysis of survival data by the proportional odds model. *Statistics in Medicine*, 2(2):273–277, 1983.
7. J. Berkson and R. Gage. Survival curve for cancer patients following treatment. *Journal of the American Statistical Association*, 47:501–515, 1952.
8. M.H. Chen, J.G. Ibrahim, and D. Sinha. A new Bayesian model for survival data with a surviving fraction. *Journal of the American Statistical Association*, 94(447):909–910, 1999.
9. M.H. Chen, J.G. Ibrahim, and D. Sinha. Bayesian inference for multivariate survival data with a cure fraction. *Journal of Multivariate Analysis*, 80(1):101–126, 2002.
10. F. Cooner, S. Banerjee, B.P. Carlin, and D. Sinha. Flexible cure rate modeling under latent activation schemes. *Journal of the American Statistical Association*, 102(478):560–572, 2007.
11. F. Corbiere and P. Joly. A SAS macro for parametric and semiparametric mixture cure models. *Computer Methods and Programs in Biomedicine*, 85(2):173–180, 2007.
12. D.R. Cox. Regression models and life-tables (with discussion). *Journal of the Royal Statistical Society, Series B (Methodological)*, 34:187–220, 1972.
13. S. Usmani, J. Crowley, A. Hoering, A. Mitchell, S. Waheed, B. Nair, Y. AlSayed, F. van Rhee, B. Barlogie. Improvement in long-term outcomes with successive total therapy trials for multiple Mycloma: Are patients now being cured? Under Review, 2011.
14. B.G.M. Durie. Role of new treatment approaches in defining treatment goals in multiple myeloma—The ultimate goal is extended survival. *Cancer Treatment Reviews*, 36:S18–S23, 2010.
15. M. Ewell and J.G. Ibrahim. The large sample distribution of the weighted log rank statistic under general local alternatives. *Lifetime Data Analysis*, 3(1):5–12, 1997.
16. V.T. Farewell. The use of mixture models for the analysis of survival data with long-term survivors. *Biometrics*, 38(4):1041–1046, 1982.
17. R.J. Gray and A.A. Tsiatis. A linear rank test for use when the main interest is in differences in cure rates. *Biometrics*, 45(3):899–904, 1989.
18. J.G. Ibrahim, M.H. Chen, and D. Sinha. Bayesian semiparametric models for survival data with a cure fraction. *Biometrics*, 57(2):383–388, 2001.
19. J.G. Ibrahim, M.H. Chen, and D. Sinha. *Bayesian Survival Analysis*. Springer Verlag, Berlin, Germany, 2001.
20. A.Y.C. Kuk and C.H. Chen. A mixture model combining logistic regression with proportional hazards regression. *Biometrika*, 79(3):531, 1992.
21. P.C. Lambert. Modeling of the cure fraction in survival studies. *Stata Journal*, 7(3):351–375(25), 2007.

22. E.M. Laska and M.J. Meisner. Nonparametric estimation and testing in a cure model. *Biometrics*, 48(4):1223–1234, 1992.
23. N.J. Law, J.M.G. Taylor, and H. Sandler. The joint modeling of a longitudinal disease progression marker and the failure time process in the presence of cure. *Biostatistics*, 3(4):547, 2002.
24. C.S. Li and J.M.G. Taylor. A semi-parametric accelerated failure time cure model. *Statistics in Medicine*, 21(21):3235–3247, 2002.
25. C. Li, J. Taylor, and J. Sy. Identifiability of cure models. *Statistics and Probability Letters*, 54:389–395, 2001.
26. Y. Li, R.C. Tiwari, and S. Guha. Mixture cure survival models with dependent censoring. *Journal of the Royal Statistical Society: Series B (Statistical Methodology)*, 69(3):285–306, 2007.
27. H. Liu and Y. Shen. A semiparametric regression cure model for interval-censored data. *Journal of the American Statistical Association*, 104(487):1168–1178, 2009.
28. W. Lu and Z. Ying. On semiparametric transformation cure models. *Biometrika*, 91:331–343, 2004.
29. S. Ma. Cure model with current status data. *Statistica Sinica*, 19:233–249, 2009.
30. R.A. Maller and S. Zhou. Testing for sufficient follow-up and outliers in survival data. *Journal of the American Statistical Association*, 89(428):1499–1506, 1994.
31. B. Nair, F. van Rhee, J.D. Shaughnessy Jr, E. Anaissie, J. Szymonifka, A. Hoering, Y. Alsayed, S. Waheed, J. Crowley, and B. Barlogie. Superior results of total therapy 3 (2003–33) in gene expression profiling-defined low-risk multiple myeloma confirmed in subsequent trial 2006–66 with VRD maintenance. *Blood*, 115(21):4168, 2010.
32. M. Othus, Y. Li, and R.C. Tiwari. A class of semiparametric mixture cure survival models with dependent censoring. *Journal of the American Statistical Association*, 104(487):1241–1250, 2009.
33. Y. Peng. Fitting semiparametric cure models. *Computational Statistics and Data Analysis*, 41(3–4):481–490, 2003.
34. Y. Peng and K.B.G. Dear. A nonparametric mixture model for cure rate estimation. *Biometrics*, 56(1):237–243, 2000.
35. Y. Peng, K.B.G. Dear, and J.W. Denham. A generalized F mixture model for cure rate estimation. *Statistics in Medicine*, 17(8):813–830, 1998.
36. Y. Peng, J.M.G. Taylor, and B. Yu. A marginal regression model for multivariate failure time data with a surviving fraction. *Lifetime Data Analysis*, 13(3):351–369, 2007.
37. R. Sposto. Cure model analysis in cancer: An application to data from the Children's Cancer Group. *Statistics in Medicine*, 21(2):293–312, 2002.
38. J.P. Sy and J.M.G. Taylor. Estimation in a Cox proportional hazards cure model. *Biometrics*, 56(1):227–236, 2000.
39. A. Tsodikov. Semiparametric models: A generalized self-consistency approach. *Journal of the Royal Statistical Society: Series B (Statistical Methodology)*, 65(3):759–774, 2003.
40. A.D. Tsodikov, B. Asselain, A. Fourque, T. Hoang, and A.Y. Yakovlev. Discrete strategies of cancer post-treatment surveillance. Estimation and optimization problems. *Biometrics*, 51(2):437–447, 1995.
41. A.D. Tsodikov, J.G. Ibrahim, and A.Y. Yakovlev. Estimating cure rates from survival data. *Journal of the American Statistical Association*, 98(464):1063–1078, 2003.
42. G. Yin and J.G. Ibrahim. A general class of Bayesian survival models with zero and nonzero cure fractions. *Biometrics*, 61(2):403–412, 2005.
43. G. Yin and J.G. Ibrahim. Cure rate models: A unified approach. *Canadian Journal of Statistics*, 33(4):559–570, 2005.

44. M. Yu, J.M.G. Taylor, and H.M. Sandler. Individual prediction in prostate cancer studies using a joint longitudinal survival-cure model. *Journal of the American Statistical Association*, 103(481):178–187, 2008.

45. B. Yu, R.C. Tiwari, K.A. Cronin, and E.J. Feuer. Cure fraction estimation from the mixture cure models for grouped survival data. *Statistics in Medicine*, 23(11):1733–1747, 2004.

46. D. Zeng, G. Yin, and J.G. Ibrahim. Semiparametric transformation models for survival data with a cure fraction. *Journal of the American Statistical Association*, 101(474):670–684, 2006.

# 22 Design and Analysis of Quality-of-Life Data

*Andrea B. Troxel and Carol M. Moinpour*

## CONTENTS

## 22.1   INTRODUCTION

The objective of this chapter is to inform those engaged in clinical trials research about the special statistical issues involved in analyzing longitudinal quality-of-life (QOL) outcome data. Since these data are collected in trials for patients with a life threatening disease, it is common to see a drop-off in submission rates for patient-reported questionnaire data, often due to death and deteriorating health. Data sets with such missing data must be analyzed appropriately in order not to arrive at misguided conclusions regarding change in QOL over the treatment course. Methods will be suggested for complete or near-complete datasets as well as for those where missing data are a concern.

### 22.1.1   ORGANIZATION OF CHAPTER

The inclusion of QOL endpoints in clinical trials must be treated as seriously as any clinical outcome. The first section of the chapter addresses QOL assessment methods, both traditional questionnaires and newer measurement approaches. Most design issues important for obtaining a credible evaluation of clinical endpoints are also important for QOL outcomes. For example, optimal timing of assessments may vary according to the treatment schedule, disease site, and other factors. Issues of clinical significance, which in turn inform sample size and power considerations, are the same, but the databases used to determine clinical significance are not as familiar to clinicians and are still being developed by QOL researchers. The use of composite variables, gaining popularity but associated with difficulties in interpretation, has also been suggested for QOL outcomes. These subjects are discussed in more detail in Section 22.3.

When QOL research is conducted in many and often widely differing institutions, quality control is critical to ensure clean, complete data. The first step is to make completion of a baseline QOL assessment a trial eligibility criterion. Enforcement of the same requirements for both clinical and QOL follow-up data communicates the importance of the QOL data for the trial. Even with the best quality control procedures, submission rates for follow-up QOL questionnaires can be less than desirable, particularly in the advanced stage disease setting. It is precisely in the treatment of advanced disease, however, that QOL data often provide key information about the extent of palliation achieved by an experimental treatment. While this is a rich source of information, data analysis is often complicated by problems of missing information. Patients sometimes fail to complete QOL assessments because of negative events they experience, such as treatment toxicities, disease progression, or death. Because not all patients are subject to these missing observations at the same rate, especially when treatment failure or survival rates differ between arms, the set of complete observations is not always representative of the total group; analyses using only complete observations are therefore potentially biased.

Several methods have been developed to address this problem. They range in emphasis from the data collection stage, where attention focuses on obtaining the missing values, to the analysis stage, where the goal is adjustment to properly account for the missing values. In Section 22.4, we first describe different types of missing data. Section 22.5 describes methods that are appropriate for complete or nearly complete data. Section 22.6 presents several methods that have been used to address incomplete datasets and informative missing data, including sensitivity analyses. Section 22.7 examines approaches for substituting scores for missing data, imputation, and methods for combining survival and QOL outcomes.

## 22.2 WHAT IS QOL AND HOW IS IT MEASURED?

### 22.2.1 General Assessment Methods

In randomized treatment trials for cancer or other chronic diseases, the primary reason for assessing QOL is to broaden the scope of treatment evaluation. We sometimes characterize QOL and cost outcomes as alternative or complementary, because they add to information provided by traditional clinical trials' endpoints such as survival, disease-free survival, tumor response, and toxicity. The challenge lies in combining this information in the treatment evaluation context. There is fairly strong consensus that, at least in the Phase III setting, QOL should be measured comprehensively [1–3]. Although a total or summary score is desirable for the QOL measure, it is equally important to have separate measures of basic domains of functioning, such as physical, emotional, social, and role functioning, as well as symptom status. Symptoms specific to the cancer site and/or the treatments under evaluation are also usually included to monitor for toxicities and to gauge the palliative effect of the treatment on disease-related symptoms. In some trials, investigators may study additional areas such as financial concerns, spirituality, family well-being, and satisfaction with care. Specific components of QOL not only provide information on specific interpretation of treatment effects but also can identify areas in which cancer survivors need assistance in their return to daily functioning. Data on specific areas of functioning can also help suggest ways to improve cancer treatments; Sugarbaker et al. [4] conducted a study in which the radiotherapy regimen was modified as a result of QOL data.

QOL data should be generated by patients in a systematic, standardized fashion. Interviews can be used to obtain these data, but self-administered questionnaires are usually more practical in the multi-institution setting of clinical trials. Selected questionnaires must be reliable and valid [5] and sensitive to change over time [6,7]; good measurement properties, along with appropriate item content, help ensure a more accurate picture of the patient's QOL. There are four QOL questionnaires that meet these measurement criteria, provide comprehensive measures of domains or areas of QOL, and are frequently used in cancer clinical trials. The Functional Assessment of Chronic Illness Therapy (FACIT), the newer name for the Functional Assessment of Cancer Therapy (FACT, version 4) [8–12], and the European Organization of Research and Therapy for Cancer (EORTC) Quality-of-Life Questionnaire-Core 30 (QLQ-C30) [13–17] are two QOL questionnaires that measure general domains or areas of QOL, the core component, along with symptom modules specific to the disease or type of treatment; see websites for currently available modules [18,19]. Others, like the Cancer Rehabilitation Evaluation System-Short Form (CARES-SF)

[20–23] and the Short Form Health Survey (SF-36, SF-12, and SF-8) [24–35], can be used with any cancer site but may require supplementation with a separate symptom measure to address concerns about prominent symptoms and side effects. The large normative database available for the SF-36 is very useful in interpreting score changes and differences; see the website for information on accessing this measure and its databases [36]. This questionnaire has been used successfully in cancer clinical trials to detect differences in treatment regimens [37].

## 22.2.2 NEW QUALITY-OF-LIFE ASSESSMENT APPROACHES

PROMIS. A new QOL assessment initiative is the Patient-Reported Outcomes Measurement Information System (PROMIS) (http://www.nihpromis.org/default. aspx). This National Institutes of Health (NIH)-supported effort developed banks of items that can be used to measure QOL more precisely (by minimizing error in the estimates) and efficiently (by requiring fewer items) across a broad range of chronic diseases including cancer [38,39]. These item banks incorporate items from existing measures (e.g., the SF-36 [40]). PROMIS domains address three main areas of health based on the World Health Organization framework [41], physical, mental, and social domains; this breakdown has been used in the development of countless QOL questionnaires. Thirty-eight subordinate domains exist under the three main areas (e.g., pain interference, emotional distress-anxiety, and discretionary social activities); new domains and subdomains are currently under development. Each domain/subdomain has a bank of items, with each item calibrated, so that scores generated by different sets of items answered by different people can be interpreted the same with respect to a person's level on the QOL domain/subdomain of interest. This domain is described as a latent trait, because we cannot measure it perfectly; item response theory methods used to create the item banks minimize error and maximize precision of measurement [42]. That is, regardless of which items a person completes from a specific bank, high scores reflect a higher level for that trait and low scores reflect a lower level for the trait. An item bank allows three general types of measurement [39,43]: static short forms, which are currently being validated by PROMIS researchers; a computer-adaptive test (CAT) [44]; and customized short forms from the item banks tailored to specific research questions. After the first item, a CAT measure determines subsequent items based on a person's response to the previous item, which allows for the most precision in measuring the latent trait with the fewest items [42,44]. Finally, part of the PROMIS technical services available to users of PROMIS measures is an assessment center, which allows individual researchers to set up studies using both PROMIS measures and non-PROMIS measures and administer these items online to study participants [45]. The assessment center is supported with NIH funding and meets all standards for protecting privacy of respondent information.

PRO-CTCAE. The National Cancer Institute (NCI) recently supported the development of a patient-reported outcomes (PRO) version of the Common Toxicity and Clinical Adverse Events rating system, the PRO-CTCAE (http://outcomes.cancer. gov/tools/pro-ctcae.html). The PRO-CTCAE ratings are being developed by Dr. Ethan Basch and colleagues at Memorial Sloan Kettering Cancer Institute.

## 22.3 DESIGN ISSUES

### 22.3.1 TIMING OF ASSESSMENTS

When adding QOL to a cancer clinical trial, it is important to think carefully about possible assessment times. Table 22.1 summarizes some of the factors that should be considered in order to select clinically meaningful time points as well as time points that are "fair" for all treatment arms under study. Most factors require discussion with clinicians involved in the trial. For example, one might want to document QOL status at known points of remission or deterioration for the particular cancer site or assess patient QOL at the earliest point when an agent could be expected to have a positive effect on the disease to see if there would be a comparable effect on QOL. The clinicians involved in the trial have likely had previous experience with the agent and can be a good source of suggestions for meaningful time points. The table notes factors affecting compliance with the QOL assessment schedule and quality control procedures. Specifying acceptable windows for the QOL assessment times in the protocol helps with quality control procedures downstream. Finally, one can base QOL assessments on events, such as the beginning of new treatment cycles, as opposed to the number of days from randomization. This decision can have implications for systems used to monitor timely submission of questionnaires. Information about delays in treatment administration often does not reach the data center in time to revise expected due dates for questionnaires; in addition, some systems may not be able to accommodate ongoing demands for due date revisions.

### 22.3.2 CLINICAL SIGNIFICANCE AND POWER

There is an increasing emphasis on the importance of addressing the clinical significance of QOL scores in cancer clinical trials and of helping clinicians and clinical trialists interpret what scores and changes in scores mean. A series of seven papers published in the Mayo Clinic Proceedings in 2002 addressed these subjects [48–54]. A protocol that includes a QOL outcome should stipulate the number of points that reflects a clinically significant difference or change for that questionnaire. Fortunately, this task is feasible using the large databases that exist for some of the more frequently used questionnaires. For example, the Functional Assessment of Cancer Therapy-Lung Cancer (FACT-L) has a separate score for the Trial Outcome Index (TOI), a measure of physical and functional well-being and symptoms/concerns. A change of 5–7 points for the TOI has been associated with differences in other clinical measures such as performance status as well as with the amount of change over time in patients with better versus worse prognosis [55]. If physical and symptom status are of primary interest in the trial, then a measure such as the TOI might be designated the primary QOL outcome variable and sample size determined based on the 5–7-point improvement for one arm versus the other. Given a trial for advanced stage disease patients, investigators might be interested in seeing if patients in one arm deteriorated by a clinically important amount such as 5–7 FACT TOI points, while the other arm remained relatively stable. Clinically important change for the EORTC QLQ-C30 varies with the subscale of interest and other

## TABLE 22.1
## Important Variables in the Determination of QOL Assessment Schedules

| Variable | Example/Rationale |
|---|---|
| Baseline assessment is mandatory | Cannot measure change without an assessment prior to the initiation of treatment. |
| Data collection prior to the administration of treatment and/or discussions with clinical staff | Compare patient experience with different regimens after recovery from previous cycle. Avoid biasing patient report based on feedback from medical staff. |
| Timing of HRQL assessments should be similar for all treatment arms | Comparable assessment times for arms problematic when regimens have different administration schedules (e.g., 3 versus 4 week cycles). Assessment time can be based on *time* (e.g., every 2 weeks from randomization/registration) or on *event* (e.g., every two treatment cycles). |
| Natural course of the disease | Known points of remission and deterioration. |
| Disease stage | 1. *Early stage disease*: longer follow-up to address survivorship issues, monitor late effects (both positive and negative), and see if patients are able to return to "normal" activities. <br> 2. *Late stage disease*: shorter follow-up period because of the potential for missing data. Median survival one basis for length of QOL follow-up. |
| Effects associated with the treatment course or administration | 1. Documentation of acute, short-term side effects or cumulative side effects such as at the end of radiotherapy (XRT). <br> 2. Minimum number of cycles required to see an effect of treatment on QOL. |
| Timing of important clinical events or monitoring | 1. Can assess QOL when patients go off treatment, such as at progression, but results in patient-specific measurement times based on event timing and the possibility of no data for patients who do not experience the event. <br> 2. Pair QOL assessments with clinical monitoring (e.g., tumor measurements) to enhance forms compliance. |
| Completion of treatment and/or a short time after completion of treatment | For example, resolution of mucositis may require 2–4 weeks postcompletion of XRT. Treatment arms might be compared at the end of XRT and 2–4 weeks later to see how much better/sooner palliation occurs. |
| Scheduling issues for special populations Example: end-of-life care | Four factors ⇒ suggested *weekly* assessment schedule [46]: (1) length of survival (~30 days for terminal patients); (2) variability in deterioration (more pronounced 1–3 weeks prior to death); (3) length of time required to observe effect of intervention; (4) burden issues. |

**TABLE 22.1 (continued)**
## Important Variables in the Determination of QOL Assessment Schedules

| Variable | Example/Rationale |
|---|---|
| Compliance with assessment schedule | 1. Respondent burden: too many assessments are burdensome and affect the patient's adherence to the QOL assessment schedule.<br>2. Institution staff burden can also affect compliance.<br>3. Data collection and management resources: frequent assessments require more personnel and data management effort and can compromise quality control procedures.<br>4. Specification of acceptable time windows: even with specified times of assessment, variability occurs in completion dates. This can affect how QOL is rated and possibly the interpretation of treatment arm comparisons [47]. |

*Source:* Adaptation from Sprangers, M.A.G. et al., the Clinical Significance Consensus Meeting Group, *Mayo Clin. Proc.*, 77, 564, 2002, Table 2.

variables such as stage of disease [56]; Osoba et al. [57] suggest that a change of 10–20 QLQ-C30 points on a 0–100 scale reflects a moderate effect.

If change for a particular questionnaire has not been documented, it is possible to use effect size as a basis for determining a clinically important difference. Effect size [58] is a measure of the change or difference in scores relative to variability in the scores. It is calculated in a number of different ways but can be summarized as follows: $\delta$ (effect size) = Mean $[\mu]_{Arm\,2}$ – Mean $[\mu]_{Arm\,1}$/Standard Deviation $[\sigma]_{Arm\,1}$. In this case, one has access to means and standard deviations for this questionnaire. The denominator can also be the standard deviation of the control arm, of a stable group, or of the difference, to name a few variations. See Sprangers et al. [48] for a summary of these formulas. Cohen [58] has described effect sizes of 0.2 as small, 0.5 as moderate, and 0.8 as large. If the number of points reflecting clinically significant change is not available, sample sizes can be estimated from standard software using effect size parameters: $\mu_1 = 0$; $\mu_2$ = the minimum $\delta$ of interest; $\sigma = 1$; $\alpha = 0.05$; and power = 0.80. One half of a standard deviation is often used as a benchmark for a moderate-sized effect or change [58,59]. However, Hays et al. [60] caution that distribution-based methods such as the standard deviation do not inform us about minimally or clinically important change for group or individual change; they only provide a standardized metric for observed change. Sloan et al. [59] noted that a difference of 10 on a 0–100 scale generally reflects a moderate effect.

If there are normative data for a questionnaire, one can characterize the meaning of a score by comparing the difference in points observed in the trial to differences reported for other groups of patients. Moinpour et al. [37] reported that a median difference of eight points was found for the SF-36 Mental Health Inventory (MHI) [25] for men receiving orchiectomy plus the antiandrogen flutamide with a median score of 76 compared to the arm treated with orchiectomy alone with a median score of 84, where a lower score reflects worse emotional well-being. Normative data for the MHI indicate that men with benign prostatic hyperplasia and hypertension had a median score of 88 while men with congestive heart failure had a median score of 80 [27]. The severity of these two medical conditions clearly differs, with men with congestive heart failure reporting more compromised emotional well-being. These data help establish the clinical meaningfulness of an eight-point difference. Even a three-point difference on the MHI is clinically important since it is associated with decreases in scores reported by individuals who have just lost their jobs [28]. It is also possible to include a single item rating of change in QOL and use this anchor to determine the number of points required for clinical significance [50].

### 22.3.3 CLINICAL SIGNIFICANCE BENCHMARKS FOR INDIVIDUAL CHANGE

Clinicians and QOL researchers are naturally interested in extending the use of PROs from clinical trials to monitoring of QOL in the clinic setting. However, we know much less about the application of the benchmarks described earlier for meaningful differences for an individual patient at one or two points in time. Donaldson [61] notes that the 95% confidence interval for a 5-point change benchmark for group comparisons would be 4.5–7.8; the 95% confidence interval for the same benchmark at the individual level would be 15–20 points. The reason is the increase in measurement error, given less information (e.g., change for other similar individuals and multiple longitudinal measures), and we are less confident that the benchmark was met. Increasing the sample size in group comparisons improves precision, as does increasing the number of longitudinal assessments for the individual; the reliability of the measure is also an important factor. The reliability of measures used at the individual level should be at least 0.90 [62,63], which is not met by all measures in use for group comparisons (where the recommendation is $\geq 0.70$). For individual change, "...the error variabilities of the two measurements combine, increasing the standard error by a factor of $\sqrt{2}$" [61]. However, while additional research to validate benchmarks for individual change continues, PRO measures can be used to improve patient/physician communication regarding QOL issues of interest to both parties.

### 22.3.4 COMPOSITE VARIABLES

Another issue that arises in cancer clinical trials with multiple traditional clinical endpoints is the advisability of creating composite variables to examine effectiveness; these composite variables can include outcomes such as hospital days, patient-reported symptoms, or general QOL (PROs). For example, Freemantle et al. [64] specified a composite variable including all-cause mortality, nonfatal myocardial infarction, and refractory ischemia. They reported that the composite variable in the four trials favored treatment with the inhibitor; however, all-cause mortality, a critical component of the composite variable, did not favor the new treatment. This shows the importance of describing effects for all components of a composite variable, so that a composite variable does not mask negative or null effects of a more clinically salient outcome. Johnson et al. [65] noted that all components of a composite variable need to be related and should have similar clinical importance in order to reflect clinical benefit. Composite variables can increase the statistical precision and efficiency of a trial when the individual components behave in the same direction. However, the results are not clinically helpful when components differ in the size and direction of the treatment effect. Freemantle et al. [64] suggested that interpretation of results for a composite variable should make clear that these results apply to the combination and not necessarily to individual components. The authors also note that the components should be treated as secondary outcomes with results reported separately for each.

### 22.3.5  COMPARATIVE EFFECTIVENESS RESEARCH

PRO measures are an important component of comparative effectiveness research (CER). CER documents benefit and harm associated with medical interventions that span the full continuum from prevention and screening, diagnosis, treatment, and survivorship [66,67]. CER usually has a more comprehensive battery of outcome measures than most clinical trials including measures of cost and health state utilities to address cost-effectiveness, resource utilization, and QOL. PRO measures (the QOL and utility outcomes) add to the information provided by more traditional measures of cost effectiveness. An example of a CER study is SWOG 1007: A Phase III, Randomized Clinical Trial of Standard Adjuvant Endocrine Therapy ± Chemotherapy in patients with one to three positive nodes, hormone receptor-positive, and HER2-Negative Breast Cancer with Recurrence Score (RS) of 25 or less. The study coordinator is Ana M. Gonzalez-Angulo, M.D. This study addresses the role of gene expression profile tests on decision making for the treatment of breast cancer for these patients. It evaluates the impact of the testing on patient levels of anxiety and decision making conflicts. The randomized trial evaluates the impact of hormonal therapy alone versus with chemotherapy for women identified as low risk for recurrence on the basis of the OncoType DX® RS. Table 22.2 and Figure 22.1 describe the study and how patients will progress through its two steps or phases. The randomized trial will evaluate whether or not women with low risk for recurrence need chemotherapy in addition to hormonal therapy.

## 22.4  TYPES OF MISSING DATA

As mentioned briefly earlier, QOL data are often subject to missingness. Depending on the nature of the mechanism producing the missing data, analyses must be adjusted differently. In the following, we list three broad classes of missing data mechanisms and provide their general descriptions along with their more formal technical names and terms.

The least problematic type of missing data is *missing completely at random* data (MCAR); this mechanism is sometimes termed "sporadic." Missing data probabilities are independent of both observable and unobservable quantities; observed data are a random subsample of complete data. This type of mechanism rarely obtains in real data.

**TABLE 22.2**

**Example of SWOG Trial with PRO and CER Outcomes**

### CANCERGEN: Center for Comparative Effectiveness Research in SWOG

| Study | Intervention | PRO Measures |
|---|---|---|
| Genomics testing to guide cancer treatment for women with one to three positive nodes, HR-positive, Her2-negative breast cancer | *Step 1*: SWOG institutions are enrolling women who discuss testing with MD, agree to receive the Oncotype DX test, and then meet with MD to learn the Recurrence Score (RS) results: a PRO assessment occurs before RS testing and after results are shared with the patient. Women with RS ≤ 25 who do not agree to randomization are administered a second PRO assessment with extra questions on their decision not to have treatment based on randomization; they receive no further follow-up. Those with RS > 25 complete a second PRO assessment and receive treatment for higher risk disease. These women receive no additional PRO follow-up. | All women, *Step 1*: PROMIS Anxiety SF,[a,b] Decisional Conflict Scale,[c] Survivor Concerns,[d] Oncotype DX testing questions,[e] and EQ-5D[f] (assessments pre and post Oncotype DX testing when results known). |
| | *Step 2*: Those with Recurrence Score (RS) ≤ 25 (low-risk) who agree to randomization receive either chemotherapy followed by hormonal treatment or hormonal treatment alone. PRO follow-up occurs at 6, 12, and 36 months. Cost of care will be determined on a subset of patients who are Medicare eligible or who have commercial health insurance from one of four health insurance groups. | Randomized study, *Step 2*: PROMIS Anxiety,[a,b] Fatigue,[a,b] Cognitive Concerns,[a,b] Decisional Conflict Scale,[c] Survivor Concerns,[d] Oncotype DX testing questions,[e] and EQ-5D[f] (four total assessments). |

[a] Garcia SF, Cella D, Clauser SB, Flynn KE, Lai J-S, Reeve BB, Wilder Smith A, Stone AA, Weinfurt K. Standardizing patient-reported outcomes assessment in cancer clinical trials: A patient-reported outcomes measurement information system initiative. *J Clin Oncol* 2007; 25:5106–5112.

[b] Personal Communications, D Cella, S Garcia, J-S Lai, 2010 and draft project summaries for the Cancer PROMIS Supplement.

[c] O'Connor AM, User Manual. Decisional Conflict Scale 1993 (updated 2005). Available from www.ohri.ca/decisionaid.

[d] Gotay CC, Pagano IS. Assessment of Survivor Concerns (ASC): A newly proposed brief questionnaire. Health Qual Life Outcomes 2007; 5:15 (http://www.hqlocom/content/5/1/15).

[e] Lo SS, Mumby PB, Norton J, Tychlik K, Smerage J, Kash J, Chew HK et al. Prospective multicenter study of the impact of the 21-gene recurrence score assay on medical oncologist and patient adjuvant breast cancer treatment selection. *J Clin Oncol* 2010; 28:1671–1676.

[f] Pickard AS, Wilke CT, Lin H-W, Lloyd A. Health utilities using the EQ-5D in studies of cancer. *Pharmacoeconomics* 2007; 25(5):365–384.

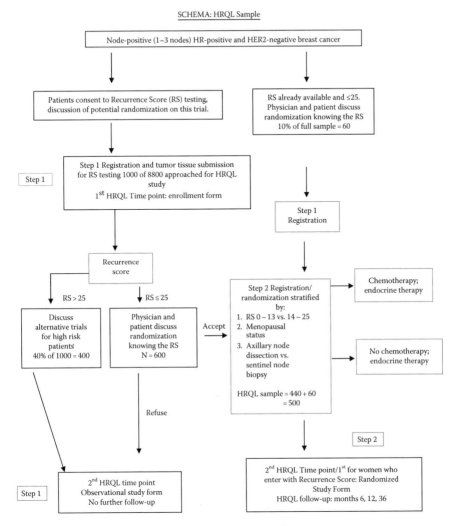

**FIGURE 22.1**    SWOG1007: SCHEMA for HRWL sample.

Data are said to be *missing at random* (MAR) when the missing data probabilities are dependent on observable quantities, such as previously measured QOL outcomes or covariates like age, sex, and stage of disease, and the analysis can generally be adjusted by weighting schemes or stratification. This type of mechanism can hold if subjects with poor baseline QOL scores are more prone to missing values later in the trial, or if an external measure of health, such as the Karnofsky performance status, completely explains the propensity to be missing. Because the missingness mechanism depends on observed data, analyses can be conducted that adjust properly for the missing observations.

The most difficult type of missing data to handle is termed *nonrandom, missing not at random* (MNAR), or *nonignorable* (NI). Here, missing data probabilities are dependent on unobservable quantities, such as missing outcome values or unobserved latent variables describing outcomes such as general health and well-being. This type of mechanism is fairly common in QOL research. One example is treatment-based differences in QOL compliance, due to worse survival on one arm of the trial. Another is when subjects having great difficulty coping with disease and treatment are more likely to refuse to complete a QOL assessment.

To determine which methods of statistical analysis will be appropriate, the analyst must first determine the patterns and amount of missing data and identify potential mechanisms that could have generated missing data. In general, there is no reliable way to test for a given type of missing data mechanism, and thus sensitivity analyses are a crucial component of any analysis; this is discussed in more detail in the following. Rubin [68] addressed the assumptions necessary to justify ignoring the missing data mechanism and established that the extent of ignorability depends on the inferential framework and the research question of interest. Under likelihood-based and Bayesian inference, the missing data are said to be *ignorable* if the missing data mechanism is MAR, and the parameters of the missing data model are distinct from those of the model of interest for the outcome. Identification of missing data mechanisms in QOL research proceeds through two complementary avenues: (1) collecting as much additional patient information as possible and applying simple graphical techniques and (2) using hypothesis testing to distinguish missing data processes, subject to modeling assumptions about the missingness mechanism.

### 22.4.1 GRAPHICAL DESCRIPTION OF MISSING DATA MECHANISMS

Graphical presentations can be crucial as a first step in elucidating the relationship of missing data to the outcome of interest and providing an overall summary of results that is easily understood by nonstatisticians. A clear picture of the extent of missing QOL assessments is necessary both for the selection of the appropriate methods of analysis and for honest reporting of the trial with respect to reliability and generalizability. In clinical trials, this means summarizing the proportions of patients in whom assessment is possible, such as surviving patients still on study, and then the pattern of assessments among these patients. Machin and Weeden [69] combine these two concepts in Figure 22.2, using the familiar Kaplan–Meier plot to indicate survival rates and a simple table describing QOL assessment compliance. For this study of palliative treatment for patients with small-cell lung cancer (SCLC) and poor prognosis, the Kaplan–Meier plot illustrates why the expected number of assessments is reduced by 60% at the time of the final assessment. The table further indicates the increase in missing data even among surviving subjects, from 25% at baseline to 71% among the evaluable patients at 6 months. If the reasons for missing assessments differ over time or across treatment groups, it may be necessary to present additional details about the missing data.

A second step is describing the missing data mechanism, especially in relation to the patients' QOL. A useful technique is to present the available data separately for patients with different amounts of and reasons for dropout. This is illustrated by Figure 22.3, due to Troxel [70], where estimates of average symptom distress in patients with advanced colorectal cancer are presented by reason for dropout and duration of follow-up. Patients who drop out due to death or illness report higher

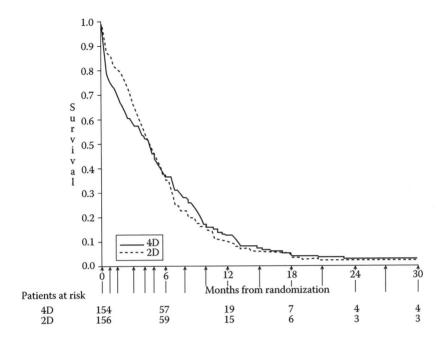

| Schedule (d) | 0 | 21 | 42 | 91 | 122 | 152 | 183 |
|---|---|---|---|---|---|---|---|
| Expected | 310 | 252 | 238 | 194 | 173 | 151 | 127 |
| window (d) | −7 to 0 | 14 to 28 | 35 to 49 | 77 to 105 | 108 to 136 | 138 to 166 | 169 to 197 |
| received | 232 | 165 | 137 | 78 | 66 | 49 | 37 |
| % | 75 | 66 | 58 | 40 | 38 | 33 | 29 |

**FIGURE 22.2** Kaplan–Meier estimates of the survival curves of patients with SCLC by treatment group (after MRC Lung Cancer Working Party, 1996). The times at which QOL assessments were scheduled are indicated beneath the time axis. The panel indicates the QOL assessments made for the seven scheduled during the first 6 months as a percentage of those anticipated from the currently living patients. (From Machin, D. and Weeden, S.: Suggestions for the presentation of quality-of-life data from clinical trials. *Stat. Med.* 1998. 17. 711–724. Copyright Wiley-VCH Verlag GmbH & Co. KGaA. Reproduced with permission.)

symptom distress and the worsening of symptom status over time is more severe for these patients as well. Patients with a decreasing QOL score may also be more likely to drop out, as demonstrated by Curran et al. [71], where a change score between two previous assessments was predictive of dropout.

## 22.4.2 COMPARING MISSING DATA MECHANISMS

Assuming a monotone pattern of missing data, Diggle [72] and Ridout [73] have proposed methods to compare MCAR and MAR dropout. The former proposal involves testing whether scores from patients who drop out immediately after a given time point are a random sample of scores from all available patients at that assessment.

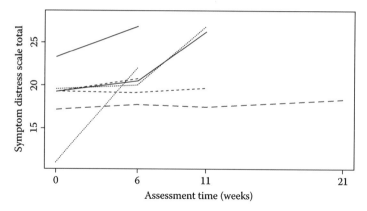

**FIGURE 22.3**  Average Symptom Distress Scale scores by type and length of follow-up. —— lost-death - - - - lost-illness – – – lost-other —— complete follow-up (From Troxel, A.B.: A comparative analysis of quality-of-life data from a Southwest Oncology Group randomized trial of advanced colorectal cancer. *Stat. Med.* 1998. 17. 767–779. Reproduced with permission.)

The latter proposal centers on logistic regression analysis to test whether observed covariates affect the probability of dropout.

Testing the assumptions of MAR against a hypothesis of MNAR is not trivial; such a procedure rests on strong assumptions that are themselves untestable [71]. When fitting an NI model, certain assumptions are made in the specification of the model about the relationship between the missing data process and unobserved data. These assumptions are fundamentally untestable. Molenberghs et al. [74] provide examples where different models produce almost similar fits to the observed data, but yield very different predictions for the unobserved data. Little [75], discussing pattern-mixture models, suggests that underidentifiability is a serious problem with MNAR missing data models and that problems may arise when estimating the parameters of the missing data mechanism simultaneously with the parameters of the underlying data model. Similar problems may exist in the selection model framework [76].

## 22.5  LONGITUDINAL ANALYSIS OPTIONS FOR "COMPLETE" DATA SETS

In general, the methods described later are applicable to both repeated measures on an individual over time and measurements of different scales or scores on a given individual at the same point in time. Many studies of course utilize both of these designs, asking patients to fill out questionnaires comprising several subscales at repeated intervals over the course of the study.

### 22.5.1  NORMAL LINEAR MIXED MODELS

The normal linear mixed model [77] is widely used in longitudinal analysis. For $i = 1, \ldots, n$ individuals, the repeated QOL measurements are organized into outcome vectors $y_i$, which are assumed to be normally distributed, and a linear function of both fixed effects $X_i$ and random effects $Z_i$, as follows:

$$y_i = X_i \alpha + Z_i b_i + e_i$$

where
   $\alpha$ is a vector of parameters linking the outcomes to the fixed effects
   The random parameters $b_i$ follow $k$-variate normal distributions with mean zero and variance-covariance matrix $D$
   $e_i$ follow multivariate normal distributions with mean zero and variance-covariance matrix $S_i$

Here, $D$ is a positive-definite covariance matrix of dimension $k$, and $S_i$ is a positive-definite covariance matrix of dimension $n_i$ whose parameters do not depend on $i$. The model can be formulated using either a classical likelihood approach or Bayesian methodology; in both cases, the EM algorithm [78] can be used for estimation. When the variance parameters in $S_i$ and $D$ are unknown, they can be estimated using either maximum likelihood (ML) or restricted maximum likelihood (REML). REML estimates avoid the downward bias of the ML estimates, which occurs because they fail to account for the degrees of freedom lost in estimating the regression parameters. Software is available to fit this model in many standard packages, including SAS and Splus [79,80].

The linear mixed model is very appealing, as it allows for individual effects on QOL in addition to fixed effects for treatment, time, and clinical variables. These effects can describe individual variation around the average outcome at different times or they can take the form of growth curve parameters for individuals. Furthermore, more traditional analysis of variance (ANOVA) and covariance (ANCOVA) models are simply special cases of the model stated here in which the $b_i = 0$.

## 22.5.2  GENERALIZED LINEAR MODELS

A second general class of models is the likelihood-based generalized linear model (GLM) [81]. This framework is attractive since it accommodates a whole class of data, rather than being restricted to continuous Gaussian measurements; it allows a unified treatment of measurements of different types, with specification of an appropriate link function that determines the form of the mean and variance. For example, binary data can be evaluated using a logistic link function, in order to evaluate the proportion of subjects experiencing a particular outcome. Estimation proceeds by solving the likelihood score equations, usually using iteratively reweighted least squares or Newton–Raphson algorithms. GLMs can be fit with GLIM [82], with Splus using the GLM function [83], or with SAS using the GLM or mixed procedures [84]. If missing data are MAR, unbiased estimates will be obtained. Generalized linear mixed models are a useful extension, allowing for the inclusion of random effects in the GLM framework. Most widely used software packages have routines available to fit these models [79,85,86].

### 22.5.3 GENERALIZED ESTIMATING EQUATIONS

Like GLMs, generalized estimating equations (GEEs) [87] provide a framework to treat disparate kinds of data in a unified way. In addition, they require specification of only the first two moments of the repeated measures, rather than the likelihood. Estimates are obtained by solving an estimating equation of the following form:

$$U = \sum_{i=1}^{n} D_i' V_i^{-1}(Y_i - \mu_i) = 0$$

where

$\mu_i = E(Y_i|X_i, \beta)$ and $D_i = \partial\mu_i/\partial\beta$ are the usual mean and derivative functions
$V_i$ is a working correlation matrix

For Gaussian measurements, the estimating equations resulting from the GEE are equivalent to the usual score equations obtained from a multivariate normal maximum likelihood model; the same estimates will be obtained from either method. Software is again widely available [85–88].

### 22.5.4 CHANGE-SCORE ANALYSIS

Analysis of individual or group changes in QOL scores over time is often of great importance in longitudinal studies. The simplest and most commonly used type of change-score analysis is to take the difference of QOL outcomes at two time points and apply a $t$-test or nonparametric test to compare treatment groups. Alternatively, one can assess the extent of change by applying a paired $t$-test to repeated measurements within a population. Change-score analysis has the advantage of inherently adjusting for the baseline score, but must also be undertaken with caution, as it is by nature sensitive to problems of regression to the mean [89]. In QOL studies in particular, a large amount of individual subject variation can overwhelm a statistically significant but small effect; changes in means scores by treatment group must be interpreted with great caution before being applied to individual patients [90].

### 22.5.5 TIME-TO-EVENT ANALYSIS

If attainment of a particular QOL score or milestone is the basis of the experiment, time-to-event or survival analysis methods can be applied. Once the event has been clearly defined, the analysis tools can be directly applied. These include Kaplan–Meier estimates of "survival" functions [91], Cox proportional hazard regression models [92] to relate covariates to the probability of the event, and logrank and other tests for differences in the event history among comparison groups. The QOL database, however, supports few such milestones at this point in time.

## 22.6 METHODS FOR ANALYSIS WITH MISSING DATA

### 22.6.1 JOINT MODELING OF MEASUREMENT AND MISSINGNESS PROCESSES

One can model the joint distribution of the underlying complete data $Y_i$ and the missingness indicators $R_i$. If conditioning arguments are used, two types of models can result; the selection model is concerned with $f(Y_i)f(R_i|Y_i)$, while the pattern mixture model is concerned with $f(R_i)f(Y_i|R_i)$. The two approaches are discussed and compared in detail by Little [75]. Pattern mixture models proceed by estimating the parameters of interest within strata defined by patterns of and/or reasons for missingness and then by combining the estimates. Selection models proceed by modeling the complete data and then modeling the behavior of the missingness probabilities conditional on the outcome data.

Selection models for continuous and event data have been used by many authors; see the following for application to QOL [74,93–95]. While the computations can be burdensome, the approach will produce unbiased estimates even in the face of MNAR processes, provided that both parts of the model are correctly specified. Most selection models assume that the complete underlying responses are multivariate normal; any parametric model, such as the logistic, can be used for the missing data probabilities. The type of missingness mechanism is controlled by the covariates and/or responses that are included in the model for the missingness probabilities. For example, Troxel et al. [93] posit a multivariate normal model for coping scores in a breast cancer trial, assuming an autoregressive covariance structure, along with a logistic model for the missing data probabilities that depends on current and possibly unobserved values of QOL:

$$Y_{it}^* \mid Y_{i,t-1}^* \sim N\left\{\mu_{it} + \rho_{t-1}\frac{\sigma_t}{\sigma_{t-1}}\left(Y_{i,t-1}^* - \mu_{i,t-1}\right), \sigma_t^2\left(1 - \rho_{t-1}^2\right)\right\}$$

$$\pi_{it} = \text{logit}\left[P(R_{it} = 0)\right] = \beta_0 + \beta_1 Y_{it}^*$$

where

$Y_{it}^*$ represents the true but potentially unobserved QOL score for subject $i$ at time $t$ $\sigma_t^2 = \text{var}\left(Y_{it}^*\right)$, $\rho_t = \text{corr}\left(Y_{it}^*, Y_{i,t+1}^*\right)$

$R_{it}$ is an indicator for subject $i$ at time $t$ taking the value 1 if $Y_{it}^*$ is observed and 0 otherwise

$\pi_{it}$ is the probability that $Y_{it}^*$ is missing

Since the probabilities depend on the current, possibly unobserved measurement $Y_{it}^*$, the model can handle MNAR data; it is possible to allow dependence on previous values as well. The observed data likelihood is obtained by integrating the complete data likelihood over the missing values, as follows:

$$\int \cdots \int f_{i1}^* \pi_{i1}^{1-R_{i1}} (1 - \pi_{i1})^{R_{i1}} \prod_{t=2}^T f_{t|t-1}^* \pi_{it}^{1-R_{it}} (1 - \pi_{it})^{R_{it}} \prod_{t=1}^T \left(dY_{it}^*\right)^{1-R_{it}}$$

where

$f_{i1}^*$ is the normal density for $Y_{i1}^*$

$f_{t|t-1}^*$ is the conditional normal density for $Y_{it}^* \mid Y_{i,t-1}^*$

$\pi_{i1}$ is the probability that the first value for subject $i$ is observed

$T$ is the last assessment time

Estimates are usually obtained through direct maximization of the likelihood surface; numerical integration is generally required. Once estimates are obtained, inference is straightforward using standard likelihood techniques. This method allows analysis of all the data, even when the missingness probabilities depend on potentially unobserved values of the response. The estimates are also likely to depend on modeling assumptions, most of which are untestable in the presence of MNAR missing data. Despite these drawbacks, these models can be very useful for investigation and testing of the missingness mechanism. In addition, the bias that results from assuming the wrong type of missingness mechanism may well be more severe than the bias that results from mis-specification of a full maximum likelihood model. Software to fit the Diggle and Kenward [76] model is available [96].

Many authors have proposed pattern-mixture models [97–100]. Pauler et al. [99] used a pattern-mixture model approach to model repeated measures conditional on death and drop-out times, with a multinomial model for the death times themselves. The QOL outcomes follow a normal linear mixed model:

$$Y_i(t) \mid (b_{0i}, b_{1i}) \sim N\left(\beta_0 + \beta_1 t + \beta_2 z + \beta_3 zt + b_{0i} + b_{1i} t, \sigma^2\right)$$

$$(b_{0i}, b_{1i})' \sim N_2\left((0,0)', D\right)$$

where

$t$ and $z$ are time and treatment effects, respectively

$b_{0i}$ and $b_{1i}$ are individual-specific intercepts and slopes

$\sigma^2$ is the conditional within-subject variation

For discrete data, methods allowing for NI missing data have also been proposed [101–106]. Often, log-linear models are used for the joint probability of outcome and response variables conditional on covariates. The models can be fit using the EM algorithm [78] treating the parameters of the missingness model as a nuisance or using estimating equations.

Several extensions to standard mixed models have been proposed in the context of longitudinal measurements in clinical trials. Zee [107] has proposed growth curve models where the parameters relating to the polynomial in time are allowed to differ according to the various health states experienced by the patient, for example, on treatment, off treatment, and postrelapse. This method requires that the missing data be MAR and may be fit with standard packages by simply creating an appropriate variable to indicate health state; in essence, it is a type of pattern mixture model.

Schluchter [108] has proposed a joint mixed effects model for the longitudinal assessments and the time to dropout, in which a vector of random effects and the log of the dropout time are jointly normally distributed. This model allows MNAR data in the sense that the time of dropout is allowed to depend on the rate of change in the underlying measurements. More recently, a number of authors have proposed sophisticated joint models for longitudinal and event-time data. Work in HIV/AIDS focused on repeated measurements of CD4 counts as predictors of recurrence or other kinds of failure and posited a measurement error model for the repeated measurements and a Cox model for the survival outcome [109–112]. Because these models account for measurement error in the repeated measures, they are readily adaptable to longitudinal values with missing data; in general, the data must be MAR for valid inference, but they can be used for MNAR mechanisms if the dropout times are determined by survival data. More recent developments include estimation via estimating equations [113], relaxation of assumptions of normality [114], and use of Bayesian methods to handle longitudinal measures with varying assessment schedules [115].

A number of authors have suggested shared parameter models, in which random effects shared between the missing data model and the outcome model accommodate NI missing data mechanisms [116–118]. In this case, the complete-data likelihood can be written as $\int f\left(Y^o, Y^m \mid b, \theta\right) f\left(R \mid b, \theta\right), f\left(b \mid \theta\right) db$. Here, the outcomes $Y$ and the missing data indicators $R$ are assumed to be independent, conditional on the random effects $b$. As noted by [75,119], SPMs are appropriate when missingness can be attributed to some latent process, such as disease progression, that the longitudinal outcomes measure imperfectly. The size of the measurement error determines the strength of the dependence of the missingness on the latent variable $b$. A shared parameter model by definition implies MNAR missing data, because the previous likelihood implies that the missing data mechanism can be written as $f\left(R \mid Y^o, Y^m, \theta\right) = \int f\left(R \mid b, \theta\right), f\left(b \mid Y^o, Y^m, \theta\right) db$; thus, the probability of nonresponse depends on the missing values through the posterior distribution of the random effects given both the observed and missing outcomes. There are several options for handling the random effects $b$. The simplest approach is to assume a multivariate normal distribution, as in the general random-effects framework, but several authors have shown that this can result in biased estimates if the assumptions are not met [120–123]. More recent work has proposed using mixtures of normal distributions [124,125] or leaving the random-effects distribution completely unspecified [118,126].

## 22.6.2 Weighted GEEs

GEEs produce unbiased estimates for data that are MCAR. Extensions to the GEE exist for data that are MAR: weighted GEEs will produce unbiased estimates provided the weights are estimated consistently [127,128]. When the missingness probabilities depend only on observed covariates, such as the stage of disease, or responses, such as the baseline QOL score, a logistic or probit model can be used to estimate missingness probabilities for every subject; the weights used in the analysis are then the inverses of these estimated probabilities. Robins et al. [128] discuss these equations and their properties in detail; presented simply, the estimating equation takes the form

$$U = \sum_{i=1}^{n} D_i' V_i^{-1} \mathrm{diag}\left(\frac{R_i}{\hat{\pi}_i}\right)(Y_i - \mu_i) = 0$$

where

$\pi_i = P(R_{ij} = 1 \mid Y_i^o, W_i, \alpha)$

$\hat{\pi}_i$ is an estimate of $\pi_i$

diag($Q$) indicates a matrix of zeroes with the vector $Q$ on the diagonal

Although software exists to fit GEEs, additional programming is usually required to fit a weighted version.

### 22.6.3 SENSITIVITY ANALYSIS

Even while more sophisticated methods for handling missing data are developed, sensitivity analysis remains an integral part of any analysis involving incomplete data. Sensitivity analyses, in which the parameters governing the missing data mechanism are varied to determine their effect on estimates of the parameters of interest, are even more crucial in settings where NI missing data may occur.

Sensitivity analyses can take several forms. Some authors have recommended global sensitivity analyses in the context of selection models for likelihood-based [56] or semiparametric inference [129]. Others have proposed analogous approaches in the context of pattern-mixture models [130,131]. These analyses can be very useful, but can sometimes still involve assumptions about the complete data distribution and require difficult computations. Another option is to study sensitivity locally, in the neighborhood of the MAR model. Copas and Li [132] describe an approach for a normal linear model, in which the correlation of error terms in the model of interest and the missing data model is treated as a sensitivity parameter. Others have suggested using ideas of local influence and likelihood displacement to assess sensitivity due to individual observations or collections of observations [133]. More recently, Troxel et al. [134] proposed a more general index of local sensitivity in the context of parametric selection models. This approach focuses on the behavior of the maximum likelihood estimate (MLE) as the nonignorability parameter moves away from its value under the MAR model (usually zero). The idea has been extended to longitudinal data, survival data, and many other specialized models [135–138] and is appealing since it requires no specialized computations and focuses on the neighborhood of the MAR model, since that is the preferred mode of analysis if the sensitivity is not extreme.

## 22.7 AVOIDING PITFALLS: SOME COMMONLY USED SOLUTIONS

### 22.7.1 SUBSTITUTION METHODS

In general, methods that rely on substitution of some value, determined in a variety of ways, are subject to bias and heavily subject to assumptions made in obtaining the substituted value. For these reasons, they should not be used to produce a primary analysis on which treatment or other decisions are based. One problem with substitution methods, especially when the worse score method is used, is that they can seriously affect the psychometric properties of a measure. These properties, such as reliability and validity, rely on variations in the scores in order to hold. A second problem is that in substituting values and then conducting analyses based on those data, the variance of estimates will be underestimated, since the missing values, had they been observed, would carry with them random variation, which the substituted values do not. Substitution methods can be useful, however, in conducting sensitivity analyses to determine the extent to which the analysis is swayed by differing data sets.

The worst score method is often used in sensitivity analyses, making the implicit assumption that subjects who did not submit an assessment are as worse off as they can possibly be with respect to QOL. This is usually an extreme assumption, so an analysis robust to worst score substitution has a strong defense.

The last value carried forward (LVCF) substitution method tries to use each patient's score to provide information about the imputed value. It assumes, however, that subjects who drop out do not have a changing QOL score, when in practice the subjects in rapid decline often tend to drop out prematurely. For this reason, LVCF should be always be avoided.

The use of the average score, either within a patient or within a group of patients, such as those on the same treatment arm, is more closely related to classic imputation methods. Again, it assumes that the imputed values are no different from the observed values, but it does not necessarily force each subject's score to remain constant.

### 22.7.2 MULTIPLE IMPUTATION

Imputation or "filling-in" of data sets is a valid way of converting an incomplete to a complete data set. This method is attractive because once the imputation is conducted, the methods for complete data described in Section 22.5 can be applied. Unlike ordinary substitution, single imputation consists of substituting a value for the missing observations and then adjusting the analysis to account for the fact that the substituted value was not obtained with the usual random variation.

Multiple imputation [139] is similar in spirit to single imputation, but with added safeguards against underestimation of variance due to substitution. Several data sets are imputed, and the analysis in question is conducted on each of them, resulting in a set of estimates obtained from each imputed data set. These several results are then combined to obtain final estimates based on the multiple sets.

Multiple imputations can be conducted in the presence of all kinds of missingness mechanisms. The usual drawback with respect to NI missingness applies, however. A model is required to obtain the imputed values, and, in the presence of NI missingness, the resultant estimates are sensitive to the chosen model; even worse, the assumptions governing that model are generally untestable.

### 22.7.3 ADJUSTED SURVIVAL ANALYSES

Some authors have proposed analyses in which survival is treated as the primary outcome, with adjustment for the QOL experience of the patients. This is an extremely appealing idea, for it clarifies the inherent trade-off between length and QOL that applies to most patients. It can be difficult to implement satisfactorily in practice, however, because of the difficulty of obtaining the appropriate weights for survival in different periods. The two methods described later have gained some popularity.

### 22.7.3.1   Quality Adjusted Life Years

This method consists of estimating a fairly simple weighted average, in which designated periods of life are weighted according to some utility describing QOL [140–144]. Because utilities are obtained using lengthy interviews or questionnaires focusing on time trade-offs or standard gambles, investigators commonly substitute utilities obtained from some standard population rather than any information obtained directly from the patient. This renders the analysis largely uninterpretable, in our view.

### 22.7.3.2   Q-TWiST

Q-TWiST [145–149], or quality-adjusted time without symptoms and toxicity, is a more detailed method of adjustment, though still one that relies on utilities. The patient's course through time is divided up into intervals in which the patient experiences toxicity due to treatment, toxicity due to disease brought on by relapse, and no toxicity. These intervals may be somewhat arbitrary, determined not by the patient's actual experience with toxicity but by predefined averages observed among patients with a given disease receiving a given treatment. To compound this arbitrariness, utilities for each period are chosen by the analyst, but the impact of different utilities can be examined in sensitivity analyses. This results in an analysis that reflects only a small amount of patient-derived data, and a large number of parameters chosen by the investigator; as with the adjusted life-years approach mentioned earlier, these attributes make it very difficult to obtain reliable inference. Indeed, data from patient rating scales and Q-TWiST analyses have been shown to differ considerably [150].

## 22.8   CONCLUSIONS

QOL data are an integral part of modern clinical studies in cancer and can provide valuable information about appropriate treatment choices to patients and caregivers. For this information to be most useful, care must be taken with every aspect of the QOL study, from questionnaire development and design, to setting measurement schedules, to minimizing missing data, to using appropriate analytic methods that accommodate the variability in individual assessments over time and the potential missing data or censoring mechanisms. Continued research into all these areas will add to our ability to accurately measure, estimate, and compare QOL in cancer patients, with the goal of enhancing their experiences and alleviating their suffering.

## REFERENCES

1. Moinpour CM, Feigl P, Metch B, Hayden KH, Meyskens FL Jr, Crowley J. Quality of life end points in cancer clinical trials: Review and recommendations. *J Natl Cancer Inst* 1989; 81:485–495.
2. Nayfield S, Ganz PA, Moinpour CM, Cella D, Hailey B. Report from a National Cancer Institute (USA) workshop on quality of life assessment in cancer clinical trials. *Qual Life Res* 1992; 1:203–210.

3. National Cancer Institute (US). Quality of life in clinical trials. *Proceedings of a workshop held at the National Institute of Health*, March 1–2, 1995. Bethesda (MD): National Institute of Health, 1996.

4. Sugarbaker PH, Barofsky I, Rosenberg SA, Gianola FJ. Quality of life assessment of patients in extremity sarcoma clinical trials. *Surgery* 1982; 9:17–23.

5. Nunnally, J. *Psychometric Theory*. New York: McGraw-Hill, 1978.

6. Kirshner B, Guyatt GH. A methodological framework for assessing health indices. *J Chronic Dis* 1985; 1:27–36.

7. Guyatt GH, Deyo RA, Charlson M, Levine MN, Mitchell A. Responsiveness and validity in health status measurement: A clarification. *J Clin Epidemiol* 1989; 42:403–408.

8. Cella DF, Tulsky DS, Gray G, Sarafian B, Linn E, Bonomi AE, Silberman M et al. The Functional Assessment of Cancer Therapy scale: Development and validation of the general measure. *J Clin Oncol* 1993; 11(3):570–579.

9. Cella DF, Bonomi AE, Lloyd ST, Tulsky DS, Kaplan E, Bonomi P. Reliability and validity of the Functional Assessment of Cancer Therapy—Lung (FACT-L) quality of life instrument. *Lung Cancer* 1995; 12:199–220.

10. Esper P, Mo F, Chodak G, Sinner M, Cella D, Pienta KJ. Measuring quality of life in men with prostate cancer using the Functional Assessment of Cancer Therapy—Prostate instrument. *Urology* 1997; 50:920–928.

11. Cella DF. Manual of the Functional Assessment of Chronic Illness Therapy (FACIT Scales)—Version 4. Outcomes, Research, and Education (CORE), Evanston Northwestern Healthcare and Northwestern University, Evanston, IL, 1997.

12. Webster K, Odom L, Peterman A, Lent L, Cella D. The Functional Assessment of Chronic Illness Therapy (FACIT) measurement system: Validation of version 4 of the core questionnaire. *Qual Life Res* 1999; 8:604.

13. Aaronson NK, Bullinger M, Ahmedzai S. A modular approach to quality of life assessment in cancer clinical trials. *Recent Results Cancer Res* 1988; 111:231–249.

14. Aaronson NK, Ahmedzai S, Bergman B, Bullinger M, Cull A, Duez NJ, Filiberti A et al. For the European Organization for Research and Treatment of Cancer Study Group on Quality of Life. The European Organization for Research and Treatment of Cancer QLQ-C30: A quality-of-life instrument for use in international clinical trials in oncology. *J Natl Cancer Inst* 1993; 85:365–376.

15. Fayers P, Aaronson N, Bjordal K, Groenvold M, Curran D, Bottomley A. On behalf of EORTC Quality of Life Study Group. *EORTC QLQ-C30 Scoring Manual*. 3rd edn. Brussels, Belgium: EORTC, 2001.

16. Fayers P, Weeden S, Curran D. On behalf of EORTC Quality of Life Study Group. *EORTC QLQ-C30 Reference Values*. Brussels, Belgium: EORTC Quality of Life Study Group, 1998.

17. Fayers P, Bottomley A. On behalf of the EORTC Quality of Life group and of the Quality of Life Unit. Quality of life research within the EORTC-the EORTC QLQ-C30. *Eur J Cancer* 2002; 38:S125–S133.

18. www.facit.org/FACITOrg/QUestionnairs (accessed May 2011).

19. www.eortc.be/home/qol/questionnaires_modules.htm (accessed May 2011).

20. Schag CAC, Ganz PA, Heinrich RL. Cancer rehabilitation evaluation system—Short Form (CARES-SF): A cancer specific rehabilitation and quality of life instrument. *Cancer* 1991; 68:1406–1413.

21. Heinrich RL, Schag CAC, Ganz PA. Living with cancer: The cancer inventory of problem situations. *J Clin Psychol* 1984; 40:972–980.

22. Schag CAC, Heinrich RL, Ganz PA. The cancer inventory of problem situations: An instrument for assessing cancer patients' rehabilitation needs. *J Psychosoc Oncol* 1983; 1:11–24.

23. Schag CAC, Heinrich RL. Development of a comprehensive quality of life measurement tool: CARES. *Oncology* 1990; 4:135–138.

24. Stewart AL, Ware JE, Jr. *Measuring Functioning and Well Being: The Medical Outcomes Approach*. Durham, NC: Duke University Press, 1992.

25. Ware JE, Jr., Sherbourne CD. The MOS 36-item short-form health survey (SF-36). I. Conceptual framework and item selection. *Med Care* 1992; 30(6):473–483.

26. McHorney C, Ware JE, Jr., Raczek A. The MOS 36-item short-form health survey (SF-36): II. Psychometric and clinical tests of validity in measuring physical and mental health constructs. *Med Care* 1993; 31(3):247–263.

27. McHorney CA, Ware JE, Jr., Lu RJF, Sherbourne CD. The MOS 36-item short-form health survey (SF-36): III. Tests of data quality, scaling assumptions, and reliability across diverse patient groups. *Med Care* 1994; 32(1):40–46.

28. Ware JE, Jr., Snow KK, Kosinski MA, Gandek B. *SF-36 Health Survey: Manual and Interpretation Guide*. Boston, MA: Nimrod Press, 1993.

29. Ware JE, Jr., Kosinski M, Keller SD. *SF-36 Physical and Mental Health Summary Scales: A User's Manual*. Boston, MA: The Health Institute, New England Medical Center, 1994.

30. Ware JE, Jr. The SF-36 health survey. In: Spilker B, ed. *Quality of Life and Pharmacoeconomics in Clinical Trials*. Philadelphia, PA: Lippincott-Raven, 1996.

31. Ware JE, Kosinski M, Dewey JE. *How to Score Version Two of the SF-36 Health Survey*. Lincoln, RI: QualityMetric Incorporated, 2000.

32. Ware JE, Kosinski M, Turner-Bowker DM, Gandek B. *How to Score Version 2 of the SF-12® Health Survey (With a Supplement Documenting Version 1)*. Lincoln, RI: QualityMetric Incorporated, 2002.

33. Turner-Bowker DM, Bartley PJ, Ware JE Jr. *SF-36® Health Survey & "SF" Bibliography: Third Edition (1998–2000)*. Lincoln, RI: QualityMetric Incorporated, 2002.

34. Ware JE, Jr., Kosinski M, Dewey JE, Gandek B. *How to Score and Interpret Single-Item Health Status Measures: A Manual for User of the SF-8™ Health Survey*. Lincoln, RI: QualityMetric Incorporated, 2001.

35. Turner-Bowker DM, Bayliss MS, Ware JE, Jr., Kosinski M. Usefulness of the SF-8™ Health Survey for comparing the impact of migraine and other conditions. *Qual Life Res* 2003; 12:1003–1012.

36. www.sf-36.org (accessed August 2004).

37. Moinpour CM, Savage MJ, Troxel AB, Lovato LC, Eisenberger M, Veith RW, Higgins B et al. Quality of life in advanced prostate cancer: Results of a randomized therapeutic trial. *J Natl Cancer Inst* 1998; 90:1537–1544.

38. Cella D, Yount S, Rothrock N, Gershon R, Cook K, Reeve B, Ader D, Fries JF, Bruce B, Matthias R, on behalf of the PROMIS cooperative group. The Patient Reported Outcomes Measurement Information System (PROMIS): Progress of an NIH Roadmap Cooperative Group during its first two years. *Med Care* 2007; 45(5):S3–S11. (NIHMSID: 166544, PMCID: Unavailable).

39. Cella D, Riley W, Stone A, Rothrock N, Reeve B, Yount S, Amtmann D et al., on behalf of the PROMIS Cooperative Group. The Patient Reported Outcomes Measurement Information System (PROMIS) developed and tested its first wave of adult self-reported health outcome item banks: 2005–2008. *J Clin Epidemiol* 2010; 63(11):1179–1194. (PMCID: In process).

40. Ware JE. Improvements in short-form measures of health status: Introduction to a series. *J Clin Epidemiol* 2008; 61(1):1–5. (PMCID: Not applicable).

41. World Health Organization. Constitution of the World Health Organization. Geneva, Switzerland: WHO, 1946.

42. Reeve B, Hays RD, Bjorner J, Cook K, Crane PK, Teresi JA, Thissen D et al. on behalf of the PROMIS cooperative group. Psychometric evaluation and calibration of health-related quality of life item banks: Plans for the Patient-Reported Outcome Measurement Information System (PROMIS). *Med Care* 2007; 45(5):S22–S31. (PMCID: Unavailable).

43. Garcia SF, Cella D, Clauser SB, Flynn KE, Lad T, Lai JS, Reeve B, Smith AW, Stone AA, Weinfurt KP. Standardizing patient-reported outcomes assessment in cancer clinical trials: A PROMIS initiative. *J Clin Oncol* 2007; 25(32):5106–5112. (PMCID: Unavailable).

44. Reeve BB. Special issues for building computerized-adaptive tests for measuring patient-reported outcomes: The National Institute of Health's investment in new technology. *Med Care* 2006; 44(11, Suppl 3):S198–S204.

45. Gershon RC, Rothrock NE, Hanrahan RT, Jansky LJ, Harniss M, Riley W. The development of a clinical outcomes survey research application: Assessment Center. *Qual Life Res* 2010; 19(5):677–685. (PMCID: In process).

46. Tang ST, McCorkle R. Appropriate time frames for data collection in quality of life research among cancer patients at the end of life. *Qual Life Res* 2002; 11:145–155.

47. Hakamies-Blomqvist L, Luoma M-L, Sjöström J, Pluzanska A, Sjödin M, Mouridsen H, Østenstad B et al. Timing of quality of life (QoL) assessments as a source of error in oncological trials. *J Adv Nurs* 2001; 35:709–716.

48. Sprangers MAG, Moinpour CM, Moynihan TJ, Patrick DL, Revicki DA, the Clinical Significance Consensus Meeting Group. Assessing meaningful change in quality of life over time: A user's guide for clinicians. *Mayo Clin Proc* 2002; 77:561–571.

49. Sloan JA, Cella D, Frost M, Guyatt GH, Springers M, Symonds T, the Clinical Significance Consensus Meeting Group. Assessing clinical significance in measuring oncology patient quality of life: Introduction to the Symposium, content overview, and definition of terms. *Mayo Clin Proc* 2002; 77:367–370.

50. Guyatt GH, Osoba D, Wu AW, Wyrwich KW, Norman GR, the Clinical Significance Consensus Meeting Group. Methods to explain the clinical significance of health status measures. *Mayo Clin Proc* 2002; 77:371–383.

51. Cella D, Bullinger M, Scott C, Barofsky I, the Clinical Significance Consensus Meeting Group. Group vs individual approaches to understanding the clinical significance of differences or changes in quality of life. *Mayo Clin Proc* 2002; 77:384–392.

52. Sloan JA, Aaronson N, Cappelleri JC, Fairclough DL, Varricchio C, the Clinical Significance Consensus Meeting Group. Assessing the clinical significance of single items relative to summated scores. *Mayo Clin Proc* 2002; 77:479–487.

53. Frost MH, Bonomi AE, Ferrans CE, Wong GY, Hays RD, the Clinical Significance Consensus Meeting Group. Patient, clinician, and population perspectives on determining the clinical significance of quality-of-life scores. *Mayo Clin Proc* 2002; 77:488–494.

54. Symonds T, Berzon R, Marquis P, Rummans TA, the Clinical Significance Consensus Meeting Group. The clinical significance of quality-of-life results: Practical considerations for specific audiences. *Mayo Clin Proc* 2002; 77:572–583.

55. Cella D, Eton DT, Fairclough DL, Bonomi P, Heyes AE, Silberman C, Wolf MK, Johnson DH. What is a clinically meaningful change on the Functional Assessment of Cancer Therapy—Lung (FACT-L) Questionnaire? Results from Eastern Cooperative Oncology Group (ECOG) Study 5592. *J Clin Epidemiol* 2002; 55:285–295.

56. King MT. The interpretation of scores from the EORTC quality of life questionnaire QLQ-C30. *Qual Life Res* 1996; 5:555–567.

57. Osoba D, Rodriques, Myles J, Zee B, Pater J. Interpreting the significance of changes in health-related quality-of-life scores. *J Clin Oncol* 1998; 16:139–144.

58. Cohen J, *Statistical Power Analysis for the Behavioral Sciences*. 2nd edn. Hillsdale, NJ: Lawrence Erlbaum Associates, 1988.

59. Sloan JA, Loprinzi CL, Kuross SA, Miser AW, O'Fallon JR, Mahoney MR, Heid IM, Bretscher ME, Vaught NL. Randomized comparison of four tools measuring overall quality of life in patients with advanced cancer. *J Clin Oncol* 1998; 16:3662–3673.

60. Hays RD, Brodsky M, Johnston MF, Spritzer KL, Hui K-K. Evaluating the statistically significance of health-related quality-of-life change in individual patients. *Eval Health Prof* 2005; 28(2):160–171.

61. Donaldson G. Patient-reported outcomes and the mandate of measurement. *Qual Life Res* 2008; 17:1303–1313.
62. Nunnally JC, Bernstein IH. *Psychometric Theory.* New York: McGraw-Hill, 1994.
63. McHorney CA, Tarlov AR. Individual-patient monitoring in clinical practice: Are available health status surveys adequate? *Qual Life Res* 1995; 4:293–307.
64. Freemantle N, Calvert M, Wood J, Eastaugh J, Griffin C. Composite outcomes in randomized trials. Greater precision but with greater uncertainty? *J Am Med Assoc* 2003; 289:2554–2559.
65. Johnson JR, Williams G, Pazdur R. End points and United States Food and Drug Administration approval of oncology drugs. *J Clin Oncol* 2003; 21:1404–1411.
66. Sox HC, Greenfield S. Comparative effectiveness research: A report from the Institute of Medicine. *Ann Intern Med* 2009; 151(3):203–205.
67. Sox HC. Comparative effectiveness research: the importance of getting is right. *Med Care* 2010; 48(Suppl 6):S7–S8.
68. Rubin DB. Inference and missing data. *Biometrika* 1976; 63:581–592.
69. Machin D, Weeden S. Suggestions for the presentation of quality of life data from clinical trials. *Stat Med* 1998; 17:711–724.
70. Troxel AB. A comparative analysis of quality of life data from a Southwest Oncology Group randomized trial of advanced colorectal cancer. *Stat Med* 1998; 17:767–779.
71. Curran D, Bacchi M, Schmitz SFH, Molenberghs G, Sylvester RJ. Identifying the types of missingness in quality of life data from clinical trials. *Stat Med* 1998; 17:697–710.
72. Diggle PJ. Testing for random dropouts in repeated measurement data. *Biometrics* 1989; 45:1255–1258.
73. Ridout M. Reader reaction: Testing for random dropouts in repeated measurement data. *Biometrics* 1991; 47:1617–1621.
74. Molenberghs G, Goetghebeur EJT, Lipsitz SR, Kenward MG. Nonrandom missingness in categorical data: Strengths and limitations. *Am Stat* 1999; 53:110–118.
75. Little RJA. Modeling the drop-out mechanism in repeated-measures studies. *J Am Stat Assoc* 1995; 90:1112–1121.
76. Diggle P, Kenward, M. Informative drop-out in longitudinal analysis (with discussion). *Appl Stat* 1994; 43:49–93.
77. Laird NM, Ware JH. Random-effects models for longitudinal data. *Biometrics* 1982; 38:963–974.
78. Dempster AP, Laird NM, Rubin DB. Maximum likelihood estimation from incomplete data via the EM algorithm (with discussion). *J R Stat Soc B* 1977; 39:1–38.
79. The SAS Institute, Cary, NC; www.sas.com/index.html (accessed August 2004).
80. TIBCO Spotfire, Somerville, MA; spotfire.tibco.com/products/s-plus/statistical-analysis-software.aspx (accessed May 2011).
81. McCullagh P, Nelder JA. *Generalized Linear Models.* 2nd edn. London, U.K.: Chapman & Hall, 1989.
82. Baker RJ, Nelder JA. *The GLIM System, Release 3, Generalized Linear Interactive Modeling.* Oxford, U.K.: Numerical Algorithms Group, 1978.
83. Hastie TJ, Pregibon D. Generalized linear models. In: Chambers JM, Hastie TJ, eds. *Statistical Models in S.* London, U.K.: Chapman & Hall, 1993.
84. Wolfinger R, Chang M. *Comparing the SAS GLM and MIXED Procedures for Repeated Measures.* Cary, NC: The SAS Institute.
85. Stata Corp, College Station, TX; www.stata.com (accessed May 2011).
86. www.r-project.org (accessed May 2011).
87. Liang KY, Zeger SL. Longitudinal data analysis using generalized linear models. *Biometrika* 1986; 73:13–22.
88. Groemping U. GEE: A SAS macro for longitudinal data analysis. Technical Report, Fachbereich Statistik, Dortmund, Germany: Universitaet Dortmund, 1994.

89. Fleiss JL. *The Design and Analysis of Clinical Experiments.* New York: John Wiley & Sons, 1986.

90. Donaldson GW, Moinpour CM. Individual differences in quality-of-life treatment response. *Med Care* 2002; 40:III-39–III-53.

91. Kaplan EL, Meier P. Nonparametric estimator from incomplete observations. *J Am Stat Assoc* 1958; 53:457–481.

92. Cox, DR. Regression models and life tables (with discussion). *J R Stat Soc B* 1972; 21:411–421.

93. Troxel AB, Harrington DP, Lipsitz SR. Analysis of longitudinal data with non-ignorable non-monotone missing values. *Appl Stat* 1998; 47:425–438.

94. Beacon HJ, Thompson SC. Multi-level models for repeated measurement data: Application to quality of life in clinical trials. *Stat Med* 1996; 15:2717–2732.

95. Michiels B, Molenberghs G, Bijnens L, Vangeneugden T, Thijs H. Selection models and pattern-mixture models to analyse longitudinal quality of life data subject to drop-out. *Stat Med* 2002; 21:1023–1041.

96. Smith DM. The Oswald manual. Technical Report, Statistics Group, Lancaster, England: University of Lancaster, 1996.

97. Little RJA. Pattern-mixture models for multivariate incomplete data. *J Am Stat Assoc* 1993; 88:125–134.

98. Little RJA. A class of pattern-mixture models for normal incomplete data. *Biometrika* 1994; 81:471–483.

99. Pauler DK, McCoy S, Moinpour C. Pattern mixture models for longitudinal quality of life studies in advanced stage disease. *Stat Med* 2003; 22:795–809.

100. Hogan JW, Laird NM. Mixture models for the joint distribution of repeated measures and event times. *Stat Med* 1997; 16:239–257.

101. Fay RE. Causal models for patterns of nonresponse. *J Am Stat Assoc* 1986; 81:354–365.

102. Baker SG, Laird NM. Regression analysis for categorical variables with outcome subject to nonignorable nonresponse. *J Am Stat Assoc* 1988; 83:62–69.

103. Conaway MR. The analysis of repeated categorical measurements subject to nonignorable nonresponse. *J Am Stat Assoc* 1992; 87:817–824.

104. Fitzmaurice GM, Molenberghs G, Lipsitz SR. Regression models for longitudinal binary responses with informative drop-outs. *J R Stat Soc B* 1995; 57:691–704.

105. Lipsitz SR, Ibrahim JG, Fitzmaurice GM. Likelihood methods for incomplete longitudinal binary responses with incomplete categorical covariates. *Biometrics* 1999; 55:214–223.

106. Horton NJ, Fitzmaurice GM. Maximum likelihood estimation of bivariate logistic models for incomplete responses with indicators of ignorable and non-ignorable missingness. *Appl Stat* 2002; 51:281–295.

107. Zee BC. Growth curve model analysis for quality of life data. *Stat Med* 1998; 17:757–766.

108. Schluchter MD. Methods for the analysis of informatively censored longitudinal data. *Stat Med* 1992; 11:1861–1870.

109. Tsiatis AA, DeGruttola V, Wulfsohn MS. Modeling the relationship of survival to longitudinal data measured with error: Applications to survival and CD4 counts in patients with AIDS. *J Am Stat Assoc* 1995; 90:27–37.

110. Wulfsohn MS, Tsiatis AA. A joint model for survival and longitudinal data measured with error. *Biometrics* 1997; 53:330–339.

111. Wang Y, Taylor JMG. Jointly modeling longitudinal and event time data with application to acquired immunodeficiency syndrome. *J Am Stat Assoc* 2001; 96:895–905.

112. Faucett CL, Schenker N, Elashoff RM. Analysis of censored survival data with intermittently observed time-dependent binary covariates. *J Am Stat Assoc* 1998; 93:427–437.

113. Lipsitz SR, Ibrahim JG. Estimating equations with incomplete categorical covariates in the Cox model. *Biometrics* 1998; 54:1002–1013.

114. Tsiatis AA, Davidian M. A semiparametric estimator for the proportional hazards model with longitudinal covariates measured with error. *Biometrika* 2001; 88:447–458.

115. Pauler DK, Finkelstein DA. Predicting time to prostate cancer recurrence based on joint models for non-linear longitudinal biomarkers and event time outcomes. *Stat Med* 2002; 21:3897–3911.

116. Wu MC, Carroll R. Estimation and comparison of changes in the presence of informative right censoring by modeling the censoring process. *Biometrics* 1988; 44:175–188.

117. Follman D, Wu M. An approximate generalized linear model with random effects for informative missing data. *Biometrics* 1995; 51:151–168.

118. Tsonaka R, Verbeke G, Lesaffre E. A semi-parametric shared parameter model to handle nonmonotone nonignorable missingness. *Biometrics* 2009; 65:81–87.

119. DeGruttola V, Tu XM. Modelling progression of CD4 lymphocyte count and its relationship to survival time. *Biometrics* 1994; 50:1003–1014.

120. Lange N, Ryan L. Assessing normality in random effects models. *Ann Statist* 1989; 17:634–643.

121. Verbeke G. The linear mixed model: A critical investigation in the context of longitudinal data analysis. PhD thesis, Faculty of Science, Department of Mathematics, Catholic University of Leuven, Leuven, Belgium.

122. Verbeke G, Lesaffre E. A linear mixed-effects model with heterogeneity in the random-effects population. *J Am Stat Assoc* 1996; 91:217–221.

123. Verbeke G, Lesaffre E. The effect of misspecifying the random effects distribution in linear mixed models for longitudinal data. *Comp Stat Data Anal* 1997; 23:541–556.

124. Lin H, McCulloch CE, Turnbull BW, Slate EH, Clark LC. 2000. A latent class mixed model for analysing biomarker trajectories with irregularly scheduled observations. *Stat Med* 2000; 19:1303–1318.

125. Beukckens C, Molenberghs G, Verbeke G, Mallinckrodt C. A latent-class mixture model for incomplete longitudinal Gaussian data. *Biometrics* 2008; 64:96–105.

126. Tsonaka R, Verbeke G, Lessafre E. Nonignorable models for intermittently missing categorical longitudinal responses. *Biometrics* 2010; 66:834–844.

127. Robins JM, Rotnitzky A. Semiparametric efficiency in multivariate regression models with missing data. *J Am Stat Assoc* 1995; 90:122–129.

128. Robins JM, Rotnitzky A, Zhao LP. Analysis of semiparametric regression models for repeated outcomes in the presence of missing data. *J Am Stat Assoc* 1995; 90:106–121.

129. Scharfstein DO, Rotnitzky A, Robin JM. Adjusting for nonignorable drop-outs using semiparametric nonresponse models. *J Am Stat Assoc* 1999; 94:1096–1120.

130. Little RJA, Wang Y. Pattern-mixture models for multivariate incomplete data with covariates. *Biometrics* 1996; 52:98–111.

131. Daniels MJ, Hogan JW. Reparameterizing the pattern mixture model for sensitivity analyses under informative dropout. *Biometrics* 2000; 56:1241–1248.

132. Copas JB, Li HG. Inference for non-random samples (with discussion). *J R Stat Soc B* 1997; 59:55–95.

133. Verbeke G, Molenberghs G, Thijs H, Lesaffre E, Kenward MG. Sensitivity analysis for nonrandom dropout: A local influence approach. *Biometrics* 2001; 57:7–14.

134. Troxel AB, Ma G, Heitjan DF. An index of local sensitivity to nonignorability. *Stat Sin* 2004; 14:1221–1237.

135. Ma G, Troxel AB, Heitjan DF. An index of local sensitivity to nonignorable drop-out in longitudinal modeling. *Stat Med* 2005; 24:2129–2150.

136. Xie H, Heitjan DF. Local sensitivity to nonignorability: Dependence on the assumed dropout mechanism. *Stat Biopharm Res* 2009; 1:243–257.

137. Xie H. A local sensitivity analysis approach to longitudinal non-Gaussian data with nonignorable dropout. *Stat Med* 2008; 27:3155–3177.

138. Mahabadi SE, Ganjali M. An index of local sensitivity to non-ignorability for multi-variate longitudinal mixed data with potential non-random dropout. *Stat Med* 2010; 29:1779–1792.

139. Rubin DB. *Multiple Imputation for Nonresponse in Surveys*. New York: John Wiley & Sons, 1987.

140. Torrance GW. Designing and conducting cost-utility analyses. In: Spilker B, ed. *Quality of Life and Pharmacoeconomics in Clinical Trials*, 2nd edn. Philadelphia, PA: Lippincott-Raven Publishers, 1996, pp. 1105–1111 (Ch 1114).

141. La Puma J, Lawlor EF. Quality-adjusted life-years. Ethical implications for physicians and policymakers. *J Am Med Assoc* 1990; 263:2917–2921.

142. Mehrez A, Gafni A. Quality-adjusted life years, utility theory, and healthy-years equiva-lents. *Med Decis Making* 1989; 9:142–149.

143. Johannesson M. QALYs, HYEs and individual preferences—A graphical illustration. *Soc Sci Med* 1994; 39:1623–1632.

144. Ramsey SD, Etzioni R, Troxel A, Urban N. Optimizing sampling strategies for estimat-ing quality-adjusted life years. *Med Decis Making* 1997; 17:431–438.

145. Glasziou PP, Simes RJ, Gelber RD. Quality adjusted survival analysis. *Stat Med* 1990; 9:1259–1276.

146. Gelber RD, Gelman RS. A quality-of-life-oriented endpoint for comparing therapies. *Biometrics* 1989; 45:781–795.

147. Gelber RD, Goldhirsch A, Cole BF for the International Breast Cancer Study Group. Parametric extrapolation of survival estimates with applications to quality of life evalu-ation of treatments. *Controlled Clin Trials* 1993; 14:485–499.

148. Goldhirsch A, Gelber RD, Simes J, Glasziou P, Coates A. Costs and benefits of adju-vant therapy in breast cancer: A quality-adjusted survival analysis. *J Clin Oncol* 1989; 7:36–44.

149. Gelber RD, Cole BF, Goldhirsch A. Comparing treatments using quality-adjusted sur-vival: The Q-TWiST method. *Am Stat* 1995; 49:161–169.

150. Fairclough DL, Fetting JH, Cella D, Wonson W, Moinpour CM. Quality of life and qual-ity adjusted survival for breast cancer patients receiving adjuvant therapy. *Qual Life Res* 2000; 8:723–731.

# 23 Economic Analyses alongside Cancer Clinical Trials

*Dean A. Regier and Scott D. Ramsey*

## CONTENTS

## 23.1 INTRODUCTION AND RATIONALE

The ever-increasing cost of cancer care, combined with the high prevalence and economic burden of cancer in economically developed societies, has fostered a strong demand for economic information regarding new technologies aimed at the prevention, detection, and treatment of cancer. As efforts to control health care spending become increasingly intense, decision makers are forced to confront the reality that adopting new, cost-increasing technologies necessitates spending less in other areas of health care, which may adversely affect health outcomes. In this context, some have argued that it is reasonable to consider health outcomes and costs for cancer treatments relative to the health outcomes and costs for other medical interventions. The most common approach to compare the relative value of different interventions in creating better health and/or longer life is cost-effectiveness analysis (CEA) [1].

Conducting cost-effectiveness analyses alongside clinical trials has two important advantages. First, it is an efficient and timely way to obtain data on clinical, economic, and humanistic outcomes simultaneously. Timely economic data will be particularly useful to those who are responsible for health care budgets and are often critical to formulary considerations. Second, performing a CEA alongside a randomized, controlled clinical trial has high internal validity and low potential for bias. Because economic considerations are unavoidable in clinical decision making, the highest quality economic evidence should be used.

Many countries now require economic information as part of applications for listing new products on national formularies. For example, the U.K. National Institute for Clinical Excellence has published a guidance document for manufacturers and sponsors that outlines best practice recommendations when submitting economic information as part of the application materials [2]. In the United States, the Academy of Managed Care Pharmacy has published its Format for Formulary Submissions, a guidance document for health insurance plans on requesting clinical and economic information on new medicines from pharmaceutical manufacturers [3]. The "AMCP Format" has been widely adopted by health plans, and many pharmaceutical companies now routinely prepare AMCP style dossiers for new products prior to marketing.

To address the regulatory requirements of many countries and to provide timely and highly robust data on economic endpoints, economic analyses are now commonly performed alongside clinical trials of new treatments. The rising popularity of these so-called piggyback economic studies poses an opportunity and a challenge for the field. Moving economic analyses in sync with clinical trials increases their value to decision makers, and consequently their influence in clinical practice policy. The challenge is for researchers to raise the standards of these analyses so that they are considered of equal quality to the trials themselves. Although standard methods for conducting and reporting economic evaluations of health care technologies are available [4,5], developing a consistent approach for conducting economic evaluation alongside clinical trials is a continuing priority for the field.

Despite broad agreement on the principles that underpin cost-effectiveness studies, there are concerns about the external validity of performing cost-effectiveness analyses alongside clinical trials. First, the clinical care which occurs in the trial is not representative of care that occurs in typical medical practice [6,7]. This problem has several manifestations: (1) the control group often differs from standard practice, for example, placebo; (2) protocol-induced procedures such as eligibility screening tests artificially raise the cost of care; (3) strict screening and selection criteria mean that trial subjects are much more homogenous and likely to comply with therapy than patients typically seen in practice; and (4) investigators conducting the trial have particular expertise in the disease.

Second, clinical trials and cost-effectiveness analyses are designed for different purposes. In short, clinical trials are designed to test whether a new intervention is efficacious (Does it work?) while cost-effectiveness analyses are designed to evaluate if the intervention provides good value for money and how it should be prioritized given a constrained health care budget (Is it worth the expenditure?). The distinction creates several potential conflicting issues: (1) clinical trials consider very narrowly defined patient populations that are treated in a highly controlled and monitored environment, while CEAs should consider the care of patients in "real-world" clinical practice settings; (2) some cancer trials are designed to test intermediate endpoints such as progression-free survival, while appropriate outcome measures for CEAs include survival and health-related quality of life, where the latter can be quantified using preference-based techniques; (3) sample size needs for clinical endpoints are likely to be insufficient for joint clinical/economic trials; and (4) the time horizon for clinical trials is usually shorter than the relevant time horizon for CEAs, which should consider the entire course of disease.

Finally, including CEA-related endpoints increases the cost of data collection in a clinical trial. It can be difficult and expensive to design forms and collect data on health care utilization, both trial and nontrial related, and costs. In addition, tracking CEA-related endpoints, such as survival, may entail enlarging the sample size or extending the period of observation beyond that which is often necessary to establish clinical effectiveness. Such additional costs can be difficult to justify when the outcome of the trial is uncertain.

## 23.2   DESIGN ISSUES FOR ECONOMIC ANALYSES ALONGSIDE CLINICAL TRIALS

### 23.2.1   Selecting Trials for Parallel Economic Evaluation

Dozens of cancer-related controlled clinical trials are started each year [8]. Not all of them warrant the cost and expense necessary to support a parallel economic evaluation. Given research budget constraints, it is important to be selective and provide adequate resources for economic analyses.

### 23.2.2   Statement of Study Objectives and Hypotheses

Most clinical trials are designed with the goal of assessing the efficacy of an experimental intervention compared to a standard treatment or placebo. Thus, a null hypothesis is set forth: $H_0$: $\mu_a = \mu_b$ versus an alternative $H_1$: $\mu_a < \mu_b$, where $\mu$ is a clinical outcome of interest, such as survival, and a and b are the competing therapies. In contrast, the aim of cost-effectiveness analyses is to characterize the trade-off between the comparative cost and health status of competing interventions; the primary endpoint of a cost-effectiveness analysis is typically expressed via the incremental cost-effectiveness ratio (ICER):

$$\text{Incremental Cost-Effectiveness}_a = R = \frac{(\text{Cost}_a - \text{Cost}_b)}{(\text{Effectiveness}_a - \text{Effectiveness}_b)} = \frac{\Delta C}{\Delta E}.$$

$$(23.1)$$

In the context of cost-effectiveness studies alongside randomized trials, treatment a is the experimental therapy and treatment b is the standard therapy for the condition. The most appropriate comparison intervention for a CEA (Effectiveness$_b$) is the most effective therapy or therapies for the condition, but unfortunately, the comparison for a clinical trial is often placebo in many cases. Cost$_a$ and Cost$_b$ are the average costs per patient for persons in the intervention and control groups, respectively, and include the cost of therapy and other related medical care such as side effects related to chemotherapy. Further, when a societal perspective is taken in the analysis, the average cost per patient can include the direct costs associated with treatment as well as any indirect costs (e.g., lost days from work) borne by other parties, including families or informal caregivers. Effectiveness can be measured in ad hoc units, such as relapse free survival, or in common metrics that facilitate comparison across interventions. The most common metrics of effectiveness are life years or quality-adjusted life years (QALYs).

In a seminal article, O'Brien et al. [9] suggested that the appropriate null and alternative hypotheses for a clinical trial evaluating cost-effectiveness should be $H_0: R = R_{max}$ versus $H_1: R < R_{max}$, where R is the incremental cost-effectiveness of the experimental intervention, given by Equation 23.1, and $R_{max}$ is a prespecified threshold that characterizes decision makers' willingness to pay for an effectiveness or health status gain. A persistent issue that haunts cost-effectiveness researchers is that there is no widely agreed upon $R_{max}$. Indeed, it is likely that $R_{max}$ varies substantially among organizations and governments that fund medical care. The probability that $R = R_{max}$ is therefore reported at different thresholds of $R_{max}$. As will be discussed in the following, the value selected for $R_{max}$ will greatly affect the sample size requirements for the study.

### 23.2.3 Sample Size and Power Estimation for Joint Clinical/Economic Trials

With regard to sample size and the appropriate threshold ($R_{max}$) for hypothesis testing, research budgetary constraints will usually dictate the number of subjects that can be enrolled in the clinical trial. It may be reasonable to take sample size as given and *solve* for $R_{max}$ using the usually accepted levels of power $(1 - \beta)$ and significance $(\alpha)$. Decision makers can then decide if the study will achieve adequate power to evaluate a cost-effectiveness threshold that is meaningful to their organization. There are certain technical challenges to calculating the power curves for cost-effectiveness studies, because more parameters must be solicited for clinical/economic trials than for typical clinical trials.

Classical RCTs without economic endpoints often have a single primary endpoint. For example, an RCT for cancer treatment may monitor 5 year survival past cancer treatment with an outcome $Y = 1$ if alive at 5 years and 0 if dead at 5 years, with effect size estimating the difference or ratio of the survival rates in treatment, $p_1 = E(Y_i | \text{Treatment})$, and control, $p_0 = E(Y_i | \text{Control})$. With economic outcomes, the difference is preferred as an effect size estimator. Power calculations for a traditional RCT are a matter of determining an adequate sample size to assure that the difference in $p_1$ and $p_0$ can be observed.

Economic studies measure the health benefit of the treatment on the total dollars expended. If D refers to the total treatment dollar expenditure, then we could summarize the effect of treatment choice on costs alone by the difference in mean treatment costs $\mu_1 - \mu_0$ where $\mu_1 = E(D | \text{Treatment})$ and $\mu_0 = E(D | \text{Control})$. Evaluating the effect of treatment choice on dollars alone would require a simple power analysis to detect the difference $\mu_1 - \mu_0$. Solicitation for detecting differences in costs would typically also include stating $\sigma_1 = \text{StdDev}(D | \text{Treated})$ and $\sigma_1 = \text{StdDev}(D | \text{Control})$.

When economic and efficacy endpoints are combined, we summarize their joint behavior in the ICER $R = (\mu_1 - \mu_0)/(p_1 - p_0)$. In addition to treatment effects on outcomes and costs, we must also characterize the *correlation* of costs and effects, $\rho = \text{cor}(D_i, Y_i)$ in order to calculate the sample size for the study. Although the correlation between costs and effects is not an explicit part of R or its estimator, $\hat{R} = (\hat{\mu}_1 - \hat{\mu}_0)/(\hat{p}_1 - \hat{p}_0)$, it does have great influence on the sampling behavior and hence power calculations. Positive correlations will tend to minimize variability compared to negative correlations [10]. Unfortunately, soliciting the correlation between costs and outcomes is nonintuitive. Because the sampling behavior of $\hat{R}$ is most dependent on the correlation between costs and outcomes, power calculations for CEA should include sensitivity analyses when evaluating power. Relatively straightforward methods to determine power are available [11].

## 23.3 DATABASE ISSUES

### 23.3.1 SELECTING OUTCOME ENDPOINTS

Possible health outcome measures for cost-effectiveness analyses include measures of averted morbidity, surrogate clinical markers, life extension, health-related quality of life, disability-adjusted survival, and quality-adjusted survival. Researchers have used treatment-specific measures such as symptom-free time, cases of disease prevented, and change in likelihood of progression of disease in the denominator of the cost-effectiveness ratio. The problem with these measures is that they are intermediate endpoints, that is, they are not linked to a final health outcome, or are treatment or disease specific. Although intermediate or treatment-specific effects are appropriate from a clinical perspective, from a productive or allocative efficiency perspective, the health policy analyst would prefer to have a common and standard measure of health outcome that extends across different diseases and treatments to facilitate comparability of cost-effectiveness studies.

Although there is no international "gold standard" regarding the outcome measure that is most appropriate for cost-effectiveness evaluations, the U.S. Panel on Cost-effectiveness in Medicine suggests using QALYs, because it links to neoclassical welfare theory and fits within a resource allocation framework when a willingness to pay for a QALY gain is hypothesized [12,13]. QALYs are defined as the duration of

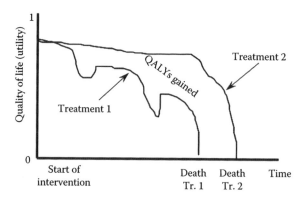

**FIGURE 23.1** QALYs gained using a new therapy. (From Ramsey, S.D. et al., *Annu. Rev. Public Health*, 22, 129, 2001.)

an individual's life as modified by the changes in health and well-being experienced over the lifetime [14]. Well-being is measured as a health state utility value, where utility is defined as the quantitative representation of individuals' preferences over different health states, and utility is maximized subject to constraints. The utility weights for the health states are anchored on 1 (perfect health) and 0 (death), where health states "worse than death" are possible. Figure 23.1 depicts this concept as the area under the curve.

There are several methods for obtaining health state utilities, including interviewer administered approaches using, for example, the standard gamble or time trade-off preference elicitation techniques [4], or multiattribute "off-the-shelf" survey instruments using the Health Utilities Index or EuroQoL 5-D [15]. In practice, multiattribute instruments are most often used in clinical trials because of their ease of administration and low respondent burden. To obtain health state utility weights using multiattribute survey methods, it is necessary to survey patients regularly over the course of the trial. In addition, if serious sequelae that influence health-related quality of life occur sporadically, it may be necessary to sample patients experiencing those outcomes and survey them to obtain utilities for those health states. This can become a complex task for clinical trialists wishing to keep the study procedures at a minimum. Finally, since trials are of finite duration and treatment effects related to cancer treatment can continue for a lifetime, it is important to consider how one will estimate these health-related quality of life outcomes after the trial. Most cost-effectiveness analysts rely on modeling techniques or other indirect methods to estimate life expectancy and health state utilities after the trial has ended [16].

### 23.3.2 EXTRAPOLATING COSTS AND OUTCOMES BEYOND THE TRIAL PERIOD

Often an intervention will affect health outcomes and costs beyond the observation period of the clinical study. These costs and outcomes should be included in the cost-effectiveness analysis. If effects beyond the observation period are anticipated at the time of the trial, steps can be taken to address this issue. It may be useful to include in study consent forms a notice that subjects will be contacted weeks, months, or years after the trial to determine how the intervention is affecting them. Arrangements can be made to collect billing records after the trial is completed, for example, Medicare claims. In most cases, some degree of mathematical modeling will be necessary to project costs and outcomes over a plausible range of scenarios. Models can be reviewed prior to the trial to determine the most relevant application [17,18]. Because many readers are skeptical of models that project outcomes into the future, and prefer to see results of the "real" data, presenting both the trial-period and lifetime cost-effectiveness ratios allows readers more flexibility in judging the outcomes of the trial.

### 23.3.3 MEASURING COSTS

Costs are a function of resources that are consumed during the course of care, multiplied by values or prices of each resource. Costs stemming from a therapy include the following costs:

1. Direct medical care costs, including the intervention itself, and follow-up care to the condition
2. Indirect patient nonmedical care related to the treatment, such as the cost of traveling to and from the clinic
3. Indirect societal costs associated with the value of time that family and friends spend caring for the patient
4. Indirect patient costs of the value of the patient's time in treatment

#### 23.3.3.1 Tracking Resources Consumed in Care

Although much of the direct medical care can be obtained directly from collection forms designed for the trial itself, it is sometimes necessary to modify the collection forms to collect data that would otherwise not be collected. In cases where clinical forms include only minimal health care utilization data, finding all relevant data can be problematic. One option is to collect billing or insurance records. This option will be viable only if the records are easily obtainable and are comprehensive with regard to capturing all relevant health utilization. Often, this is not the case. For example, Medicare records do not include drug information and some nursing and home care. In cases where billing or insurance records are unobtainable or incomplete, health care utilization tracking forms may need to be designed. Research coordinators can fill in these forms during interviews at scheduled visits or they can be filled in periodically by subjects themselves. While no study has compared collection methods directly, researchers must be aware of the potential for recall bias in either form of recording. Short time intervals between collection intervals are necessary to minimize recall problems [19]. For economic data, we recommend monthly data collection.

Tracking nonmedical care resources related to treatment and the value of time lost to treatment, for example, the cost of lost work while seeking medical care, can be especially problematic. Many times, these data are imputed; estimates are made based on interviews with samples of patients or from national databases such as wage rates from the U.S. Bureau of Labor Statistics. Many researchers choose to explicitly delete nonmedical care from the analyses. In this case, the perspective of the study is no longer societal, but rather closer to the health insurance payer perspective. The U.K. National Institute for Clinical Excellence recommends including only direct costs in the primary analysis and both direct and indirect costs in deterministic sensitivity analysis [2].

### 23.3.3.2 Protocol-Induced Costs

Protocol-induced costs are costs incurred for patient care related to the clinical trial that will not be incurred once the intervention is used in practice. There are two types of protocol-induced costs: direct and indirect. Direct protocol costs are costs incurred for tests that are included in a trial for regulatory, scientific, or other reasons beyond clinical care. Direct protocol-induced costs are relatively easy to identify and eliminate from the analysis. Leaders from centers involved in the trial can be polled to identify resources that are unlikely to be utilized outside the clinical trial setting.

Indirect protocol-induced costs are costs incurred when investigators respond to abnormalities found during protocol testing, if these abnormalities would not have been identified otherwise. For example, if a protocol for a clinical trial of an exercise intervention for emphysema patients calls for preintervention fine resolution computed tomography (CT) scanning of the chest, evaluation costs will occur when scanning identifies pulmonary nodules that would be missed during screening of these patients in nonexperimental settings. Indirect protocol-induced costs can be quite difficult to identify *ex ante*. If such costs are expected, it is useful to first consider whether there will be differences in these costs between study arms. If not, then there is less concern, because the costs will be eliminated in the incremental analysis (Equation 23.1), although the average cost of treatment in any one arm will be artificially inflated. If indirect protocol costs are likely to be different between arms, for example, due to differences in protocol evaluation for each arm, then special measures must be taken to identify them. In extreme cases, chart auditing may be necessary to identify the events and associated resources incurred following the trial.

### 23.3.3.3 Assigning Values to Resources Consumed

After resources are collected, they must be valued, ideally using nationally representative price weights. When considering prices, it is important to distinguish between charges, reimbursements, and true costs. Charges are the bills that hospitals and health care providers send to payers and patients for health care services. Reimbursement is the amount that is actually paid to the health care providers by patients and the insurer. True costs are what health care providers actually expend, including overhead costs, to provide the services, before markup or profit. Charges, reimbursement levels, and true costs can differ substantially. When the perspective of the study is societal, true costs are most appropriate. If an insurer's viewpoint is used, reimbursements are most appropriate. In all cases, using charges to value health resources is inappropriate, because charges almost always greatly overstate the value of the service relative to what it actually costs to provide the service and to what most parties in today's market are willing to pay.

## 23.4  ANALYSIS OF FINDINGS

### 23.4.1  ANALYSIS OF COSTS

The analysis of medical care costs raises two methodologically challenging issues. First, analyses are difficult to perform when the proper interval for the cost-effectiveness analysis exceeds the length of the follow-up period for most or all of the study subjects. Second, cost data are difficult to analyze using standard normality assumptions because of their typically nonstandard statistical distribution. For example, medical cost distributions often exhibit a mass at zero representing nonusers of medical resources, and right skewness, representing relatively small numbers of extremely high users. Historically, the methods developed to deal with costs were not designed to accommodate censored data [20]. In recent years, nonparametric bootstrapping methods have been described to estimate medical care costs. Nonparametric methods do not impose a particular statistical distribution on costs. Lin et al. proposed a method for estimating costs as follows [21]:

$$\hat{C} = \sum_{j=1}^{J} C_j S_j, \tag{23.2}$$

where

$C_j$ is the observed mean cost in month j among survivors to month j
$S_j$ is the Kaplan–Meier estimate of survival to month j
the summation is over months or some other interval after the start of the trial

This estimator uses data from every patient during each month for which he or she is under observation. For validity, it requires independent censoring in time and representativeness of the observed mean monthly cost. A second nonparametric method by Bang and Tsiatis [22] does not pose any restrictions on the distribution of censoring times. The estimator uses cost information from uncensored individuals only and weights these observations by the inverse of the probability of not being censored at the point of death. This estimator is defined as

$$\hat{C} = \frac{1}{n} \sum_{i=1}^{n} \frac{\delta_i M_i}{K(T_i)}, \tag{23.3}$$

where

$K(T_i)$ is the probability that the individual i has survived to $T_i$ without being censored
$M_i$ denotes the total cost of the patient during the specified time
$\delta$ takes the value of 1 when the observation is uncensored and 0 otherwise [22]

Raikou and McGuire find that both the Lin et al. and Bang and Tsiatis methods produce consistent estimators of average cost; however, the Bang and Tsiatis method becomes less stable at very high levels of censoring [23]. The choice of a method therefore should depend on the degree of censoring observed in the clinical trial.

Stratification is used in RCTs to reduce potential confounding factors that could impact clinical outcomes between the treatment and control groups, but may not necessarily address factors that could influence *economic* outcomes. Multivariate methods [24,25] can be employed to produce adjusted cost estimates in cases where unequal stratification of factors influencing costs is suspected.

### 23.4.2 PER PROTOCOL VERSUS INTENT TO TREAT ANALYSES

To preserve the benefits of the randomization process in RCTs, the "intent-to-treat" approach analyzes individuals in their assigned groups regardless of treatment actually received [26]. In most cases, the intent-to-treat design is also appropriate for the economic analysis, but in some cases, special circumstances related to the trial or discrepancies between how the intervention is being used in the trial and how it is likely to be used in practice may warrant attention during the design phase. For example, trial investigators for the National Emphysema Treatment Trial, a randomized trial of lung volume reduction surgery versus medical therapy for patients with severe emphysema, expected that some patients who are randomized to the medical therapy arm would obtain surgery outside the clinical trial [27]. Including these patients as originally randomized for analysis under "intent-to-treat" would bias both the final cost and outcome estimates. In this case, out-of-protocol use of surgery should be identified and related resource use must be tracked. If the proportion of out-of-protocol use is small, it is reasonable to include costs and outcomes for those patients as assigned in the trial. If a substantial proportion of patients in the medical therapy arm obtain surgery outside the trial, an additional analysis should be performed excluding such patients and compared to results from the intent-to-treat analysis.

### 23.4.3 MISSING DATA

Missing data are inevitable in clinical trials and can be handled by a variety of approaches depending on the type of missingness; see Little and Rubin [28] and Chapter 22. Missing data are also common in economic analyses conducted alongside trials, particularly if researchers for the clinical trial view the extra work of collecting cost or specialized outcome variables as burdensome, or when patients record resource utilization as part of a monthly diary. In this case, the degree of missingness for the economic information typically exceeds that for the clinical information. Recently, researchers have begun to address the issues of missing data in economic analyses alongside clinical trials. The issues that one must consider for missing economic data are not necessarily different to other forms of missing data, with the exception that cost data are often highly skewed. In analyzing datasets with missing data, one must determine the nature of the missing data and then define an approach for dealing with the missing data.

The researcher can address missing data by imputation, replacing the missing field with an estimate of the value. Commonly used methods for imputation include using the mean value from available data, regression analysis using complete variables, "hot deck" imputation, and maximum likelihood approaches. In a recent paper, Briggs et al. outline the advantages and potential problems with these methods for cost data [29]. The primary problem with these "deterministic" methods is that they reduce the variance of the imputed data set. Missing variables are often from severely ill persons on the skewed end of the distribution so that symmetric parametric methods yield inappropriate imputations. Multiple imputation approaches introduce a random component into each imputed value, reflecting the uncertainty that is inherent in missing data [30]. Nonparametric bootstrapping is an attractive method for generating such "stochastic" imputed data for costs. Bayesian simulation methods are also available to address these issues [31,32]. Most of the commonly used statistical software packages include programs for imputation of missing data. A review of these programs can be found at Multiple Imputation Online [33,34].

### 23.4.4 ADJUSTMENT TO CONSTANT DOLLARS AND DISCOUNTING OF FUTURE COSTS AND OUTCOMES

In cases where costs are collected over a number of years or in several geographic regions, prices must be adjusted to constant nationally representative dollars. Prices can be adjusted to constant dollars for a year of reference using the medical care component of the consumer price index [35].

Costs and outcomes stemming from medical interventions should be discounted to a present value to reflect the idea that individuals prefer immediate over delayed monetary gains or health benefits. The present value of future costs and outcomes can be calculated as follows:

$$C_{present} = \sum_{j=1}^{J} \frac{c_j}{(1+r)^{1-j}}, \tag{23.4}$$

where
  $C_{present}$ represents the cost in current dollars
  $j$ is the year of the study (year 1 is the first year of the intervention and year J is the final year of observation)
  $c_j$ is the cost in year $j$
  $r$ is the discount rate

Note that the equation is the same when discounting outcomes (e.g., QALYs), simply substitute $O_{present}$ for $C_{present}$ and $o_j$ for $c_j$.

There is ongoing debate regarding the appropriateness of using the same discount rate for health outcomes and costs versus differential discounting for costs and health benefits, and in constant versus time-varying discount rates, such as 5% over the first 5 years and 3% for later years. The discounting approach chosen can have a substantial impact on the cost-effectiveness estimates of health care programs where most of the costs are incurred in the near future and health benefits occur in the distant future. Uniform discounting of costs and outcomes leads to prioritizing of treatments with immediate benefit over those with effects that occur in the future, for example, chemotherapy for cancer versus smoking cessation programs.

Ideally, the discount rate for the costs and health outcomes from health care interventions should be based on actual measures of the social rate of time preference, that is, the rate at which society is willing to trade off present for future consumption. Unfortunately, estimating the actual social time preference is difficult and itself controversial [36–38]. As a result, the discount rate is usually chosen by panels. In the United States, the U.S. Panel on Cost Effectiveness and Medicine has chosen a 3% discount rate for costs and outcomes [5].

### 23.4.5 SUMMARY MEASURES

Equation 23.1 summarizes the results of a CEA as a ratio of the difference of costs to the difference in outcomes. It is common to place bootstrapped ICER estimates on the cost-effectiveness (CE) plane shown in Figure 23.2 [39]. The CE plane plots the difference in effectiveness per patient against the difference in cost per patient on a Cartesian coordinate system. Placing the effectiveness difference on the horizontal axis and the cost difference on the vertical axis allows the slope of a line that joins any point on the plane to the origin to be equal to the ICER. Using the four quadrants of the plane, the possible trade-offs between cost and consequences are depicted. Results in the northeast quadrant (higher costs, greater outcomes) are most common. In the positive quadrants, low ICERs are preferred to high ICERs. The CE plane was developed because of three potential problems that can arise for the

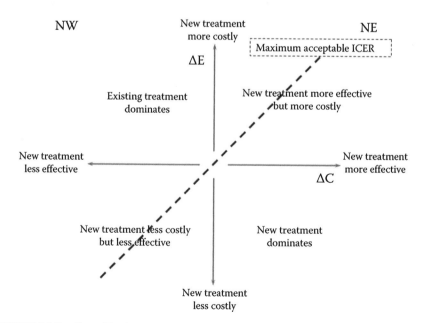

**FIGURE 23.2** Cost-effectiveness plane. (From Black, W.C., *Med. Decis. Making*, 10, 212, 1990.)

analyst when only the summary or mean ICER estimate is presented. The first is when either the difference in costs or effectiveness is negative, such as lower costs or worse outcome for the intervention group. Unlike situations where the difference in costs and outcomes are both positive, interpreting negative ratios can be misleading. In the northwest quadrant, for example, "less negative" values (smaller difference in effects) are preferable, while in the southeast quadrant, "more negative" values (greater difference in costs) are preferred.

A second potential problem arises when either the cost difference or the effect difference is not statistically significantly different from zero. In either case, it is common to focus on one dimension of the CE plane. In the more common case where costs are different but the effect is not, such analyses are called *cost-minimization* analyses. Briggs and O'Brien have argued that the problem with this simple approach to decision making in situations where either cost or effect is not statistically significant is that it is based on simple and sequential tests of hypotheses [40].

A third problem with summarizing cost-effectiveness results as a ratio involves evaluation of the joint uncertainty of costs and effect. While it is straightforward to use the bootstrapping technique to create confidence intervals around the ICER, problems of interpretation arise when one end of the confidence bounds cross zero. As we have discussed earlier, another possible problem can occur when the difference in effect is very small even when statistically significant. In this case, the denominator causes instability in the cost-effectiveness ratio and large or infinite confidence intervals are possible [10]. As will be discussed later, methods have been developed to address the problems inherent in ratio-based summary measures.

### 23.4.6 Cost-Effectiveness Acceptability Curves

Cost-effectiveness researchers have addressed the problems with ratio-based summary measures by replacing the ratio with a decision rule: If the estimated ICER lies below some ceiling ratio $\lambda$, reflecting the maximum that decision makers (or society) are willing to invest to achieve a unit of effectiveness, then the new technology should be implemented. On the CE plane, we could summarize uncertainty by determining the proportion of the bootstrap replications that fall below and to the right of a line with slope equal to $\lambda$. If there is disagreement about the value of $\lambda$, one can report the proportion of bootstrap replications falling below $\lambda$ as it is varied across a range. Assuming joint normality of cost and effect differences, one can plot the probability that the intervention falls on the cost-effective side of the cost-effectiveness plane as $\lambda$ varies from zero to infinity. Such a plot has been termed a cost-effectiveness acceptability curve [41]. Figure 23.3 shows examples of these curves for a cost-effectiveness evaluation of lung volume reduction surgery for severe emphysema [42]. The curve represents the probability that the intervention is associated with an ICER that is the same or less than the corresponding cost-effectiveness ratios displayed on the x-axis. Note that the median value ($p = 0.5$) corresponds to the base-case ICER. The curve thus allows the analyst to determine the likelihood that the intervention is cost-effective under a wide range of threshold values. The shape of the curve itself also allows the analyst to gauge the level of

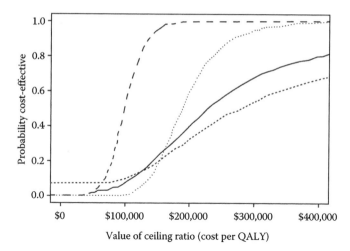

**FIGURE 23.3**   Cost-effectiveness acceptability curves for lung volume reduction surgery versus medical therapy for all patients and for three subgroups with significantly improved clinical outcomes in the lung volume reduction surgery arm (either reduced mortality, improved quality of life, or both). The curve represents the probability that lung volume reduction surgery is associated with a cost per QALY gained that is lower than the corresponding cost-effectiveness ratios displayed on the x-axis. The value of the ceiling ratio at a probability of 0.5 is the median cost per QALYs for lung volume reduction surgery. Solid horizontal lines denote 95% confidence limits for the projections. Overall (- - - - -) upper-lobe emphysema and low exercise capacity; (........) upper-lobe emphysema and high exercise capacity; (—) non-upper-lobe emphysema and low exercise capacity (– –). (From Ramsey, S.D. et al., *N. Engl. J. Med.*, 348(21), 2092, 2003.)

uncertainty surrounding the results (across all point estimates). Flatter curves denote more uncertainty, while more S-shaped curves suggest less uncertainty surrounding the estimates.

### 23.4.7   NET HEALTH BENEFIT APPROACH

Another approach analysts have used to address the problem of ratio-based summary measures is to eliminate the ratio altogether. Assuming that λ represents a threshold ICER, one can rearrange the equation $ICER = \Delta C / \Delta E \leq \lambda$ as follows:

$$NMB = \lambda \Delta E - \Delta C, \qquad (23.5)$$

where NMB is the net monetary benefit of investing resources in the new technology rather than the established technology. If the NMB > 0, the new intervention is cost-effective; if NMB < 0, greater health improvement could be attained by investing resources elsewhere [43]. The variance for the NHB can be estimated as follows:

$$var\,NMB = \lambda^2 \, var(\Delta E) + var(\Delta C) - 2\lambda \, cov(\Delta E, \Delta C). \qquad (23.6)$$

One can compute net benefit statistics as a function of $\lambda$, and in this case, the interpretation is similar to the cost-effectiveness acceptability curve. In fact, each point of the acceptability curve can be calculated from the p-value of the net-benefit being positive [44].

## 23.4.8  Value of Information Analysis

When the decision to adopt a health technology is based on current information derived from a single clinical trial, the outcome metric informing the decision will be subject to statistical uncertainty. Consequently, there is some probability that the wrong course of action will be pursued. Choosing the incorrect course of action will impose opportunity costs in the form of health benefit and/or health care resources forgone. Conceptually, the "cost" of uncertainty can be considered as jointly determined by the probability that a decision is incorrect, and the health benefit and resource consequences of an incorrect decision. Decision makers may consider collecting additional data to reduce statistical uncertainty, which will reduce the opportunity cost of making an incorrect decision. Value of information analysis can help inform the maximum decision makers that they should be willing to pay to decrease uncertainty through collecting additional evidence [45].

A common approach to value of information analysis is the expected value of perfect information (EVPI) approach. EVPI is based on the idea that perfect information will eliminate the probability of making a wrong decision because the decision maker knows how any uncertainty is resolved *before* the decision is made. Consequently, the cost of imperfect information in EVPI can be framed as the difference between making the decision to adopt an alternative j when the uncertainty surrounding a vector of parameters, $\theta$, has been resolved, and making the decision to pursue the kth alternative based on currently available information and unresolved uncertainty around parameters. EVPI is calculated as follows:

$$EVPI = E_\theta \max NMB(k,\theta) - \max_k E_\theta NMB(k,\theta), \qquad (23.7)$$

where
   $\max_k E_\theta NMB(k,\theta)$ indicates that the best decision under limited information is
      the kth alternative that results in the maximum expected NMB
   $E_\theta \max NMB(k,\theta)$ is the expected value of the optimal decision when $\theta$ is known
      with certainty [45]

Analytically, Equation 23.7 can be obtained using iterations obtained from the non-parametric bootstrapping procedure. That is, under the constraint of solely using current information, a decision maker's optimal choice is the alternative with highest mean NMB over all bootstrapped iterations ($\max_k E_\theta NMB(k,\theta)$), while under perfect information, the decision maker could choose the alternative with the maximum NMB for each iteration (when the uncertainty for each iteration is resolved). $E_\theta \max NMB(k,\theta)$ is simply the average, over all iterations, of the best alternative for each bootstrap iteration.

EVPI estimates the cost of making an incorrect decision each time a decision is needed, that is, at the patient level. Population EVPI incorporates the cost of making the incorrect decision for all current and future patients:

$$\text{EVPI for the population} = \text{EVPI} \times \sum_{j=1}^{J} \frac{I_j}{(1+r)^j}, \tag{23.8}$$

where

J is the time horizon over which the technology is used
I is the incidence in each time period of the disease
r is the discount rate [45]

Population EVPI is the metric that commonly informs the potential value of conducting additional research. If Equation 23.8 exceeds the expected costs of collecting additional data, then it may be cost-effective to pursue additional research.

## REFERENCES

1. Weinstein, M.C. and W.B. Stason, Foundations of cost-effectiveness analysis for health and medical practices. *N Engl J Med*, 1977, 296(13): 716–721.
2. National Institute for Clinical Excellence, NICE Guide to the methods of technology appraisal. June 2008.
3. Fry, R., S. Avey, and S. Sullivan, The Academy of Managed Care Pharmacy Format for Formulary Submissions—A Foundation for Managed Care Pharmacy Task Force report. *Value Health*, 2003, 6: 505–521.
4. Drummond, M.F. et al., *Methods for the Economic Evaluation of Health Care Programmes*. 2nd edn., 1997, Oxford, U.K.: Oxford University Press.
5. Weinstein, M.C. et al., Recommendations of the panel on cost-effectiveness in health and medicine. *J Am Med Assoc*, 1996, 276(15): 1253–1258.
6. Adams, M.E. et al., Economic analysis in randomized control trials. *Med Care*, 1992, 30(3): 231–243.
7. Drummond, M.F. and G.L. Stoddart, Economic analysis and clinical trials. *Control Clin Trials*, 1984, 5(2): 115–128.
8. National Institutes of Health, ClinicalTrials.gov, N.L.o. Medicine, ed. 2011 http://www.clinicaltrials.gov/ct.
9. O'Brien, B.J. et al., In search of power and significance: Issues in the design and analysis of stochastic cost-effectiveness studies in health care. *Med Care*, 1994, 32(2): 150–163.
10. McIntosh, M. et al., Parameter solicitation for planning cost effectiveness studies with dichotomous outcomes. *Health Econ*, 2001, 10(1): 53–66.
11. Briggs, A.H. and A.M. Gray, Power and sample size calculations for stochastic cost-effectiveness analysis. *Med Decis Making*, 1998, 18(2 Suppl): S81–S92.
12. Garber, A.M. and C.E. Phelps, Economic foundations of cost-effectiveness analysis. *J Health Econ*, 1997, 16(1): 1–31.
13. Gold, M.R. et al., eds. *Cost-Effectiveness in Health and Medicine*. 1996, New York: Oxford University Press.
14. Patrick, D.L. and P. Erickson, eds. *Health Status and Health Policy: Quality of Life in Health Care Evaluation and Resource Allocation*. 1993, New York: Oxford University Press.

Economic Analyses alongside Cancer Clinical Trials **385**

15. Torrance, G.W., Measurement of health state utilities for economic appraisal. *J Health Econ*, 1986, 5(1): 1–30.

16. Weinstein, M.C. et al., Principles of good practice for decision analytic modeling in health-care evaluation: Report of the ISPOR Task Force on Good Research Practices—Modeling studies. *Value Health*, 2003, 6(1): 9–17.

17. Eddy, D.M., Selecting technologies for assessment. *Int J Technol Assess Health Care*, 1989, 5(4): 485–501.

18. Habbema, J.D. et al., The MISCAN simulation program for the evaluation of screening for disease. *Comput Methods Programs Biomed*, 1985, 20(1): 79–93.

19. Mauskopf, J. et al., A strategy for collecting pharmacoeconomic data during phase II/III clinical trials. *Pharmacoeconomics*, 1996, 9(3): 264–277.

20. Duan, N., Smearing estimate: A nonparametric retransformation method. *J Am Stat Assoc*, 1983, 78: 605–610.

21. Lin, D.Y. et al., Estimating medical costs from incomplete follow-up data. *Biometrics*, 1997, 53(2): 419–434.

22. Bang, H. and A.A. Tsiatis, Estimating costs with censored data. *Biometrika*, 2000, 87(2): 329–343.

23. Raikou, M. and A. McGuire, Estimating medical care costs under conditions of censoring. *J Health Econ*, 2004, 23(3): 443–470.

24. Lin, D., Linear regression analysis of censored medical costs. *Biostatistics*, 2000, 1(1): 35–47.

25. Lin, D.Y., Regression analysis of incomplete medical cost data. *Stat Med*, 2003, 22(7): 1181–1200.

26. Fisher, L.D. et al., Intention to treat in clinical trials, in *Statistical Issues in Drug Research and Development*, K.E. Peace, ed. 1990, Dekker: New York, pp. 331–350.

27. Rationale and design of The National Emphysema Treatment Trial: A prospective randomized trial of lung volume reduction surgery. The National Emphysema Treatment Trial Research Group. *Chest*, 1999, 116(6): 1750–1761.

28. Little, R.J.A. and D.B. Rubin, *Statistical Analysis with Missing Data*. 1987, New York: John Wiley & Sons.

29. Briggs, A. et al., Missing… presumed at random: Cost-analysis of incomplete data. *Health Econ*, 2003, 12(5): 377–392.

30. Rubin, D.B., *Multiple Imputation for Nonresponse in Surveys*. 1987, New York: John Wiley.

31. Tanner, M.A. and W.H. Wong, The calculation of posterior distributions by data augmentation. *J Am Stat Assoc*, 1987, 82: 528–550.

32. Gelfand, A.E. and A.F.M. Smith, Sampling-based approaches to calculating marginal densities. *J Am Stat Assoc*, 1990, 85: 398–409.

33. van Buuren, S., Multiple Imputation Online. 2004, Leiden, The Netherlands: The Department of Statistics of TNO Prevention and Health. http://web.inter.nl.net/users/S.van.Buuren/mi/. Accessed July 23, 2004.

34. Horton, N.J. and S.R. Lipsitz, Multiple imputation in practice: Comparison of software packages for regression models with missing variables. *Am Stat*, 2001, 55(3): 244–254.

35. U.S. Department of Labor and Bureau of Labor Statistics, Consumer Price Indexes. 2004. http://www.bls.gov/cpi.

36. Feldstein, M.S., The inadequacy of weighted discount rates, in *Cost-Benefit Analysis*, R. Layard, ed. 1972, London, U.K.: Penguin, pp. 140–155.

37. Bradford, D.F., Constraints on government investment opportunities and the choice of discount rate. *Am Econ Rev*, 1975, 65: 887–895.

38. Bonneux, L. and E. Birnie, The discount rate in the economic evaluation of prevention: A thought experiment. *J Epidemiol Community Health*, 2001, 55(2): 123–125.

39. Black, W.C., The CE plane: A graphic representation of cost-effectiveness. *Med Decis Making*, 1990, 10(3): 212–214.

40. Briggs, A.H. and B.J. O'Brien, The death of cost-minimization analysis? *Health Econ*, 2001, 10(2): 179–184.

41. van Hout, B.A. et al., Costs, effects and C/E-ratios alongside a clinical trial. *Health Econ*, 1994, 3(5): 309–319.

42. Ramsey, S.D. et al., Cost effectiveness of lung-volume-reduction surgery for patients with severe emphysema. *N Engl J Med*, 2003, 348(21): 2092–2102.

43. Stinnett, A.A. and J. Mullahy, Net health benefits: A new framework for the analysis of uncertainty in cost-effectiveness analysis. *Med Decis Making*, 1998, 18(2 Suppl): S68–S80.

44. Briggs, A.H., B.J. O'Brien, and G. Blackhouse, Thinking outside the box: Recent advances in the analysis and presentation of uncertainty in cost-effectiveness studies. *Annu Rev Public Health*, 2002, 23: 377–401.

45. Briggs, A.H. et al., *Decision Modelling for Health Economic Evaluation*. 1st edn., 2006, Oxford, U.K.: Oxford University Press.

# 24 Structural and Molecular Imaging in Cancer Therapy Clinical Trials

*Brenda F. Kurland and David A. Mankoff*

## CONTENTS

## 24.1 IMAGING DATA IN ONCOLOGY MAY BE QUALITATIVE OR QUANTITATIVE, STRUCTURAL OR FUNCTIONAL

Imaging has a long history in cancer diagnosis and staging, and is increasingly used to evaluate therapeutic response (Eisenhauer et al., 2009; Wen et al., 2010). Molecular imaging is being developed for rapid characterization of response (especially for targeted therapy), with the long-term goal of more individualized therapies (Weber, 2006; Mankoff et al., 2007b).

The use of imaging to help direct and evaluate cancer therapy falls under the general category of use as a cancer biomarker. The aims for the use of qualitative and quantitative imaging biomarkers are similar to the aims for biomarkers from tissue and serum. To develop and apply appropriate statistical methods for analysis of these markers, it is important to understand the similarities and differences between tissue and imaging biomarkers (Table 24.1). It is also important to acknowledge that in many circumstances for clinical application and for design of clinical trials, information from both modalities (tissue and imaging biomarkers) may be available. Depending on the nature of overlap between tissue and imaging biomarkers, they may be used as confirmatory or complementary.

Imaging biomarkers may be used to overcome two significant limitations of tissue biomarkers (Mankoff et al., 2007b). First, tissue assays are prone to sampling

---

**TABLE 24.1**

**Overview of Characteristics of Tissue/Blood, Structural Imaging, and Functional Imaging as Sources of Biomarker Data**

| | Tissue/Blood | Structural Imaging | Functional Imaging |
|---|---|---|---|
| Can probe many features with one sample (also allows ease of patient and clinician blinding for selected results) | Yes | No | No |
| Can provide information about multiple disease sites with one probe | No | Yes | Yes |
| Batch processing available | Yes | No | No |
| Retrospective studies possible with new probe | Yes | No | No |
| Can provide information about interactions among drug, tumor, transport mechanisms such as the circulatory system, and host tissue | No | No | Yes |

error, especially when minimally invasive procedures are chosen for patient comfort. A small portion of a tumor may not be representative of the tumor as a whole. Some cancers, such as sarcomas, characteristically display heterogeneity in cellular characteristics and functional behavior (O'Sullivan et al., 2003). Other cancers, such as early stage breast cancer, may be less prone to tissue sampling error (Barry et al., 2010). However, when multiple disease sites are present, a single tissue sample from one tumor may not fully characterize the burden of disease or the molecular and structural properties of other tumors (Fisher et al., 2008; Kurland et al., 2011). Second, perturbation by tissue sampling may disturb the complex tumor microenvironment. Finally, serial tissue samples will not describe drug metabolism, drug delivery, and other key aspects of tumor response to therapy. In vivo imaging can address these limitations of tissue biomarkers.

In turn, the limitations of various in vivo imaging modalities, as discussed later (Section 24.2.3), may often be compensated for by the use of tissue sampling or other imaging modalities. Our goal in this chapter is to alert analysts to the strengths and weaknesses of current applications of in vivo imaging, to guide the design and analysis of clinical trials using these promising modalities for drug development and treatment selection.

### 24.1.1 Imaging May Yield Structural or Functional Information

Until recently, clinical imaging for cancer has been largely structural (anatomical) in nature, designed to identify tumor structural characteristics such as size, shape, and density. Tumors are recognized by abnormal shape or density compared to expected structures; tumors may also reveal abnormal features after the administration of intravenous contrast material. Changes in tumor size measured by structural imaging are commonly used to assess response in clinical trials. More recently, imaging has expanded to include functional and molecular imaging methods such as functional magnetic resonance imaging (fMRI) and positron emission tomography (PET), which may offer more specific measures of tumor response on the basis of change at the molecular and biochemical level. This chapter examines the use of both structural and functional imaging in cancer clinical trials. Sample images are shown in Figure 24.1.

### 24.1.2 Structural Imaging Modalities Used in Oncology Clinical Trials

#### 24.1.2.1 Computed Tomography

Computed tomography (CT) scanning measures projections of radiographic density (the ability of tissue to attenuate x-rays) at various scanned angles. Since different tissues have different radiographic densities, these projections may be reconstructed into high-resolution 3D images of bodily structures. Oral or intravenous contrast is often used to help delineate normal gastrointestinal organs (the stomach and intestines) as well as other structures, including blood vessels (Barentsz et al., 2006).

CT scanning is relatively rapid (about 5–15 min depending upon the extent of the body imaged and protocols used), but exposes the patient to a dose of radiation, as high as 15 mSv for body surveys (Mettler et al., 2008; Spiegelhalter, 2011).

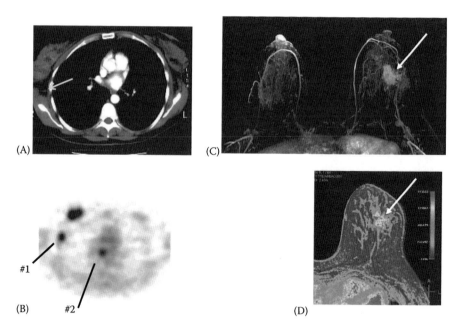

**FIGURE 24.1** Imaging examples: (A) CT scan to examine extent of disease for a patient diagnosed with breast cancer. (B) FDG PET scan paired with CT scan in panel (A). Lesion #1, axillary metastases from a breast cancer primary tumor, was visible on CT (arrow in panel (A)). Lesion #2, a mediastinal lesion, was not visible on CT. (C) Breast MRI with gadolinium contrast. Morphological characteristics of tumor (arrow) are demonstrated. (D) Map of MRI kinetics for the same scan. Shading reflects area under the contrast enhancement curve, showing how contrast signal intensity changes over the time of the scan. Rapid uptake followed by washout (arrow) is a characteristic of tumors.

By comparison, the ambient radiation dose for U.S. residents has been estimated as 3 mSv/year (National Research Council, 1990), and therapeutic doses are typically 1000 mSv or considerably more. Although risks of radiation exposure from medical imaging have not been demonstrated, greater use of serial CT for screening (Aberle et al., 2011) and restaging have led to the need for refinements in order to reduce exposure, especially for children (Hricak et al., 2011).

### 24.1.2.2 Magnetic Resonance Imaging

Magnetic resonance imaging (MRI), as widely used in medicine, uses magnetic fields and radiofrequency waves to perturb and detect signals arising from nuclei, mostly hydrogen in water. These signals are translated into a high-resolution image of bodily structures. Gadolinium chelates, which affect MRI signal intensity, are often injected (akin to contrast for CT), in order to delineate vascular structures and tissue perfusion. The use of MRI in cancer has increased considerably in the past 10–15 years. For example, MRI is becoming established as a valuable tool to screen for breast cancer in high-risk women (Warner et al., 2004; Lehman et al., 2007) and is the imaging modality of choice for neuro-oncology, given its unique ability to image the brain and central nervous system structures (Wen et al., 2010). MRI does not expose the patient to ionizing radiation. Although most routine MRI imaging focuses on structural information, MRI may also yield functional information such as quantitative tumor perfusion, as discussed later (Section 24.1.3.3).

### 24.1.3 FUNCTIONAL IMAGING MODALITIES USED IN ONCOLOGY CLINICAL TRIALS

Imaging has been extended beyond traditional structural/anatomical imaging to measure functional and molecular processes. Functional imaging lacks the regional structural precision of anatomical imaging, but carries quantitative information about regional physiology and biochemistry. The modalities most frequently used in current clinical practice and cancer clinical trials include PET and functional MRI, discussed in this section. Other functional molecular imaging modalities, such as optical imaging and microbubble ultrasound, are under development (Kelloff et al., 2005) and will not be discussed in the context of clinical trials.

#### 24.1.3.1 FDG PET

PET is a radionuclide imaging method: the PET scanner detects emissions arising from radioactive nuclei in radiopharmaceuticals administered intravenously to the patient. PET uses a special class of radioisotopes that emit a positron (antielectron). Emitted positrons annihilate with electrons within short distance (typically a few mm or less) of the emission site and generate two collinear annihilation photons, which are detected by the PET scanner. Detection of these annihilation photon pairs yield estimates of projections of positron-emitter concentration, akin to projection of radiographic density for CT. Using mathematics similar to CT, an image of regional radiopharmaceutical concentration is generated. PET has several advantages over other radionuclide imaging methods (such as single-photon emission computed tomography, or SPECT) for applications in oncology: higher spatial resolution (though considerably lower than CT or MRI), a wide range of radiopharmaceuticals designed to probe biochemical and molecular pathways, and the ability to measure absolute regional radiopharmaceutical concentration in 3D. PET tomographs are now generally packaged together with CT scanners to yield PET/CT devices, which can provide co-registered molecular and structural images. The effective radiation dose to the patient for PET scans depends mostly on the injected dose and is generally 4–6 mSv (Hays et al., 2002; Mankoff et al., 2002). PET/CT scans have higher effective doses of radiation (up to 25 mSv) due to increased radiation from the CT component, although additional exposure can be reduced to <5 mSv without much loss of CT image quality (Brix et al., 2005). Although a patient may spend as few as 5 min in the PET scanner (or as long as 120 min), it is sometimes necessary to wait between injection and scanning for the injected matter to go through the bloodstream and be metabolized by tissues, including tumors.

Currently, the most commonly used PET radiotracer is FDG ($^{18}$F-fluorodeoxyglucose), which is a radiolabeled glucose analog and a tracer of glucose metabolism. Tumors have been shown to be highly glycolytic, with a high rate of glycolysis compared to most normal tissues (Warburg, 1956). FDG is transported into cells using the same transport system as glucose, where it undergoes the first committed step of glucose metabolism, namely phosphorylation by hexokinase to FDG-6-phosphate

(FDG-6-P). However, FDG-6-P cannot continue on the glycolysis pathway, and thus is "metabolically trapped" in cells with active glucose metabolism. The rate of FDG-6-P (henceforth abbreviated as FDG) accumulation can be measured as a quantitative estimate of the regional glucose metabolic rate through kinetic analysis of dynamic uptake imaging by PET.

The most common method of quantifying FDG uptake uses a static measure obtained at a fixed time after injection (typically 60 min) (Shankar et al., 2006), known as the standardized uptake value (SUV):

$$ SUV = \frac{tissue\ activity \left[ kBq/mL \right]}{\left( injected\ dose/patient\ mass \right)\left[ MBq/kg \right]}. $$

Regional tissue activity is measured by the PET scanner, and then normalized by the injected radioactivity dose per patient weight. The SUV is a simple uptake ratio. It has density units and is unitless under the assumption of water density (1 g/mL), a reasonable assumption in most tissues. An SUV of 1 represents uniform distribution of the tracer in the tissue region, while values greater than 1 indicate tissue retention of FDG and thus glucose metabolism.

While the FDG SUV is the primary quantitative PET measure used in clinical practice and under development for use in clinical trials, a more detailed analysis is possible by applying tissue compartmental modeling using dynamic FDG PET imaging data and the FDG blood clearance curve, instead of relying on injected dose and patient mass to approximate distribution of the tracer (Mankoff et al., 2006). Dynamic imaging can provide more detailed information on regional biochemical kinetics, by separating the contributions of FDG and FDG-6P to the imaging, which are indistinguishable on simple static images. This approach can provide a more sensitive measure for discerning changes in metabolism in response to therapy (Doot et al., 2007), but is considerably more complex than an SUV and requires the patient to spend more time in the scanner (although the length of the clinic visit and radiation dose are unchanged).

Further methods for analyzing PET images have also been developed. These include parametric imaging methods that provide an image of tracer kinetic parameters at the voxel (volumetric pixel) level (O'Sullivan, 2006). In addition, measures taking into account the level of FDG uptake and the volume of metabolically active tumor have also been investigated as alternative measures of tumor burden (Larson et al., 1999).

### 24.1.3.2 Other PET Tracers

Currently the only approved PET imaging agents for cancer are FDG and [18]F-fluoride, an agent for imaging bone and bone metastases. A number of other radiopharmaceuticals, currently investigational, hold promise for cancer biomarker imaging (Kelloff et al., 2005; Mankoff et al., 2007a). Among these, some are being incorporated into multicenter therapy clinical trials. [18]F-fluorothymidine (FLT) is a thymidine analog used to assess regional cellular proliferation. Like FDG, the FLT tracer is trapped in the cell after phosphorylation along the thymidine salvage pathway for incorporation into newly synthesized DNA. Its accumulation is therefore a marker of the rate of DNA synthesis and, as such, a measure of cellular proliferation. FLT PET provides an in vivo measure of proliferation analogous to the Ki-67 tissue assay, where the overall rate of FLT accumulation in tissue has been correlated to Ki-67 levels (Buck et al., 2002; Vesselle et al., 2002; Muzi et al., 2005). Measuring changes in cellular proliferation may be especially advantageous for assessing therapeutic response. For example, if a treatment induces cell cycle arrest rather than tumor cell death, a successful response to therapy may not be reflected by changes in tumor size or metabolism, but may display change in cellular proliferation. Previous studies have assessed FLT PET as an early indicator of therapeutic response for both cytotoxic and cytostatic cancer drugs (Sohn et al., 2008; Kenny et al., 2009). The American College of Radiology Imaging Network (ACRIN) is evaluating FLT PET in an ongoing multicenter trial to measure early response to breast cancer neoadjuvant chemotherapy (ACRIN 6688) (Jolles et al., 2011).

### 24.1.3.3 Functional Applications of MRI in Oncology

Although MRI is used primarily to identify structural features, there are also functional applications for MRI. The kinetics of dynamic contrast-enhanced (DCE) MRI in tissue early after injection of MRI contrast agents reflect blood flow and capillary permeability. Semiquantitative measures of kinetics are typically incorporated into MRI assessments for breast cancer screening (Erguvan-Dogan et al., 2006). A variety of methods have been used to estimate the rate of early transport of the contrast from blood to tissue, often called the $K_{trans}$. This measure provides a quantitative indication of capillary transport, related to both blood flow and capillary permeability, since the movement of most MRI contrast agents across the capillary walls is limited by capillary permeability. Increased blood flow and capillary permeability is a hallmark of the vessels resulting from tumor angiogenesis, and therefore serial DCE-MRI has been used in a number of studies to assess the effect of antiangiogenic drugs (O'Connor et al., 2007). However, pseudoresponse is a concern, since the changes to tumor enhancement with antiangiogenic agents may not reflect a true antitumor effect (Wen et al., 2010). Serial DCE-MRI may also measure response to standard chemotherapy, likely through the direct effects on the tumor and on tumor vasculature (Padhani and Khan, 2010).

Other functional MRI measures are under development for use in clinical trials. For example, diffusion-weighted imaging (DWI) MRI measures water motility through extracellular spaces and therefore can provide a measure of tumor cellularity. Some studies have shown that serial DWI can provide a measure of early response to treatment, seen as a decline in tissue cellularity (increase in diffusion) accompanying tumor cell death in response to treatment (Theilmann et al., 2004; Hamstra et al., 2008). The imaging magnets used for MRI can also be used for magnetic resonance spectroscopy (MRS), which provides regional estimates of the concentration of specific tissue molecules that may provide an indication of active tumor. For example, the ability to measure changes in the level of choline, a component of cell membranes found in many tumor cells, appears to provide an early measure of response for some tumors, including breast cancer (Meisamy et al., 2004).

## 24.2 CLINICAL TRIAL DESIGN AND ANALYSIS CONSIDERATIONS

This section is divided based on potential uses of imaging as a quantitative biomarker. We first consider imaging as a proxy for clinical response, since this is the area where imaging is most widely applied. We next summarize current thinking about standardization and calibration, crucial prerequisites for the use of imaging modalities in multicenter trials. Finally, we discuss the process of validating molecular imaging biomarkers, and describe a case study of an experimental imaging procedure investigated as a predictive assay.

### 24.2.1 IMAGING MAY BE USED AS A PROXY FOR CLINICAL RESPONSE (SURROGATE ENDPOINTS)

#### 24.2.1.1 RECIST is a Consensus Standard for Response in Solid Tumor Oncology

In a phase II trial examining activity of a new therapy or combination of therapies, it is often infeasible to wait for a "hard" clinical endpoint such as overall survival or even progression-free survival. Objective response criteria were sought for early phase clinical trials, for the purpose of comparing therapies and planning follow-up studies. The World Health Organization (WHO) published tumor response criteria in 1981, using change from baseline in bidimensional tumor measurements (Miller et al., 1981). These criteria were refined and simplified by an International Working Party, resulting in the original Response Evaluation Criteria in Solid Tumors (RECIST) criteria (Therasse et al., 2000), based on unidimensional measurements. Further development through data warehouse analyses, simulation studies, and literature reviews led to the updated RECIST 1.1 guidelines (Eisenhauer et al., 2009).

The underlying concept of response by RECIST is simple: tumors treated effectively will reduce in size. Prior to therapy, radiologists identify target lesions and sum their longest diameters to quantify tumor burden at baseline. Objective criteria for complete response (CR), partial response (PR), progressive disease (PD), and stable disease (SD) can then be defined for these target lesions (Table 24.2). Statistical analysis of response by RECIST is usually summarized as a binomial proportion (with confidence interval): "response" (CR+PR versus SD+PD) or "clinical benefit" (CR+PR+SD versus PD) (Shankar et al., 2009).

Several factors complicate the classification of tumor response by RECIST. First, a PR at the first follow-up (such as 8 weeks) followed by PD at 16 weeks would

---

**TABLE 24.2**

**RECIST 1.1 Criteria for Target Lesions**

| | |
|---|---|
| Complete response | Disappearance of all target lesions |
| Partial response | At least 30% decrease in sum of diameters of target lesions |
| Progressive disease | At least 5 mm and 20% increase from the smallest recorded sum of diameters of target lesions, or appearance of at least one new lesion |
| Stable disease | Responses that are not categorized as CR, PR, or PD |

---

generally not be interpreted as a successful therapy. RECIST criteria generally require that a response is confirmed by achieving a result in the same class (i.e., PR or CR) at least 4 weeks after the previous scan. Once PR and CR in Table 24.2 are further classified as confirmed versus unconfirmed, the simplicity of the response criteria (their major benefit) is jeopardized. Further, not all lesions are eligible as target lesions. Some may be too small, not localized (such as pleural effusion), or not easily measurable on imaging modalities used for RECIST criteria (such as bone metastases).

Scans are often performed at regular intervals for clinical monitoring and for establishing radiographic progression in a clinical trial. Response by RECIST criteria at a specified timepoint may not account for variability in the time until maximum treatment benefit. Therefore, best overall response is often proposed as a trial endpoint. For decision criteria to determine best overall response in the context of all patient response data, refer to the RECIST 1.1 guidelines (Eisenhauer et al., 2009).

The burden for radiologists and clinical trial staff involved in measuring and tracking multiple lesions is a legitimate reason to investigate limiting the number of lesions for which data are collected. RECIST 1.0 criteria were based on the sum of longest diameters of up to 10 lesions. Simulation studies (Moskowitz et al., 2009) and reanalysis of clinical trial results (Hillman et al., 2009) both suggest that RECIST response criteria will still adequately classify patients as responders or non-responders when assessed for no more than five lesions (Moskowitz et al., 2009) or even two (Hillman et al., 2009). The criteria for RECIST 1.1 are based on five lesions for phase II and three lesions for phase III trials, reflecting the partly exploratory nature of phase II trials and the need to simplify data collection procedures for randomized phase III trials. However, even if all lesions are not measured in detail, all visible lesions must be documented since appearance of new lesions is a criterion for PD.

Informatics infrastructure used by radiologists in clinical practice has made it feasible to conduct centralized assessment of images such as CT results. Although in some settings the increased costs and delays that are likely to occur with centralized assessment are unlikely to be justified by improved accuracy (Dodd et al., 2008), centralized review has intuitive appeal for standardization of study protocols (Shankar et al., 2009). Centralized imaging core laboratories are worthwhile, but may most effectively improve trial data collection through a well-designed audit strategy (Dodd et al., 2011).

### 24.2.1.2 RECIST Has Limitations, Especially for Tumor-Treatment Combinations for Which Response is Not Characterized by Tumor Shrinkage

Although reduction in tumor size is attractive as an objective measure, there are many limitations to its use as an endpoint in clinical trials. A treatment that is cytostatic, rather than cytotoxic, may interfere with cell metabolism and proliferation without resulting in cancer cell death (Ratain et al., 2006). Even when tumor shrinkage is an expected result of therapy, cancer cell death and clearance as detected by CT/MRI are the result of a cascade of events and are not an early response to treatment (Yu and Mankoff, 2007). Volumetric CT may be more sensitive to early changes (Zhao et al., 2010) but is not implemented for clinical practice. The RECIST criteria also categorize data (size measurements) that are inherently continuous. This abstraction may be necessary for phase III trials to guide clinical practice; however, in phase II trials, quantitative summaries and waterfall plots of percent reduction in tumor diameter or tumor metabolism are complementing or replacing overall response by RECIST criteria (Herbst et al., 2007; Karrison et al., 2007; Tutt et al., 2010).

RECIST response criteria are also clearly impractical to apply without modification in specific cases of disease characteristics and/or mechanisms of treatment. Gastrointestinal stromal tumors and other sarcomas may result in tumor necrosis rather than tumor shrinkage, and long-term response to targeted therapies such as imatinib may not be represented well by RECIST criteria (Antoch et al., 2004). In response to these limitations, the Choi criteria for response in gastrointestinal stromal tumors defined response as a ≥10% decrease in size or a ≥15% decrease in density on contrast-enhanced CT (Benjamin et al., 2007). Other extensions of or alternatives to RECIST may incorporate functional imaging such as PET, for sarcoma (Benz et al., 2009) or for solid tumors in general, as discussed later (Wahl et al., 2009).

Another well-characterized example of limitations of RECIST to measure response is high-grade gliomas. Clinically relevant changes can occur in the short term, so increases or decreases in the use of corticosteroids (to reduce swelling and ease symptoms) and changes in neurologic status (alertness, ability to perform daily activities, etc.) have been incorporated into response criteria (Macdonald et al., 1990). Treatments for high-grade gliomas also affect tumor imaging in manners that may or may not reflect tumor response. Chemoradiation may cause psuedoprogression (transient increase in tumor enhancement), and rapid decrease in contrast enhancement under antiangiogenic treatment is due to reduced vascular permeability to contrast agents rather than antitumor effect. Corticosteroids also affect enhancement in contrast-enhanced CT and MRI scans. Response Assessment in Neuro-Oncology (RANO) response criteria (Wen et al., 2010) acknowledge these phenomena when defining criteria for response, mostly by repeated emphasis of the requirement that CR and PR be confirmed by a repeat follow-up scan at least 4 weeks later. The RANO response criteria also clarify that PD can be apparent from nonenhancing lesions. The Macdonald criteria and the 2010 RANO updates both rely on bidimensional lesion measurements. This is not due to differences in brain tumors, but reflects the early adoption of the Macdonald criteria (published 10 years before RECIST 1.0) and a desire to allow comparisons to historical controls (Wen et al., 2010).

### 24.2.1.3 FDG PET is Being Investigated as an Endpoint for Chemotherapy Response

Although PET is not widely accepted as a surrogate endpoint in clinical trials, specific cases have been identified where FDG PET offers advantages over structural imaging. For example, in lymphoma, a mass may persist on CT after treatment, but not contain viable tumor. This can be detected by PET as an absence of uptake post-therapy (often termed a complete metabolic response) (Juweid et al., 2007).

Complete metabolic response by FDG PET has been incorporated qualitatively into response criteria for lymphoma trials.

The PERCIST criteria (PET Response Criteria in Solid Tumors) are an effort to offer response criteria based on functional imaging to complement the RECIST criteria based on structural imaging (Wahl et al., 2009). While acknowledging that efforts are continuing to standardize and optimize PET measures, the PERCIST criteria make evidence-based recommendations for response categories. The SUV measure of choice is the "SUL peak," the mean lean-body-mass adjusted SUV of a 1.2 cm diameter spherical region of interest in the part of a lesion with the highest uptake. Change in FDG uptake is measured as the percentage difference between the lesion with the highest SUV peak at baseline, and the lesion with the highest SUV peak at follow-up (not necessarily the same lesion). Measures based on the summed uptake for several lesions are suggested as exploratory.

In the PERCIST criteria, CR, or "complete metabolic response" is defined as the visual disappearance of all metabolically active tumor. PR is defined as a ≥30% decrease in uptake and a ≥0.8 SUV unit decrease in the SUL peak. PD is defined as confirmed new lesions, a ≥ 30% increase in uptake and a ≥ 0.8 SUV unit increase in the SUL peak, or a 75% increase in total lesion glycolysis (mean SUV of tumor times total tumor volume in mL) (Larson et al., 1999) for the most active tumor. Other responses are categorized as SD.

The cutoff value of 30% change for PR or PD is larger than other thresholds based on doubling the test-retest repeatability standard deviation (Weber et al., 1999) or retrospective studies of clinical benefit. The rationale for this decision is partly illustrated in Figure 24.2, reproduced from the manuscript introducing PERCIST (and in turn reproduced from an earlier review [Kasamon et al., 2007]). The assumptions of Figure 24.2 are the minimal size of cancers at diagnosis ($10^{10}$–$10^{11}$ cells) and that cell kill occurs as a percentage of the tumor, not an absolute number of cells. Lines A, B, and C represent the cell kill trajectories of effective therapies with "brisk," intermediate, and slower tumor response. Due to the limitations of spatial resolution in PET scanners, PET will not be able to discriminate between microscopic residual tumor and no tumor burden. This is apparent in Figure 24.2 (which shows a lower limit of detection for PET) and from clinical studies (Crippa et al., 2004). However, the positive conclusion of Figure 24.2 is that metabolic response due to tumor cell death and to more direct effects of treatment will be apparent after 1–3 cycles of chemotherapy for most promising therapies. Serial FDG PET appears to hold promise for monitoring the therapeutic response of individual patients (as will be discussed later) and shows promise as a surrogate endpoint for progression-free survival or overall survival, with proper validation for specific diseases and classes of therapy. Such studies will need to be carried out in prospective trials.

### 24.2.2 STANDARDIZATION AND CALIBRATION PROCEDURES ARE PREREQUISITES TO MULTICENTER CLINICAL TRIALS USING FUNCTIONAL IMAGING

Standards to reduce bias and measurement error have been suggested to address some known issues in application of PET in clinical trials (Shankar et al., 2006; Boellaard, 2009; Boellaard et al., 2010), but the combined impact of these

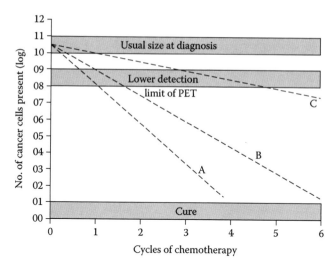

**FIGURE 24.2** Kinetics of tumor cell kill and PET limits of detection suggest a role for PET in detecting early response to therapy. Lines A and B represent brisk and moderate rates of tumor cell kill, leading to cure in four and six cycles of chemotherapy, respectively. Line C represents a therapy that is not curative, but has clinical benefit. Metabolic response to therapy should be apparent after one to three cycles of chemotherapy for most promising therapies. (From Kasamon et al., *J. Nucl. Med.*, 48(Suppl 1), 19S, 2007, Figure 4. Reprinted with permission from the Society of Nuclear Medicine.)

standards has not been evaluated. Standardization of patient preparation protocols (Shankar et al., 2006) may be feasible, but standardization of image acquisition and analysis is difficult due to inherent differences between brands of PET scanners and physiological differences between patients (e.g., it is easier to localize a positron emission in a smaller body). Furthermore, individual institutions may use scanner and image analysis settings to optimize performance for certain clinical or research applications, and changing the settings between scans is infeasible. Scanner hardware, reconstruction algorithms, and region of interest definition may contribute to additional measurement error or bias (Krak et al., 2005; Westerterp et al., 2007).

Studies using pseudo-patient phantoms (Fahey et al., 2010) and patient test-retest with no intervening treatment (Weber et al., 1999; Velasquez et al., 2009) suggest that under ideal conditions (same scanner, same technician), instrumentation is precise enough to produce <5% measurement error for phantom studies and about 10% for the SUV of in vivo tumors. However, even for closely monitored trials, errors in recording or transcribing factors such as patient weight and the interval between injection and scanning may occur and result in considerable mismeasurement of SUVs (Scheuermann et al., 2009). The 10% measurement error estimate for individual FDG PET SUV values has been cited as a reason to accept 20% change or greater as "significant" (Weber et al., 1999). However, it should be noted that Weber's data also supported measurement error as an absolute value (i.e., 0.5 SUV unit) rather than a percentage (Weber et al., 1999). Furthermore, even if the same scanner is used for all of one patient's scans, scanner drift or calibration errors could occur over those weeks and months that would not be evident in a test–retest study (Lockhart et al., 2011).

Efforts for standardization and harmonization of quantitative imaging biomarkers for use in multicenter clinical trials are ongoing (Meyer et al., 2009; Scheuermann et al., 2009). Statistical input is needed to design these studies and to interpret and implement the results.

### 24.2.3  DEVELOPMENT OF MOLECULAR IMAGING AS A BIOMARKER

Several steps are necessary for validation as a biomarker before functional imaging such as PET could be used to direct therapy or evaluate response in early stage clinical trials (McShane et al., 2005; Krohn et al., 2007; Pepe et al., 2008; Sargent et al., 2009; Dancey et al., 2010). Most guidelines for biomarker development were developed with the strengths and limitations of blood and tissue biomarkers in mind, such as false discovery rate issues for high throughput assays. Also, the focus of most consensus statements has been cancer screening or endpoints for pivotal trials. Considerations for early phase trials, where molecular imaging shows great promise for facilitating drug development, have drawn less attention. Although these guidelines for biomarker development are general enough to apply to other modalities such as functional imaging, it is incumbent upon researchers who use imaging to identify the strengths to exploit and the weaknesses to overcome. This section discusses technical strengths and limitations of many imaging biomarkers, and explores study designs to exploit the promise of these biomarkers.

#### 24.2.3.1  How is Imaging Different from Tissue or Blood Assays?

One strength of functional imaging is the ability to study molecular processes over time without disturbing the tumor microenvironment, which allows for creative designs using imaging biomarkers in drug development and treatment selection. Functional imaging can also characterize the entire disease burden, rather than the limited sample from a tissue or blood assay tissue or blood assay (Table 24.1).

A limitation of functional imaging is that there are several irreversible steps in image generation that preclude centralized processing for many phases of analysis. Thus, standardization of imaging protocols and calibration of imaging technologies has been a focus of efforts to validate quantitative imaging for use in multicenter clinical trials (see Section 24.2.2). For tissue and blood assays, a single sample may yield many clinical results. The treating clinician and patient may not feel anything is "missing" if the results from an experimental technique (performed on the available sample) are omitted from clinical reports. In contrast, blinding of patients and clinicians to functional imaging results is challenging. There may be temptation to act upon results from experimental techniques, making it difficult to conduct studies with objective assessments.

Unlike some tissue assays, which can be validated using banked samples (Pepe et al., 2008), molecular imaging must be performed prospectively. Radiation safety concerns for novel PET tracers are another barrier to thorough well-powered validation studies. Additional logistical challenges include the short half-life of many radiopharmaceuticals (the half-life of $^{18}$F is 110 min, but the half-life of $^{15}$O is only 2 min), and the availability of an on-site cyclotron to generate novel radiopharmaceuticals and tracers with a very short half-life. These considerations, as well as overall cost and patient burden, constrain the size of clinical trials involving novel molecular imaging such as FDG PET.

The role of the analyst is to recognize the necessity of limited sample sizes for novel molecular imaging, and to participate in planning a design and analysis strategy that will make the best use of a limited number of scans. These design and analysis considerations are not fundamentally different from considerations for any clinical trial, but the goal here is to provide guidance for statisticians encountering the challenges that are important, and sometimes unique, to molecular imaging.

### 24.2.3.2 Potential Applications for Molecular Imaging as a Biomarker

Imaging may be used to screen patients for study enrollment in an enrichment design (Chapter 17; Simon, 2010) (Figure 24.3A). One example is using FDG PET uptake as a study entry criterion, to identify thyroid cancer patients with aggressive disease for a phase II study of systemic therapy (Carr et al., 2010). If imaging is only used in the screening phase, the cost of imaging will be the same as if all patients were enrolled and treated. However, if an enrichment (or "targeted"/"marker positive") design is

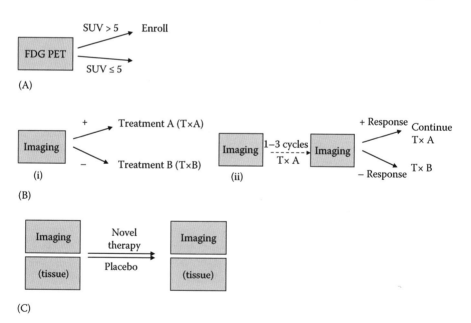

**FIGURE 24.3** Designs using quantitative imaging as a biomarker in early stage clinical trials. (A) Targeted (enrichment) design (prognostic marker for high risk of recurrence). (B) Predictive marker: (i) single scan as predictive marker and (ii) early response as predictive marker. (C) Proof of mechanism studies (pharmacodynamic marker), single arm or randomized placebo-controlled. Imaging and tissue may each be fit-for-purpose (directly related to hypothesized mechanism of therapy) or general antitumor response.

warranted (see Chapter 17), quantitative or qualitative imaging may be used as part of entry criteria.

Imaging may also be used as a predictive marker. A single pretreatment measurement could be used to direct therapy (Figure 24.3Bi), or serial measurements over a short period of therapy (Figure 24.3Bii), could inform whether a therapy is productive or futile. As an example, evaluation of [18]F-fluoroestradiol (FES) PET as a predictive marker is described later (Section 24.2.4).

Serial imaging over a short period of time has particular promise in proof of mechanism studies (Figure 24.3C). Dramatic changes in tumor metabolism may be detected as changes in FDG PET SUV in as few as 8 days, as for the response of gastrointestinal stromal tumors to imatinib (Stroobants et al., 2003). These changes in tumor metabolism occur more quickly than changes related to cell death, such as change in tumor size. Although it is possible that these pharmacodynamic changes may not lead to clinically meaningful results, the subsequent success of imatinib in randomized trials with sound clinical endpoints such as recurrence-free survival (DeMatteo et al., 2009) encourages the exploration of functional imaging as a pharmacodynamic endpoint. Although serial biopsy is feasible, serial imaging may be seen as less invasive, and does not change the tumor as biopsy would.

## 24.2.4 EXAMPLE: DEVELOPMENT OF FES PET IMAGING AS A PREDICTIVE MARKER

To illustrate design and analysis considerations for evaluating functional imaging as a predictive marker, we describe the development of [18]F-fluoroestradiol (FES) PET, which produces in vivo quantitative measures of regional estrogen receptor (ER) binding in breast cancer tumors. Over 70% of breast cancers are ER positive, and ER-directed adjuvant therapy is credited as a key factor in the recent decline in breast cancer mortality (EBCTCG, 2005). However, only 50%–85% of newly diagnosed patients with ER+ tumors respond to primary endocrine therapy (Ravdin et al., 1992), and many patients who initially respond to endocrine therapy later become refractory (Buzdar et al., 1996). There is evidence from tissue assays that higher quantitative ER expression is associated with a greater chance for response to endocrine therapy (Dowsett et al., 2008). However, many patients considering endocrine therapy have tumors that make biopsy difficult or painful. FES PET could be used to help direct treatment selection for patients with advanced breast cancer. Patients with high ER expression could be directed to endocrine therapy, while patients with low or absent FES uptake could be directed to alternative treatment, such as cytotoxic chemotherapy.

Early studies examined criterion validity of FES PET through comparisons to tissue assays with ER expression measured by immunohistochemistry (IHC) (Mintun et al., 1988; Peterson et al., 2008). As a side note, this "validation" was mostly assessed as correlation coefficient for the linear relationship between quantitative levels of ER functioning by FES PET and tissue assay, demonstrating the need for application of more appropriate methods for agreement between assays (Bland and Altman, 1986).

Other analyses from these early clinical studies suggested that the response rate to endocrine therapy could be improved by selection based on quantitative FES

PET SUV (Mortimer et al., 2001; Linden et al., 2006). A simplified version of one such analysis (Linden et al., 2006) follows. Clinical records for patients scanned under several developmental protocols were examined to identify patients whose scans occurred shortly before initiating or changing endocrine therapy (N=46) (Figure 24.4A). FES PET results were summarized by the average SUV for up to three lesions. The distribution of FES SUV values is shown in Figure 24.5, separately for those who responded and did not respond to endocrine therapy. (We assumed that the endpoint "response to endocrine therapy" was a gold standard measured without error.) Eleven of 46 patients (24%) were responders. While responders on average had higher average FES SUV than non-responders, there is considerable overlap between the average FES SUV values for responders and non-responders. However, there are many mechanisms of resistance for advanced breast cancer to endocrine therapy (Johnston, 2009): FES PET cannot be expected to be a perfect classifier of responders from non-responders, just as ER expression by IHC is not. Rather than considering overall classification or the positive predictive value (chance of response for high values of FES SUV), we examine the negative predictive value (chance of non-response for low values of FES SUV). Observing the horizontal line on Figure 24.5 at SUV = 1.5, we see that the response rate is extremely low for patients with FES SUV ≤ 1.5, approximately the threshold distinguishing ER+ and ER− tumors in studies in which imaging was paired with IHC. None of the 15 patients with an SUV ≤ 1.5 responded to therapy, whereas 11 of 31 patients (35%) with SUV > 1.5 responded. The association between response and FES PET and other categorical predictors was

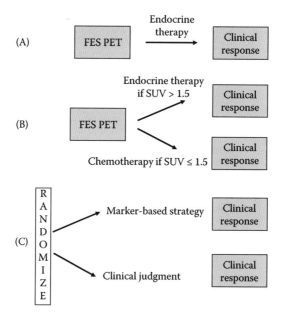

**FIGURE 24.4** Studies to develop FES PET as a predictive biomarker for response to endocrine therapy. (A) Heterogeneous patient population (newly diagnosed breast cancer through nth line metastatic), n=46. (B) Newly diagnosed metastatic breast cancer, n=50. (C) Newly diagnosed metastatic breast cancer, n=500.

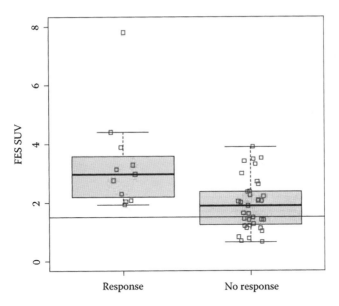

**FIGURE 24.5**    Distribution of FES SUV by clinical response (n = 46).

assessed using the mid-P adjustment to Fisher's exact test (Lancaster, 1961). Both one-sided and two-sided (based on minimum likelihood) mid-P values have Type I error rates closer to nominal rates than Fisher's exact test or classical asymptotic tests when used to compare binomial probabilities in groups that differ in sample size (Hirji et al., 1991; Agresti, 2001). Using a two-sided mid-P test, we concluded that the response rate to endocrine therapy was higher in the patients with SUV > 1.5 (p = 0.006).

We next consider possible studies that might follow the previously published studies to test FES PET as a means for selecting therapy for breast cancer patients. One possible pilot study to test the feasibility of using FES PET to direct patient treatment is illustrated in Figure 24.4B. Participants would have metastatic breast cancer from an ER+ primary tumor, and be candidates for endocrine therapy but considering both endocrine therapy and systemic chemotherapy. Patients with average FES SUV higher than the previously measured threshold for response (tentatively FES SUV > 1.5) would be directed to endocrine therapy, and patients with low FES SUV (tentatively ≤ 1.5) would be directed to alternative therapy such as chemotherapy. Since the PET-directed strategy will presumably lead to a change in therapy (chemotherapy instead of endocrine therapy) in only about 1/3 of participants, it may be difficult to demonstrate that the FES-directed population had a higher overall response rate. The study would be powered to rule out a low response rate (25%) to endocrine therapy in the high-FES-SUV group, and to provide support for a response rate of 40% or greater. In the range of expected sample size for the FES SUV >1.5 group (32–36 patients of n = 50 total), the number of responses to rule out a response rate of 25% is the same as the number of responses to achieve an observed rate over 40%. For example, if 13 of 33 patients with FES SUV > 1.5 respond to endocrine therapy (39%), the 95% Wilson (score) confidence interval for response would be (0.25, 0.56). The study power would be about 0.64 if the FES-selected response rate is 44% (as observed for HER2-negative patients in preliminary data), and about 0.85 if the FES-selected response rate is 50%. The study will also provide further preliminary data for the response to chemotherapy in patients with low FES SUV, and the percentage of patients with low FES SUV (estimated as 33%).

If preliminary studies provide consistent support for imaging as means for selecting endocrine therapy in the salvage setting, a definitive multicenter randomized two-arm trial could use a strategy design (Chapter 17), in which therapy is directed by imaging in one arm, and by clinical judgment without imaging in the other arm (Figure 24.4C). The sample size would have to be about n = 500 to have 90% power to detect a 15% point difference in overall response rate between the imaging-directed strategy and clinical judgment. Imaging would not be performed in the clinical judgment arm, so the treatment outcomes could not be compared across arms for groups defined by FES SUV. However, the definitive trial as proposed in Figure 24.4C would effectively compare an imaging-based strategy to the standard of care, and could include assessments of cost-effectiveness and patient discomfort and distress due to both procedures (imaging and biopsy) and treatment. FES PET may have a role as a predictive marker primarily in patients who are unable or unwilling to undergo biopsy of metastatic lesions.

In summary, the example of the emerging evaluation of FES PET as a predictive marker illustrates the need to keep the next study in mind when designing the current study, and taking into account changes in technologies and clinical practice that occur during the development of an agent, marker, or modality.

## 24.3 NOVEL APPROACHES AND FUTURE DIRECTIONS

### 24.3.1 Co-Development of Agents, Tissue/Blood Biomarkers, and Imaging Biomarkers, and Novel Designs

In the pursuit of personalized medicine, technology to assess biomarkers, proposed mechanisms of action described by biomarkers, and therapeutic agents targeted at those mechanisms of action are continuously under development. Reassessment is also desirable when a marker or agent is proposed for use in a new tumor type, for a new purpose (i.e., as a predictive marker to guide therapy, rather than as a response measure to a particular therapy), or a different patient population (such as early stage disease for markers or agents developed in late stage settings). In development of a new drug or combination of drugs, or a new predictive marker to guide therapy selection, study designs to accommodate "co-development" must be considered.

Clearly, co-development of markers and therapies "increases the complexity of all stages of the development process" (Simon, 2010). Draft guidance for co-development of drugs and in vitro diagnostic markers for Food and Drug Administration (FDA) approval (of drugs or markers) emphasize clarity of reporting, validation of instrumentation, and prespecification of assay cutoff values (FDA, 2005). A possible area for exploration is the use in early phase studies of biomarkers that address similar targets, but through a different modality (i.e., imaging versus tissue) or as an embedded validation study (Suman et al., 2008; Dancey et al., 2010). To avoid "fishing expeditions" that waste resources (Ratain and Glassman, 2007), the studies should be designed to ensure that the details of the results will be useful in planning future studies.

For example, consider a randomized phase II trial to evaluate different doses or schedules of combined antiangiogenic and cytotoxic chemotherapy. The study could be designed to evaluate dose–response relationships for both fit-for-purpose markers (DCE-MRI perfusion measures, plasma vascular endothelial growth factor measures) and for general tumor response markers (FDG PET SUV, response by RECIST). If both markers show a dose–response relationship, the mechanism of action is as surmised. If the fit-for-purpose marker shows a dose–response relationship but the tumor response marker does not, this is evidence that the antiangiogenic target has been hit, but tumor response is limited: perhaps downstream effects must also be accounted for in treatment, or the tumor response marker may be inadequate. Or, if there is strong tumor response for all dose levels, the extent of action measured by the fit-for-purpose marker may not be necessary for therapeutic effect. We emphasize that the markers must be chosen carefully and the possible outcomes considered ahead of time. Specific fit-for-purpose imaging markers are discussed by Kelloff et al. (2005), and genomic biomarkers associated with drug development are discussed by Chau et al. (2008).

A possible flow chart for including functional imaging in clinical trials is shown in Figure 24.6. FDG PET is emerging as a widely applicable marker for measuring tumor metabolic response (Wahl et al., 2009). Depending on hypothesized mechanisms of action, additional PET tracers or imaging modalities may be used to measure effects on perfusion (DCE-MRI or $^{15}$O water PET), proliferation (FLT PET), or binding to specific receptors.

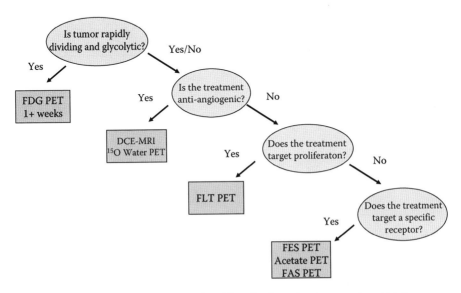

**FIGURE 24.6** Potential uses for functional imaging in early phase treatment trials.

### 24.3.2 NOVEL APPROACHES TO THE ANALYSIS OF IMAGING DATA IN CANCER CLINICAL TRIALS

Imaging offers the opportunity to analyze the entire tumor burden for a patient. This may be achieved by summary measures such as total lesion glycolysis (Larson et al., 1999) or summing the FDG SUV from individual lesions (an exploratory endpoint proposed for PERCIST [Wahl et al., 2009]), or by analysis of individual lesions within a person as correlated data (Gonen et al., 2001; Kurland et al., 2011). Lesion level response to therapy may be analyzed, and within-patient and between-patient heterogeneity may be described to gain insight regarding the development of metastatic lesions.

Data from multiple imaging probes (and/or multiple other biomarkers) may also be combined to evaluate tumor characteristics (Krohn et al., 2007; Strauss et al., 2008). Two examples are examining simple ratio of imaging parameters as novel measures. Mismatch of tumor blood flow (measured by $^{15}O$ water PET or DCE-MRI) and tumor metabolism (measured by FDG PET) may identify subsets of tumors susceptible and resistant to cytotoxic chemotherapy and identify targets for targeted therapy (Specht et al., 2010). A high FES/FDG ratio, indicating high ER activity and low tumor glycolytic activity, could identify indolent breast cancer lesions susceptible to endocrine therapy (Mankoff and Dehdashti, 2009).

In summary, incorporation of functional imaging, quantitative imaging measures, and other imaging biomarkers into cancer clinical trials is a multidisciplinary effort requiring patience and diligence, as well as technical innovation. Statisticians have a role in collaboration with physicians, physicists, bioinformaticians, and other clinical trialists to develop these promising modalities effectively.

## ACKNOWLEDGMENTS

This work was supported in part by NIH grants CA138293 and CA148131, and uses data from projects funded by CA42045, CA72064, CA148131, and DOD W81XWH-04-01-0675. The authors thank Mark Muzi, Savannah Partridge, Hannah Linden, and Xiaoyu Chai for their contributions.

## REFERENCES

Aberle, D. R., Berg, C. D., Black, W. C., Church, T. R., Fagerstrom, R. M., Galen, B., Gareen, I. F. et al. 2011. The National Lung Screening Trial: Overview and study design. *Radiology*, 258, 243–253.

Agresti, A. 2001. Exact inference for categorical data: Recent advances and continuing controversies. *Stat Med*, 20, 2709–2722.

Antoch, G., Kanja, J., Bauer, S., Kuehl, H., Renzing-Koehler, K., Schuette, J., Bockisch, A., Debatin, J. F., and Freudenberg, L. S. 2004. Comparison of PET, CT, and dual-modality PET/CT imaging for monitoring of imatinib (STI571) therapy in patients with gastrointestinal stromal tumors. *J Nucl Med*, 45, 357–365.

Barentsz, J., Takahashi, S., Oyen, W., Mus, R., De Mulder, P., Reznek, R., Oudkerk, M., and Mali, W. 2006. Commonly used imaging techniques for diagnosis and staging. *J Clin Oncol*, 24, 3234–3244.

Barry, W. T., Kernagis, D. N., Dressman, H. K., Griffis, R. J., Hunter, J. D., Olson, J. A., Marks, J. R. et al. 2010. Intratumor heterogeneity and precision of microarray-based predictors of breast cancer biology and clinical outcome. *J Clin Oncol*, 28, 2198–2206.

Benjamin, R. S., Choi, H., Macapinlac, H. A., Burgess, M. A., Patel, S. R., Chen, L. L., Podoloff, D. A., and Charnsangavej, C. 2007. We should desist using RECIST, at least in GIST. *J Clin Oncol*, 25, 1760–1764.

Benz, M. R., Czernin, J., Allen-Auerbach, M. S., Tap, W. D., Dry, S. M., Elashoff, D., Chow, K. et al. 2009. FDG-PET/CT imaging predicts histopathologic treatment responses after the initial cycle of neoadjuvant chemotherapy in high-grade soft-tissue sarcomas. *Clin Cancer Res*, 15, 2856–2863.

Bland, J. M. and Altman, D. G. 1986. Statistical methods for assessing agreement between two methods of clinical measurement. *Lancet*, 1, 307–310.

Boellaard, R. 2009. Standards for PET image acquisition and quantitative data analysis. *J Nucl Med*, 50 (Suppl 1), 11S–20S.

Boellaard, R., O'Doherty, M. J., Weber, W. A., Mottaghy, F. M., Lonsdale, M. N., Stroobants, S. G., Oyen, W. J. et al. 2010. FDG PET and PET/CT: EANM procedure guidelines for tumour PET imaging: Version 1.0. *Eur J Nucl Med Mol Imaging*, 37, 181–200.

Brix, G., Lechel, U., Glatting, G., Ziegler, S. I., Munzing, W., Muller, S. P., and Beyer, T. 2005. Radiation exposure of patients undergoing whole-body dual-modality 18F-FDG PET/CT examinations. *J Nucl Med*, 46, 608–613.

Buck, A. K., Schirrmeister, H., Hetzel, M., Von der Heide, M., Halter, G., Glatting, G., Mattfeldt, T., Liewald, F., Reske, S. N., and Neumaier, B. 2002. 3-Deoxy-3-[(18)F]fluorothymidine-positron emission tomography for noninvasive assessment of proliferation in pulmonary nodules. *Cancer Res*, 62, 3331–3334.

Buzdar, A., Jonat, W., Howell, A., Jones, S. E., Blomqvist, C., Vogel, C. L., Eiermann, W. et al. 1996. Anastrozole, a potent and selective aromatase inhibitor, versus megestrol acetate in postmenopausal women with advanced breast cancer: Results of overview analysis of two phase III trials. Arimidex Study Group. *J Clin Oncol*, 14, 2000–2011.

Carr, L. L., Mankoff, D. A., Goulart, B. H., Eaton, K. D., Capell, P. T., Kell, E. M., Bauman, J. E., and Martins, R. G. 2010. Phase II study of daily sunitinib in FDG-PET-positive, iodine-refractory differentiated thyroid cancer and metastatic medullary carcinoma of the thyroid with functional imaging correlation. *Clin Cancer Res*, 16, 5260–5268.

Chau, C. H., Rixe, O., Mcleod, H., and Figg, W. D. 2008. Validation of analytic methods for biomarkers used in drug development. *Clin Cancer Res*, 14, 5967–5976.

Crippa, F., Gerali, A., Alessi, A., Agresti, R., and Bombardieri, E. 2004. FDG-PET for axillary lymph node staging in primary breast cancer. *Eur J Nucl Med Mol Imaging*, 31 (Suppl 1), S97–S102.

Dancey, J. E., Dobbin, K. K., Groshen, S., Jessup, J. M., Hruszkewycz, A. H., Koehler, M., Parchment, R. et al. 2010. Guidelines for the development and incorporation of biomarker studies in early clinical trials of novel agents. *Clin Cancer Res*, 16, 1745–1755.

DeMatteo, R. P., Ballman, K. V., Antonescu, C. R., Maki, R. G., Pisters, P. W., Demetri, G. D., Blackstein, M. E. et al. 2009. Adjuvant imatinib mesylate after resection of localised, primary gastrointestinal stromal tumour: A randomised, double-blind, placebo-controlled trial. *Lancet*, 373, 1097–1104.

Dodd, L. E., Korn, E. L., Freidlin, B., Gray, R., and Bhattacharya, S. 2011. An audit strategy for progression-free survival. *Biometrics*, 67, 1092–1099.

Dodd, L. E., Korn, E. L., Freidlin, B., Jaffe, C. C., Rubinstein, L. V., Dancey, J., and Mooney, M. M. 2008. Blinded independent central review of progression-free survival in phase III clinical trials: Important design element or unnecessary expense? *J Clin Oncol*, 26, 3791–3796.

Doot, R. K., Dunnwald, L. K., Schubert, E. K., Muzi, M., Peterson, L. M., Kinahan, P. E., Kurland, B. F., and Mankoff, D. A. 2007. Dynamic and static approaches to quantifying 18F-FDG uptake for measuring cancer response to therapy, including the effect of granulocyte CSF. *J Nucl Med*, 48, 920–925.

Dowsett, M., Allred, C., Knox, J., Quinn, E., Salter, J., Wale, C., Cuzick, J. et al. 2008. Relationship between quantitative estrogen and progesterone receptor expression and human epidermal growth factor receptor 2 (HER-2) status with recurrence in the arimidex, tamoxifen, alone or in combination trial. *J Clin Oncol*, 26, 1059–1065.

Early Breast Cancer Trialists' Collaborative Group (EBCTCG). 2005. Effects of chemotherapy and hormonal therapy for early breast cancer on recurrence and 15-year survival: An overview of the randomised trials. *Lancet*, 365, 1687–1717.

Eisenhauer, E. A., Therasse, P., Bogaerts, J., Schwartz, L. H., Sargent, D., Ford, R., Dancey, J. et al. 2009. New response evaluation criteria in solid tumours: Revised RECIST guideline (version 1.1). *Eur J Cancer*, 45, 228–247.

Erguvan-Dogan, B., Whitman, G. J., Kushwaha, A. C., Phelps, M. J., and Dempsey, P. J. 2006. BI-RADS-MRI: A primer. *AJR Am J Roentgenol*, 187, W152–W160.

Fahey, F. H., Kinahan, P. E., Doot, R. K., Kocak, M., Thurston, H., and Poussaint, T. Y. 2010. Variability in PET quantitation within a multicenter consortium. *Med Phys*, 37, 3660–3666.

FDA. 2005. Drug–diagnostic co-development concept paper. http://www.fda.gov/downloads/Drugs/ScienceResearch/ResearchAreas/Pharmacogenetics/UCM116689.pdf.

Fisher, B., Redmond, C. K., and Fisher, E. R. 2008. Evolution of knowledge related to breast cancer heterogeneity: A 25-year retrospective. *J Clin Oncol*, 26, 2068–2071.

Gonen, M., Panageas, K. S., and Larson, S. M. 2001. Statistical issues in analysis of diagnostic imaging experiments with multiple observations per patient. *Radiology*, 221, 763–767.

Hamstra, D. A., Galban, C. J., Meyer, C. R., Johnson, T. D., Sundgren, P. C., Tsien, C., Lawrence, T. S. et al. 2008. Functional diffusion map as an early imaging biomarker for high-grade glioma: Correlation with conventional radiologic response and overall survival. *J Clin Oncol*, 26, 3387–3394.

Hays, M. T., Watson, E. E., Thomas, S. R., and Stabin, M. 2002. MIRD dose estimate report no. 19: Radiation absorbed dose estimates from (18)F-FDG. *J Nucl Med*, 43, 210–214.

Herbst, R. S., Davies, A. M., Natale, R. B., Dang, T. P., Schiller, J. H., Garland, L. L., Miller, V. A. et al. 2007. Efficacy and safety of single-agent pertuzumab, a human epidermal receptor dimerization inhibitor, in patients with non small cell lung cancer. *Clin Cancer Res*, 13, 6175–6181.

Hillman, S. L., An, M. W., O'Connell, M. J., Goldberg, R. M., Schaefer, P., Buckner, J. C., and Sargent, D. J. 2009. Evaluation of the optimal number of lesions needed for tumor evaluation using the Response Evaluation Criteria in Solid Tumors: A North Central Cancer Treatment Group investigation. *J Clin Oncol*, 27(19), 3205–3210.

Hirji, K. F., Tan, S. J., and Elashoff, R. M. 1991. A quasi-exact test for comparing two binomial proportions. *Stat Med*, 10, 1137–1153.

Hricak, H., Brenner, D. J., Adelstein, S. J., Frush, D. P., Hall, E. J., Howell, R. W., Mccollough, C. H. et al. 2011. Managing radiation use in medical imaging: A multifaceted challenge. *Radiology*, 258, 889–905.

Johnston, S. R. 2009. Enhancing the efficacy of hormonal agents with selected targeted agents. *Clin Breast Cancer*, 9 (Suppl 1), S28–S36.

Jolles, P. R., Kostakoglu, L., Bear, H. D., Idowu, M. O., Kurdziel, K. A., Shankar, L., Mankoff, D. A., Duan, F., and L'Heureux, D. 2011. ACRIN 6688 phase II study of fluorine-18 3-deoxy-3 fluorothymidine (FLT) in invasive breast cancer. *J Clin Oncol*, 29, abstract TPS125.

Juweid, M. E., Stroobants, S., Hoekstra, O. S., Mottaghy, F. M., Dietlein, M., Guermazi, A., Wiseman, G. A. et al. 2007. Use of positron emission tomography for response assessment of lymphoma: Consensus of the Imaging Subcommittee of International Harmonization Project in Lymphoma. *J Clin Oncol*, 25, 571–578.

Karrison, T. G., Maitland, M. L., Stadler, W. M., and Ratain, M. J. 2007. Design of phase II cancer trials using a continuous endpoint of change in tumor size: Application to a study of sorafenib and erlotinib in non small-cell lung cancer. *J Natl Cancer Inst*, 99, 1455–1461.

Kasamon, Y. L., Jones, R. J., and Wahl, R. L. 2007. Integrating PET and PET/CT into the risk-adapted therapy of lymphoma. *J Nucl Med*, 48 (Suppl 1), 19S–27S.

Kelloff, G. J., Krohn, K. A., Larson, S. M., Weissleder, R., Mankoff, D. A., Hoffman, J. M., Link, J. M. et al. 2005. The progress and promise of molecular imaging probes in oncologic drug development. *Clin Cancer Res*, 11, 7967–7985.

Kenny, L. M., Contractor, K. B., Stebbing, J., Al-Nahhas, A., Palmieri, C., Shousha, S., Coombes, R. C., and Aboagye, E. O. 2009. Altered tissue 3′-deoxy-3′-[18F]fluoro-thymidine pharmacokinetics in human breast cancer following capecitabine treatment detected by positron emission tomography. *Clin Cancer Res*, 15, 6649–6657.

Krak, N. C., Boellaard, R., Hoekstra, O. S., Twisk, J. W., Hoekstra, C. J., and Lammertsma, A. A. 2005. Effects of ROI definition and reconstruction method on quantitative outcome and applicability in a response monitoring trial. *Eur J Nucl Med Mol Imaging*, 32, 294–301.

Krohn, K. A., O'Sullivan, F., Crowley, J., Eary, J. F., Linden, H. M., Link, J. M., Mankoff, D. A. et al. 2007. Challenges in clinical studies with multiple imaging probes. *Nucl Med Biol*, 34, 879–885.

Kurland, B. F., Peterson, L. M., Lee, J. H., Linden, H. M., Schubert, E. K., Dunnwald, L. K., Link, J. M., Krohn, K. A., and Mankoff, D. A. 2011. Between-patient and within-patient (site-to-site) variability in estrogen receptor binding, measured *in vivo* by [18]F-fluoroestradiol (FES) PET. *J Nucl Med*, 52(10), 1541–1549.

Lancaster, H. O. 1961. Significance tests in discrete distributions. *J Am Stat Assoc*, 56, 223–234.

Larson, S. M., Erdi, Y., Akhurst, T., Mazumdar, M., Macapinlac, H. A., Finn, R. D., Casilla, C. et al. 1999. Tumor treatment response based on visual and quantitative changes in global tumor glycolysis using PET-FDG imaging. The visual response score and the change in total lesion glycolysis. *Clin Positron Imaging*, 2, 159–171.

Lehman, C. D., Gatsonis, C., Kuhl, C. K., Hendrick, R. E., Pisano, E. D., Hanna, L., Peacock, S. et al. 2007. MRI evaluation of the contralateral breast in women with recently diagnosed breast cancer. *N Engl J Med*, 356, 1295–1303.

Linden, H. M., Stekhova, S. A., Link, J. M., Gralow, J. R., Livingston, R. B., Ellis, G. K., Petra, P. H. et al. 2006. Quantitative fluoroestradiol positron emission tomography imaging predicts response to endocrine treatment in breast cancer. *J Clin Oncol*, 24, 2793–2799.

Lockhart, C. M., Macdonald, L. R., Alessio, A. M., Mcdougald, W. A., Doot, R. K., and Kinahan, P. E. 2011. Quantifying and reducing the effect of calibration error on variability of PET/CT standardized uptake value measurements. *J Nucl Med*, 52, 218–224.

Macdonald, D. R., Cascino, T. L., Schold, S. C., JR., and Cairncross, J. G. 1990. Response criteria for phase II studies of supratentorial malignant glioma. *J Clin Oncol*, 8, 1277–1280.

Mankoff, D. A. and Dehdashti, F. 2009. Imaging tumor phenotype: 1 plus 1 is more than 2. *J Nucl Med*, 50, 1567–1569.

Mankoff, D. A., Dunnwald, L. K., Gralow, J. R., Ellis, G. K., Charlop, A., Lawton, T. J., Schubert, E. K., Tseng, J., and Livingston, R. B. 2002. Blood flow and metabolism in locally advanced breast cancer: Relationship to response to therapy. *J Nucl Med*, 43, 500–509.

Mankoff, D. A., Eary, J. F., Link, J. M., Muzi, M., Rajendran, J. G., Spence, A. M., and Krohn, K. A. 2007a. Tumor-specific positron emission tomography imaging in patients: [18F] fluorodeoxyglucose and beyond. *Clin Cancer Res*, 13, 3460–3469.

Mankoff, D. A., Muzi, M., and Zaidi, H. 2006. Quantitative analysis in nuclear oncologic imaging. In: Zaidi, H. (ed.) *Quantitative Analysis in Nuclear Medicine Imaging*. New York: Springer.

Mankoff, D. A., O'Sullivan, F., Barlow, W. E., and Krohn, K. A. 2007b. Molecular imaging research in the outcomes era: Measuring outcomes for individualized cancer therapy. *Acad Radiol*, 14, 398–405.

McShane, L. M., Altman, D. G., Sauerbrei, W., Taube, S. E., Gion, M., and Clark, G. M. 2005. Reporting recommendations for tumor marker prognostic studies (REMARK). *J Natl Cancer Inst*, 97, 1180–1184.

Meisamy, S., Bolan, P. J., Baker, E. H., Bliss, R. L., Gulbahce, E., Everson, L. I., Nelson, M. T. et al. 2004. Neoadjuvant chemotherapy of locally advanced breast cancer: Predicting response with in vivo (1)H MR spectroscopy—A pilot study at 4 T. *Radiology*, 233, 424–431.

Mettler, F. A. Jr., Huda, W., Yoshizumi, T. T., and Mahesh, M. 2008. Effective doses in radiology and diagnostic nuclear medicine: A catalog. *Radiology*, 248, 254–263.

Meyer, C. R., Armato, S. G., Fenimore, C. P., Mclennan, G., Bidaut, L. M., Barboriak, D. P., Gavrielides, M. A. et al. 2009. Quantitative imaging to assess tumor response to therapy: Common themes of measurement, truth data, and error sources. *Transl Oncol*, 2, 198–210.

Miller, A. B., Hoogstraten, B., Staquet, M., and Winkler, A. 1981. Reporting results of cancer treatment. *Cancer*, 47, 207–214.

Mintun, M. A., Welch, M. J., Siegel, B. A., Mathias, C. J., Brodack, J. W., Mcguire, A. H., and Katzenellenbogen, J. A. 1988. Breast cancer: PET imaging of estrogen receptors. *Radiology*, 169, 45–48.

Mortimer, J. E., Dehdashti, F., Siegel, B. A., Trinkaus, K., Katzenellenbogen, J. A., and Welch, M. J. 2001. Metabolic flare: Indicator of hormone responsiveness in advanced breast cancer. *J Clin Oncol*, 19, 2797–2803.

Moskowitz, C. S., Jia, X., Schwartz, L. H., and Gonen, M. 2009. A simulation study to evaluate the impact of the number of lesions measured on response assessment. *Eur J Cancer*, 45, 300–310.

Muzi, M., Vesselle, H., Grierson, J. R., Mankoff, D. A., Schmidt, R. A., Peterson, L., Wells, J. M., and Krohn, K. A. 2005. Kinetic analysis of 3'-deoxy-3'-fluorothymidine PET studies: Validation studies in patients with lung cancer. *J Nucl Med*, 46, 274–282.

National Research Council, C. O. T. B. E. O. I. R. 1990. Health Effects of Exposure to Low Levels of Ionizing Radiation, BEIR V. Washington, DC: National Academy Press.

O'Connor, J. P., Jackson, A., Parker, G. J., and Jayson, G. C. 2007. DCE-MRI biomarkers in the clinical evaluation of antiangiogenic and vascular disrupting agents. *Br J Cancer*, 96, 189–195.

O'Sullivan, F. 2006. Locally constrained mixture representation of dynamic imaging data from PET and MR studies. *Biostatistics*, 7, 318–338.

O'Sullivan, F., Roy, S., and Eary, J. 2003. A statistical measure of tissue heterogeneity with application to 3D PET sarcoma data. *Biostatistics*, 4, 433–448.

Padhani, A. and Khan, A. 2010. Diffusion-weighted (DW) and dynamic contrast-enhanced (DCE) magnetic resonance imaging (MRI) for monitoring anticancer therapy. *Targeted Oncol*, 5, 39–52.

Peterson, L. M., Mankoff, D. A., Lawton, T., Yagle, K., Schubert, E. K., Stekhova, S., Gown, A., Link, J. M., Tewson, T., and Krohn, K. A. 2008. Quantitative imaging of estrogen receptor expression in breast cancer with PET and 18F-fluoroestradiol. *J Nucl Med*, 49, 367–374.

Pepe, M. S., Feng, Z., Janes, H., Bossuyt, P. M., and Potter, J. D. 2008. Pivotal evaluation of the accuracy of a biomarker used for classification or prediction: Standards for study design. *J Natl Cancer Inst*, 100, 1432–1438.

Ratain, M. J., Eisen, T., Stadler, W. M., Flaherty, K. T., Kaye, S. B., Rosner, G. L., Gore, M. et al. 2006. Phase II placebo-controlled randomized discontinuation trial of sorafenib in patients with metastatic renal cell carcinoma. *J Clin Oncol*, 24, 2505–2512.

Ratain, M. J. and Glassman, R. H. 2007. Biomarkers in phase I oncology trials: Signal, noise, or expensive distraction? *Clin Cancer Res*, 13, 6545–6548.

Ravdin, P. M., Green, S., Dorr, T. M., Mcguire, W. L., Fabian, C., Pugh, R. P., Carter, R. D. et al. 1992. Prognostic significance of progesterone receptor levels in estrogen receptor-positive patients with metastatic breast cancer treated with tamoxifen: Results of a prospective Southwest Oncology Group study. *J Clin Oncol*, 10, 1284–1291.

Sargent, D. J., Rubinstein, L., Schwartz, L., Dancey, J. E., Gatsonis, C., Dodd, L. E., and Shankar, L. K. 2009. Validation of novel imaging methodologies for use as cancer clinical trial end-points. *Eur J Cancer*, 45, 290–299.

Scheuermann, J. S., Saffer, J. R., Karp, J. S., Levering, A. M., and Siegel, B. A. 2009. Qualification of PET scanners for use in multicenter cancer clinical trials: The American College of Radiology Imaging Network experience. *J Nucl Med*, 50, 1187–1193.

Shankar, L. K., Hoffman, J. M., Bacharach, S., Graham, M. M., Karp, J., Lammertsma, A. A., Larson, S. et al. 2006. Consensus recommendations for the use of 18F-FDG PET as an indicator of therapeutic response in patients in National Cancer Institute Trials. *J Nucl Med*, 47, 1059–1066.

Shankar, L. K., Van den Abbeele, A., Yap, J., Benjamin, R., Scheutze, S., and Fitzgerald, T. J. 2009. Considerations for the use of imaging tools for phase II treatment trials in oncology. *Clin Cancer Res*, 15, 1891–1897.

Simon, R. 2010. Clinical trial designs for evaluating the medical utility of prognostic and predictive biomarkers in oncology. *Per Med*, 7, 33–47.

Sohn, H. J., Yang, Y. J., Ryu, J. S., Oh, S. J., Im, K. C., Moon, D. H., Lee, D. H., Suh, C., Lee, J. S., and Kim, S. W. 2008. [18F]Fluorothymidine positron emission tomography before and 7 days after gefitinib treatment predicts response in patients with advanced adenocarcinoma of the lung. *Clin Cancer Res*, 14, 7423–7429.

Specht, J. M., Kurland, B. F., Montgomery, S. K., Dunnwald, L. K., Doot, R. K., Gralow, J. R., Ellis, G. K. et al. 2010. Tumor metabolism and blood flow as assessed by positron emission tomography varies by tumor subtype in locally advanced breast cancer. *Clin Cancer Res*, 16, 2803–2810.

Spiegelhalter, D. 2011. Fear and numbers in Fukushima. *Significance*, 8(3), 100–103.

Strauss, L. G., Koczan, D., Klippel, S., Pan, L., Cheng, C., Willis, S., Haberkorn, U., and Dimitrakopoulou-Strauss, A. 2008. Impact of angiogenesis-related gene expression on the tracer kinetics of 18F-FDG in colorectal tumors. *J Nucl Med*, 49, 1238–1244.

Stroobants, S., Goeminne, J., Seegers, M., Dimitrijevic, S., Dupont, P., Nuyts, J., Martens, M. et al. 2003. 18FDG-positron emission tomography for the early prediction of response in advanced soft tissue sarcoma treated with imatinib mesylate (Glivec). *Eur J Cancer*, 39, 2012–2020.

Suman, V. J., Dueck, A., and Sargent, D. J. 2008. Clinical trials of novel and targeted therapies: Endpoints, trial design, and analysis. *Cancer Invest*, 26, 439–444.

Theilmann, R. J., Borders, R., Trouard, T. P., Xia, G., Outwater, E., Ranger-Moore, J., Gillies, R. J., and Stopeck, A. 2004. Changes in water mobility measured by diffusion MRI predict response of metastatic breast cancer to chemotherapy. *Neoplasia*, 6, 831–837.

Therasse, P., Arbuck, S. G., Eisenhauer, E. A., Wanders, J., Kaplan, R. S., Rubinstein, L., Verweij, J. et al. 2000. New guidelines to evaluate the response to treatment in solid tumors. European Organization for Research and Treatment of Cancer, National Cancer Institute of the United States, National Cancer Institute of Canada. *J Natl Cancer Inst*, 92, 205–216.

Tutt, A., Robson, M., Garber, J. E., Domchek, S. M., Audeh, M. W., Weitzel, J. N., Friedlander, M. et al. 2010. Oral poly(ADP-ribose) polymerase inhibitor olaparib in patients with BRCA1 or BRCA2 mutations and advanced breast cancer: A proof-of-concept trial. *Lancet*, 376, 235–244.

Velasquez, L. M., Boellaard, R., Kollia, G., Hayes, W., Hoekstra, O. S., Lammertsma, A. A., and Galbraith, S. M. 2009. Repeatability of 18F-FDG PET in a multicenter phase I study of patients with advanced gastrointestinal malignancies. *J Nucl Med*, 50, 1646–1654.

Vesselle, H., Grierson, J., Muzi, M., Pugsley, J. M., Schmidt, R. A., Rabinowitz, P., Peterson, L. M., Vallieres, E., and Wood, D. E. 2002. In vivo validation of 3′deoxy-3′-[(18)F]fluorothymidine ([(18)F]FLT) as a proliferation imaging tracer in humans: Correlation of [(18)F]FLT uptake by positron emission tomography with Ki-67 immunohistochemistry and flow cytometry in human lung tumors. *Clin Cancer Res*, 8, 3315–3323.

Wahl, R. L., Jacene, H., Kasamon, Y., and Lodge, M. A. 2009. From RECIST to PERCIST: Evolving considerations for PET response criteria in solid tumors. *J Nucl Med*, 50 (Suppl 1), 122S–150S.

Warburg, O. 1956. On the origin of cancer cells. *Science*, 123, 309–314.

Warner, E., Plewes, D. B., Hill, K. A., Causer, P. A., Zubovits, J. T., Jong, R. A., Cutrara, M. R. et al. 2004. Surveillance of BRCA1 and BRCA2 mutation carriers with magnetic resonance imaging, ultrasound, mammography, and clinical breast examination. *JAMA*, 292, 1317–1325.

Weber, W. A. 2006. Positron emission tomography as an imaging biomarker. *J Clin Oncol*, 24, 3282–3292.

Weber, W. A., Ziegler, S. I., Thodtmann, R., Hanauske, A. R., and Schwaiger, M. 1999. Reproducibility of metabolic measurements in malignant tumors using FDG PET. *J Nucl Med*, 40, 1771–1777.

Wen, P. Y., Macdonald, D. R., Reardon, D. A., Cloughesy, T. F., Sorensen, A. G., Galanis, E., Degroot, J. et al. 2010. Updated response assessment criteria for high-grade gliomas: Response assessment in neuro-oncology working group. *J Clin Oncol*, 28, 1963–1972.

Westerterp, M., Pruim, J., Oyen, W., Hoekstra, O., Paans, A., Visser, E., Van Lanschot, J., Sloof, G., and Boellaard, R. 2007. Quantification of FDG PET studies using standardised uptake values in multi-centre trials: Effects of image reconstruction, resolution and ROI definition parameters. *Eur J Nucl Med Mol Imaging*, 34, 392–404.

Yu, E. Y. and Mankoff, D. A. 2007. Positron emission tomography imaging as a cancer biomarker. *Expert Rev Mol Diagn*, 7, 659–726.

Zhao, B., Oxnard, G. R., Moskowitz, C. S., Kris, M. G., Pao, W., Guo, P., Rusch, V. M., Ladanyi, M., Rizvi, N. A., and Schwartz, L. H. 2010. A pilot study of volume measurement as a method of tumor response evaluation to aid biomarker development. *Clin Cancer Res*, 16, 4647–4653.

# Part IV

**Exploratory and High-Dimensional Data Analyses**

# 25 Prognostic Factor Studies

*Martin Schumacher, Norbert Holländer, Guido Schwarzer, Harald Binder, and Willi Sauerbrei*

## CONTENTS

## 25.1 INTRODUCTION

Besides investigations on etiology, epidemiology, and the evaluation of therapies, the identification and assessment of prognostic factors constitutes one of the major tasks in clinical cancer research. Studies on prognostic factors attempt to determine survival probabilities, or, more generally, a prediction of the course of the disease for groups of patients defined by the values of prognostic factors, and to rank the relative importance of various factors. In contrast to therapeutic studies, however, where statistical principles and methods are well developed and generally accepted, this is not the case for the evaluation of prognostic factors. Although some efforts toward an improvement of this situation have been undertaken (Infante-Rivard et al. 1989; McGuire 1991; Clark 1992; Simon and Altman 1994; Altman and Lyman 1998), most of the studies investigating prognostic factors are based on historical data lacking precisely defined selection criteria. Furthermore, sample sizes are often far too small to serve as a basis for reliable results. As far as the statistical analysis is concerned, a proper multivariate analysis simultaneously considering the influence of various potential prognostic factors on overall or event-free survival (EFS) of the patients is not always attempted. Missing values in some or all of the prognostic factors constitute a serious problem which is often underestimated.

In general, the evaluation of prognostic factors based on historical data has the advantage that baseline and follow-up data of patients might be readily available in a database, and that the values of new prognostic factors obtained from stored tissue or blood samples may be added retrospectively. However, such studies are particularly prone to some of the deficiencies mentioned earlier, including insufficient quality of data on prognostic factors and follow-up data and heterogeneity of the patient population due to different treatment strategies. These issues are often not considered in the publication of prognostic studies but might explain, at least to some extent, why prognostic factors are controversial and why prognostic models derived from such studies are often not accepted for practical use (Wyatt 1995).

There have been some "classic" articles on statistical aspects of prognostic factors in oncology (Armitage and Gehan 1974; Byar 1982, 1984; Simon 1984; George 1988) that describe the statistical methods and principles that should be used to analyze prognostic factor studies. However, these articles do not fully address the issue that statistical methods and principles are not adequately applied when analyzing and presenting the results of a prognostic factor study (Altman et al. 1994, 2004; Simon and Altman 1994; Wyatt and Altman 1995). We therefore aim to not only present updated statistical methodology but also point out the possible pitfalls when applying these methods to prognostic factor studies. Statistical aspects of prognostic factor studies are also discussed in the monograph on prognostic factors in cancer (Gospodarowicz et al. 2001), in some textbooks on survival analysis (Marubini and Valsecchi 2004; Machin et al. 2004; Hosmer et al. 2008) and in some recent monographs (Royston and Sauerbrei 2008b; Steyerberg 2009; Andersen and Skovgaard 2010).

Two main aims should be distinguished when creating a prognostic model (Sauerbrei et al. 2007a). The first is prediction, with little consideration of the model structure; the second is explanation, where researchers try to identify influential predictors and gain insight into the relationship between the predictors and the outcome through the model structure. In prediction, model fit and mean square prediction error are the main criteria for model adequacy. However, more often studies are done to investigate whether particular variables are prognostically important. For continuous predictors, the shape of the function is often of interest, for example, whether there is an increasing trend or a plateau at high values of the variable. In observational studies such assessments must be done in a multivariable context. Usually, many variables may be considered as potential predictors, but only a few will have a relevant effect. The task is to identify them. Often, generalizability and practical usefulness are important components of a good model and should be kept in mind when developing a model.

In order to illustrate important statistical aspects in the evaluation of prognostic factors and to examine the problems associated with such an evaluation in more detail, data from two prognostic factor studies in breast cancer shall serve as illustrative examples. Even before the results of gene expression analyses have been reported on a large-scale basis, the effects of more than 200 potential prognostic factors were controversially discussed; about 1000 papers were published in 2001. This illustrates the importance of and the unsatisfactory situation in prognostic factors research. An evidence-based approach is clearly needed. It is usually difficult to ascertain the benefit of a marker from a single published study, which may be overly optimistic owing to small sample size and selective reporting, and a clear view is only likely to emerge from examining multiple studies (Riley et al. 2009).

A substantial improvement of this situation is possible only with an improvement in the application of statistical methodology, and in better reporting single studies (comparable to the CONSORT statement [Altman et al. 2001] for randomized controlled trials) which provides a more suitable basis for a systematic review of studies for a specific marker of interest. An international working group has developed the REMARK reporting recommendations for prognostic studies (McShane et al. 2005).

As exploratory analyses play an important role, several analyses are usually conducted, only some of which have been completely reported, with the results of others mentioned only briefly in the text (and easily overlooked) or not reported at all. Therefore, a two-part REMARK profile was proposed whose first part gives details about how the marker of interest was handled in the analysis and which further variables were available for multivariable modeling (Mallett et al. 2010). In the second part of the REMARK profile, an overview of all analyses conducted is given. Severe weaknesses of reporting methods and results of prognostic factor studies have been well known (Altman 2001; Riley et al. 2003, 2009; Mallett et al. 2010). To improve future research in prognostic factors several recommendations are given in these papers; however, none of them focuses on statistical aspects of single studies.

Throughout this chapter we assume that the reader is familiar with standard statistical methods for survival data to the extent as is presented in more practically oriented textbooks (Harris and Albert 1991; Therneau and Grambsch 2000; Collett 2003; Lee and Wang 2003; Marubini 2004; Machin et al. 2006; Hosmer et al. 2008). For a deeper understanding of those methods, we refer to the more theoretically oriented textbooks on survival analysis and counting processes (Andersen et al. 1993; Kalbfleisch and Prentice 2002; Fleming and Harrington 2005). As compared with the previous editions of the handbook, this chapter contains new sections on treatment–covariate interactions and on regularized estimation in the presence of high-dimensional predictors. References on reporting standards and on new developments have been updated where needed.

## 25.2 "DESIGN" OF PROGNOSTIC FACTOR STUDIES

The American Joint Committee on Cancer (AJCC) has established three major criteria for prognostic factors. Factors must be significant, independent, and clinically important (Burke and Henson 1993). According to Gospodarowicz et al. (2001), significance implies that the prognostic factor rarely occurs by chance; independent means that the prognostic factor retains its prognostic value despite the addition of other prognostic factors; and clinically important implies clinical relevance, such as being capable (at least in principle) of influencing patient management and thus outcome.

From these criteria, it is apparent that statistical aspects will play an important role in the investigation of prognostic factors (Fielding et al. 1992; Henson 1992; Fielding and Henson 1993; Gospodarowicz et al. 2001). That is also emphasized by Simon and Altman (1994) who give a concise and thoughtful review of statistical aspects of prognostic factor studies in oncology. Recognizing that these will be observational studies, the authors argue that they should be carried out in a way that the same careful design standards are adopted as are used in clinical trials, except for randomization. For confirmatory studies that may be seen comparable to phase III studies in therapeutic research, they listed 11 important requirements that are given in a somewhat shortened version in Table 25.1. From these requirements, it can be deduced that prognostic factors should be investigated in carefully planned, prospective studies with sufficient numbers of patients and sufficiently long follow-up to observe the endpoint of interest (typically event-free or overall survival). Thus, a prospective observational study, where treatment is standardized and everything is planned in advance, emerges as the most desirable study design. A slightly different

---

**TABLE 25.1**

**Requirements for Confirmatory Prognostic Factor Studies according to Simon and Altman (1994)**

1. Documentation of intra- and inter-laboratory reproducibility of assays
2. Blinded conduct of laboratory assays
3. Definition and description of a clear inception cohort
4. Standardization or randomization of treatment
5. Detailed statement of hypotheses (in advance)
6. Justification of sample size based on power calculations
7. Analysis of additional prognostic value beyond standard prognostic factors
8. Adjustment of analyses for multiple testing
9. Avoidance of outcome-oriented cut-off values
10. Reporting of confidence intervals for effect estimates
11. Demonstration of subset-specific treatment effects by an appropriate statistical test

---

design is represented by a randomized controlled clinical trial where in addition to some therapeutic modalities various prognostic factors are investigated. It is important in such a setting that the prognostic factors of interest are measured either in all patients enrolled into the clinical trial or in those patients belonging to a predefined subset. Both designs, however, usually require enormous resources and a long time until results will be available. Thus, a third type of "design" is used in the vast majority of prognostic factor studies, which can be termed a "retrospectively defined historical cohort," where stored tumor tissue or blood samples are available and baseline as well as follow-up data of the patients is already documented in a database. To meet the requirements listed in Table 25.1 in such a situation, it is clear that inclusion and exclusion criteria have to be carefully applied. In particular, treatment has to be given in a standardized manner, at least to some sufficient extent. Otherwise, patients for whom these requirements are not fulfilled have to be excluded from the study. If the requirements are followed in a consistent manner, this will usually lead to a drastic reduction in the number of patients eligible for the study compared to the number of patients available in the original database. In addition, follow-up data are often not of sufficient quality as should be the case in a well-conducted clinical trial or prospective study. Thus, if this "design" is applied, special care is necessary in order to arrive at correct and reproducible results regarding the role of potential prognostic factors.

The types of designs described earlier will also be illustrated in the prognostic studies in breast cancer that we will use as examples and that will be dealt with in more detail in the next section. It is interesting to note that other types of designs, for example, nested case-control studies, case-cohort studies, or other study types often used in epidemiology (Rothman et al. 2008), have only rarely been used for the investigation of prognostic factors. Their role and potential use for prognostic factor research has not yet been fully explored. There is one situation where the randomized controlled clinical trial should be the design type of choice: the investigation of so-called predictive factors that indicate whether a specific treatment works in a particular subgroup of patients defined by the predictive factor but not in another subgroup of patients, where it may be harmful. Since this is clearly an investigation of treatment–covariate interactions, it should ideally be performed in the setting of a large-scaled randomized trial where information on the potential predictive factor is recorded and analyzed by means of appropriate statistical methods (Simon 1982; Byar 1985; Gail and Simon 1985; Schmoor et al. 1993; Royston and Sauerbrei 2004a).

## 25.3  EXAMPLES: PROGNOSTIC STUDIES IN BREAST CANCER

### 25.3.1  Freiburg DNA Study

The first study is based on an observational database consisting of data of all patients with primary, previously untreated node positive breast cancer who received surgery between 1982 and 1987 in the Department of Gynecology at the University of Freiburg and whose tumor material was available for DNA investigations. Some exclusion criteria were defined retrospectively, including history of malignoma, $T_4$ and/or $M_1$ tumors according to the TNM classification system of the Union for International Cancer Control (UICC) (Gospodarowicz et al. 2001), without adjuvant therapy after primary surgery, and older than 80 years. This excluded 139 patients of 218 originally investigated for the analysis. This study will be referred to as the Freiburg DNA study in the sequel.

Eight patient characteristics were investigated. In addition to age, the number of positive lymph nodes and the size of the primary tumor, the grading score according to Bloom and Richardson (1957), and estrogen and progesterone receptor status were recorded. DNA flow cytometry was used to measure ploidy status of the tumor using a cutpoint of 1.1 for the DNA index and S-phase fraction (SPF), which is the percentage of tumor cells in the DNA synthesizing phase obtained by cell cycle analysis. The distribution of these characteristics in the patient population is displayed in Table 25.2.

The median follow-up was 83 months. At the time of analysis, 76 events were observed for EFS, which was defined as the time from surgery to the first of the

---

**TABLE 25.2**

**Patient Characteristics in the Freiburg DNA Breast Cancer Study**

| Factor | Category | n | (%) |
|---|---|---|---|
| Age | ≤50 years | 52 | (37) |
|  | >50 years | 87 | (63) |
| No. of positive lymph nodes | 1–3 | 66 | (48) |
|  | 4–9 | 42 | (30) |
|  | ≥10 | 31 | (22) |
| Tumor size | ≤2 cm | 25 | (19) |
|  | 2–5 cm | 73 | (54) |
|  | >5 cm | 36 | (27) |
|  | Missing | 5 |  |
| Tumor grade | 1 | 3 | (2) |
|  | 2 | 81 | (59) |
|  | 3 | 54 | (39) |
|  | Missing | 1 |  |
| Estrogen receptor | ≤20 fmol | 32 | (24) |
|  | >20 fmol | 99 | (76) |
|  | Missing | 8 |  |
| Progesterone receptor | ≤20 fmol | 34 | (26) |
|  | >20 fmol | 98 | (74) |
|  | Missing | 7 |  |
| Ploidy status | Diploid | 61 | (44) |
|  | Aneuploid | 78 | (56) |
| S-phase fraction | <3.1 | 27 | (25) |
|  | 3.1–8.4 | 55 | (50) |
|  | >8.4 | 27 | (25) |
|  | Missing | 30 |  |

*Source:* Pfisterer, J. et al. *Anal. Quant. Cytol. Histol.*, 17, 406, 1995.

following events: occurrence of locoregional recurrence, distant metastasis, second malignancy, or death. EFS was estimated as 50% at 5 years. Further details of the study can be found in the work of Pfisterer et al. (1995).

## 25.3.2  GBSG-2-Study

The second study is a prospective controlled clinical trial on the treatment of node positive breast cancer patients conducted by the German Breast Cancer Study Group (GBSG) (Schumacher et al. 1994); this study will be referred to as the GBSG-2-study in the sequel.

The principal eligibility criterion was a histologically verified primary breast cancer of stage T1a-3aN+M0, that is, positive regional lymph nodes but no distant metastases. Primary local treatment was by a modified radical mastectomy (Patey) with en bloc axillary dissection with at least six identifiable lymph nodes. Patients were not older than 65 years of age and presented with a Karnofsky index of at least 60. The study was designed as a comprehensive cohort study (Schmoor et al. 1996). That is, randomized as well as nonrandomized patients who fulfilled the entry criteria were included and followed according to the study procedures.

The study had a $2 \times 2$ factorial design with four adjuvant treatment arms: three versus six cycles of chemotherapy with and without hormonal treatment. Prognostic factors evaluated in the trial include patient's age, menopausal status, tumor size, estrogen and progesterone receptors, tumor grading according to Bloom and Richardson (1957), histological tumor type, and the number of involved lymph nodes. Histopathologic classification was reexamined, and grading was performed centrally by one reference pathologist for all cases. EFS was defined as time from mastectomy to the first occurrence of either locoregional or distant recurrence, contralateral tumor, secondary tumor, or death.

During 6 years 720 patients were recruited, of whom about two-thirds gave consent to randomization. Complete data on the seven standard prognostic factors as given in Table 25.3 were available for 686 (95.3%) patients, who were taken as the basic patient population for this study. After a median follow-up time of nearly 5 years, 299 events for EFS and 171 deaths were observed. EFS was about 50% at 5 years. Data of the GBSG-2-study are available from http://www.imbi.uni-freiburg. de/biom/Royston-Sauerbrei-book/.

## 25.4  CUTPOINT MODEL

In prognostic factor studies, values of the factors considered are often categorized in two or three categories. This may be done according to medical or biological reasons or may just reflect some consensus in the scientific community. When a "new" prognostic factor is investigated, the choice of such a categorization represented by one or more cutpoints is by no means obvious. Thus, often an attempt is made to derive such cutpoints from the data and to take those cutpoints that give the best separation in the data at hand. In the Freiburg DNA breast cancer study we consider SPF as a "new" prognostic factor, which it indeed was some years ago (Altman et al. 1994). For simplicity, we restrict ourselves to the problem of selecting only one cutpoint

**TABLE 25.3**

**Patient Characteristics in GBSG-2-Study**

| Factor | Category | n | (%) |
|---|---|---|---|
| Age | ≤45 years | 153 | (22) |
| | 46–60 years | 345 | (50) |
| | >60 years | 188 | (27) |
| Menopausal status | Pre | 290 | (42) |
| | Post | 396 | (58) |
| Tumor size | ≤20 mm | 180 | (26) |
| | 21–30 mm | 287 | (42) |
| | >30 mm | 219 | (32) |
| Tumor grade | 1 | 81 | (12) |
| | 2 | 444 | (65) |
| | 3 | 161 | (24) |
| No. of positive lymph nodes | 1–3 | 376 | (55) |
| | 4–9 | 207 | (30) |
| | ≥10 | 103 | (15) |
| Progesterone receptor | <20 fmol | 269 | (39) |
| | ≥20 fmol | 417 | (61) |
| Estrogen receptor | <20 fmol | 262 | (38) |
| | ≥20 fmol | 424 | (62) |

*Source:* Schumacher M. et al., for the German Breast Cancer Study Group, *J. Clin. Oncol.*, 12, 2086, 1994.

based on a univariate analysis. Let Z denote the covariate of interest, in the Freiburg DNA breast cancer data the SPF, as a potential prognostic factor. If this covariate has been measured on a quantitative scale, the proportional hazards (Cox 1972) cutpoint model is defined as

$$\lambda(t \mid Z > \mu) = \exp(\beta)\lambda(t \mid Z \leq \mu), t > 0$$

where $\lambda(t \mid \cdot) = \lim_{h \to 0}(1/h)\Pr(t \leq T < t + h \mid T \geq t, \cdot)$ denotes the hazard function of the EFS time random variable T. The parameter $\theta = \exp(\beta)$ is referred to as the hazard ratio of observations with $Z > \mu$ with respect to observations with $Z \leq \mu$ and is estimated by $\hat{\theta} = \exp(\hat{\beta})$ by maximizing the corresponding partial likelihood (Cox 1972) with given cutpoint $\mu$. The fact that $\mu$ is usually unknown makes this a problem of model selection where the cutpoint $\mu$ also has to be estimated from the data. A popular approach for this type of data-dependent categorization is the minimum p-value method where, within a certain range of the distribution of Z called the selection interval, the cutpoint $\hat{\mu}$ is chosen such that the p-value for the comparison of observations below and above the cutpoint is a minimum. Applying this method to SPF in the Freiburg DNA breast cancer

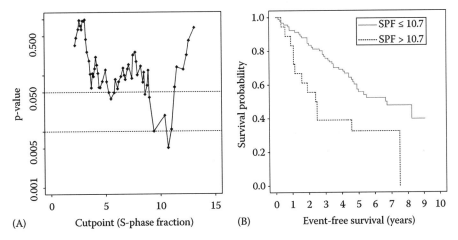

**FIGURE 25.1**   p-Values of the logrank test as a function of all possible cutpoints for S-phase fraction (A) and Kaplan–Meier estimates of event-free survival probabilities by S-phase fraction (B) in the Freiburg DNA study.

data we obtain, based on the logrank test, a cutpoint of $\hat{\mu} = 10.7$ and a minimum p-value of $p_{min} = 0.007$ when using the range between the 10% and 90% quantile of distribution of Z as the selection interval. Figure 25.1A shows the resulting p-values as a function of the possible cutpoints considered; Figure 25.1B displays the Kaplan–Meier estimates of the EFS functions of the groups defined by the estimated cutpoint $\hat{\mu} = 10.7$. The difference in EFS looks rather impressive and the estimated hazard ratio with respect to the dichotomized covariate $I(Z > \hat{\mu})$ using the "optimal" cutpoint $\hat{\mu} = 10.7$, $\hat{\theta} = 2.37$, is quite large; the corresponding 95% confidence interval is [1.27; 4.44].

Simulating the null hypothesis of no prognostic relevance of SPF with respect to EFS ($\beta = 0$), we illustrate that the minimum p-value method may lead to a drastic overestimation of the absolute value of the log-hazard ratio (Schumacher et al. 1996a). By a random allocation of the observed values of SPF to the observed survival times, we simulate independence of these two variables, which is equivalent to the null hypothesis $\beta = 0$. This procedure was repeated a 100 times and in each repetition we selected a cutpoint by using the minimum p-value method, which is often also referred to as an "optimal" cutpoint. In the 100 repetitions, we obtained 44 significant ($p_{min} < 0.05$) results for the logrank test corresponding well to theoretical results outlined in Lausen and Schumacher (1992).

The estimated "optimal" cutpoints of the 100 repetitions and the corresponding estimates of the log-hazard ratio are shown in Figure 25.2A. We obtained no estimates near the null hypothesis $\beta = 0$ as a result of the optimization process of the minimum p-value approach. Due to the well-known problems resulting from multiple testing, it is obvious that the minimum p-value method cannot lead to correct results of the logrank test. However, this problem can be solved by using a corrected p-value $p_{cor}$ as proposed in Lausen and Schumacher (1992), developed by taking the minimization process into account. The formula reads

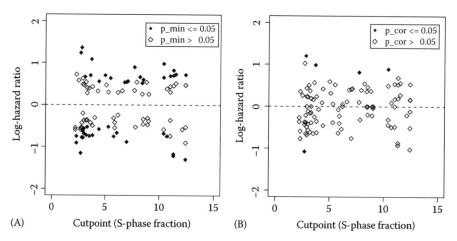

**FIGURE 25.2**   Estimates of cutpoints and log-hazard ratio in 100 repetitions of randomly allocated observed SPF values to event-free survival times in the Freiburg DNA study before (A) and after (B) correction.

$$p_{cor} = \varphi(u)\left[u - \frac{1}{u}\right]\log\left[\frac{(1-\varepsilon)^2}{\varepsilon^2}\right] + 4\frac{\varphi(u)}{u}$$

where

$\varphi$ denotes the probability density function

u is the $(1 - p_{min}/2)$ quantile of the standard normal distribution

The selection interval is characterized by the proportion $\varepsilon$ of smallest and largest values of Z that are not considered as potential cutpoints. It should be mentioned that other approaches of correcting the minimum p-value could be applied; a comparison of three approaches can be found in a paper by Hilsenbeck and Clark (1996). In particular, if there are only a few cutpoints, an improved Bonferroni inequality can be applied (Worsley 1982; Lausen et al. 1994; Lausen and Schumacher 1996) or the p-value correction can be derived from the exact distribution of the maximally selected logrank test (Hothorn et al. 2003). Using the correction formula given previously in the 100 repetitions of our simulation experiment, we obtained five significant results ($p_{cor} < 0.05$) corresponding to the significance level of $\alpha = 0.05$. Four significant results were obtained with the usual p-value when using the median of the empirical distribution of SPF in the original data as a fixed cutpoint in all repetitions.

In order to correct for overestimation, it has been proposed (Verweij and Van Houwelingen 1993) to shrink the parameter estimates by a shrinkage factor c. Considering the cutpoint model, the log-hazard ratio should then be estimated by

$$\hat{\beta}_{cor} = \hat{c} \cdot \hat{\beta}$$

where

$\hat{\beta}$ is based on the minimum p-value method

$\hat{c}$ is the estimated shrinkage factor

Values of $\hat{c}$ close to 1 indicate a minor degree of overestimation whereas small values of $\hat{c}$ reflect a substantial overestimation of the log-hazard ratio. Obviously, with maximum partial likelihood estimation of c in a model

$$\lambda\left(t \mid SPF > \mu\right) = \exp(c\hat{\beta}\,)\lambda\left(t \mid SPF \leq \mu\right)$$

using the original data we get $\hat{c}=1$ since $\hat{\beta}$ is the maximum partial likelihood estimate. Schumacher et al. (1997) compared several methods to estimate $\hat{c}$. In Figure 25.2B, the results of the correction process in the 100 simulated studies are displayed when a heuristic estimate $\hat{c}=(\hat{\beta}^2 - var(\hat{\beta}))/\hat{\beta}^2$ was applied where $\hat{\beta}$ and $var(\hat{\beta})$ are resulting from the minimum p-value method (Van Houwelingen and Le Cessie 1990). This heuristic estimate performed quite well when compared to more elaborated cross-validation and resampling approaches (Schumacher et al. 1997).

In general, minimum p-value method leads to a dramatic inflation of the type I error rate. The chance of declaring a quantitative factor as prognostically relevant when in fact it does not have any influence on EFS is about 50% when a level of 5% has been intended. Thus, correction of p-values is essential but leaves the problem of overestimation of the hazard ratio in absolute terms. The latter problem, which is especially relevant when sample sizes and/or effect sizes are small to moderate, could at least partially be solved by applying some shrinkage method. In the Freiburg DNA breast cancer data, we obtain a corrected p-value of $p_{cor}=0.123$ that provides no clear indication that S-phase is of prognostic relevance for node-positive breast cancer patients. The correction of the hazard ratio estimate leads to a value of $\hat{\theta}_{cor}=2.1$ for the heuristic method and to $\hat{\theta}_{cor}=2$ for the cross-validation and bootstrap approaches. Unfortunately, confidence intervals are not straight forward to obtain; bootstrapping the whole model building process including the estimation of a shrinkage factor would be one possibility (Holländer et al. 2004).

In the 100 repetitions of our simulation experiment, 39 confidence intervals calculated from the model after cutpoint selection did not contain the value $\beta=0$ (Figure 25.3A), corresponding to the number of significant results according to the minimum p-value. Although shrinkage is capable of correcting for overestimation of the log-hazard ratio (Figure 25.2B), confidence intervals calculated with the estimated model-based standard error do not obtain the desired coverage. In our simulation, there are still 17 out of 100 intervals that do not contain the value $\beta=0$ (Figure 25.3B). Using the shrunken risk estimate $\hat{c}\hat{\beta}$ and its empirical variance calculated from 100 bootstrap samples in each repetition of the simulation experiment instead leads to the correct coverage; only five repetitions do not contain $\beta=0$. This agrees with the p-value correction and corresponds to the significance level of $\beta=0.05$. It should be noted, however, that the optimal cutpoint approach still has disadvantages. One of these is that different studies will most likely yield different cutpoints, making comparisons across studies extremely difficult or even impossible.

Altman et al. (1994) point out this problem for studies of the prognostic relevance of SPF in the breast cancer literature; they identified 19 different cutpoints, some of them motivated only as the "optimal" cutpoint in a specific dataset. Although dichotomization has advantages such as simplifying an analysis, Royston et al. (2006) argue strongly against dichotomization as it may create rather than avoid problems,

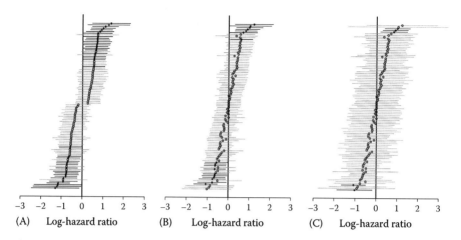

-3  -2  -1   0   1   2   3        -3  -2  -1   0   1   2   3        -3  -2  -1   0   1   2   3
(A)    Log-hazard ratio         (B)    Log-hazard ratio         (C)    Log-hazard ratio

**FIGURE 25.3**  Ninety-five percent confidence intervals for the log-hazard ratio of the S-phase fraction in 100 repetitions of randomly re-allocated S-phase values to the observed survival time: estimate based on "optimal" cutpoints, naïve model-based variance (A); shrunk estimate, naïve model-based variance (B); and shrunk estimate, empirical variance from 100 bootstrap samples (C). Confidence intervals not including $\beta=0$ are marked with filled circles, and the samples are ordered according to the values of $\hat{\beta}$ from smallest to largest.

notably a considerable loss of power, residual confounding, and a serious bias if a data derived "optimal" cutpoint is used. Thus, other approaches, such as regression modeling, might be preferred. Taking, for example, S-phase as a continuous covariate in a Cox regression model, with baseline hazard function $\lambda_0(t)$:

$$\lambda(t \mid Z) = \lambda_0(t)\exp(\tilde{\beta}Z)$$

yields a p-value of $p=0.061$ for testing the null hypothesis $\tilde{\beta}=0$.

## 25.5  REGRESSION MODELING AND RELATED ASPECTS

The Cox proportional hazards regression model (Cox 1972; Andersen 1991) is the standard statistical tool to simultaneously analyze multiple prognostic factors. If we denote the prognostic factors under consideration by $Z_1, Z_2, \ldots, Z_k$ then the model is given by

$$\lambda(t \mid Z_1, Z_2 \ldots, Z_k) = \lambda_0(t)\exp(\beta_1 Z_1 + \beta_2 Z_2 + \cdots + \beta_k Z_k)$$

where

   $\lambda(t|\cdot)$ denotes the hazard function of the event-free or overall survival time random variable t

   $\lambda_0(t)$ is the unspecified baseline hazard

The estimated log-hazard ratios $\hat{\beta}_j$ can then be interpreted as estimated "effects" of the factors $Z_j(j=1, \ldots, k)$. If $Z_j$ is measured on a quantitative scale, then $\exp(\hat{\beta}_j)$

represents the increase or decrease in risk if $Z_j$ is increased by one unit; if $Z_j$ is a binary covariate, then $\exp(\hat{\beta}_j)$ is simply the hazard ratio of category 1 to the reference category ($Z_j = 0$), which is assumed to be constant over the time range considered. It has to be noted that the "final" multivariate regression model is often the result of a more or less extensive model building process which may involve the categorization and/or transformation of covariates as well as the selection of variables in an automatic or a subjective manner. This model building process should in principle be taken into account when judging the results of a prognostic study; in practice, it is often neglected. We will come back to this problem at several occasions later, especially in Sections 25.7 and 25.8.

We will demonstrate various approaches with the data of the GBSG-2-study. The factors listed in Table 25.3 are investigated with regard to their prognostic relevance. Since all patients received adjuvant chemotherapy in a standardized manner and there appeared to be no difference between three and six cycles (Schumacher et al. 1994), chemotherapy is not considered any further. Because of the patients' preference in the nonrandomized part and because of a change in the study protocol concerning premenopausal patients, only about a third of the patients received hormonal treatment. Age and menopausal status had a strong influence on whether this therapy was administered. Since hormonal treatment was not of primary interest, all analyses were stratified by it. That is, the baseline hazard was allowed to vary between the two groups defined by hormonal treatment.

### 25.5.1   ASSUMING A LOG-LINEAR RELATIONSHIP FOR CONTINUOUS COVARIATES

In a first attempt, all quantitative factors are included as continuous covariates. Age is taken in years, tumor size in mm, lymph nodes as the number of involved nodes, and progesterone and estrogen receptors in fmol/mL. Menopausal status is a binary covariate coded "0" for premenopausal and "1" for postmenopausal. Grade is considered as a quantitative covariate in this approach, that is, the risk between grade categories 1 and 2 is the same as between grade categories 2 and 3. The results of this Cox regression model are given in Table 25.4 in terms of estimated hazard ratios and p-values of the corresponding Wald tests under the heading "Full model." In a publication, this should at least be accompanied by confidence intervals for the hazard ratios that we have omitted here for brevity. From this full model, it can be seen that tumor size, tumor grade, the number of positive lymph nodes, and the progesterone receptor have a significant impact on EFS, when a significance level of 5% is used. Age, menopausal status, and the estrogen receptor do not exhibit prognostic relevance.

A key issue is the choice between a full, a prespecified, or a selected model. As a theoretical construct, the full model avoids several complications and biases introduced by model building. In practice, the full model would require prespecification of all aspects of the model. This is possible when analyzing a randomized trial; in an observational study, however, prespecifying all aspects of a full model is unrealistic (Sauerbrei et al. 2007a; Royston and Sauerbrei 2008). The gain of removing bias by avoiding data-dependent model building is offset by the high cost of ignoring models which may fit the data much better than the prespecified one. Also, what needs

**TABLE 25.4**

**Estimated Hazard Ratio (HR) and Corresponding p-Value in the Cox Regression Models for the GBSG-2-Study; Quantitative Prognostic Factors Are Taken as Continuous Covariates Assuming a Log-Linear Relationship**

| | Full Model | | BE (0.157) | | BE (0.05) | | BE (0.01) | |
|---|---|---|---|---|---|---|---|---|
| Factor | HR | p-Value | HR | p-Value | HR | p-Value | HR | p-Value |
| Age | 0.991 | 0.31 | — | — | — | — | — | — |
| Menopausal status | 1.310 | 0.14 | — | — | — | — | — | — |
| Tumor size | 1.008 | 0.049 | 1.007 | 0.061 | — | — | — | — |
| Tumor grade | 1.321 | 0.009 | 1.325 | 0.008 | 1.340 | 0.006 | 1.340 | 0.006 |
| Lymph nodes | 1.051 | <0.001 | 1.051 | <0.001 | 1.057 | <0.001 | 1.057 | <0.001 |
| Progesterone receptor | 0.998 | <0.001 | 0.998 | <0.001 | 0.998 | <0.001 | 0.998 | <0.001 |
| Estrogen receptor | 1.000 | 0.67 | — | — | — | — | — | — |
| AIC = −2logL + 2p | 3120.18 | | 3116.59 | | 3117.93 | | 3117.93 | |
| BIC = −2logL + log(ñ)p | 3146.09 | | 3131.39 | | 3129.03 | | 3129.03 | |

p denotes the number of covariates in the model and ñ denotes effective sample size, ñ = 299.

to be done if assumptions of the prespecified model are violated, for example, the assumed log-linear relationship for quantitative factors may be in sharp contrast to the real situation. Another disadvantage is that irrelevant factors are included that will not be needed in subsequent steps, for example, in the formation of risk groups defined by the prognostic factors. In addition, correlation between various factors may lead to undesirable statistical properties of the estimated regression coefficients, such as inflation of standard errors or problems of instability caused by multicollinearity. That is less critical if the aim is to derive a prediction model; however, for explanatory models it is desirable to arrive at a simple and parsimonious final model that contains only those prognostic factors that strongly affect EFS (Sauerbrei 1999; Sauerbrei et al. 2007a; Royston and Sauerbrei 2008). The other three columns of Table 25.4 contain the results of the Cox regression models obtained after backward elimination (BE) for three different selection levels (Miller 1990). A single factor BE with selection level 15.7% (BE(0.157)) corresponds asymptotically to the well-known Akaike information criterion (AIC), whereas selection levels of 5% or even 1% lead to a more stringent selection of factors (Teräsvirta and Mellin 1986). In general, BE can be recommended because of several advantages compared to other stepwise variable selection procedures (Mantel 1970; Sauerbrei 1993; Sauerbrei 1999; Royston and Sauerbrei 2008).

In the GBSG-2-study, tumor grade, lymph nodes, and progesterone receptor are selected for all three selection levels considered; when using 15.7% as the selection level, tumor size is included in addition. The AIC or the Bayesian information criterion (BIC) (Schwarz 1978), which depends on sample size and puts more penalty on each covariate in the selected model than the AIC, may be used for model assessment. Then, the smallest value of AIC or BIC corresponds to the best model.

For the two different selected models, the values of AIC and BIC and their order are similar, and at least for AIC the full model seems to be only slightly worse. Thus, the results of the full model and the three BE procedures do not differ too much for these data. However, this should not be expected in general. One reason might be that there is a relatively clear-cut difference between the three strong factors (and perhaps tumor size) and the others that show only a negligible influence on EFS in this study.

## 25.5.2 CATEGORIZING CONTINUOUS COVARIATES

The previous approach implicitly assumes that the influence of a prognostic factor on the hazard function follows a log-linear relationship. By taking lymph nodes as the covariate Z, for example, this means that the risk is increased by the factor $exp(\hat{\beta})$ if the number of positive lymph nodes is increased from m to m + 1 for m = 1,2 and so on. This could be a questionable assumption at least for large numbers of positive lymph nodes. For other factors even monotonicity of the log-hazard ratio may be violated which could result in overlooking an important prognostic factor. Because of this uncertainty, the prognostic factors under consideration are often categorized and replaced by dummy variables for the different categories.

In a second analysis of the GBSG-2-study, the categorizations in Table 25.3 are used, which were prespecified in accordance with the literature (Schumacher et al. 1994). For those factors with three categories, two binary dummy variables were defined contrasting the corresponding category with the reference category chosen as that with the lowest values. So, for example, lymph nodes were categorized into 1–3, 4–9, and ≥10 positive nodes; 1–3 positive nodes serve as the reference category. Table 25.5 displays the results of the Cox regression model for the categorized covariates, where again, the results of the full model are supplemented by those obtained after BE with three selection levels. Elimination of only one dummy variable corresponding to a factor with three categories corresponds to an amalgamation of categories (Byar 1984). In these analyses, tumor grade, lymph nodes, and progesterone receptor again show the strongest effects. Age and menopausal status are marginally significant and are included in the BE(0.157) model. For age, there is some indication that linearity or even monotonicity of the log-hazard ratio may be violated. Grade categories 2 and 3 do not seem well separated as is suggested by the previous approaches presented in Table 25.4, where grade was treated as a continuous covariate; compared to grade 1, the latter one would lead to estimated hazard ratios of 1.321 and $1.745 = (1.321)^2$ for grades 2 and 3, respectively, in contrast to values of 1.723 and 1.746 when using dummy variables. The use of dummy variables with the coding used here may also be the reason that grade is no longer included by BE with a selection level of 1%. In Table 25.5 we have given the p-values of the Wald tests for the two dummy variables separately; alternatively, we could also test the two-dimensional vector of corresponding regression coefficients to be zero.

**TABLE 25.5**

**Estimated Hazard Ratio and Corresponding p-Values in the Cox Regression Models for the GBSG-2-Study; Prognostic Factors Are Categorized as in Table 25.3**

| Factor | | Full Model HR | p-Value | BE (0.157) HR | p-Value | BE (0.05) HR | p-Value | BE (0.01) HR | p-Value |
|---|---|---|---|---|---|---|---|---|---|
| Age | ≤45 | 1 | — | 1 | — | — | — | — | — |
| | 45–60 | 0.672 | 0.026 | 0.679 | 0.030 | — | — | — | — |
| | 60 | 0.687 | 0.103 | 0.692 | 0.108 | — | — | — | — |
| Menopausal | Pre | 1 | — | 1 | — | — | — | — | — |
| status | Post | 1.307 | 0.120 | 1.304 | 0.120 | — | — | — | — |
| Tumor size | ≤20 | 1 | — | — | — | — | — | — | — |
| | 21–30 | 1.240 | 0.165 | — | — | — | — | — | — |
| | >30 | 1.316 | 0.089 | — | — | — | — | — | — |
| Tumor grade | 1 | 1 | — | 1 | — | 1 | — | — | — |
| | 2 | 1.723 | 0.031 | 1.718 | 0.032 | 1.709 | 0.033 | — | — |
| | 3 | 1.746 | 0.045 | 1.783 | 0.036 | 1.778 | 0.037 | — | — |
| Lymph nodes | 1–3 | 1 | — | 1 | — | 1 | — | 1 | — |
| | 4–9 | 1.976 | <0.001 | 2.029 | <0.001 | 2.071 | <0.001 | 2.110 | <0.001 |
| | ≥10 | 3.512 | <0.001 | 3.687 | <0.001 | 3.661 | <0.001 | 3.741 | <0.001 |
| Progesterone | <20 | 1 | — | 1 | — | 1 | — | 1 | — |
| receptor | ≥20 | 0.545 | <0.001 | 0.545 | <0.001 | 0.536 | <0.001 | 0.494 | <0.001 |
| Estrogen | <20 | 1 | — | — | — | — | — | — | — |
| receptor | ≥20 | 0.994 | 0.97 | — | — | — | — | — | — |
| AIC =−2logL + 2p | | 3087.24 | | 3084.49 | | 3083.58 | | 3085.05 | |
| BIC =−2logL + log(ñ)p | | 3128.05 | | 3114.09 | | 3102.09 | | 3096.15 | |

p denotes the number of covariates in the model and ñ denotes effective sample size, ñ = 299.

In any case, this needs two degrees of freedom whereas when treating grade as a quantitative covariate one degree of freedom would be sufficient. The data of the GBSG-2-study suggest that grade categories 2 and 3 could be amalgamated into one category (grade 2–3); this would lead to an estimated hazard ratio of 1.728 and a corresponding p-value of 0.019. Investigating goodness of fit in terms of AIC and BIC, BE leads to an improvement but differences are rather small. For a more detailed discussion on model building with categorical predictors, see Royston and Sauerbrei (2008).

### 25.5.3 DETERMINING FUNCTIONAL RELATIONSHIPS FOR CONTINUOUS COVARIATES

The results of the two approaches presented in Tables 25.4 and 25.5 show that model building within the framework of a prognostic study has to find a compromise between sufficient flexibility with regard to the functional shape of the underlying log-hazard ratio functions and simplicity of the derived model to avoid problems with serious overfitting and instability. From this point of view, the first approach assuming all relationships to be log-linear may be not flexible enough and may not capture important features of the relationship between various prognostic factors and EFS. On the other hand, the categorization used in the second approach can always be criticized because of some degree of arbitrariness and subjectivity concerning the number of categories and the specific cutpoints chosen. In addition, it will not fully exploit the information available and will be associated with some loss in efficiency. For a more flexible modeling of the functional relationship, a larger number of cutpoints and corresponding dummy variables would be needed. We will therefore sketch a third approach that will provide more flexibility while preserving simplicity of the final model to an acceptable degree.

The method was originally developed by Royston and Altman (1994) and is termed the "fractional polynomial (FP)" approach. For a quantitative covariate Z, it uses functions $\beta_0 + \beta_1 Z^p + \beta_2 Z^q$ to model the log-hazard ratio; the powers p and q are taken from the set $\{-2, -1, -0.5, 0, 0.5, 1, 2, 3\}$ and $Z^0$ is defined as log Z. For practical purposes, the use of two terms is sufficient and the resulting function is termed a FP of degree 2. This simple extension of ordinary polynomials generates a considerable range of curve shapes while still preserving simplicity when compared to smoothing splines or other nonparametric techniques, for example. Furthermore, Holländer and Schumacher (2006) showed in a simulation study that the data driven selection process, which is used to select the best FP, maintains the type I error rate, and generally ends up with a log-linear relationship if it is present. This is in contrast to the optimal cutpoint selection procedure outlined in Section 25.4.

Sauerbrei et al. (1999) have extended the FP approach, proposing a model building strategy consisting of FP-transformations and selection of variables by BE called the multivariable FP (MFP) approach. Omitting details of this model building process, which are reported elsewhere (Sauerbrei et al. 1999; Royston and Sauerbrei 2008b), we have summarized the results in Table 25.6. For age, the powers −2 and −0.5 have been estimated and provide significant contributions to the log-hazard ratio as a function of Z. This function is displayed in Figure 25.4A in comparison with the corresponding functions derived from the two other approaches. It provides further indication that there is a nonmonotonic relationship that would be overlooked by the log-linear approach. Grade categories 2 and 3 have been amalgamated as has been pointed out previously. A further restriction has been incorporated for lymph nodes by assuming that the relationship should be monotone with an asymptote for large numbers of positive nodes. This was achieved by using the simple primary transformation exp(−0.12* Lymph nodes) where the factor 0.12 was estimated from the data (Sauerbrei and Royston 1999). The estimated power for this transformed variable was equal to one and a second power was not needed. Likewise, for progesterone receptor a power of 0.5 was estimated that gives a significant contribution to the log-hazard ratio functions. For the latter, an improvement in the log-likelihood of about 7.47 was achieved as compared to the inclusion of a linear term only. Figures 25.4B and C show these functions for lymph nodes and progesterone receptor, respectively,

**TABLE 25.6**

**Estimated Regression Coefficients and Corresponding p-Values in the Final Cox Regression Model for the GBSG-2-Study Using the Fractional Polynomial Approach**

| Factor/Function | Regression Coefficient | p-Value |
|---|---|---|
| $(Age/50)^{-2}$ | 1.742 | — |
| $(Age/50)^{-0.5}$ | −7.812 | <0.001* |
| Tumor grade 1 | 0 | — |
| Tumor grade 2–3 | 0.517 | 0.026 |
| exp (−0.12×Lymph nodes) | −1.981 | <0.001 |
| (Progesterone Receptor + 1)$^{0.5}$ | −0.058 | <0.001 |

*p-Value for both terms of age function.

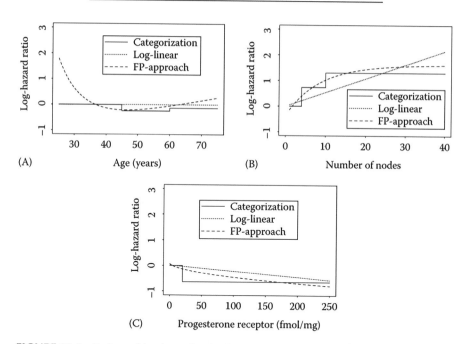

(A) Age (years)  (B) Number of nodes  (C) Progesterone receptor (fmol/mg)

**FIGURE 25.4**  Estimated log-hazard ratios functions for age (A), lymph nodes (B), and progesterone receptor (C) obtained by the FP, categorization, and log-linear approaches in the GBSG-2-study.

in comparison with those derived from the log-linear and from the categorization approach. For lymph nodes, it suggests that the log-linear approach underestimates the increase in risk for small numbers of positive nodes whereas it substantially overestimates it for very large numbers. The categorization approach seems to provide a reasonable compromise for this factor.

### 25.5.4 INTERACTIONS BETWEEN TREATMENT AND CONTINUOUS COVARIATES

Rather than assuming that "one-size-fits-all" clinicians aim to improve patient management by optimized, stratified treatment based on knowledge of markers (Simon 2005). In statistical terms, that means consideration of interactions between treatment and several variables with differential treatment effects across subgroups. In some areas in medicine (mainly in cancer) such factors are termed "predictive" markers. The statistical community is generally skeptical of the existence of interactions and often neglects to investigate them; an exception is a small number of predefined hypotheses in the protocol of a randomized controlled trial. Tests for interaction are necessary (see also the last point in Table 25.1), but often have low power. That is due to the fact that a trial is usually powered to test for a main effect of interest in all patients, not for an interaction.

Separate analyses of treatment effects in subgroups are popular, not always followed by a formal test for an interaction. Analyses in subgroups are appropriately criticized and overinterpretation of results is a critical issue (Assmann et al. 2000; Rothwell 2005). Caused by searching for "significant" treatment–covariate interactions among many candidates, multiple testing with the correspondingly increased type I error is often considered as a major issue. In order to preserve the type I error, many statisticians argue to adjust for multiple testing.

The type II error, which means to miss identifying that a treatment effect varies in subgroups or depends on the value of a continuous covariate, is rarely discussed as a serious deficiency. Furthermore, despite severe weaknesses (e.g., dependence on specific cutpoints, loss of power, biologically implausible step functions), categorization of a continuous covariate into two (sometimes three or four) groups is the standard approach to investigate interactions between treatment and continuous covariates (Wang et al. 2007). Probably, the main reason for this insufficient technique is the simplicity in prespecifying subgroups to investigate for interactions and that a standard test for an interaction can be used.

Given the enormous amount of resources spent on conducting a large randomized trial, it is surprising that greater efforts are not made to try to extract more information from these data. Therefore, Sauerbrei and Royston (2007b) consider exploratory analyses and the search for interactions between treatment and continuous variables as an important activity. To improve power and to overcome the problems caused by categorization, Royston and Sauerbrei (2004a) proposed the MFPI algorithm, an extension of MFP, to model interactions between treatment and continuous covariates by using FP. They distinguish the two cases with a prespecified hypothesis and hypothesis generation. The heart of the MFPI algorithm is the same for the two situations, the main difference is the consideration of multiple testing and the interpretation of results.

The MFPI algorithm models the prognostic effect of a continuous covariate Z by separate FP transformations within treatment groups, but under the constraint of the same powers. It can be used in a univariate setting, or by adjusting for a model depending on other covariates. Influence of the covariate Z on the estimated treatment effect is determined by the difference between the estimated functions for the prognostic effect in the two treatment groups. The resulting plot with the corresponding pointwise confidence interval is called the treatment effect plot. Comparing the model with a different function for Z in each treatment group with that with the same function in each group constitutes a test of interaction based on deviances. A detailed application to the GBSG-2-study, which is not replicated here, is given in the original publication (Royston and Sauerbrei 2004a).

A small simulation study showed that the type I error of the MFPI procedure is close (5.4% instead of 5%) to its nominal level (Sauerbrei et al. 2007b). MFPI was shown in several examples to be able to identify treatment/covariate interactions which may be missed by methods which do not use the full information from a continuous covariate (Royston and Sauerbrei 2004a). It is obvious that such results from data-dependent modeling have to be interpreted carefully and need validation in independent data.

Another technique to investigate for treatment interactions with continuous covariates is the subpopulation treatment effect pattern plot (STEPP) (Bonetti and Gelber 2000, 2004; Lazar et al. 2010). It involves dividing the observations into subgroups defined with respect to the covariate Z of interest and estimating the treatment effect separately within each subpopulation. To increase the number of patients that contribute to each point estimate, subpopulations are allowed to overlap. To create subpopulations, sliding window and tail-oriented variants are used and several tests for interactions have been proposed. The influence of a varying number of subpopulations, the difference between the two variants, and stability investigations using bootstrap replications have been illustrated by re-analysis of a randomized trial in kidney cancer. Results are also compared to MFPI. Based on these limited experiences, Royston and Sauerbrei (2008a) argue in an editorial that STEPP is an appropriate exploratory technique and a suitable method to check interactions detected by MFPI.

Approaches to investigate for interactions between treatment and continuous covariates are an area of active research. Several others have been proposed recently, for example, Cai et al. (2011).

### 25.5.5 FURTHER ISSUES

Some other important issues have not been explicitly mentioned so far. One is model checking with regard to the specific assumptions to be made; for this issue, we refer to textbooks and review articles on survival analysis (Marubini and Valsecchi 1995; Harrell et al. 1996; Valsecchi and Silvestri 1996; Therneau and Grambsch 2000; Harrell 2001). A second issue is concerned with other flexible statistical methods, such as generalized additive models (Hastie and Tibshirani 1990); a comparison of such methods and the FP approach using the data of the GBSG-2-study is presented in the work of Sauerbrei et al. (1999).

Another issue is stability and addresses the question whether we could replicate the selected final model having different data. Bootstrap resampling has been applied in order to investigate this issue (Chen and George 1985; Altman and Andersen 1989; Hastie and Tibshirani 1990; Sauerbrei and Schumacher 1992). In each bootstrap sample, the whole model selection or building process is repeated and the results are summarized over the bootstrap samples. We illustrate this procedure for BE with a

**TABLE 25.7**
**Inclusion Frequencies over 1000 Bootstrap**
**Samples Using the Backward Elimination**
**Method with a Selection Level of 5%**
**(BE (0.05)) in the GBSG-2-Study**

| Factor | Inclusion Frequency (%) |
|---|---|
| Age | 18.2 |
| Menopausal status | 28.8 |
| Tumor size | 38.1 |
| Tumor grade | 62.3 |
| Lymph nodes | 100 |
| Progesterone receptor | 98.1 |
| Estrogen receptor | 8.1 |

selection level of 5% in the Cox regression model with quantitative factors included as continuous covariates and assuming a log-linear effect (Table 25.4). In Table 25.7, the inclusion frequencies over 1000 bootstrap samples are given for the prognostic factors under consideration. These frequencies underline that tumor grade, lymph nodes, and progesterone receptor are by far the strongest factors; lymph nodes is always included, progesterone receptor in 98% and tumor grade in 62% of the bootstrap samples, respectively. The percentage of bootstrap samples where exactly this model—containing these three factors only—is selected is 26.1%. In 60.4% of the bootstrap samples, a model is selected that contains these three factors possibly with other selected factors. These figures might be much lower in other studies where more factors with a weaker effect are investigated. This bootstrap approach has been adapted by Royston and Sauerbrei (2003) who investigate the stability of the multivariable FP approach. It also provides insight into the interdependencies between different factors or functions selected by inspecting the bivariate or multivariate dependencies between models selected (Sauerbrei and Schumacher 1992; Royston and Sauerbrei 2003). These investigations underline the nonlinear effect of age on disease-free survival in the GBSG-2-study.

## 25.6 CLASSIFICATION AND REGRESSION TREES

Hierarchical trees are one approach for nonparametric modeling of the relationship between a response variable and several potential prognostic factors. The book of Breiman et al. (1984) gives a comprehensive description of the method of classification and regression trees (CART) that has been modified and extended in various directions (Zhang et al. 1998). We concentrate solely on the application to survival data (Gordon and Olshen 1985; LeBlanc and Crowley 1992, 1993; Segal 1988, 1998) and will use the abbreviation CART as a synonym for different types of tree-based analyses. CART is a prominent example of so-called machine learning methods.

Briefly, the idea of CART is to construct subgroups which are internally as homogeneous as possible with regard to the outcome and externally as separated as possible. Thus, the method leads directly to prognostic subgroups defined by the potential prognostic factors. This is achieved by a recursive tree building algorithm. As in Section 25.5, we start with k potential prognostic factors $Z_1, Z_2, ..., Z_k$ that may have an influence on the survival time random variable T. We define a minimum number of patients within a subgroup, $n_{min}$ say, and prespecify an upper bound for the p-values of the logrank test statistic, $p_{stop}$. Then the tree building algorithm is defined by the following steps (Lausen et al. 1994):

1. The minimal p-value of the logrank statistic is computed for all k factors and all allowable splits within the factors. An allowable split is given by a cutpoint of a quantitative or an ordinal factor within a given range of the distribution of the factor or some bipartition of the classes of a nominal factor.
2. The whole group of patients is split into two subgroups based on the factor and the corresponding cutpoint with the minimal p-value, if the minimal p-value is smaller than or equal to $p_{stop}$.
3. The partition procedure is stopped if there exists no allowable split, if the minimal p-value is greater than $p_{stop}$ or because the size of the subgroup is smaller than $n_{min}$.
4. For each of the two resulting subgroups the procedure is repeated.

This tree building algorithm yields a binary tree with a set of patients, a splitting rule, and the minimal p-value at each interior node. For patients in the resulting final nodes, various quantities of interest can be computed, such as Kaplan–Meier estimates of EFS or hazard ratios with respect to specific references or amalgamated groups.

Since prognostic factors are usually measured on different scales, the number of possible partitions will also be different, leading to the problems that have already been extensively discussed in Section 25.4. Thus, correction of p-values and/or restriction to a set of few prespecified cutpoints may be useful to overcome the problem that factors allowing more splits have a higher chance of being selected by the tree building algorithm. Because of multiple testing, the algorithm may be biased in favor of these factors over binary factors with prognostic relevance.

We will illustrate the procedure by means of the GBSG-2-study. If we restrict the possible splits to the range between the 10% and 90% quantile of the empirical distribution of each factor, then the factor age, for example, will allow 25 splits whereas the binary factor menopausal status will allow for only one split. Likewise, tumor size will allow for 32 possible splits, tumor grade for only 2. Lymph nodes will allow for 10 possible splits; progesterone and estrogen receptors offer 182 and 177 possible cutpoints, respectively. Thus, we decide to use the p-value correction as outlined in Section 25.4, and we define $n_{min} = 20$ and $p_{stop} = 0.05$. As a splitting criterion, we use the logrank test statistic; for simplicity, not stratified for hormonal therapy.

The result of the tree-building procedure is summarized in Figure 25.5. In this graphical representation, the size of the subgroups is taken proportional to the width

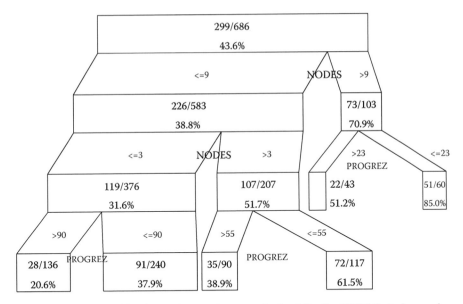

**FIGURE 25.5** Classification and regression tree obtained for the GBSG-2-study; p-value correction but no prespecification of cutpoints was used.

of the boxes whilst the centers of the boxes correspond to the observed event rates. This presentation allows an immediate visual impression about the resulting prognostic classification obtained by the final nodes of the tree.

We start with the whole group of 686 patients (the "root") where a total of 299 events (event rate 43.6%) have been observed. The factor with the smallest corrected p-value is the number of lymph nodes and the whole group is split at an estimated cutpoint of nine positive lymph nodes ($p_{cor} < 0.0001$), yielding a subgroup of 583 patients with less than or equal to nine positive lymph nodes and a subgroup of 103 patients with more than nine positive lymph nodes. The procedure is then repeated with the left and right tree nodes. At this level, in the left tree node, the number of lymph nodes again appeared to be the strongest factor, with a cutpoint of three positive lymph nodes ($p_{cor} < 0.0001$). For the right tree node, progesterone receptor is associated with the smallest corrected p-value and the cutpoint is obtained as 23 fmol ($P_{cor} = 0.0003$). In these two subgroups, no further splits are possible because of the $p_{stop}$ criterion.

In subgroups of patients with 1–3 and 4–9 positive nodes, progesterone receptor is again the strongest factor with cutpoints of 90 fmol ($p_{cor} = 0.006$) and 55 fmol ($p_{cor} = 0.0018$), respectively. Because of the $p_{stop}$ criterion, no further splits are possible.

There exist a variety of definitions of CART-type algorithms that usually consist of tree building, pruning, and amalgamation (Breiman et al. 1984; Ciampi et al. 1992; Tibshirani and LeBlanc 1992; Zhang et al. 1998). In order to protect against serious overfitting of the data, which in other algorithms is accomplished by tree pruning, we have defined various restrictions, such as the $p_{stop}$ and the $n_{min}$ criteria, and used corrected p-values. Applying these restrictions, we have obtained the tree displayed in Figure 25.5, which is parsimonious in the sense that only the strongest factors, lymph nodes and the progesterone receptor, are selected for the splits. However, the values of the cutpoints obtained for progesterone receptor (90, 55, and 23 fmol) are somewhat arbitrary and may not be reproducible or comparable to those obtained in other studies. Another useful restriction may be the definition of a set of prespecified possible cutpoints for each factor. In the GBSG-2-study, we specified 35, 40, 45, 50, 55, 60, 65, 70 years for age, 10, 20, 30, 40 mm for tumor size, and 5, 10, 20, 100, 300 fmol for progesterone and estrogen receptors. The resulting tree is displayed in Figure 25.6A. It only differs from the one without this restriction in the selected cutpoints for the progesterone receptor in the final nodes. For comparison, trees without the p-value correction and with and without prespecification of a set of possible cutpoints are presented in Figures 25.6B and C. Since lymph nodes and progesterone receptor are the dominating prognostic factors in this patient population, the resulting trees are identical at the first two levels to those where the p-values have been corrected. The final nodes in the latter ones, however, are again split leading to a larger number of final nodes. In addition, other factors like age, tumor size, and estrogen receptor are now used for the splits at subsequent nodes. A more detailed investigation of the influence of p-value correction and prespecification of possible cutpoints on resulting trees and their stability is given by Sauerbrei (1997).

To improve the predictive ability of trees, stabilizing methods based on resampling, such as bagging, have been proposed (Breiman 1996; Diettrich 2000; Friedman and Hastie 2000; Breiman 2001a; Hothorn et al. 2004). However, interpretation of the results is difficult, which limits their value for practical applications. It is important to carefully consider advantages and disadvantages of statistical versus machine learning methods (Breiman 2001b).

## 25.7  FORMATION AND VALIDATION OF RISK GROUPS

While the final nodes of a regression tree define a prognostic classification scheme, some combination of final nodes to a prognostic subgroup might be indicated. This is especially important if the number of final nodes is large and/or if the prognosis of patients in different final nodes is comparable. So, for example, from the regression tree presented in Figure 25.6A the simple prognostic classification given in Table 25.8 can be derived, which is broadly in agreement with current knowledge about the prognosis of node-positive breast cancer patients. The results in terms of estimated EFS are displayed in Figure 25.7A; the Kaplan–Meier curves show a good separation of the four prognostic subgroups. Since in other studies or in clinical practice progesterone receptor may often be only recorded as positive (PR > 20) or negative, the prognostic classification scheme in Table 25.8 may be modified in a way that the definition of subgroups I and II are replaced, respectively, by

$$I^* : (LN \leq 3 \text{ and } PR > 20)$$

and

$$II^* : (LN \leq 3 \text{ and } PR \leq 20) \text{ or } (LN \ 4-9 \text{ and } PR > 20)$$

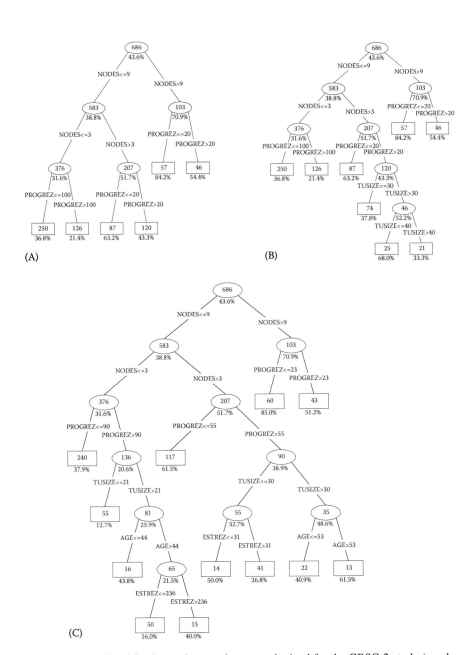

**FIGURE 25.6** Classification and regression trees obtained for the GBSG-2-study (p-value correction and prespecification of cutpoints (A); no p-value correction with (B) and without (C) prespecification of cutpoints).

**TABLE 25.8**

**Prognostic Classification Scheme Derived from the Regression Tree (p-Value Correction and Predefined Cutpoints) in the GBSG-2-Study**

| Prognostic Subgroup | Definition of Subgroup (LN: No. of Positive Lymph Nodes; PR: Progesterone Receptor) |
|---|---|
| I | (LN ≤ 3 and PR > 100) |
| II | (LN ≤ 3 and PR ≤ 100) or (LN 4–9 and PR > 20) |
| III | (LN 4–9 and PR ≤ 20) or (LN > 9 and PR > 20) |
| IV | (LN > 9 and PR ≤ 20) |

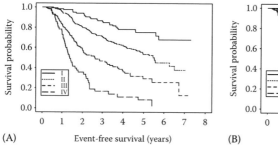 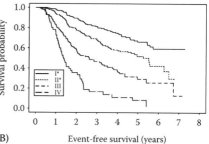

(A)  Event-free survival (years)     (B)  Event-free survival (years)

**FIGURE 25.7**  Kaplan–Meier estimates of event-free survival probabilities for the prognostic subgroups derived from the CART approach (A) and the modified CART approach (B) in the GBSG-2-study.

where

    LN are the lymph nodes

    PR is the progesterone receptor

The resulting Kaplan–Meier estimates of EFS are depicted in Figure 25.7B.

For two of the regression approaches in Section 25.5, prognostic subgroups have been formed by dividing the distribution of the prognostic index, $\hat{\beta}_1 Z_1 + \cdots + \hat{\beta}_k Z_k$, into quartiles; the stratified EFS curves are displayed in Figures 25.8A (Cox regression model with continuous factors, BE(0.05), Table 25.4) and 8B (Cox regression model with categorized covariates, BE(0.05), Table 25.5). As a reminder, in the definition of the corresponding subgroups tumor grade also enters in addition to lymph nodes and progesterone receptor.

For comparison, Figure 25.8C shows the Kaplan–Meier estimates of EFS for the well-known Nottingham Prognostic Index (Haybittle et al. 1982; Galea et al. 1992), the only prognostic classification scheme based on standard prognostic factors that enjoys widespread acceptance (Balslev et al. 1994). This index is defined as

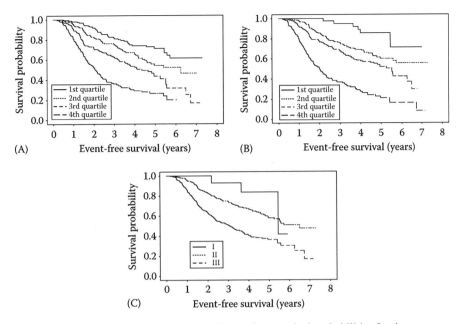

**FIGURE 25.8**   Kaplan–Meier estimates of event-free survival probabilities for the prognostic subgroups derived from a Cox model with continuous (A) and categorized (B) covariates and according to the Nottingham Prognostic Index (C) in the GBSG-2-study.

$$\text{NPI} = 0.02 \times \text{size (in mm)} + \text{lymph node stage} + \text{tumor grade},$$

where lymph node stage is equal to 1 for node-negative patients, 2 for patients with one to three positive lymph nodes, and 3 if four or more lymph nodes were involved. It is usually divided into three prognostic subgroups NPI-I (NPI $< 3.4$), NPI-II ($3.4 \leq$ NPI $\leq 5.4$), and NPI-III (NPI $> 5.4$). Since it was developed for node-negative and node-positive patients, there seems room for improvement by taking other factors, such as progesterone receptor, into account (Collett et al. 1998).

Since the Nottingham Prognostic Index has been validated in various other studies (Balslev et al. 1994; Blamey et al. 2007; Van Belle et al. 2010), we can argue that the degree of separation that is displayed in Figure 25.8C could be achieved in general. This, however, is by no means true for the other proposals derived by regression modeling or CART techniques, where some shrinkage has to be expected (Van Houwelingen and Le Cessie 1990; Copas 1997; Vach 1997a; Sauerbrei 1999). We therefore attempted to validate the prognostic classification schemes defined earlier with the data of an independent study that in more technical terms is often referred to as a "test set" (Ripley 1996). As a test set, we take the Freiburg DNA study that covers the same patient population and prognostic factors as in the GBSG-2-study. Only progesterone and estrogen receptor status (positive: $>20$ fmol and negative: $\leq 20$ fmol) is recorded in the Freiburg DNA study and the original values are not available. Thus, only those classification schemes where progesterone receptor enters as positive or negative can be considered for validation. Furthermore, we restrict ourselves

**TABLE 25.9**

**Estimated Hazard Ratios for Various Prognostic Classification Schemes Derived in the GBSG-2-Study and Validated in the Freiburg DNA Study**

| | | Estimated Hazard Ratios (No. of Patients) | | | |
|---|---|---|---|---|---|
| Prognostic Groups | | GBSG-2-Study | | Freiburg DNA Study | |
| Cox | I | 1 | (52) | 1 | (33) |
| | II | 2.68 | (218) | 1.78 | (26) |
| | III | 3.95 | (236) | 3.52 | (58) |
| | IV | 9.92 | (180) | 7.13 | (14) |
| CART | I* | 1 | (243) | 1 | (50) |
| | II* | 1.82 | (253) | 1.99 | (38) |
| | III | 3.48 | (133) | 3.19 | (33) |
| | IV | 8.20 | (57) | 4.34 | (11) |
| NPI | II | 1 | (367) | 1 | (46) |
| | III | 2.15 | (301) | 2.91 | (87) |

to those patients where the required information on prognostic factors is complete. Table 25.9 shows the estimated hazard ratios for the prognostic groups derived from the categorized Cox model and from the modified CART classifications scheme defined earlier. The hazard ratios have been estimated by using dummy variables defining the risk groups and by taking the group with the best prognosis as reference. When applying the classification schemes to the data of the Freiburg DNA study, the definitions and categorization derived in the GBSG-2-study are used. Note that the categorization into quartiles of the prognostic index does not yield groups with equal number of patients since the prognostic index from the categorized Cox model takes only few different values.

From the values given in Table 25.9, it can be seen that there is some shrinkage in the hazard ratios when estimated in the Freiburg DNA test set. This shrinkage is more pronounced in the modified CART classification scheme (reduction by 47% in the relatively small high risk group) as compared with the categorized Cox model (reduction by 28% in the high risk group).

In order to get some idea of the amount of shrinkage that has to be anticipated in a test set, based on the "training set" (Ripley 1996) where the classification scheme has been developed, cross-validation or other resampling methods can be used. Similar techniques as in Section 25.4 can be used, which essentially estimate a shrinkage factor for the prognostic index (Van Houwelingen and Le Cessie 1990; Verweij and Van Houwelingen 1993). The hazard ratios for the prognostic subgroups are then estimated by categorizing the shrinked prognostic index according to the cutpoints used in the original data. In the GBSG-2-study, we obtained an estimated shrinkage factor of $\hat{c}=0.95$ for the prognostic index derived from the categorized Cox model indicating that we would not expect a serious shrinkage of the hazard ratios between the prognostic subgroups. Compared to the estimated hazard ratios in the Freiburg

DNA study (Table 25.9), it is clear that the shrinkage effect in the test set can only be predicted to a limited extent. This deserves at least two comments. First, we have used leave-one-out cross-validation that possibly could be improved by bootstrap or other resampling methods (Schumacher et al. 1997); second, we did not take the variable selection process into account. By doing so, we would expect more realistic estimates of the shrinkage effect in an independent study. Similar techniques can also be applied to classification schemes derived by CART methods. Further approaches to assess the predictive ability of prognostic classification schemes will be presented in Section 25.10.

## 25.8 ARTIFICIAL NEURAL NETWORKS

The application of artificial neural networks (ANNs) for prognostic and diagnostic classification in clinical medicine has attracted growing interest in the medical literature. So, for example, a "mini-series" on neural networks that appeared in the Lancet contained three more or less enthusiastic review articles (Baxt 1995; Cross et al. 1995; Dybowski and Gant 1995) and an additional commentary expressing some scepticism (Wyatt 1995). In particular, feed-forward neural networks have been used extensively, often accompanied by exaggerated statements of their potential. In a review article (Schwarzer et al. 2000) we identified a substantial number of articles with application of ANNs to prognostic classification in oncology.

The relationship between ANNs and statistical methods, especially logistic regression models, has been described in several articles (Ripley 1993; Cheng and Titterington 1994; Penny and Frost 1996; Schumacher et al. 1996b; Stern 1996; Warner and Misra 1996). Briefly, the conditional probability that a binary outcome variable Y is equal to 1, given the values of k prognostic factors $Z_1 Z_2, \ldots, Z_k$ is given by a function $f(Z,w)$. In feed-forward neural networks, this function is defined by

$$f(Z,w) = \Lambda\left( W_0 + \sum_{j=1}^{r} W_j \cdot \Lambda\left( w_{0j} + \sum_{i=1}^{k} w_{ij} Z_i \right) \right)$$

where
  $w = (w_0, \ldots, w_r, w_{01}, \ldots, w_{kr})$ are the unknown parameters called "weights"
  $\Lambda(\cdot)$ denotes the logistic function, $\Lambda(u) = (1 + \exp(-u))^{-1}$, called "activation-function"

The weights w can be estimated from the data via maximum likelihood although other optimization procedures are often used in this framework. The ANN is usually introduced by a graphical representation like that in Figure 25.9. This figure illustrates a feed-forward neural network with one hidden layer. The network consists of k input units, r hidden units denoted by $h_1, \ldots, h_r$, and one output unit and corresponds to the ANN with $f(Z,w)$ defined before. The arrows indicate the "flow of information." The number of weights is $(r + 1) + (k + 1)$ because every input unit is connected with every hidden unit and the latter are all connected to the output unit. If there is no hidden layer ($r = 0$), the ANN reduces to a common logistic regression model which is also called the "logistic perceptron."

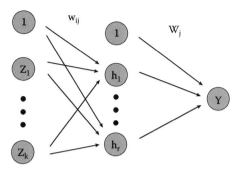

**FIGURE 25.9** Graphical representation of an artificial neural network with one input layer, one hidden layer, and one output layer.

In general, feed-forward neural networks with one hidden layer are universal approximators (Hornik et al. 1989) and thus can approximate any function defined by the conditional probability that Y is equal to one given Z with arbitrary precision by increasing the number of hidden units. This flexibility can lead to serious over-fitting which can again be compensated by introducing some weight decay (Ripley 1996, 1998), for example, by adding a penalty term

$$-\lambda \left( \sum_{j=1}^{r} W_j^2 + \sum_{j=1}^{r} \sum_{i=1}^{k} w_{ij}^2 \right)$$

to the log-likelihood. The smoothness of the resulting function is then controlled by the decay parameter $\lambda$. It is interesting to note that in our literature review of articles published between 1991 and 1995, we have not found any application in oncology where weight decay has been used (Schwarzer et al. 2000).

Extension to survival data with censored observations is associated with various problems. Although there is a relatively straightforward extension of ANNs to handle grouped survival data (Liestøl et al. 1994), several naïve proposals can be found in the literature. In order to predict outcome (death or recurrence) of individual breast cancer patients, Ravdin et al. (1992) and Ravdin and Clark (1992) use a network with only one output unit but using the number j of the time interval as additional input. Moreover, they consider the unconditional probability of dying before $t_j$ rather than the conditional one as output. Their underlying model then reads

$$P(T < t_j | Z) = \Lambda \left( w_0 + \sum_{i=1}^{k} w_i Z_i + w_{k+1} \cdot j \right)$$

for $j = 1, \ldots, J$. T denotes the survival time random variable, and the time intervals are defined by $t_{j-1} \leq t < t_j, \ 0 = t_0 < t_1 < \cdots < t_J < \infty$. This parameterization not only ensures monotonicity of the survival probabilities but also implies a rather stringent and unusual shape of the survival distribution, since in the case of no covariates this equation reduces to

$$P(T < t_j) = \Lambda(w_0 + w_{k+1} \cdot j)$$

for $j = 1, \ldots, J$. Obviously, the survival probabilities do not depend on the length of the time intervals, which is a rather strange and undesirable feature. Including a hidden layer in this expression is a straightforward extension retaining all the features summarized previously. De Laurentiis and Ravdin (1994) call this type of neural networks "time coded models." Another form of neural networks that has been applied to survival data are the so-called "single time point models" (De Laurentiis and Ravdin 1994). Since they are identical to a logistic perceptron or a feed-forward neural network with a hidden layer, they correspond to fits of logistic regression models or their generalizations to survival data. In practice, a single time point $t^*$ is fixed and the network is trained to predict the survival probability. The corresponding model is given by

$$P(T < t^* | Z) = \Lambda\left(w_0 + \sum_{i=1}^{k} w_i z_i\right)$$

or its generalization when introducing a hidden layer. This approach is used by Burke (1994) to predict 10 year survival of breast cancer patients based on various patient and tumor characteristics at time of primary diagnosis. McGuire et al. (1992) utilized this approach to predict 5 year EFS of patients with axillary node-negative breast cancer based on seven potentially prognostic variables. Kappen and Neijt (1993) used it to predict 2 year survival of patients with advanced ovarian cancer obtained from 17 pretreatment characteristics. The neural network they actually used reduced to a logistic perceptron.

The aforementioned procedure can be repeatedly applied for the prediction of survival probabilities at fixed time points $t^* = t_1 < t_2 < \cdots < t_j$, replacing $w_0$ by $w_{0j}$ and $w_i$ by $w_{ij}$ for $j = 1, \ldots, J$ (Kappen and Neijt 1993). But without restriction on the parameters such an approach does not guarantee that the probabilities $P(T < t_j | Z)$ increase with $j$, and hence may result in life-table estimators suggesting a nonmonotone survival function. Closely related are "multiple time point models" (De Laurentiis and Ravdin 1994) where one neural network with J output units with or without a hidden layer is used.

A common drawback of these naïve approaches is that they do not allow incorporating censored observations in a straightforward manner, which is closely related to the fact that they are based on unconditional survival probabilities instead of conditional survival probabilities. Neither omission of the censored observations, as suggested by Burke (1994), nor treating censored observations as uncensored are valid approaches, but a serious source of bias, which is well known in the statistical literature. De Laurentiis and Ravdin (1994) and Ripley (1998) propose to impute estimated conditional survival probabilities for the censored cases from a Cox regression model.

Faraggi and Simon (1995) and others (Biganzoli et al. 1998; Ripley and Ripley 2001; Biganzoli et al. 2002; Ripley et al. 2004) proposed a neural network generalization of the Cox regression model defined by

$$\lambda(t \mid Z_1,\ldots,Z_k) = \lambda_0(t)\exp(f_{FS}(Z,w))$$

where

$$f_{FS}(Z,w) = \sum_{j=1}^{r} W_j \Lambda \left( w_{0j} + \sum_{i=1}^{k} w_{ij} Z_i \right)$$

Note that the constant $W_0$ is omitted in the framework of the Cox model. Estimation of weights is then done by maximizing the partial likelihood. Although the problem of censoring is satisfactorily solved in this approach there remain problems with potentially serious overfitting of the data, especially if the number r of hidden units is large.

For illustration, we consider factors included in the final FP model of the GBSG-2-study (Section 25.5, Table 25.6). Thus, we used the four factors, age, grade, lymph nodes, and progesterone receptor (all scaled to the interval [0;1]), and hormone therapy as inputs for the Faraggi and Simon network. Figure 25.10 shows the results for various Faraggi and Simon networks compared to the FP approach in terms of Kaplan–Meier estimates of EFS in the prognostic subgroups defined by the quartiles of the corresponding prognostic indices. It should be noted that the Faraggi and Simon network contains $5 + (6 \times 5) = 35$ parameters when five hidden units are used and $20 + (6 \times 20) = 140$ when 20 hidden units are used. The latter one must be suspected of serious overfitting with a high chance that the degree of separation

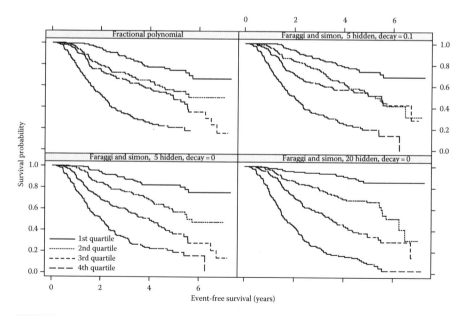

**FIGURE 25.10**   Kaplan–Meier estimates of event-free survival probabilities for the prognostic subgroups derived from various Faraggi and Simon networks and from the FP approach in the GBSG-2-study.

achieved could never be reproduced in other studies. In order to highlight this phenomenon, we trained a slightly different Faraggi and Simon (F&S) network where, in addition to age, tumor size, tumor grade, and the number of lymph nodes, estrogen and progesterone status (positive: >20 fmol, negative: ≤20 fmol) were used as inputs. This network contained 20 hidden units $(20 + (7 \times 20) = 160$ parameters) and showed a similar separation to the one where estrogen and progesterone receptors entered as quantitative inputs. Table 25.10 contrasts the results from the GBSG-2-study used as training set and the Freiburg DNA study used as test set in terms of estimated hazard ratios, where the predicted EFS probabilities are categorized in quartiles. In the training set, we observe a 20-fold increase in risk between the high-risk and the low-risk group. But in the test set, the F&S network turns out to yield a completely useless prognostic classification scheme; the estimated hazard ratios are not even monotone increasing. It is obvious that some restrictions, either in terms of a maximum number of parameters or a weight decay, are absolutely necessary to avoid such overfitting. The results for a network with five hidden units are comparable to the FP

### TABLE 25.10
### Estimated Hazard Ratios for Various Prognostic Classification Schemes Based on Faraggi and Simon Neural Networks Derived in the GBSG-2-Study and Validated in the Freiburg DNA Study

| | | Estimated Hazard Ratios (No. of Patients) | | | |
|---|---|---|---|---|---|
| Prognostic Groups | | GBSG-2-Study | | Freiburg DNA Study | |
| F&S[a] | I | 1 | (179) | 1 | (37) |
| | II | 3.24 | (178) | 0.34 | (16) |
| | III | 7.00 | (159) | 0.98 | (38) |
| | IV | 22.03 | (170) | 1.39 | (35) |
| F&S[b] | I | 1 | (171) | 1 | (23) |
| | II | 1.45 | (172) | 1.57 | (25) |
| | III | 2.62 | (171) | 3.09 | (32) |
| | IV | 5.75 | (172) | 4.27 | (46) |
| F&S[c] | I | 1 | (172) | 1 | (20) |
| | II | 1.64 | (171) | 1.03 | (31) |
| | III | 3.27 | (171) | 1.89 | (28) |
| | IV | 8.49 | (172) | 2.72 | (47) |
| F&S[d] | I | 1 | (172) | 1 | (23) |
| | II | 1.46 | (171) | 1.57 | (25) |
| | III | 2.62 | (171) | 3.22 | (33) |
| | IV | 5.77 | (172) | 4.14 | (45) |

[a] 20 hidden units, weight decay = 0.
[b] 20 hidden units, weight decay = 0.1.
[c] 5 hidden units, weight decay = 0.
[d] 5 hidden units, weight decay = 0.1.

approach, especially when some weight decay is introduced. It should be noted that the FP approach contains at most eight parameters if we ignore the preselection of the four factors.

## 25.9 REGULARIZED ESTIMATION

In recent years, datasets with high-dimensional molecular measurements have increasingly become available, resulting in development of regularization techniques for estimating prognostic models when the number of candidate prognostic factors is larger than the number of observations. Some of these regularization techniques have their origin in low-dimensional applications, that is, their relative success in high-dimensional applications might lead toward reconsidering them even if the number of factors is smaller than the number of observations (Porzelius et al. 2010b). Therefore, we will discuss these techniques for both low- and high-dimensional applications in the following, at some points hinting toward specific modeling challenges in the latter setting.

### 25.9.1 GENERAL PRINCIPLES

In the previous sections, the need for controlling complexity or over-optimism has already been hinted at several times. For example, shrinkage factors were introduced in Section 25.4 for scaling a prognostic index toward a realistic level, or weight decay was used for avoiding overfitting in neural networks. When dealing with a large number of covariates, overfitting becomes an even more severe issue. For example, a large number of molecular measurements will nowadays often be available for a patient, in principle allowing for perfect separation in the training data, while potentially providing only limited prognostic value for new patients. Furthermore, if the number of covariates is larger than the number of events, standard maximum likelihood techniques no longer work. A large number of techniques have been developed for addressing such modeling problems. For a comprehensive overview see Hastie et al. (2009). Common to all these techniques is the need to provide some form of regularization, subject to similar statistical principles. In the following, we will first review some of these general principles. After that, some exemplary regularization techniques will be discussed.

As indicated in Section 25.1, two aims can be distinguished when building a prognostic model: prediction, that is, obtaining good prediction performance, and explanation, that is, identifying important prognostic factors, or identifying a signature, that is, a set of factors that appropriately represents the disease process of interest. In low-dimensional settings, these two can often be obtained simultaneously. If a model provides a prognostic signature, this signature will typically comprise the most important factors, and their combination will provide reasonable prediction performance. In contrast, in a high-dimensional setting, typically not all of these goals can be obtained simultaneously, and different approaches target different aims. For example, a prognostic signature might contain a factor that is only representative for a group of highly correlated factors. With slightly different data, a different factor from that group might be selected. Therefore, the signature will be rather unstable. While prediction performance may not be affected much, interpretation will be different. Consequently, it can no longer be assumed that a signature contains all important prognostic factors. For obtaining optimal prediction performance, it may even be reasonable to give up on identifying a signature, but to include all factors to some degree.

For interpreting the effect of a covariate in a prognostic model, confidence intervals for the estimated effect are typically deemed essential. However, whenever some kind of variable selection is performed, these confidence intervals may become unreliable. In particular, shrinkage approaches are affected that provide variable selection, where it may no longer be possible to obtain reasonable confidence intervals (Leeb and Pötscher 2006).

## 25.9.2 Tuning Parameters/Selection of Tuning Parameters

A common theme to all shrinkage approaches in this context is that some kind of tuning parameter is available and needs to be selected for controlling the degree of shrinkage. Following the aim of optimizing for prediction performance, these tuning parameters are typically selected according to estimates of prediction performance. The latter are obtained from resampling approaches, such as cross-validation or the bootstrap.

Before describing specific resampling approaches, the number of tuning parameters required by a modeling approach should be considered. Besides the main tuning parameter that controls the overall degree of shrinkage, more sophisticated approaches may introduce further parameters. For example, underestimation of effects by the lasso approach (Tibshirani 1997), which uses only one tuning parameter, can be corrected by a second tuning parameter (Zou 2006). In principle, the same resampling procedure that is employed for selecting the value for one tuning parameter could be extended for several tuning parameters. However, the grid search, required for determining an optimal combination of a larger number of tuning parameters, is not only computationally expensive but may also stop at suboptimal solutions due to the variability of resampling estimates. The difficulty of selecting several tuning parameters for translating the theoretical advantages of more sophisticated modeling approaches is, for example, illustrated in Benner et al. (2010). For example, underestimation of effects by the lasso approach can only be successfully corrected if the data provide enough information for adequately choosing a second tuning parameter. Otherwise, the resulting estimates might even be worse.

For cross-validation, the original data are repeatedly split into training and test data. The prognostic model is fitted to the training data for each value of the tuning parameter, and evaluated in the test data. For the Cox proportional hazards model, the predictive partial likelihood is determined, where time structure carefully has to be taken into account, as outlined in Verweij and Van Houwelingen (1993). The partial likelihood is specific for the Cox proportional hazards model. For other approaches, and also for comparing Cox models to other approaches, a different criterion is needed. In Section 25.10, the Brier score will be introduced for comparing models regardless of the likelihood structure. This criterion, which determines the average square difference between the predicted survival probability and the true 0/1 survival status at a specific time, can also be employed for model selection (Porzelius et al. 2010a).

While formally the same criteria can be employed for selecting tuning parameters and for evaluating and comparing different prognostic models, these two applications should not be confused. For example, if cross-validation is first employed for selecting the value of a tuning parameter that results in an optimal Brier score, the value of the latter will no longer be an unbiased estimate of the Brier score for new patients. This can only be avoided by a nested approach, for example, performing cross-validation for tuning parameter selection nested within the training data sets of an outer cross-validation, used for estimating prediction performance. Another frequent mistake is to select the tuning parameter only once in the original data and then determining prediction performance by resampling using that fixed parameter value. The severe bias that can result from such an approach in a high-dimensional setting has, for example, been illustrated in Simon et al. (2003): Artificial data were generated such that there is no connection between the covariates and the endpoint. Despite this, a set of "best" covariates, preselected on the original data, exhibit excellent predicting performance in resampling. The true prediction performance is only seen when using a nested approach, that is, selecting covariates within each resampling training data set.

### 25.9.3 POST-ESTIMATION SHRINKAGE

Different strategies have been developed for dealing with large variability and potential instability, arising, for example, when building prognostic models with high-dimensional data. Bagging (Breiman 1996), for increasing stability, has already been mentioned in previous sections. Briefly, bootstrap samples of the original data are generated by drawing from the empirical distribution, that is, by drawing observations from the original data with replacement. Models are then built in these bootstrap data sets. The estimators from these models are then averaged over all bootstrap samples. Bagging is a strategy for post-model building modification. In principle, this idea is similar to the post-estimation shrinkage factor introduced in Section 25.4. Instead of a global shrinkage factor (Van Houwelingen and Le Cessie 1990), parameterwise shrinkage factors can be determined by a resampling approach (Sauerbrei 1999).

The random forest approach (Breiman 2001a) can be considered as a more advanced implementation of such post-estimation model modification, where bagging is extended by deliberately introducing random elements into regression tree building on the bootstrap samples. At each node, not all covariates, but only a random subset is considered for splitting. This increases the variety of trees generated for combination after model fitting. The downside of such an approach is that the role of a single prognostic factor can no longer easily be seen. While importance measures for identifying the most important factors are available (see, e.g., Ishwaran et al. 2010), the convenient interpretation of a single tree is lost.

### 25.9.4 SIMULTANEOUS ESTIMATION AND SHRINKAGE

Instead of applying some form of shrinkage after estimation, the shrinkage idea can also be directly built into estimation of prognostic models by imposing constraints on the estimates, for example, by attaching a penalty term to the likelihood used for estimation. One advantage of doing this is that estimation becomes feasible even in settings where the number of covariates is larger than the number of events. For a more comprehensive overview of such approaches see Binder et al. (2011). One of the earliest of these penalized likelihood approaches is ridge regression (Hoerl and Kennard 1970). In this approach, the penalty term comprises the sum of the squared regression coefficients. This shrinks parameter estimates toward zero and decreases variability. While ridge regression does not provide selection of important prognostic factors, it might provide superior prediction performance (Bøvelstad et al. 2007). The garotte (Breiman 1995) is an example of a simultaneous approach that also provides a shrinkage factor for each single regression coefficient of a prognostic model.

Alternatively, the lasso approach (Tibshirani 1997) uses a penalty term comprising the sum of the absolute values of the regression coefficients. This typically results in several estimates equal to zero, thus providing selection of prognostic factors. This comes at the cost of no longer being able to determine reliable confidence intervals and p-values. This is a more general problem with data-driven model building (Leeb and Pötscher 2006), but has specifically been investigated for the lasso, as it is one of the most prominent approaches for variable selection by shrinkage. Furthermore, the estimated effects will be biased toward zero, even if the true effect of a prognostic factor is large. There are several proposals how this bias could be reduced, for example, the adaptive lasso (Zou 2006). All of these approaches depend on a second tuning parameter. As already discussed, selection of such a second parameter might be difficult. For example, the results in Benner et al. (2010) indicate that the theoretical advantage of approaches that improve the lasso might be lost due to empirical tuning parameter selection, and the results might even be worse compared to the lasso.

The nature of the lasso estimates can be illustrated, by reformulating it as a stagewise regression approach (Efron et al. 2004). Starting from a model that does not contain any prognostic factor, the regression coefficients of the prognostic factors are updated, one factor at a time, in a large number of model building steps. In each step, that prognostic factor which improves the fit the most receives an update. This update comprises only a fraction of the full maximum likelihood estimate, leaving room for improvement in later steps. The estimates for all other prognostic factors are kept fixed during that step. This is in contrast to the classic stepwise regression approach, where after each inclusion or exclusion of a covariate the effects of all prognostic factors are re-estimated. By fixing all other components, variability is reduced. Componentwise likelihood-based boosting generalizes this stagewise regression idea toward generalized linear models (Tutz and Binder 2007) and the Cox proportional hazards model (Binder and Schumacher 2008). For a comprehensive overview of (componentwise) boosting techniques see Bühlmann and Hothorn (2007).

Figure 25.11 shows the coefficient paths obtained by componentwise likelihood-based boosting for the GBSG-2-study, that is, the stagewise build-up of the regression coefficients in the course of the model building steps. The boosting steps correspond to the degree of regularization, that is, a small number of boosting steps correspond to a large degree of regularization, and a large number of boosting steps correspond to a small degree of regularization. The coefficient paths show the estimated regression coefficients corresponding to these different degrees of

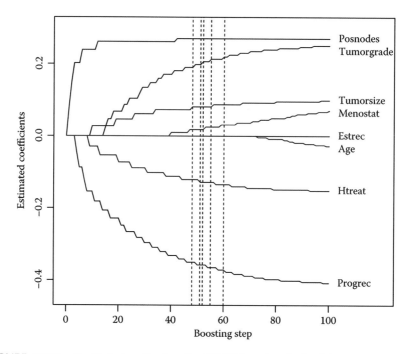

**FIGURE 25.11** Coefficient paths for the GBSG-2-study obtained by componentwise likelihood-based boosting for the Cox proportional hazards model. Continuous covariates have been centered and standardized, and binary and ordinal covariates have been transformed toward the range [−1;1], to provide a similar amount of regularization. Treatment has not been used for stratification, but is included as a covariate ("Htreat"). The boosting steps selected by five repetitions of 10-fold cross-validation are indicated by vertical dashed lines.

regularization. Similar coefficient paths could be obtained from the lasso, where a large value of the lasso tuning parameter corresponds to a small number of boosting steps, and a large value of the lasso parameter corresponds to a large number of boosting steps. As seen from Figure 25.11, very strong regularization will result in a model where all estimates are equal to zero, that is, all factors are excluded from the model, while all factors are included for a small degree of regularization. Therefore, selecting the degree of regularization is critical for determining which factors are important. Often, 10-fold cross-validation is used for selecting the number of boosting steps, that is, the degree of regularization, for the final prognostic model. This approach relies on resampling estimates of prediction performance and therefore is subject to random variability. To illustrate this, we repeat cross-validation five times with different random splits. The models selected in these repetitions are indicated by vertical dashed lines in Figure 25.11. The same set of prognostic factors with nonzero estimates is seen to be selected in all five repetitions in this example. However, slightly more variability could, for example, have led to exclusion of "menostat" (menopausal status). On the other hand, "menostat" might be only included because "age" is excluded, potentially due to ignoring its nonlinear effect in the present model. This illustrates that careful model checking is needed when useful prognostic models are to be developed by regularized approaches, where potential nonlinear effects should be considered in low-dimensional as well as in high-dimensional settings.

## 25.10 ASSESSMENT OF PROGNOSTIC CLASSIFICATION SCHEMES

Once a prognostic classification scheme is developed, the question arises as to how its predictive ability can be assessed and compared to competitors. There is no commonly agreed upon approach and most measures are somewhat ad-hoc. Suppose that a prognostic classification scheme consists of g prognostic groups, called risk strata or risk group, then one common approach is to present the Kaplan–Meier estimates for event-free or overall survival in the g groups. This is the way we presented the results of prognostic classification schemes in previous sections. The resulting figures are often accompanied by p-values of the logrank test for the null hypothesis that the survival functions in the g risk strata are equal. It is clear that a significant result is a necessary but not sufficient condition for good predictive ability. Sometimes, a Cox model using dummy variates for the risk strata is fitted and the log-likelihood and/or estimated hazard ratios of risk strata with respect to a reference are given. Based on this, we have proposed a summary measure of separation (Sauerbrei et al. 1998) defined as

$$ SEP = \exp\left[ \sum_{j=1}^{g} \frac{n_j}{n} |\hat{\beta}_j| \right], $$

where
  $n_j$ denotes the number of patients in risk stratum j
  $\hat{\beta}_j$ is the estimated log-hazard ratio of patients in risk stratum j with respect to a baseline reference

Models are favored which have large SEP values. Although SEP was designed for use with survival data, it is also applicable to binary data. Algebraically, for survival data SEP turns out to be essentially an estimate of the standard deviation of the predicted log-hazard ratios according to a model with a dummy variable for each group. SEP is fairly independent of the number of groups employed. It has the advantage that it can be calculated for models which generate only groups and no risk score, such as tree-based methods (CART), simple schemes based on counting adverse risk factors, or expert subjective opinion. SEP has some drawbacks which motivated Royston and Sauerbrei (2004b) to propose improved measures of separation taking the risk ordering across individual patients into account.

We now briefly outline another approach complementing the measure of separation; a detailed description can be found elsewhere (Graf et al. 1999; Schumacher et al. 2003). First, it is important to recognize that the time-to-event itself cannot adequately be predicted (Parkes 1972; Forster and Lynn 1988; Henderson 1995; Henderson and Jones 1995; Maltoni et al. 1995; Henderson and Keiding 2005). The best one can do at baseline (t=0) is to try to estimate the probability that the event of interest will not occur until a prespecified time horizon represented by some time point t*. Consequently, a measure of inaccuracy that is aimed to assess the value of a given prognostic classification scheme should compare the estimated event-free probabilities with the observed ones.

Assume for now there is no censoring. The aim is to compare estimated event-free probabilities $\hat{S}(t^*|Z=z)$ for patients with covariates $Z=z$ to observed indicators of survival $I(T>t^*)$ leading to

$$BS(t^*) = \frac{1}{n} \sum_{i=1}^{n} \left( I(T_i > t^*) - \hat{S}(t^* \mid Z = z_i) \right)^2$$

where the sum is over all n patients. This quantity is also known as the quadratic score. Multiplication by a factor of 2 yields the Brier score, which was originally developed for judging the inaccuracy of probabilistic weather forecasts (Brier 1950; Hilden et al. 1978; Hand 1997). The expected value of the Brier score may be interpreted as a mean square error of prediction if the event status at t* is predicted by the estimated event-free probabilities. The Brier score takes values between zero and one; a trivial, constant prediction $\hat{S}(t^*)=0.5$ for all patients yields a Brier score equal to 0.25.

If some closer relationship to the likelihood is intended, the so-called logarithmic score may be preferred, given by

$$LS(t^*) = -\frac{1}{n} \sum_{i=1}^{n} \left\{ I(T_i > t^*) \log \hat{S}(t^* \mid Z = z_i) + I(T_i \leq t^*) \log(1 - \hat{S}(t^* \mid Z = z)) \right\}$$

where we adopt conventions "$0.\log 0 = 0$" and "$1.\log 0 = -\infty$" (Hand 1997; Shapiro 1997). Again, models are preferred which minimize this score.

If we do not wish to restrict ourselves to one fixed time point t*, we can consider the Brier and logarithmic scores as a function of time for $0 \leq t \leq t^*$. In case of the Brier score, we use the term "prediction error curve" for this function. If one wants a single number summary, this function can also be averaged over time, by integrating it with respect to some weight function W(t) over $t \in [0,t^*]$ (Graf et al. 1999).

Censoring can be accommodated by reweighting the individual contributions in a similar way as in the calculation of the Kaplan–Meier estimator, so that consistency of estimates is preserved. The reweighting of uncensored observations and of observations censored after t is done by the reciprocal of the Kaplan–Meier estimate of the censoring distribution, whereas observations censored before t get weight zero. With this weighting scheme, a Brier or a logarithmic score under random censorship can be defined that enjoys the desirable statistical properties (Graf et al. 1999). $R^2$-type measures (Korn and Simon 1991; Schemper 1990; Schemper and Stare 1996; Schemper and Henderson 2000; Graf and Schumacher 1995) can also be readily defined by relating the Brier or logarithmic scores to the pooled Kaplan–Meier estimate, which is used as a "universal" prediction for all patients. A $R^2$-type measure based on the measure of separation (Sauerbrei et al. 1998) has also been developed.

We calculated the Brier score for the data of the GBSG-2-study. In Figure 25.12A, the estimated prediction error curves of the classification schemes considered in

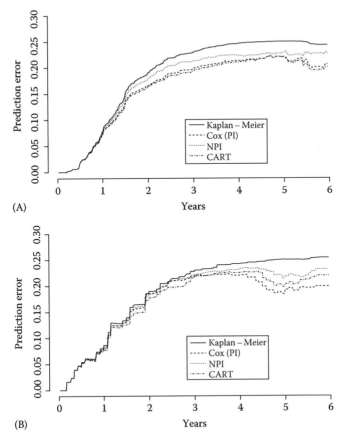

**FIGURE 25.12** Estimated prediction error curves for various prognostic classification schemes derived in the data of the GBSG-2-study (A) and validated in the Freiburg DNA study (B).

Section 25.7 (Table 25.9) are contrasted to the estimated prediction error curve based on the pooled Kaplan–Meier estimator. Because the latter prediction ignores all covariate information, it yields a benchmark value. It is found that the simplified COX index performs better than the NPI, and some further improvement is achieved by the CART index. Relative to the prediction with the pooled Kaplan–Meier estimate for all patients, there is only a moderate gain of accuracy.

In general, it has to be acknowledged that measures of inaccuracy tend to be large reflecting that predictions are far from being perfect (Ash and Schwartz 1999). In addition, it has to be mentioned that there will be overoptimism when a measure of inaccuracy is calculated from the same data where the prognostic classification scheme was derived, such as the case for the curves in Figure 25.12A. To demonstrate this, Figure 25.12B shows prediction error curves using the external Freiburg DNA study for the same prognostic factors. As already indicated in Table 25.9, there is almost no discrimination between the various classification schemes in this independent test data at least for values of t up to about 3 years. Afterward, the

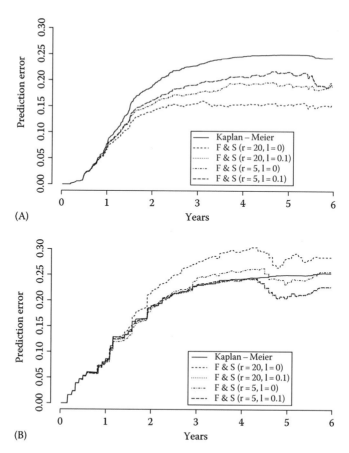

**FIGURE 25.13** Estimated prediction error curves for various Faraggi–Simon neural networks derived in the data of the GBSG-2-study (A) and validated in the Freiburg DNA study (B).

classification scheme based on the COX model has slightly lower prediction error than the other ones.

In order to expand on that issue further, we estimated prediction error curves for the various neural networks discussed in Section 25.8. The prediction error curves corresponding to the neural networks presented in Table 25.10 are displayed in Figure 25.13. The neural network with 20 hidden nodes and no weight decay has the lowest prediction error (Figure 25.13A), whereas the other three neural networks have a prediction error of similar magnitude to the other prognostic classification schemes. The resulting overoptimism can best be illustrated by inspection of Figure 25.13B where the Freiburg DNA study is used for validation. Here, the prediction error curve of the neural network with 20 hidden nodes and no weight decay used is highest, even exceeding the pooled Kaplan–Meier estimate. The two neural networks where weight decay is used have similar prediction error as the other prognostic classification schemes displayed in Figure 25.12B.

To reduce the inherent overoptimism, cross-validation and resampling techniques (Gerds and Schumacher 2007) can be employed in a similar way as for the estimation of error rates (Efron 1983; Efron and Tibshirani 1997; Wehberg and Schumacher 2004), which can also be used in high-dimensional data situations (Schumacher et al. 2007). For definitive conclusions, however, the determination of measures of inaccuracy in an independent test data set is absolutely necessary (Ripley 1996). An overview on various approaches to quantify the predictive accuracy of prognostic models has recently been given (Gerds et al. 2008; Steyerberg et al. 2010) including also the use of ROC curves methodology (Heagerty et al. 2000).

## 25.11 SAMPLE SIZE CONSIDERATIONS

To investigate the role of a new prognostic factor, careful planning of an appropriate study is required. Sample size and power formulae in survival analysis have been developed for randomized treatment comparisons, but in the analysis of prognostic factors, the covariates included are expected to be correlated with the factor of primary interest. In this situation, the existing sample size and power formulae are not valid and may not be applied. In this section, we give an extension of Schoenfeld's formula (Schoenfeld 1983) to the situation where a correlated factor is included in the analysis.

Suppose we wish to study the prognostic relevance of a certain factor, denoted by $Z_1$, in the presence of a second factor $Z_2$, where either can be a composite score based on several factors. The criterion of interest is overall or EFS of the patients. We assume that the analysis of the main effects of $Z_1$ and $Z_2$ is performed with the Cox proportional hazards model given by

$$\lambda(t \mid Z_1, Z_2) = \lambda_0(t) \exp(\beta_1 Z_1 + \beta_2 Z_2)$$

where

$\lambda_0(t)$ denotes an unspecified baseline hazard function

$\beta_1$ and $\beta_2$ are the unknown regression coefficients representing the effects of $Z_1$ and $Z_2$

For simplicity, we assume that $Z_1$ and $Z_2$ are binary with $p = P(Z_1 = 1)$ denoting the prevalence of $Z_1 = 1$. Assume that the effect of $Z_1$ shall be tested by an appropriate two-sided test based on the partial likelihood derived from the Cox model with significance level $\alpha$ and power $1 - \beta$ to detect an effect which is given by a hazard ratio of $\theta_1 = \exp(\beta_1)$.

For independent $Z_1$ and $Z_2$, it was shown by Schoenfeld (1983) that the total number of patients required is given by

$$N = \frac{(u_{1-\alpha/2} + u_{1-\beta})^2}{(\log \theta_1)^2 \psi(1-p)p}$$

where

$\psi$ is the probability of an uncensored observation

$u_\gamma$ denotes the $\gamma$-quantile of the standard normal distribution with $y = \lambda - \alpha/2$ and $y = \lambda - \beta$, respectively

This is the same formula as that used by George and Desu (1974), Bernstein and Lagakos (1978) and Schoenfeld (1981) in related problems.

The sample size formula depends on p, the prevalence of $Z_1 = 1$. The expected number of events, often also called the "effective sample size," to achieve a prespecified power is minimal for $p = 0.5$, the situation of a randomized clinical trial with equal probabilities for treatment allocation. By using the same approximations as Schoenfeld (1983), one can derive a formula for the case when $Z_1$ and $Z_2$ are correlated with correlation coefficient $\rho$; for details we refer to Schmoor et al. (2000). This formula reads

$$N = \frac{(u_{(1-\alpha)/2} + u_{1-\beta})^2}{(\log \theta_1)^2 \psi(1-p)p} \left( \frac{1}{1-\rho^2} \right)$$

where the factor $1/(1 - \rho^2)$ is the variance inflation factor (VIF).

This formula is identical to a formula derived by Lui (1992) for the exponential regression model in the case of no censoring and to that developed by Palta and Amini (1985) for the situation that the effect of $Z_1$ is analyzed by a stratified logrank test where $Z_2 = 0$ and $Z_2 = 1$ define the two strata. Table 25.11 gives, for some situations, the value of the VIF and the effective sample size $N\psi$, that is, the number of events required to obtain a power of 0.8 to detect an effect to $Z_1$ of magnitude $\theta_1$. It shows that the required number of events for the case of two correlated factors may increase up to a factor of 50% in situations realistic in practice.

The aforementioned sample size formulae will now be illustrated by means of the GBSG-2-study. Suppose we want to investigate the influence of the progesterone

---

**TABLE 25.11**

**Variance Inflation Factors and Effective Sample Size Required to Detect an Effect of $Z_1$ of Magnitude $\theta_1$ with Power 0.8 as Calculated by the Approximate Sample Size Formula for Various Values of p, $\rho$, $\theta_1$ ($\alpha = 0.05$)**

| | | | $N\psi$ | | |
|---|---|---|---|---|---|
| p | $\rho$ | VIF | $\theta_1 = 1.5$ | $\theta_1 = 2$ | $\theta_1 = 4$ |
| 0.5 | 0 | 1 | 191 | 65 | 16 |
| | 0.2 | 1.04 | 199 | 68 | 17 |
| | 0.4 | 1.19 | 227 | 78 | 19 |
| | 0.6 | 1.56 | 298 | 102 | 26 |
| 0.3 | 0 | 1 | 227 | 78 | 19 |
| | 0.2 | 1.04 | 237 | 81 | 20 |
| | 0.4 | 1.19 | 271 | 93 | 23 |
| | 0.6 | 1.56 | 355 | 122 | 30 |

**TABLE 25.12**

**Distribution of Progesterone Receptor by Tumor Grade and Estrogen Receptor in the GBSG-2-Study**

| | | Tumor Grade | | Estrogen Receptor | |
|---|---|---|---|---|---|
| | | 1 | 2 + 3 | <20 | ≥20 |
| Progesterone receptor | <20 | 5 | 264 | 190 | 79 |
| | ≥20 | 76 | 341 | 72 | 345 |
| Correlation coefficient | | −0.248 | | 0.536 | |

receptor in the presence of tumor grade. The Spearman correlation coefficient of these two factors is $\rho = -0.377$; if they are categorized as binary variables, we obtain $\rho = -0.248$ (Table 25.12). Taking the prevalence of progesterone-positive tumors, $p = 60\%$, into account, 213 events are required to detect a hazard ratio of 0.67, and 74 events are required to detect a hazard ratio of 0.5 with power 80% and significance level $\alpha = 5\%$. In this situation, the variance inflation factor is equal to 1.07 indicating that the correlation between the two factors has only little influence on power and required sample sizes.

If we want to investigate the prognostic relevance of progesterone receptor in the presence of estrogen receptor, a higher correlation must be considered. The Spearman correlation coefficient is $\rho = 0.598$ if both factors are measured on a quantitative scale and $\rho = 0.536$ if they are categorized into positive (>20 fmol) and negative (≤20 fmol) as given in Table 25.12. This leads to a variance inflation factor of 1.41 and a number of events of 284 and 97 required to detect a hazard ratio of 0.67 and 0.5, respectively (power = 80%, significance level $\alpha = 5\%$). This has to be contrasted with the situation that both factors under consideration are uncorrelated; in this case, the required number of events is 201 to detect a hazard ratio of 0.67, and 69 to detect a hazard ratio of 0.5, both with a power of 80% at a significance level of 5%.

Based on their calculations, the GBSG-2-study with 299 events does not seem too small to investigate the relevance of prognostic factors that exhibit at least a moderate effect (hazard ratio of 0.67 or 1.5). The question is whether it is large enough to permit the investigation of several prognostic factors. There use some recommendations in the literature, based on practical experience or on results from simulation studies, regarding the event per variable relationship (Harrell et al. 1984, 1985, 1996; Concato et al. 1995; Peduzzi et al. 1995). More precisely, it is the number of events per model parameter that matters which is often overlooked. These recommendations range from 10 to 25 events per model parameter to ensure stability of the selected model and of corresponding parameter estimates and to avoid serious overfitting. Sometimes the primary focus is estimation of the marker effect after adjustment for a set of standard variables, and correctly identifying which of the other variables are really important contributors to the model is of less concern. In this situation, sample size need not be as large as the 10–25 events per variable rule would recommend (Vittinghoff and McCulloch 2007).

The sample size formula given earlier addresses the situation of two binary factors. For more general situations, such as factors occurring on several levels or factors with continuous distributions, the required sample size may be calculated using a more general formula that can be developed along the lines of Lubin and Gail (1990). The anticipated situation needs then to be specified in terms of the joint distribution of the factors under study and the size of corresponding effects on survival. It may be more difficult to pose the necessary assumptions than in the situation of only two binary factors. Numerical integration techniques are then required to perform the necessary calculation.

If there are several factors in the analysis, one practical solution is to prespecify a prognostic score based on the existing standard factors as the second covariate to be adjusted for. Another possibility would be to adjust for the prognostic factor with the largest effect on survival and for which the highest correlation is anticipated. Finally, it should be mentioned that a sample size formula for the investigation of interactive effects of two prognostic factors is also available (Olschewski et al. 1992; Peterson and George 1993; Schmoor et al. 2000).

## 25.12 CONCLUDING REMARKS

There is a large concern about the quality of prognostic studies, and progress is needed to produce clinically relevant results (Hinestrosa et al. 2007). It is evident that prognostic marker studies are often badly designed (Simon and Altman 1994; Altman and Lyman 1998), inappropriately analyzed (Sauerbrei et al. 2006), poorly reported (Riley et al. 2003), and subject to numerous biases, such as selective reporting (Kyzas et al. 2007). Bad quality of design, analysis, and reporting of individual studies results in confusion regarding the prognostic value of a new marker (Sauerbrei 2005). To assess the value of a prognostic marker in a systematic review, problems from the individual studies will cause critical issues when trying to derive an overall estimate of the effect of a marker (Riley et al. 2009). To improve in general upon the current situation, a Prognosis Methods Group was established within the Cochrane Collaboration (http://prognosismethods.cochrane.org/).

In this chapter we considered statistical aspects of the evaluation of prognostic factors. Some general conclusions can be summarized as follows: A multivariate approach is absolutely essential. Thoughtful application of model building techniques should help to obtain models that are as simple and parsimonious as possible and to avoid serious overfitting in order to achieve generalizability for future patients. Thus, validation in an independent study is a further essential step. Some insight into the stability and generalizability of the derived models can be gained by cross-validation and resampling methods; however, these methods cannot completely replace an independent validation study. For a concrete study, the statistical analysis should be carefully planned step by step and the model building process should at least in principal be fixed in advance in a statistical analysis plan as is required in much more detail for clinical trials according to international guidelines.

There are a number of important topics that have not or have only been mentioned in passing in this chapter. One of these topics is concerned with the handling of missing values in prognostic factors (Robins et al. 1994; Vach 1994, 1997b; Lipsitz and Ibrahim 1998; Buuren van et al. 1999; Sterne et al. 2009). We have also assumed that effects of prognostic factors are constant over time and that prognostic factors are recorded and known at time of diagnosis. These assumptions do not cover the situation of time-varying effects and of time-dependent covariates. If multiple endpoints or different events are of interest, the use of competing risk and multi-state models may be necessary. For these topics, which are also of importance for prognostic factor studies we refer to more advanced textbooks in survival analysis (Andersen et al. 1993; Kalbfleisch and Prentice 2002; Klein and Moeschberger 2003; Marubini and Valsecchi 2004) and current research papers. In general, the methods and approaches presented in this contribution have at least in part been selected and assessed according to the subjective views of the authors. Thus, other approaches may be viewed as useful and adequate, too. What should not be a matter of controversy, however, is the need for a careful planning, conducting and analyzing of prognostic factor studies in order to arrive at generalizable and reproducible results that could contribute to a better understanding and possibly to an improvement of the prognosis of cancer patients.

## ACKNOWLEDGMENTS

We thank our colleagues Thomas Gerds, Erika Graf, and Claudia Schmoor for valuable contributions and Regina Gsellinger for her assistance in preparing the manuscript.

## REFERENCES

Altman DG. Systematic reviews of studies of prognostic variables. In: Egger M, Davey S, Altman D, eds. *Systematic Reviews in Health Care: Meta Analysis in Context*. London, U.K.: BMJ Books, pp. 228–247, 2001.

Altman DG, Andersen PK. Bootstrap investigation of the stability of a Cox regression model. *Stat Med* 1989; 8:771–783.

Altman DG, De Stavola BL, Love SB et al. Review of survival analyses published in cancer journals. *Br J Cancer* 1995; 72:511–518.

Altman DG, Lausen B, Sauerbrei W et al. Dangers of using "optimal" cutpoints in the evaluation of prognostic factors. Commentary. *J Natl Cancer Inst* 1994; 86:829–835.

Altman DG, Lyman GH. Methodological challenges in the evaluation of prognostic factors in breast cancer. *Breast Cancer Res Treat* 1998; 52:289–303.

Altman DG, Schulz KF, Moher D et al. for the CONSORT Group. The revised CONSORT statement for reporting randomized trials: Explanation and elaboration. *Ann Intern Med* 2001; 134:663–694.

Andersen PK. Survival analysis 1982–1991: The second decade of the proportional hazards regression model. *Stat Med* 1991; 10:1931–1941.

Andersen PK, Borgan O, Gill RD et al. *Statistical Methods Based on Counting Processes*. New York: Springer, 1993.

Andersen PK, Skovgaard LT. *Regression with Linear Predictors*. Berlin, Germany: Springer, 2010.

Armitage P, Gehan EA. Statistical methods for the identification and use of prognostic factors. *Int J Cancer* 1974; 13:16–36.

Ash A, Schwartz M. $R^2$: A useful measure of model performance when predicting a dichotomous outcome. *Stat Med* 1999; 18:375–384.

Assmann SE, Pocock SJ, Enos LE et al. Subgroup analysis and other (mis)uses of baseline data in clinical trials. *Lancet* 2000; 355:1064–1069.

Balslev I, Axelsson CK, Zedeler K et al. The Nottingham Prognostic Index applied to 9149 patients from the studies of the Danish Breast Cancer Cooperative Group (DBCG). *Breast Cancer Res Treat* 1994; 32:281–290.

Baxt WG. Application of artificial neural networks to clinical medicine. *Lancet* 1995; 346:1135–1138.

Benner A, Zucknick M, Hielscher T et al. High-dimensional Cox models: The choice of penalty as part of the model building process. *Biom J* 2010; 52(1):50–69.

Bernstein D, Lagakos SW. Sample size and power determination for stratified clinical trials. *J Stat Comput Simul* 1978; 8:65–73.

Biganzoli E, Boracchi P, Mariani L et al. Feed forward neural networks for the analysis of censored survival data: A partial logistic regression approach. *Stat Med* 1998; 17:1169–1186.

Biganzoli E, Boracchi P, Marubini E. A general framework for neural network models on censored survival data. *Neural Networks* 2002; 15:209–218.

Binder H, Porzelius C, Schumacher M. An overview of techniques for linking high-dimensional molecular data to time-to-event endpoints by risk prediction models. *Biom J* 2011; 53(2):170–189.

Binder H, Schumacher M. Allowing for mandatory covariates in boosting estimation of sparse high-dimensional survival models. *BMC Bioinf* 2008; 9:14.

Blamey RW, Ellis IO, Pinder SE et al. Survival of invasive breast cancer according to the Nottingham Prognostic Index in cases diagnosed in 1990–1999. *Eur J Cancer* 2007; 43:1548–1555.

Bloom HJG, Richardson WW. Histological grading and prognosis in primary breast cancer. *Br J Cancer* 1957; 2:359–377.

Bonetti M, Gelber RD. A graphical method to assess treatment-covariate interactions using the Cox model on subsets of data. *Stat Med* 2000; 19:2595–2609.

Bonetti M, Gelber RD. Patterns of treatment effects in subsets of patients in clinical trials. *Biostatistics* 2004; 5:465–481.

Bøvelstad HM, Nygård S, Størvold HL et al. Predicting survival from microarray data—A comparative study. *Bioinformatics* 2007; 23(16):2080–2087.

Breiman L. Better subset regression using the nonnegative garrote. *Technometrics* 1995; 37(4):373–384.

Breiman L. Bagging predictors. *Mach Learn* 1996; 24(2):123–140.

Breiman L. Random forests. *Mach Learn* 2001a; 45:5–32.

Breiman L. Statistical modeling: The two cultures (with comments and a rejoinder by the author). *Stat Sci* 2001b; 16:199–231.

Breiman L, Friedman JH, Olshen R et al. *Classification and Regression Trees*. Wadsworth, IL: Monterey, 1984.

Brier GW. Verification of forecasts expressed in terms of probability. *Monthly Weather Rev* 1950; 78:1–3.

Bühlmann P, Hothorn T. Boosting algorithms: Regularization, prediction and model fitting. *Stat Sci* 2007; 22(4):477–505.

Burke HB. Artificial neural networks for cancer research: Outcome prediction. *Semin Surg Oncol* 1994; 10:73–79.

Burke HB, Henson DE. Criteria for prognostic factors and for an enhanced prognostic system. *Cancer* 1993; 72:3131–3135.

Buuren van S, Boshuizen HC, Knook DL. Multiple imputation of missing blood pressure covariates in survival analysis. *Stat Med* 1999; 18:681–694.

Byar DP. Analysis of survival data: Cox and Weibull models with covariates. In: Mike V, Stanley KE, eds. *Statistics in Medical Research*. New York: Wiley, pp. 365–401, 1982.

Byar DP. Identification of prognostic factors. In: Buyse ME, Staquet MJ, Sylvester RJ, eds. *Cancer Clinical Trials: Methods and Practice*. Oxford, U.K.: Oxford University Press, pp. 423–443, 1984.

Byar DP. Assessing apparent treatment covariate interactions in randomized clinical trials. *Stat Med* 1985; 4:255–263.

Cai T, Tian L, Wong PH, Wei LJ. Analysis of randomized comparative clinical trial data for personalized treatment selections. *Biostatistics* 2011; 12(2):270–282.

Chen CH, George SL. The bootstrap and identification of prognostic factors via Cox's proportional hazards regression model. *Stat Med* 1985; 4:39–46.

Cheng B, Titterington DM. Neural networks: A review from a statistical perspective (with discussion). *Stat Sci* 1994; 9:2–54.

Ciampi A, Hendricks L, Lou Z. Tree-growing for the multivariate model: The RECPAM approach. In: Dodge Y, Whittaker J, eds. *Computational Statistics*, Vol. 1. Heidelberg, Germany: Physica-Verlag, 1992.

Clark GM (ed). Prognostic factor integration. Special issue. *Breast Cancer Res Treat* 1992; 22:185–293.

Collett D. *Modelling Survival Data in Medical Research*, 2nd edn. London, U.K.: Chapman & Hall, 2003.

Collett K, Skjaerven R, Machle BO. The prognostic contribution of estrogen and progesterone receptor status to a modified version of the Nottingham Prognostic Index. *Breast Cancer Res Treat* 1998; 48:1–9.

Concato J, Peduzzi P, Holford TR et al. Importance of events per independent variable in proportional hazards analysis. I. Background, goals and general strategy. *J Clin Epidemiol* 1995; 48:1495–1501.

Copas JB. Using regression models for prediction: Shrinkage and regression to the mean. *Stat Methods Med Res* 1997; 6:167–183.

Cox DR. Regression models and life tables (with discussion). *J R Stat Soc, Ser B* 1972; 34:187–220.

Cross SS, Harrison RF, Kennedy RL. Introduction to neural networks. *Lancet* 1995; 346:1075–1079.

De Laurentiis M, Ravdin PM. Survival analysis of censored data: Neural network analysis detection of complex interactions between variables. *Breast Cancer Res Treat* 1994; 32:113–118.

Diettrich TG. An experimental comparison of three methods for constructing ensembles of decision trees: Bagging, boosting, and randomization. *Mach Learn* 2000; 40:139–157.

Dybowski R, Gant V. Artificial neural networks in pathology and medical laboratories. *Lancet* 1995; 346:1203–1207.

Efron B. Estimating the error rate of prediction rule: Improvement on cross-validation. *J Am Stat Assoc* 1983; 78:316–330.

Efron B, Hastie T, Johnstone I et al. Least angle regression. *Ann Stat* 2004; 32(2):407–499.

Efron B, Tibshirani R. Improvement on cross-validation: The .632+ bootstrap method. *J Am Stat Assoc* 1997; 92:548–560.

Faraggi D, Simon R. A neural network model for survival data. *Stat Med* 1995; 14:73–82.

Fielding LP, Fenoglio-Preiser CM, Freedman LS. The future of prognostic factors in outcome prediction for patients with cancer. *Cancer* 1992; 70:2367–2377.

Fielding LP, Henson DE. Multiple prognostic factors and outcome analysis in patients with cancer. *Cancer* 1993; 71:2426–2429.

Fleming TR, Harrington DP. *Counting Processes and Survival Analysis*, 2nd edn. New York: Wiley, 2005.

Forster LA, Lynn J. Predicting life span for applicants to inpatient hospice. *Arch Intern Med* 1988; 148:2540–2543.

Friedman J, Hastie T, Tibshirani R. Additive logistic regression: A statistical view of boosting. *Ann Stat* 2000; 2:334–374.

Gail M, Simon R. Testing for qualitative interactions between treatment effects and patient subsets. *Biometrics* 1985; 41:361–372.

Galea MH, Blamey RW, Elston CE et al. The Nottingham Prognostic Index in primary breast cancer. *Breast Cancer Res Treat* 1992; 22:207–219.

George SL. Identification and assessment of prognostic factors. *Semin Oncol* 1988; 5:462–471.

George SL, Desu MM. Planning the size and duration of a clinical trial studying the time to some critical event. *J Chronic Dis* 1974; 27:15–24.

Gerds TA, Cai T, Schumacher M. The performance of risk prediction models. *Biom J* 2008; 50:457–479.

Gerds TA, Schumacher M. Efron-type measures of prediction error for survival analysis. *Biometrics* 2007; 63:1283–1287.

Gordon L, Olshen R. Tree-structured survival analysis. *Cancer Treat Rep* 1985; 69:1065–1069.

Gospodarowicz MK, Henson DE, Hutter RVP et al. *Prognostic Factors in Cancer*, 2nd edn. Heidelberg, Germany: Springer, 2001.

Graf E, Schmoor C, Sauerbrei W et al. Assessment and comparison of prognostic classification schemes for survival data. *Stat Med* 1999; 18:2529–2545.

Graf E, Schumacher M. An investigation on measures of explained variation in survival analysis. *Statistician* 1995; 44:497–507.

Hand DJ. *Construction and Assessment of Classification Rules*. Chichester, U.K.: Wiley, 1997.

Harrell FE Jr. *Regression Modelling Strategies: With Applications to Linear Models, Logistic Regression, and Survival Analysis*. New York: Springer, 2001.

Harrell FE, Lee KL, Califf RM et al. Regression modeling strategies for improved prognostic prediction. *Stat Med* 1984; 3:143–152.

Harrell FE, Lee KL, Mark DB. Multivariable prognostic models: Issues in developing models, evaluating assumptions and adequacy, and measuring and reducing errors. *Stat Med* 1996; 15:361–387.

Harrell FE, Lee KL, Matchar DB et al. Regression models for prognostic prediction: Advantages, problems and suggested solutions. *Cancer Treat Rep* 1985; 69:1071–1077.

Harris EK, Albert A. *Survivorship Analysis for Clinical Studies*. New York: Marcel Dekker, 1991.

Hastie TJ, Tibshirani RJ. *Generalized Additive Models*. New York: Chapman & Hall, 1990.

Hastie T, Tibshirani R, Friedman J. *The Elements of Statistical Learning,* 2nd edn. New York: Springer, 2009.

Haybittle JL, Blamey RW, Elston CW et al. A prognostic index in primary breast cancer. *Br J Cancer* 1982; 45:361–366.

Heagerty PJ, Lumley T, Pepe MS. Time-dependent ROC curves for censored survival data and a diagnostic marker. *Biometrics* 2000; 56:337–344.

Henderson R. Problems and prediction in survival-data analysis. *Stat Med* 1995; 3:143–152.

Henderson R, Jones M. Prediction in survival analysis. Model or medic. In: Jewell NP, Kimber AC, Ting Lee ML, Withmore GA, eds. *Lifetime Data: Models in Reliability and Survival Analysis*. Dordrecht, the Netherlands: Kluwer Academic Publishers, 1995.

Henderson R, Keiding N. Individual survival time prediction using statistical models. *J Med Ethics* 2005; 31:703–706.

Henson DE. Future directions for the American Joint Committee on Cancer. *Cancer* 1992; 69:1639–1644.

Hilden J, Habbema JDF, Bjerregard B. The measurement of performance in probabilistic diagnosis III: Methods based on continuous functions of the diagnostic probabilities. *Methods Inform Med* 1978; 17:238–246.

Hilsenbeck SG, Clark GM. Practical P-value adjustment for optimally selected cutpoints. *Stat Med* 1996; 15:103–112.

Hinestrosa MC, Dickersin K, Klein P et al. Shaping the future of biomarker research in breast cancer to ensure clinical relevance. *Nat Rev Cancer* 2007; 7:309–315.

Hoerl AE, Kennard RW. Ridge regression: Biased estimation for nonorthogonal problems. *Technometrics* 1970; 12(1):55–67.

Holländer N, Sauerbrei W, Schumacher M. Confidence intervals for the effect of a prognostic factor after selection of an 'optimal' cutpoint. *Stat Med* 2004; 23:1701–1713.

Holländer N, Schumacher M. Estimating the functional form of a continuous covariate's effect on survival time. *Comput Stat Data Anal* 2006; 50:1131–1151.

Hornik K, Stinchcombe M, White H. Multilayer feedforward networks are universal approximators. *Neural Networks* 1989; 2:359–366.

Hosmer DW, Lemeshow S, May S. Applied survival analysis: Regression modelling of time to event data. New York: Wiley, 2008.

Hothorn T, Lausen B. On the exact distribution of maximally selected rank statistics. *Comput Stat Data Anal* 2003; 121–137.

Hothorn T, Lausen B, Benner A et al. Bagging survival trees. *Stat Med* 2004; 23: 77–91.

Infante-Rivard C, Villeneuve J-P, Esnaola S. A framework for evaluating and conducting prognostic studies: An application to cirrhosis of the liver. *J Clin Epidemiol* 1989; 42:791–805.

Ishwaran H, Kogalur UB, Gorodeski EZ et al. High-dimensional variable selection for survival data. *J Am Stat Assoc* 2010; 105(489):205–217.

Kalbfleisch JD, Prentice RL. *The Statistical Analysis of Failure Time Data*, 2nd edn. New York: Wiley, 2002.

Kappen HJ, Neijt JP. Neural network analysis to predict treatment outcome. *Ann Oncol* 1993; 4(suppl):31–34.

Klein JP, Moeschberger ML. *Survival Analysis: Techniques for Censored and Truncated Data*, 2nd edn. New York: Springer, 2003.

Korn EJ, Simon R. Explained residual variation, explained risk and goodness of fit. *American Statistician* 1991; 45:201–206.

Kyzas PA, Denaxa-Kyza D, Ioannidis JP. Almost all articles on cancer prognostic markers report statistically significant results. *Eur J Cancer* 2007; 43: 2559–2579.

Lausen B, Sauerbrei W, Schumacher M. Classification and regression trees (CART) used for the exploration of prognostic factors measured on different scales. In: Dirschedl P, Ostermann R, eds. *Computational Statistics*. Heidelberg, Germany: Physica-Verlag, pp. 1483–1496, 1994.

Lausen B, Schumacher M. Maximally selected rank statistics. *Biometrics* 1992; 48:73–85.

Lausen B, Schumacher M. Evaluating the effect of optimized cutoff values in the assessment of prognostic factors. *Comput Stat Data Anal* 1996; 21:307–326.

Lazar AA, Cole BF, Bonnetti M et al. Evaluation of treatment-effect heterogeneity using biomarkers measured on a continuous scale: Subpopulation treatment effect pattern plot. *J Clin Oncol* 2010; 28:4539–4544.

LeBlanc M, Crowley J. Relative risk regression trees for censored survival data. *Biometrics* 1992; 48:411–425.

LeBlanc M, Crowley J. Survival trees by goodness of split. *J Am Stat Assoc* 1993; 88:457–467.

Lee ET, Wang GW. *Statistical Methods for Survival Data Analysis*, 3rd edn. New York: Wiley, 2003.

Leeb H, Pötscher BM. Can one estimate the conditional distribution of post-model-selection estimators? *Ann Stat* 2006; 34(5):2555–2591.

Liestøl K, Andersen PK, Andersen U. Survival analysis and neural nets. *Stat Med* 1994; 13:1189–1200.

Lipsitz SR, Ibrahim JG. Estimating equations with incomplete categorical covariates in the Cox model. *Biometrics* 1998; 54:1002–1013.

Lubin JH, Gail MJ. On power and sample size for studying features of the relative odds of disease. *Am J Epidemiol* 1990; 131:551–566.

Lui K-J. Sample size determination under an exponential model in the presence of a confounder and type I censoring. *Control Clin Trials* 1992; 13:446–458.

Machin D, Cheung YB, Parmar MKB. *Survival Analysis: A Practical Approach*, 2nd edn. Chichester, U.K.: Wiley, 2006.

Mallett S, Timmer A, Sauerbrei W, Altman DG. Reporting of prognostic studies of tumor markers: A review of published articles in relation to REMARK guidelines. *Br J Cancer* 2010; 102:173–180.

Maltoni M, Pirovano M, Scarpi E et al. Prediction of survival of patients terminally ill with cancer. *Cancer* 1995; 75:2613–2622.

Mantel N. Why stepdown procedures in variable selection? *Technometrics* 1970; 12:621–625.

Marubini E, Valsecchi MG. *Analysing Survival Data from Clinical Trials and Observational Studies.* Chichester, U.K.: Wiley, 2004.

McGuire WL. Breast cancer prognostic factors: Evaluation guidelines. *J Natl Cancer Inst* 1991; 83:154–155.

McGuire WL, Tandon AK, Allred, DC et al. Treatment decisions in axillary node-negative breast cancer patients. *J Natl Cancer Inst Monogr* 1992; 11:173–180.

McShane LM, Altman DG, Sauerbrei W et al. Reporting recommendations for tumor marker prognostic studies. *J Natl Cancer Inst* 2005; 97:1180–1184.

Miller AJ. *Subset Selection in Regression.* London, U.K.: Chapman & Hall, 1990.

Olschewski M, Schumacher M, Davis K. Analysis of randomized and nonrandomized patients in clinical trials using the comprehensive cohort follow-up study design. *Control Clin Trials* 1992; 13:226–239.

Palta M, Amini SB. Consideration of covariates and stratification in sample size determination for survival time studies. *J Chronic Dis* 1985; 38:801–809.

Parkes MC. Accuracy of predictions of survival in later stages of cancer. *BMJ* 1972; 264:29–31.

Peduzzi P, Concato J, Feinstein AR et al. Importance of events per independent variable in proportional hazards analysis. II. Accuracy and precision of regression estimates. *J Clin Epidemiol* 1995; 48:1503–1510.

Penny W, Frost D. Neural networks in clinical medicine. *Med Decis Making* 1996; 16:386–398.

Peterson B, George SL. Sample size requirements and length of study for testing interaction in a $2 \times k$ factorial design when time-to-failure is the outcome. *Control Clin Trials* 1993; 14:511–522.

Pfisterer J, Kommoss F, Sauerbrei W et al. DNA flow cytometry in node positive breast cancer: Prognostic value and correlation to morphological and clinical factors. *Anal Quant Cytol Histol* 1995; 17:406–412.

Porzelius C, Schumacher M, Binder H. A general, prediction error-based criterion for selecting model complexity for high-dimensional survival models. *Stat Med* 2010a; 29(7–8):830–838.

Porzelius C, Schumacher M, Binder H. Sparse regression techniques in low-dimensional survival settings. *Stat Comput* 2010b; 20(2):151–163.

Ravdin PM, Clark GM. A practical application of neural network analysis for predicting outcome on individual breast cancer patients. *Breast Cancer Res Treat* 1992; 22:285–293.

Ravdin PM, Clark GM, Hilsenbeck SG et al. A demonstration that breast cancer recurrence can be predicted by neural network analysis. *Breast Cancer Res Treat* 1992; 21:47–53.

Riley RD, Abrams KR, Sutton AJ et al. Reporting of prognostic markers: Current problems and development of guidelines for evidence based practice in the future. *Br J Cancer* 2003; 88:1191–1198.

Riley RD, Sauerbrei W, Altman DG. Prognostic markers in cancer: The evolution of evidence from single studies to meta-analysis, and beyond. *Br J Cancer* 2009; 100:1219–1229.

Ripley BD. Statistical aspects of neural networks. In: Barndorff-Nielsen OE, Jensen JL, eds. *Networks and Chaos—Statistical and Probabilistic Aspects.* London, U.K.: Chapman & Hall, 1993.

Ripley BD. *Pattern Recognition and Neural Networks.* Cambridge, U.K.: University Press, 1996.

Ripley RM. Neural network models for breast cancer prognosis. PhD dissertation, University of Oxford, Department of Engineering Science, Oxford, U.K., 1998.

Ripley RM, Harris AL, Tarassenko L. Non-linear survival analysis using neural networks. *Stat Med* 2004; 23:825–842.

Ripley BD, Ripley RM. Neural networks as statistical methods in survival analysis. In: Dybowski R, Gant V, eds. *Clinical Application of Artificial Neural Networks*. New York: Cambridge University Press, 2001.

Robins JM, Rotnitzky A, Zhao LD. Estimation of regression coefficients when some regressors are not always observed. *J Am Stat Assoc* 1994; 89:846–866.

Rothman KJ, Greenland S, Lash TL. *Modern Epidemiology*, 3rd edn. Philadelphia, PA: Lippincott Williams & Wilkins, 2008.

Rothwell PM. Treating Individuals 2. Subgroup analysis in randomised controlled trials: Importance, indications, and interpretation. *Lancet* 2005; 365:176–186.

Royston P, Altman DG. Regression using fractional polynomials of continuous covariates: Parsimonious parametric modelling (with discussion). *Appl Stat* 1994; 43:429–467.

Royston P, Sauerbrei W. Stability of multivariable fractional polynomial models with selection of variables and transformations: A bootstrap investigation. *Stat Med* 2003; 22:639–659.

Royston P, Sauerbrei W. A new approach to modelling interactions between treatment and continuous covariates in clinical trials by using fractional polynomials. *Stat Med* 2004a; 23:2509–2525.

Royston P, Sauerbrei W. A new measure of prognostic separation in survival data. *Stat Med* 2004b; 23:723–748.

Royston P, Altman DG, Sauerbrei W. Dichotomizing continuous predictors in multiple regression: A bad idea. *Stat Med* 2006; 25:127–141.

Royston P, Sauerbrei W. Interactions between treatment and continuous covariates—A step towards individualizing therapy (Editorial). *J Clin Oncol* 2008a; 26:1397–1399.

Royston P, Sauerbrei W. *Multivariable Model-Building. A Pragmatic Approach to Regression Analysis Based on Fractional Polynomials for Modelling Continuous Variables*. Chichester, U.K.: John Wiley & Sons Ltd., 2008b.

Sauerbrei W. Comparison of variable selection procedures in regression models—A simulation study and practical examples. In: Michaelis J, Hommel G, Wellek S, eds. Europäische Perspektiven der Medizinischen Informatik, Biometrie und Epidemiologie. München, Germany: MMV, pp. 108–113, 1993.

Sauerbrei W. On the development and validation of classification schemes in survival data. In: Klar R, Opitz O, eds. *Classification and Knowledge Organization*. Berlin, Germany: Springer, pp. 509–518, 1997.

Sauerbrei W. The use of resampling methods to simplify regression models in medical statistics. *Appl Stat* 1999; 48:313–329.

Sauerbrei W. Prognostic factors—Confusion caused by bad quality of design, analysis and reporting of many studies. In: Bier H, ed. *Current Research in Head and Neck Cancer: Advances in Oto-Rhino-Laryngology*, Vol. 62. Basel, Switzerland: Karger, pp. 184–200, 2005.

Sauerbrei W, Holländer N, Riley RD, Altman DG. Evidence-based assessment and application of prognostic markers: The long way from single studies to meta-analysis. *Commun Stat Theory Methods* 2006; 35:1333–1342.

Sauerbrei W, Hübner K, Schmoor C et al. for the German Breast Cancer Study Group. Validation of existing and development of new prognostic classification schemes in node negative breast cancer. *Breast Cancer Res Treat* 1997; 42:149–163; Correction. *Breast Cancer Res Treat* 1998; 48:191–192.

Sauerbrei W, Royston P. Building multivariable prognostic and diagnostic models: Transformation of the predictors by using fractional polynomials. *J R Stat Soc Ser A* 1999; 162:71–94.

Sauerbrei W, Royston P, Binder H. Selection of important variables and determination of functional form for continuous predictors in multivariable model building. *Stat Med* 2007a; 26:5512–5528.

Sauerbrei W, Royston P. Modelling to extract more information from clinical trials data: On some roles of the bootstrap. *Stat Med* 2007b; 26:4989–5001.

Sauerbrei W, Royston P, Bojar H et al. and the German Breast Cancer Study Group (GBSG). Modelling the effects of standard prognostic factors in node positive breast cancer. *Br J Cancer* 1999; 79:1752–1760.

Sauerbrei W, Royston P, Zapien K. Detecting an interaction between treatment and a continuous covariate: A comparison of two approaches. *Comput Stat Data Anal* 2007b; 51:4054–4063.

Sauerbrei W, Schumacher M. A bootstrap resampling procedure for model building: Application to the Cox regression model. *Stat Med* 1992; 11:2093–2109.

Schemper M. The explained variation in proportional hazards regression. *Biometrika* 1990; 77:216–218; Correction. *Biometrika* 1994; 81:631.

Schemper M, Henderson R. Predictive accuracy and explained variation in Cox regression. *Biometrics* 2000; 56:249–255.

Schemper M, Stare J. Explained variation in survival analysis. *Stat Med* 1996; 15:1999–2012.

Schmoor C, Olschewski M, Schumacher M. Randomized and non-randomized patients in clinical trials: Experiences with comprehensive cohort studies. *Stat Med* 1996; 15:263–271.

Schmoor C, Sauerbrei W, Schumacher M. Sample size considerations for the evaluation of prognostic factors in survival analysis. *Stat Med* 2000; 19:441–452.

Schmoor C, Ulm K, Schumacher M. Comparison of the Cox model and the regression tree procedure in analyzing a randomized clinical trial. *Stat Med* 1993; 12:2351–2366.

Schoenfeld DA. The asymptotic properties of nonparametric tests for comparing survival distributions. *Biometrika* 1981; 68:316–319.

Schoenfeld DA. Sample size formula for the proportional-hazard regression model. *Biometrics* 1983; 39:499–503.

Schumacher M, Bastert G, Bojar H et al. for the German Breast Cancer Study Group. Randomized $2 \times 2$ trial evaluating hormonal treatment and the duration of chemotherapy in node-positive breast cancer patients. *J Clin Oncol* 1994; 12:2086–2093.

Schumacher M, Binder H, Gerds T. Assessment of survival prediction models based on microarray data. *Bioinformatics* 2007; 23:1768–1774.

Schumacher M, Graf E, Gerds T. How to assess prognostic models for survival data: A case study in oncology. *Methods Inform Med* 2003; 42:564–571.

Schumacher M, Holländer N, Sauerbrei W. Reduction of bias caused by model building. *Proceedings of the Statistical Computing Section*, Alexandria, VA: American Statistical Association, 1996a; pp. 1–7.

Schumacher M, Holländer N, Sauerbrei W. Resampling and cross-validation techniques: A tool to reduce bias caused by model building. *Stat Med* 1997; 16:2813–2827.

Schumacher M, Rossner R, Vach W. Neural networks and logistic regression: Part I. *Comput Stat Data Anal* 1996b; 21:661–682.

Schwarz G. Estimating the dimension of a model. *Ann Stat* 1978; 6:461–464.

Schwarzer G, Vach W, Schumacher M. On the misuses of artificial neural networks for prognostic and diagnostic classification in oncology. *Stat Med* 2000; 19:541–561.

Segal MR. Regression trees for censored data. *Biometrics* 1988; 44:35–47.

Segal MR. Tree-structured survival analysis in medical research. In: Everitt BS, Dunn G, eds. *Statistical Analysis of Medical Data: New Developments*. London, U.K.: Arnold, pp. 101–125, 1998.

Shapiro AR. The evaluation of clinical predictions. *N Engl J Med* 1997; 296:1509–1514.

Simon R. Patients subsets and variation in therapeutic efficacy. *Br J Cancer* 1982; 14:473–482.

Simon R. Use of regression models: Statistical aspects. In: Buyse ME, Staquet MJ, Sylvester RJ, eds. *Cancer Clinical Trials: Methods and Practice*. Oxford, U.K.: Oxford University Press, pp. 444–466, 1984.

Simon R. Roadmap for developing and validating therapeutically relevant genomic classifiers. *J Clin Oncol* 2005; 23(29):7332–7341.

Simon R, Altman DG. Statistical aspects of prognostic factor studies in oncology. *Br J Cancer* 1994; 69:979–985.

Simon R, Radmacher M., Dobbin K et al. Pitfalls in the use of DNA microarray data for diagnostic and prognostic classification. *J Natl Cancer Inst* 2003; 95(1):14–18.

Stern HS. Neural networks in applied statistics (with discussion). *Technometrics* 1996; 38:205–220.

Sterne JAC, White IR, Carlin JB et al. Multiple imputation for missing data in epidemiological and clinical research: Potential and pitfalls. *BMJ* 2009; 338:b2393.

Steyerberg EW. *Clinical Prediction Models: A Practical Approach to Development, Validation, and Updating.* Berlin, Germany: Springer 2009.

Steyerberg EW, Vickers AJ, Cook NR et al. Assessing the performance of prediction models: A framework for traditional and novel measures. *Epidemiology* 2010; 21:128–138.

Teräsvirta T, Mellin I. Model selection criteria and model selection tests in regression models. *Scand J Stat* 1986; 13:159–171.

Therneau TM, Grambsch PM. *Modeling Survival Data.* New York: Springer, 2000.

Tibshirani R. The lasso method for variable selection in the Cox model. *Stat Med* 1997; 16(4):385–395.

Tibshirani R, LeBlanc M. A strategy for binary description and classification. *J Comput Graph Stat* 1992; 1:3–20.

Tutz G, Binder H. Boosting ridge regression. *Comput Stat Data Anal* 2007; 51(12):6044–6059.

Vach W. *Logistic Regression with Missing Values in the Covariates.* Lecture Notes in Statistics 86. New York: Springer, 1994.

Vach W. On the relation between the shrinkage effect and a shrinkage method. *Comput Stat* 1997a; 12:279–292.

Vach W. Some issues in estimating the effect of prognostic factors from incomplete covariate data. *Stat Med* 1997b; 16:57–72.

Valsecchi MG, Silvestri D. Evaluation of long-term survival: Use of diagnostics and robust estimators with Cox's proportional hazards model. *Stat Med* 1996; 15:2763–2780.

Van Belle V, Van Calster B, Brouckaert O et al. Qualitative assessment of the progesterone receptor and HER2 improves the Nottingham Prognostic Index up to 5 years after breast cancer diagnosis. *J Clin Oncol* 2010; 28:4129–4134.

Van Houwelingen HC, Le Cessie S. Predictive value of statistical models. *Stat Med* 1990; 9:1303–1325.

Verweij P, Van Houwelingen HC. Cross-validation in survival analysis. *Stat Med* 1993; 12:2305–2314.

Vittinghoff E, McCulloch CE. Relaxing the rule of ten events per variable in logistic and Cox regression. *Am J Epidemiol* 2007; 165:710–718.

Wang R, Lagakos SW, Ware JH et al. Statistics in medicine—Reporting of subgroup analyses in clinical trials. *N Engl J Med* 2007; 357:2189–2194.

Warner B, Misra M. Understanding neural networks as statistical tools. *American Statistician* 1996; 50:284–293.

Wehberg S, Schumacher M. A comparison of nonparametric error rate estimation methods in classification problems. *Biom J* 2004; 46:35–47.

Worsley KJ. An improved Bonferroni inequality and applications. *Biometrika* 1982; 69:297–302.

Wyatt J. Nervous about artificial neural networks? *Lancet* 1995; 346:1175–1177.

Wyatt JC, Altman DG. Prognostic models: Clinically useful or quickly forgotten? Commentary. *BMJ* 1995; 311:1539–1541.

Zhang H, Crowley J, Sox HC et al. Tree-structured statistical methods. In: Armitage P, Colton T, eds. *Encyclopedia of Biostatistics.* Chichester, U.K.: Wiley, pp. 4561–4573, 1998.

Zou H. The adaptive lasso and its oracle properties. *J Am Stat Assoc* 2006; 101(476):1418–1429.

# 26 Predictive Modeling of Gene Expression Data

*Alexander Hapfelmeier, Waheed Babatunde
Yahya, Robert Rosenberg, and Kurt Ulm*

## CONTENTS

## 26.1 INTRODUCTION

The treatment of cancer has changed over the past centuries, moving away from the administration of broadly acting cytotoxic drugs toward the use of more specific therapies (van't Veer and Bernards [33]). There is a shift from a "one-size" or "one-dose-fits-all" approach to a more personalized medicine. The idea behind this is to give the right dose of the right drug for the right indication for the right patient in the right time. Hamburg and Collins [12] called this approach a path to personalized medicine and described the need for the Food and Drug Administration (FDA) and National Institutes of Health (NIH) to support its growth. They gave three examples of FDA-approved drugs and diagnostics.

Such an approach requires the discovery and development of biomarkers. The identification of prognostic and/or predictive biomarkers is a great challenge for statisticians. For instance, the number of patients available is much smaller than the number of biomarkers. In order to evaluate the impact of certain markers, special methods of statistical modeling have to be applied.

In the following, we want to present some of the methods available for the selection of relevant predictive biomarkers by the example of microarray data from a study about neoadjuvant radiochemotherapy for colorectal cancer.

## 26.2 METHODS

### 26.2.1 PRELIMINARY VARIABLE SELECTION

Many statistical methods used for classification do not provide intrinsic variable selection. Among them are popular approaches like linear discriminant analysis (LDA), support vector machines (SVM), $k$-nearest neighbors ($k$-NN), and neural networks (NN). However, it is well known that the performance and interpretability of such methods can benefit from a reduction of the input space (Hastie et al. [14]). Therefore, the objective is to find a suitable subset of the entire variable space $X = \{X_1, X_2, ..., X_p\}$ a prediction method of choice should be fitted to. One possibility is to base this decision on the univariate (marginal) discriminatory power of the variables which can be measured by means of $t$-tests, Mann–Whitney $U$ tests, the area under the ROC curve (AUC), Bayesian approaches, among many others. Having examined the corresponding statistics or $p$-values, one is able to rank the variables by their strength of association to the response which leads to $X_{rank} = \{X_{(1)}, X_{(2)}, ..., X_{(p)}\}$. Assuming a descending order $X_{(1)}$ and $X_{(p)}$ are the variables with the strongest and weakest associations, respectively. Based on this ranking, two selection procedures can be differentiated.

One algorithm simply chooses the first $r$ variables, while $r$ denotes a certain fraction. The aim is to limit the number of variables to the ones with the largest discriminatory power in a marginal, univariate sense. The corresponding subset is $X_{first} = \{X_{(1)}, ..., X_{(\lfloor p \times r \rfloor)}\}$, with $\lVert \rVert$ being any measure that rounds to an integer. In some datasets with highly correlated variables, which is a known feature of microarray data, this approach can lead to a profound loss of information. Due to strong relations, selected variables might only provide very similar information. By contrast, the omitted ones, though they are weaker predictors on their own, could very well contribute additional information.

Another algorithm suggested by Jaeger et al. [17] tries to overcome this pitfall by limiting the selection to variables with correlations below a specified threshold $r$. As it incorporates bivariate correlations, this approach is not termed "univariate" but "semi-multivariate." Following the ranking order and starting with the strongest variable, the selection is built up by sequentially adding variables that have no stronger correlation than $r$ with already selected ones. The resulting set of variables $X_{uncor} = \{X_{(1)}, ..., X_{(u)}\}$ may not have performed equally well in univariate analysis but may contribute different kinds of information. The pseudoalgorithm to determine $X_{uncor}$ is as follows:

1. Set $i = 1$ and $X_{uncor} = X_{(1)}$.
2. If $i = p$ then stop and return $X_{uncor}$, else proceed.
3. Set $i = i + 1$.
4. If any $\rho(X_{uncor}, X_{(i)}) > r$ then go back to step 2, else proceed.
5. Set $X_{uncor} = \{X_{uncor}, X_{(i)}\}$ and go back to step 2.

with $\rho(X_{uncor}, X_{(i)})$ denoting Pearson's correlation coefficients between all elements of $X_{uncor}$ and $X_{(i)}$. Step 1 indicates that the entire process starts with the selection of $X_{(1)}$, producing a result that highly depends on this particular choice.

The different features of both approaches can be seen as advantageous and disadvantageous at the same time depending on the objective of research. Thus, Nicodemus et al. [21] stated that in large-scale screening studies like genome-wide association studies, a selection of correlated markers may help to uncover physical proximities and causal variants. By contrast, when it comes to prediction, it can prove beneficial to use uncorrelated predictors as shown by Hapfelmeier and Horsch [13] for the example of cancer classification in mammographic screenings. In summary, one should choose $X_{first}$ to explicitly aim at the identification of correlated structures with strong marginal associations to the response. For prediction purposes, $X_{uncor}$ has shown to lead to a higher accuracy and is therefore considered to be more appropriate. As the latter is consistent with the objective of this chapter, it is preferred in the following examples.

## 26.2.2 DIMENSION REDUCTION

Roughly speaking, dimension reduction methods like principal component analysis (PCA) and partial least squares (PLS) try to reduce the variable space $X \in \mathbb{R}^{n \times p}$ by concentrating its information in a few components $C \in \mathbb{R}^{n \times q}$, $q \ll p$. These are subsequently used for the fitting of classification methods, which could not deal with the original high-dimensional variable space. A corresponding example is given by Boulesteix and Strimmer [3] who combine PLS with LDA. Prior research of Nguyen and Rocke [19,20] has already shown that this combination is well suited for tumor classification using microarray data. However, due to the fact that the information of all variables is aggregated in a few components, it is difficult to perform variable selection. The latter is known to improve performance as shown by works of Statnikov et al. [29] and Lee et al. [18]. Yet it is not an intrinsic property of dimension reduction. In addition, the amount of components $m$ has to be determined by the user. However, a main objective of this chapter is to provide an overview of common and popular approaches that enable variable selection and sound prediction performances. Thus dimension reduction methods are excluded from further consideration in the following.

### 26.2.2.1 Linear Discriminant Analysis

After the reduction of the variable space, either by preliminary variable selection or dimension reduction, many common statistical classification methods, which by themselves are not able to deal with the $n \ll p$ problem, become applicable again.

Examples are SVM, NN, logistic regression, and linear discriminant analysis (LDA). The latter will be used as a representative of this technique in the following.

The LDA, as described by Hastie et al. [14], provides estimations of class probabilities dependent on the input vector of an observation $x \in \mathbb{R}^p$. Using Bayes theorem, the posteriori probability for a class $Y$ can be expressed as

$$P(Y = k \mid X = x) = \frac{f_k(x)\pi_k}{\sum_{l=1}^{K} f_l(x)\pi_l},$$  (26.1)

with $\pi_k$ denoting the prior probability of the class labels $k$, $k=1, \ldots, K$. Thus LDA is applicable to a multiclass problem and reduces to $k=0,1$ in the case of a binary response. The class-conditional density of $X$,

$$f_k(x) = \frac{1}{(2\pi)^{p/2} |\Sigma|^{1/2}} e^{(-1/2)(x-\mu_k)^\top \Sigma^{-1}(x-\mu_k)},$$  (26.2)

is assumed to follow a multivariate Gaussian distribution with a unique covariance matrix $\Sigma$ for all classes. As the true prior class probabilities and parameters of the Gaussian distribution are unknown, they have to be estimated by means of their empirical analogs. The decision for a class label of a new observation may now be based on the maximum posterior probability.

### 26.2.3 PENALIZATION AND SHRINKAGE

Another approach closely related to regression analysis is given by shrinkage methods. Corresponding models are estimated under the constraint of a penalty on the size of the regression coefficients which enables implicit variable selection. Popular examples are ridge regression and least absolute shrinkage and selection operators (LASSO). According to Tibshirani [32], the latter produces coefficient estimates under the assumption of standardized data $x_{ij}$ such that $\sum_i x_{ij}/n = 0$ and $\sum_i x_{ij}^2/n = 1$. For linear regression purposes, the estimation is given by

$$\hat{\beta} = \text{argmin} \left\{ \sum_{i=1}^{n} \left( y_i - \beta_0 - \sum_{j=1}^{p} \beta_j x_{ij} \right)^2 \right\} \quad \text{subject to} \quad \sum_{j=1}^{p} |\beta_j| \leq t.$$  (26.3)

Similarly generalized regression models can be constructed by maximizing the log-likelihood $l(\beta)$ such that

$$\hat{\beta} = \text{argmax}\{l(\beta)\} \quad \text{subject to} \quad \sum_{j=1}^{p} |\beta_j| \leq t.$$  (26.4)

By contrast to ridge regression, which uses a constraint of $\sum_j \beta_j^2 \leq t$, the penalty $\sum_j |\beta_j| \leq t$ ensures that some of the coefficients are exactly shrunk to zero, which implies an intrinsic variable selection. In equivalence to logistic regression, class probabilities can be estimated using its logit-link to the linear predictor $X^T \beta$:

$$P(Y = 1 \mid X = x) = \frac{e^{x^T \beta}}{1 + e^{x^T \beta}}. \tag{26.5}$$

### 26.2.4 MACHINE LEARNING APPROACHES

A popular machine learning approach, is recursive partitioning. A famous representative is given by classification and regression trees (CART) of Breiman et al. [7]. Its rationale is to repeatedly split data into binary subsets that are as homogeneous as possible in respect to the response. The split itself is performed by optimal cutpoints in single variables of the data. There are several criteria for the determination of the quality of a split. Thus for binary responses the Gini-Gain, or for regression the reduction of the residual sum of squares, can be used to evaluate the improvement of homogeneity between the data and its subsets. The splitting continues until a stopping rule is reached. This might be the minimum number of observations in a subset, a threshold for the split criterion or a certain size that leads to the best accuracy as assessed by cross-validation. An alternative approach for the creation of trees given by Hothorn et al. [16] is based on a conditional inference framework. It grows trees until the variables in a subset show no significant relation to the response. The binary splitting provides decision rules along the corresponding cutpoints, which guide an observation $x_i$ to a prediction $\hat{y}_i$. The latter is derived from the majority vote of classes or the average of responses given in a final subset. Using a $(0,1)$-vector of case weights $w(x)$ that indicates which observation is contained in the same subset as $x$ the probability estimate for a binary response becomes

$$P_{tree}(Y = 1 \mid X = x) = \left( w(x)^T 1 \right)^{-1} w(x)^T y, \tag{26.6}$$

which is simply the mean. A big advantage of this method is its ability to deal with the $n \ll p$ problem as each variable is assessed individually as a candidate for a split. Likewise, it automatically performs variable selection by choosing a certain set of variables. The structure of subsequent binary divisions makes it possible to automatically form interacting relations between the variables. This last property is a big advantage over regression analysis, for which interaction terms have to be explicitly modeled.

Breiman [5] enhanced the tree methodology by "bagging," which leads to an improved prediction accuracy. Trees are fit to bootstrapped samples of the data to build an ensemble. Random Forests as introduced by Breiman [6] extend this approach by choosing splits in a random selection of variables. Thus even highly correlated variables are able to equally contribute to a Random Forest. The single trees are grown to a maximal size until the final subsets are pure (i.e., contain only one class) or reach a minimal size. Averaged values or majority votes of the outputs given by each single tree are used as predictions:

$$P_{Forest}(Y = 1 \mid X = x) = \frac{1}{N_{trees}} \sum_{t=1}^{N_{trees}} P_t(Y = 1 \mid X = x). \tag{26.7}$$

Although the property of variable selection gets lost by consolidating several trees the strength of a variable's contribution to a Random Forest can still be measured by means of importance measures. For instance, the permutation importance measure is computed as the error of a tree is compared to the error it produces when a variable is randomly permuted. Thus it checks for differences of a tree's accuracy when a variable loses its relation to the response and therefore its predictive value. In alignment to a formulation given by Strobl et al. [30], the permutation importance is

$$VI(X_j) = \frac{1}{N_{trees}} \sum_{t=1}^{N_{trees}} \left( \frac{\sum_{i \in \bar{B}^{(t)}} I(y_i = \hat{y}_i^{(t)})}{|\bar{B}^{(t)}|} - \frac{\sum_{i \in \bar{B}^{(t)}} I(y_i = \hat{y}_{i,\pi j}^{(t)})}{|\bar{B}^{(t)}|} \right), \tag{26.8}$$

while

$\pi_j$ denotes the random permutation of $X_j$

$I()$ is a function indicating whether the prediction equals the true response status

$\bar{B}^{(t)}$ is the out of bag sample (OOB) of tree $t$

The OOB sample is made up of the observations of the bootstrap sample, which are not used for the fitting of a tree. It therefore enables an unbiased estimation of a variable's importance.

### 26.2.5 ALTERNATIVE: THE *k*-SS METHOD

The *k*-sequential feature selection and response class prediction (*k*-SS) method (Yahya et al. [36]) provides a fast and flexible algorithm that sequentially selects relevant gene predictors to classify tumor conditions in any binary response microarray problems. It represents a stepwise feature selection method that adopts the misclassification error rate (MER), which is based on the absolute error loss function:

$$\hat{\vartheta} = \frac{1}{n} \sum_{i=1}^{n} I(y_i = \hat{y}_i), \tag{26.9}$$

where $I()$ is a function indicating whether a prediction $\hat{y}_i$ equals the true response status with $y_i$

In a preliminary step, the discriminatory power of each gene variable $X_j$, $j = 1, \ldots, p$, is assessed as logistic regression models (in general any decision rule can be applied) are fit and evaluated in a Monte Carlo cross-validation (MCCV) scheme.

This resampling technique is adopted by repeatedly drawing ($s$ user specified times) a certain fraction ($m < n$) of samples as training set without replacement. By fitting a classifier to these training sets and computing its MER $\hat{\vartheta}_l$, $l = 1, \ldots, s$, on the remaining ($n - m$) test samples, one is able to assess the average performance $\widehat{\vartheta}$ of a classifier over $s$ repetitions.

The gene variable $X_{(1)}$ that yields the least of the average MER values $\left(\widehat{\vartheta}_{(1)}\right)$ among all values $\widehat{\vartheta}_j, j = 1, \ldots, p$ is selected at the first gene selection step as it showed the highest discriminatory power. To select the second best gene predictor $X_{(2)}$ at the second feature selection and classification step, a set of $p - 1$ pairs of genes is formed with the first selected gene and the remaining $p - 1$ left out genes. A logistic regression model is constructed on each gene pair and the average MER is computed following the same MCCV procedure described earlier. At the end of this exercise, the gene pair that yielded the least average MER $\widehat{\vartheta}_{(2)}$ is selected.

In the $k$th selection step the marginal gain in prediction strength $\hat{\Delta}_k = \widehat{\vartheta}_{(k)} - \widehat{\vartheta}_{(k+1)}$ due to the inclusion of $X_{(k+1)}$ into the classification model is examined by testing the hypothesis $H_{0k}:\Delta_k = 0$ vs. $H_{1k}:\Delta_k > 0$ via the test statistic

$$Z_{\hat{\Delta}_k} = \frac{\hat{\Delta}_k - E\left(\hat{\Delta}_k\right)}{\sqrt{v\left(\hat{\Delta}_k\right)}}, \tag{26.10}$$

while $v$ denotes the empirical variance. $Z_{\hat{\Delta}_k}$ follows a skew-normal distribution with shape parameter $\lambda = 4.0398$. When the null $H_{0k}$ cannot be rejected, the $(k+1)$th gene $X_{(k+1)}$ under consideration is dropped from the classification model and the $k$-SS algorithm terminates assuming that no other gene variable among the remaining $p - k$ genes is strong enough to improve the prediction strength of the current classification model. However, if $H_{1k}$ is accepted, this shows that $X_{(k+1)}$ has significantly enhanced the prediction strength of the preceding classification model and should therefore be included.

Lastly, the $k$-SS algorithm performs backward checks at each feature selection step. It enables any selected gene to be checked for its redundancy anytime a new feature is introduced into the classification model. Therefore, a model is fit by removing each of the previously selected features at any one time. If $\widehat{\vartheta}_{remove} \leq \widehat{\vartheta}_{full}$, it shows that the removed feature is now redundant in the presence of a newly selected feature, and it is subsequently removed from the model. If no gene is rejected this way after a terminating forward step the set of $k$ marker genes for classification, for example, by logistic regression, becomes the selected $k$-SS classifiers.

## 26.3 PERFORMANCE EVALUATION

Investigating a model's prediction accuracy on the same data it was fit to leads to overoptimistic results and thus to a bias. This procedure is also called "resubstitution" and is prone to overfitting a classifier to the data at hand. Especially when there are many predictor variables, which is usually the case for microarray data, it is easy to construct a model that perfectly discriminates the response classes. However, this kind of classifier only conforms to the learning data and will hardly perform as well on new observations. There are several approaches that try to simulate the latter scenario and are supposed to provide less biased estimates of performance measures. An elaborate listing and description of sampling schemes can be found in Boulesteix et al. [4]. They give a fast overview of applications to microarray data analysis without limitation of generalizability. A more profound investigation of corresponding properties is given by Hastie et al. [14].

A popular approach simply splits the data into a learning and a test set. Now any model can be fit to the learning set while the test set is left untouched and is only used for validation purposes. Another similar approach is given by $f$-fold cross-validation, which splits the data in $f$ parts. Taking $f$ turns, the $f$th part is used as the test set while the model is fit to the remaining observations. The average performance is returned as final result. There are some disadvantages like a high variability and a too pessimistic assessment of results as only a fraction of the available information is used for the training of the classifier. The latter property also holds for the popular bootstrap approach. It repeatedly draws observations with replacement from the data to build up the training set. On average this leads to a selection of $1 - (1 - 1/n)^n \approx 1 - e^{-1} = 63.2\%$ of observations. Again the remaining observations are used as evaluation set. Facing the problem of biased estimates, Efron and Tibshirani [10] introduced the .632+ estimator. It returns a weighted sum of the overoptimistic resubstitution estimate and the too pessimistic bootstrap estimate. Thus a less biased estimate of the AUC is given by

$$\widehat{AUC}_{.632+} = .368 \cdot \widehat{AUC}_{resub} + .632 \cdot \widehat{AUC}_{boot}. \tag{26.11}$$

The .632+ estimator of the AUC will also be used in the following example. Measuring the area under the curve (AUC) of the corresponding ROC curve is a well-suited means to assess the predictive power of a classification method. For each possible cutpoint in a model's prediction output (e.g., linear predictor, response probabilities), the sensitivity is plotted against 1-specificity and displayed by a step function to build the ROC curves. The AUC is simply the area between this graph and the abscissa. A value that tends to 1 indicates a model with strong discriminative power, while a value of .5 indicates no power at all (random guessing). The latter case is represented by the diagonal in the coordinate system. As shown by Bamber [2], the AUC also equals the probability that the value of a model's prediction is higher for an observation belonging to the response class of concern (e.g., malignant tissue) than for an observation belonging to the reference class (e.g., benign tissue).

## 26.4 RECTAL CANCER EXAMPLE

### 26.4.1 DESCRIPTION OF THE DATA

The application of neoadjuvant radiochemotherapy is a common treatment of locally advanced rectal cancer. It supports a complete resection of the tumor by shrinking its size. However, not every patient seems to be responsive to this therapy, which in such a case can be harmful as it induces possible side effects and delays surgery or further adjuvant treatment. Consequently, there is a strong need for a personalized treatment that is adapted to the response prediction of a patient. The analysis of microarray data, containing transcription profiles of responders and nonresponders, can be used to identify differentially expressed genes. Furthermore statistical models can be fit to obtain estimations of response probabilities.

This study is based on 43 biopsy specimens (observations) of patients treated in the Department of Surgery, Klinikum rechts der Isar, Munich, Germany. Expression profiles of 24,026 genes were assessed. Tissue samples with less than 10% viable tumor cells after radiochemotherapy were classified as responders. There are 29 responders and 14 nonresponders in the data. More detailed information about patient and treatment characteristics as well as tissue and data preparation can be found in Rimkus et al. [24] originally using the data for prediction of response status.

### 26.4.2 ANALYSIS SETTINGS

All computations were performed with the R system for statistical computing [23]. The analysis of the data is based on four different predictive modeling strategies. These are LDA with preliminary variable selection, LASSO, Random Forests, and the $k$-SS approach. The performance of each method is assessed by the $\widehat{AUC}_{.632+}$ estimator using 100 bootstrap samples. For computational reasons, all analyses are restricted to 300 genes, which provide the highest AUC values in a univariate analysis. This approach extremely reduces computation time while it is unlikely to affect classification performance by a significant extent as shown by Yahya et al. [36].

To examine different kinds of thresholds $r$ for the preliminary variable selection, a sequence of values between 0 and 1 was chosen to fit several models. Generally, a broad span ensures that the resulting variable sets range from as much as a few single features up to all available features. However, as the data at hand consist of a huge number of variables, low values of $r$ are chosen to produce sparse models, which are supposed to yield preferable performance results. In order to produce four LDA models, $r$ is set to .1, .2, .3, and .4. An implementation of LDA is given by the function lda(), which is part of the package MASS (Venaples and Ripley [34]).

The LASSO approach is realized by the function cv.glmnet() belonging to the package glmnet (Friedman et al. [11]). The default settings use 10-fold cross-validation to determine the optimal penalization for the construction of the model. Following the 1se rule, the sparsest model that provides a cross-validated error, which is within a range of one standard error (1se) from the lowest mean error given by the best model is chosen.

Random Forests were constructed to contain 100 trees. In each node, a random subset of 17 variables is tested to find eligible split criteria. This number equals the square root of 300 available variables, which is reported to be optimal in many situations (Díaz-Uriarte and Alvarez de Andrés [8]). An implementation of conditional inference based Random Forests is given by the function cforest(), which is part of the package party (Hothorn et al. [15]).

The $k$-SS approach was realized by the authors' own implementation. Within a range of 20 values for the alpha error reaching from .001 to .999, it uses 10-fold cross-validation to determine a subset of variables leading to the lowest cross-validated error.

## 26.4.3 RESULTS

### 26.4.3.1 Performance

Table 26.1 shows bootstrap-, resubstitution-, and .632+-estimators of the AUC as well as the number of selected genes for the investigated classifiers. In terms of $\widehat{\text{AUC}}_{boot}$, these values reach from .747 for the $k$-SS approach to .910 for LDA ($r=.4$). An examination of the variability is given by corresponding 2.5% and 97.5% percentiles, which, according to extensive studies of the bootstrap by Efron and Tibshirani [9], can be used for the computation of 95% confidence intervals. Although there are differences in the mean bootstrapped AUC values, the strong overlap of confidence intervals makes it difficult to identify a method that acts clearly superior. It has to be pointed out that the $k$-SS approach achieves these results using only 2.4 genes on average while the LDA ($r=.4$) makes use of the information of about 14.3 genes. For the computation of the $\widehat{\text{AUC}}_{.632+}$ (see Equation 26.11) one has to determine the $\widehat{\text{AUC}}_{resub}$, which reflects the performance a classifier achieves on the same data it was fit to. The lowest value of .951 can be observed for the LDA ($r=.1$) meaning that all classifiers perform extremely well in this case. Surprisingly even the $k$-SS approach, which tends to produce sparse models and is therefore not prone to overfitting, is able to produce an $\widehat{\text{AUC}}_{resub}$ of 1 with only three genes. Other classifiers like the

---

**TABLE 26.1**

**Bootstrap-, Resubstitution- and .632+-Estimators of the AUC for the Investigated Classifiers**

|  | LDA | | | | | | |
|---|---|---|---|---|---|---|---|
|  | $r=0.1$ | $r=0.2$ | $r=0.3$ | $r=0.4$ | LASSO | Forest | $k$-SS |
| $\widehat{\text{AUC}}_{boot}$ | 0.816 | 0.857 | 0.901 | 0.910 | 0.813 | 0.892 | 0.747 |
| Percentile 97.5% | 0.973 | 1.000 | 1.000 | 1.000 | 0.987 | 1.000 | 0.955 |
| 2.5% | 0.590 | 0.619 | 0.698 | 0.698 | 0.621 | 0.722 | 0.546 |
| Genes selected | 3.0 | 4.3 | 7.6 | 14.3 | 11.7 | 300 | 2.4 |
| $\widehat{\text{AUC}}_{resub}$ | 0.951 | 0.993 | 0.998 | 1.000 | 1.000 | 1.000 | 1.000 |
| Genes selected | 3 | 4 | 9 | 20 | 20 | 300 | 3 |
| $\widehat{\text{AUC}}_{.632+}$ | 0.866 | 0.907 | 0.937 | 0.943 | 0.882 | 0.932 | 0.840 |

Variability of the bootstrap-estimator is represented by 2.5%- and 97.5%-quantiles. In addition, the complexity of models is given by the average number of chosen variables based on 100 bootstrap samples and for a single fit on the entire data.

---

LASSO incorporate 20 genes to reach such a high classification accuracy. Finally the .632+-estimators of the AUC reach from .840 for the $k$-SS approach to .943 for the LDA ($r = .40$).

### 26.4.3.2    Gene Selection

It is a well-known approach to evaluate the stability of a model by the application of variable selection to several bootstrap samples while counting the number of times a variable is chosen. Many examples for stepwise selection methods in linear, logistic, or Cox regression models have been investigated by Sauerbrei [26] and Austin and Tu [1]. Another aim is the improvement of prediction accuracy by fitting models to the most frequently chosen variables. Both matters are also addressed in an extensive work about modeling strategies by Sauerbrei et al. [27]. Further examples for microarray data can also be found in Qiu et al. [22]. Table 26.2 shows the five most frequently selected genes for each classification method.

There are many genes that are commonly chosen by the models (e.g., USP48, TMC8 etc.) and thus indicate strong and stable predictors. This even holds for different kinds of model strategies like regression, discriminant analysis, and recursive partitioning. There is also some diversity, pointing to a certain instability of the selected gene sets. In summary, the application of bootstrapping as well as the comparison of several classifiers renders a broad view on potentially relevant genes possible by the assessment of selection frequencies within and between models.

**TABLE 26.2**

**Five Highest Selection Frequencies (#) of Genes in 100 Bootstrap Samples**

|  |  |  | 1 | 2 | 3 | 4 | 5 |
|---|---|---|---|---|---|---|---|
| LDA | $r = 0.1$ |  | USP48 | MKRN2 | SF3A1a | SF3A1b | DCUN1D2 |
|  |  | # | 18 | 11 | 9 | 9 | 8 |
|  | 0.2 |  | USP48 | ISCA1 | MKRN2 | NKTR | DCUN1D2 |
|  |  | # | 18 | 16 | 13 | 13 | 11 |
|  | 0.3 |  | LZTR | ISCA1 | USP48 | DCUN1D2 | NFATC3 |
|  |  | # | 31 | 25 | 21 | 15 | 15 |
|  | 0.4 |  | LZTR | ISCA1 | JUN | FAM89A | DCUN1D2 |
|  |  | # | 47 | 38 | 36 | 30 | 29 |
| LASSO |  |  | TMC8 | RBM18 | JUN | TFEC | MAF |
|  |  | # | 55 | 42 | 33 | 31 | 29 |
| Forest |  |  | TMC8 | SF3A1a | SF3A1b | USP48 | RBM18 |
|  |  | $\overline{VI}$ | 4.9e−5 | 4.7e−5 | 3.7e−5 | 3.5e−5 | 3.3e−5 |
| $k$-SS |  |  | USP48 | CASP1 | SF3A1b | TMC8 | SF3A1a |
|  |  | # | 21 | 12 | 12 | 12 | 11 |

The average variable importance ($\overline{VI}$) is given for random forests.

**TABLE 26.3**

**Genes Selected by the Classification Models on the Entire Data**

| Model | | Gene | | | | |
|---|---|---|---|---|---|---|
| LDA | $r=0.1$ | USP48 | ISCA1 | HERC4 | | |
| | 0.2 | USP48 | AP4S1 | LZTR | ISCA1 | |
| | 0.3 | USP48 | RBM18 | CCL3 | SERINC3 | LYRM4 |
| | | ISCA1 | SNRPA1 | FA2H | GLYATL1 | |
| | 0.4 | USP48 | M-RIP | CCL3 | LETM2 | LZTR |
| | | NKTR | RALGPS1 | SERINC3 | FAM89A | PIPOX |
| | | LYRM4 | TFEC | ISCA1 | TACC1 | ITGB1BP1 |
| | | DCUN1D2 | ACP6 | NFATC3 | RNF38 | TMEM43 |
| LASSO | | SF3A1a | TMC8 | BLVRAa | SDHC | TOE1 |
| | | MFN1 | RBM18 | TNFRSF1B | KPNB1 | AW34207 |
| | | MAF | AA889954 | LETM2 | LZTR | AI370381 |
| | | JUN | LYRM4 | TFEC | TBC1D4 | DCUN1D2 |
| Forest | (Top 10 of 300) | TMC8 | USP48 | SF3A1b | ZNF652 | RBM18 |
| | | STAT2 | ETS2 | BLVRAb | SDHC | MAF |
| $k$-SS | | USP48 | ETV6 | C21ORF91 | | |

Using the entire data for model fitting ensures that parameter estimation and variable selection is based on as much information as available. Table 26.3 shows the corresponding genes. Although each of the selections provides useful information on its own, it is also possible to make direct comparisons and assess the agreement. Either with or without additional information, for example, about stability, gained by bootstrapping, these findings can be used for further investigations.

## 26.5 CONCLUSION

In this chapter, we propose several methods for the identification of relevant genes and predictive models. The former ones can be found by selection methods like preliminary variable selection, based on semi-multivariate associations or intrinsic variable selection provided by some statistical classifiers. The selection can be based on the entire data or checked for consistency by sampling methods like bootstrapping.

Predictive modeling can be performed by a preferred application or by a comparison of multiple approaches. However, Slawski et al. [28] pointed out that a simultaneous evaluation of several models always risks to produce a "severe optimistic bias" by "reporting only the best results" as they might represent simple "noise discovery" and random findings. They recommend to "report all the obtained results or validate the best classifier using independent fresh validation data" instead of "fishing for low prediction errors." Consequently a fair comparison of all models is given in this study as all results are presented without excessive ratings. Two options to estimate the performance of single models, like the best one, are to evaluate it on new observations or within a combination of internal and external cross-validation.

There are some characteristics of the models that need to be pointed out. The $k$-SS approach shows a competitive performance although it uses extremely few genes for the model fit. Random Forests perform very well without any variable selection. Many authors like Tang et al. [31], Yang and Gu [37], Rodenburg et al. [25], and Díaz-Uriarte and Alvarez de Andrés [8] have investigated selection approaches based on variable importance measures to improve the prediction accuracy of Random Forests in the field of genome studies. Similarly, Wu et al. [35] give recommendations for the application of LASSO in genome-wide association studies. They discuss model optimization techniques, predictor pre-selection, and the identification of interaction effects.

In conclusion, there are diverse ways to find predictive genes and classifiers. The rectal cancer example shows that each of them may provide information that differs to a certain extend but is equally useful. By contrast, on some occasions, one might also observe an exceptionally best performing model. Either way a proper application of statistical methods followed by careful investigations are the most important steps leading to a valid interpretation and future applications.

## REFERENCES

1. P. C. Austin and J. V. Tu. Bootstrap methods for developing predictive models. *The American Statistician*, 58(2):131–137, 2004.
2. D. Bamber. The area above the ordinal dominance graph and the area below the receiver operating characteristic graph. *Journal of Mathematical Psychology*, 12(4):387–415, 1975.
3. A.-L. Boulesteix and K. Strimmer. Partial least squares: A versatile tool for the analysis of high-dimensional genomic data. *Briefings in Bioinformatics*, 8(1):32–44, 2007.
4. A.-L. Boulesteix, C. Strobl, T. Augustin, and M. Daumer. Evaluating microarray-based classifiers: An overview. *Cancer Information*, 6:77–97, 2008.
5. L. Breiman. Bagging predictors. *Machine Learning*, 24(2):123–140, 1996.
6. L. Breiman. Random forests. *Machine Learning*, 45(1):5–32, 2001.
7. L. Breiman, J. H. Friedman, R. A. Olshen, and C. J. Stone. *Classification and Regression Trees*. Chapman & Hall/CRC, Boca Raton, FL, 1984.
8. R. Díaz-Uriarte and S. Alvarez de Andrés. Gene selection and classification of microarray data using random forest. *BMC Bioinformatics*, 7(1):3, 2006.
9. B. Efron and R. J. Tibshirani. *An Introduction to the Bootstrap*. Chapman & Hall/CRC, Boca Raton, FL, May 1994.
10. B. Efron and R. J. Tibshirani. Improvements on cross-validation: The .632+ bootstrap method. *Journal of the American Statistical Association*, 92(438):548–560, 1997.
11. J. H. Friedman, T. Hastie, and R. J. Tibshirani. Regularization paths for generalized linear models via coordinate descent. *Journal of Statistical Software*, 33(1):1–22, 2010.
12. M. A. Hamburg and F. S. Collins. The path to personalized medicine. *The New England Journal of Medicine*, 363(4):301–304, 2010.
13. A. Hapfelmeier and A. Horsch. Image feature evaluation in two new mammography cad prototypes. *International Journal of Computer Assisted Radiology and Surgery*, 1–15, 2011. 10.1007/s11548-011-0549-5.
14. T. Hastie, R. J. Tibshirani, and J. H. Friedman. *The Elements of Statistical Learning*. Springer, Berlin, Germany, corrected edition, February 2009.
15. T. Hothorn, K. Hornik, C. Strobl, and A. Zeileis. Party: A laboratory for recursive part(y)itioning, 2008. R package version 0.9-9993.

16. T. Hothorn, K. Hornik, and A. Zeileis. Unbiased recursive partitioning. *Journal of Computational and Graphical Statistics*, 15(3):651–674, 2006.

17. J. Jaeger, R. Sengupta, and W. Ruzzo. Improved gene selection for classification of microarrays. In *Proceedings of Pacific Symposium on Biocomputing*, Lihue, HI, pp. 53–64, 2003.

18. J. W. Lee, J. B. Lee, M. Park, and S. H. Song. An extensive comparison of recent classification tools applied to microarray data. *Computational Statistics and Data Analysis*, 48(4):869–885, 2005.

19. D. V. Nguyen and D. M. Rocke. Tumor classification by partial least squares using microarray gene expression data. *Bioinformatics*, 18(1):39–50, 2002.

20. D. V. Nguyen and D. M. Rocke. On partial least squares dimension reduction for microarray-based classification: A simulation study. *Computational Statistics and Data Analysis*, 46(3):407–425, 2004.

21. K. Nicodemus, J. Malley, C. Strobl, and A. Ziegler. The behaviour of random forest permutation-based variable importance measures under predictor correlation. *BMC Bioinformatics*, 11(1):110+, February 2010.

22. X. Qiu, Y. Xiao, A. Gordon, and A. Yakovlev. Assessing stability of gene selection in microarray data analysis. *BMC Bioinformatics*, 7(1):50, 2006.

23. R Development Core Team. *R: A Language and Environment for Statistical Computing. R Foundation for Statistical Computing*, Vienna, Austria, 2011. ISBN 3-900051-07-0.

24. C. Rimkus, J. Friederichs, A.-L. Boulesteix, J. Theisen, J. Mages, K. Becker, H. Nekarda, R. Rosenberg, K.-P. Janssen, and J. R. Siewert. Microarray-based prediction of tumor response to neoadjuvant radiochemotherapy of patients with locally advanced rectal cancer. *Clinical Gastroenterology and Hepatology*, 6(1):53–61, 2008.

25. W. Rodenburg, A. G. Heidema, J. M. A. Boer, I. M. J. Bovee-Oudenhoven, E. J. M. Feskens, E. C. M. Mariman, and J. Keijer. A framework to identify physiological responses in microarray-based gene expression studies: Selection and interpretation of biologically relevant genes. *Physiological Genomics*, 33(1):78–90, 2008.

26. W. Sauerbrei. The use of resampling methods to simplify regression models in medical statistics. *Journal of the Royal Statistical Society. Series C (Applied Statistics)*, 48(3):313–329, 1999.

27. W. Sauerbrei, P. Royston, and H. Binder. Selection of important variables and determination of functional form for continuous predictors in multivariable model building. *Statistics in Medicine*, 26(30):5512–5528, 2007.

28. M. Slawski, M. Daumer, and A.-L. Boulesteix. CMA-a comprehensive bioconductor package for supervised classification with high dimensional data. *BMC Bioinformatics*, 9(1):439, 2008.

29. A. Statnikov, C. F. Aliferis, I. Tsamardinos, D. Hardin, and S. Levy. A comprehensive evaluation of multicategory classification methods for microarray gene expression cancer diagnosis. *Bioinformatics*, 21(5):631–643, 2005.

30. C. Strobl, J. Malley, and G. Tutz. An introduction to recursive partitioning: Rationale, application, and characteristics of classification and regression trees, bagging, and random forests. *Psychological Methods*, 14(4):323–348, 2009.

31. R. Tang, J. Sinnwell, J. Li, D. Rider, M. de Andrade, and J. Biernacka. Identification of genes and haplotypes that predict rheumatoid arthritis using random forests. *BMC Proceedings*, 3(Suppl 7):S68, 2009.

32. R. J. Tibshirani. Regression shrinkage and selection via the lasso. *Journal of the Royal Statistical Society. Series B (Methodological)*, 58(1):267–288, 1996.

33. L. J. van't Veer and R. Bernards. Enabling personalized cancer medicine through analysis of gene-expression patterns. *Nature*, 452:564–570, 2008.

34. W. N. Venables and B. D. Ripley. *Modern Applied Statistics with S*. Springer, Berlin, Germany, 4th edn., September 2003.

35. T. T. Wu, Y. F. Chen, T. Hastie, E. Sobel, and K. Lange. Genome-wide association analysis by lasso penalized logistic regression. *Bioinformatics*, 25(6):714–721, 2009.

36. W. B. Yahya, K. Ulm, L. Fahrmeir, and A. Hapfelmeier. k-SS: A sequential feature selection and prediction method in microarray study. *International Journal of Artificial Intelligence*, 6(S11):19–47, 2011.

37. W. Yang and C. C. Gu. Selection of important variables by statistical learning in genome-wide association analysis. *BMC Proceedings*, 3(Suppl 7):S70, 2009.

# 27 Explained Variation and Explained Randomness for Proportional Hazards Models

*John O'Quigley and Ronghui Xu*

## CONTENTS

## 27.1 INTRODUCTION

### 27.1.1 GOAL

The purpose of explained variation and explained randomness is to be able to provide a quantifying measure of a model's predictability. We would like to know how strong are predictive effects. Such a measure is immediately available via the regression coefficients themselves but, since these depend on the scale of the covariates, it is not possible to make simple comparisons on the basis of their magnitude. We would like to be able to make statements such as the following: treatment explains approximately 20% of survival but that, once we have taken account of some known prognostic factors, this figure drops to 5%, or that adding, say, tumor size to a model in which the main prognostic factors are already included the explained variation, or explained randomness, increases, say, from 32% to 33%. Simple situations may not be describable via nested models, for instance, how much do we lose (or gain) in terms of predictability by recoding some continuous prognostic variable into discrete classes on the basis of cutpoints.

The problem is more complex than it may appear and, for most of the suggested approaches in the literature, it is not even possible to assert that a population value of an explained variation coefficient of 0.57, say, indicates stronger regression effects, or indicates stronger predictability, than a value 0.15. This renders their use as a tool to order the relative importance of prognostic variables problematic to say the least. We can derive measures that reflect predictive strength but we need to keep in mind that strength will also depend on the distribution of the covariate and not just the covariate's impact on survival time. When discussing the utility of such measures, a fact that is often overlooked is that any index of predictive performance will do better when a binary covariate is balanced than when there are more in one group than the other. In consequence, for two binary covariates, $Z_1$ and $Z_2$, we are unable to state, on the basis of explained variation (called $R^2$) or some similar measure, which is the more prognostically important without consideration of their marginal distributions. Added to this difficulty is the fact that a simple change in the response variable itself can affect $R^2$, so that, when studying $T$, we would anticipate $T$ and log $T$ to result in different values of $R^2$. A sharp illustration of this is given in Section 27.1.3.

In order to take account of these difficulties where we are unable to even order values of $R^2$ in terms of prognostic importance, it can help to consider more than explained variation alone. In particular, it is useful to examine how far is one distribution from another, more precisely how far is a model in which regression effects are absent from one in which they are present. This can be described in terms of explained randomness, a quantity which itself will often be interpretable as a measure of explained variation, although not necessarily in terms of the most obvious response variable. More than one candidate measure may present itself and, in the specific case of proportional hazards regression, we may prefer a suitable measure to meet certain requirements. We would like the estimated percentages to be meaningful and directly related to predictability of the ranks of the failure times. Absence of effect should translate as 0%, perfect prediction of the survival ranks should translate as 100%, and intermediate values should be interpretable. Since the regression coefficient $\beta$ in the Cox model is unaffected by monotonic transformations on time, an appropriate measure would also have such a property. The measure introduced by O'Quigley and Flandre (1994), viewable as an index of prediction, a correlation measure or a measure of explained variation satisfies these properties. However, in order to be able to recommend the measure for general use, we establish further properties, both statistical and interpretative. The measure can be viewed as a measure of explained randomness and of explained variation, although not for $T$ given $Z$ but rather for $Z$ given $T$. One interesting and practically useful property is the ability to accommodate time-dependent covariates. We study more deeply the motivation and interpretation of the index, which besides satisfying the desirable properties mentioned earlier also has the property that increasing values of its population counterpart $\Omega^2$ correspond to increasing predictability of the ranks of the survival times. It remains invariant to linear transformation of the covariates and to increasing monotonic transformations of time and also enjoys a concrete interpretation in terms of sums of squares decompositions. Furthermore $\Omega^2$ can be shown not to be affected by independent censorship. Extension to the stratified proportional hazards model and to other relative risk models is straightforward.

## 27.1.2 MODEL AND NOTATION

In a survival study, denote $T$ the potential failure time and $C$ the potential censoring time. Let $X = \min(T, C)$, $\delta = I(T <= C)$ where $I(\cdot)$ is the indicator function and $Y(t) = I(X >= t)$. Associated with $T$ is the vector of possibly time-dependent covariates $Z(t)$. For our mathematical development, assume $(T_i, C_i, Z_i(\cdot))$, $i = 1, 2, \ldots, n$, to be i.i.d. from the distribution of $(T, C, Z(\cdot))$. We will also use the counting process notation: let $N_i(t) = I\{T_i <= t, T_i <= C_i\}$ and $\bar{N}(t) = \sum_1^n N_i(t)$. For most of this work, we assume a conditional independent censorship model. However, under the stronger assumption of independent censorship, where $C$ is assumed to be independent of $T$ and $Z$, we obtain further properties and interpretation and these are described in the following. The Cox (1972) proportional hazards model assumes that the conditional hazard function

$$\lambda\big(t \mid Z(t)\big) = \lambda_0(t) \exp\big\{\beta Z(t)\big\}, \tag{27.1}$$

where
  $\lambda_0(t)$ is an unknown "baseline" hazard
  $\beta$ is the relative risk parameter

Denote

$$\pi_i(\beta, t) = \frac{Y_i(t) \exp\big\{\beta Z_i(t)\big\}}{\sum_{j=1}^n Y_j(t) \exp\big\{\beta Z_j(t)\big\}}, \tag{27.2}$$

the conditional probability of subject $i$ being chosen to fail, given all the individuals at risk at time $t$ and that one failure occurs. The product of the $\pi$'s over the observed failure times gives Cox's (1972, 1975) partial likelihood. When $\beta = 0$, $\{\pi_i(0, t)\}_{i=1}^n$ is simply the empirical distribution, assigning equal weight to each sample subject in the risk set. Denote the expectation of a variable with respect to $\{\pi_i(\beta, t)\}_{i=1}^n$ by $\varepsilon_\beta(\cdot t)$. In particular,

$$\mathcal{E}_{\beta}(Z \mid t) = \sum_{j=1}^{n} Z_j(t)\pi_j(\beta,t) = \frac{\sum_{j=1}^{n} Y_j(t)Z_j(t)\exp\{\beta Z_j(t)\}}{\sum_{j=1}^{n} Y_j(t)\exp\{\beta Z_j(t)\}}, \qquad (27.3)$$

is the expectation of $Z(t)$ with respect to $\{\pi_i(\beta,t)\}_i$, and

$$r_i(\hat{\beta}) = Z_i(X_i) - \mathcal{E}_{\hat{\beta}}(Z \mid X_i), \qquad (27.4)$$

for $\delta_i = 1$ is the Schoenfeld (1982) residual where $\hat{\beta}$ is usually obtained by solving the estimating equation provided by the first derivative of the log-partial-likelihood, $U(\beta) = 0$. It is interesting to note that $U(\beta) = \sum_{i=1}^{n} \delta_i r_i(\beta)$. Analogous to ordinary regression, we make the sum of the residuals equal to zero in order to estimate the unknown parameter. We consider the sum of squared residuals to study predictability. This sum corresponds to an estimate of the Fisher information, not only a quantity which can be viewed as indicating how much information an observed sample conveys about a parameter but also—more importantly from our viewpoint—a quantity indicating how great the distance between distributions is. Since, under the model, the residuals $r_i$ are asymptotically orthogonal to one another (Cox, 1975), we can write

$$EU^2(\beta) = \sum_i \delta_i Er_i^2(\beta) = -\sum_i \delta_i E\left\{\frac{\partial r_i(\beta)}{\partial \beta}\right\},$$

where, again, all quantities are evaluated under the model.

### 27.1.3  EXPLAINED VARIATION

For the random pair $(T,Z)$,

$$\mathrm{Var}(T) = E\{\mathrm{Var}(T \mid Z)\} + \mathrm{Var}\{E(T \mid Z)\}. \qquad (27.5)$$

This elementary breakdown always holds, only needing the assumption that the variances exist. The variance of the response variable of interest, in our case usually time $T$, can be expressed in terms of a signal, $\mathrm{Var}\{E(T|Z)\}$ and a remaining, residual variance, or noise, $E\{\mathrm{Var}(T|Z)\}$, once the signal has been accounted for. The greater the signal or the weaker the residual noise, the stronger the predictive effect. Formally, explained variation $\Omega^2$ is defined from

$$\Omega^2 = \frac{\mathrm{Var}(T) - E\,\mathrm{Var}(T \mid Z)}{\mathrm{Var}(T)}, \qquad (27.6)$$

as the amount of variation in $T$ explained by conditioning upon $Z$. We sometimes use the notation $\Omega_T^2(Z)$ where the subscript indicates the variable that we are trying to explain, the argument $Z$ then indicates the variable being used to explain the variability in $T$. The quantity $\Omega_Z^2(T)$ is defined by interchanging the symbols and, interestingly, in the case of a bivariate normal pair $(T,Z)$, we can see that $\Omega_T^2(Z)$ and $\Omega_Z^2(T)$ are the same quantity.

When there is no reduction in variance given $Z$, $\mathrm{Var}(T) = E\{\mathrm{Var}(T|Z)\}$ and $\Omega^2 = 0$. If, given $Z = z$, $T$ assumes some given value with probability 1, then $\mathrm{Var}(T|Z) = 0$ and $\Omega^2 = 1$. In general, the more we reduce the variance then the greater we might consider the model's predictability. Unfortunately, things are not quite so straightforward when the random variables of interest are linked via some type of regression model. When models are assumed to link $T$ and $Z$, apart from the multivariate normal linear model where, as always, pretty much everything works out as we would like, it can be very difficult to interpret $\Omega^2$. In fact, unless we can interpret $\Omega^2$ as a measure of explained randomness, it is not really possible to give it a practical interpretation. As described in the following, explained randomness measures how far away the null model (when the regression coefficients are equal to zero) is from the model considered to generate the observations. In specific cases, explained variation and explained randomness coincide. The multivariate normal linear model is one such example. Another example is that of Cox regression. However, in this latter case, in order to maintain such an interpretation, it is necessary to consider the explained variation in the covariate value $Z$, given $T$ and, not as our intuition may suggest, to consider the explained variation of $T$ given $Z$.

Although it would seem natural to work with the conditional variances of $T$ given $Z$, this can lead us seriously astray, and progress can only be made by taking explicit account of any model structure. In order to highlight this point, consider a very simple example in which we have two binary variables $A$ and $B$. Survival is exponentially distributed given that $A = a$ for $a = 0,1$. The same is the case for $B$. The regression coefficient for $A$ is $\beta_A = 2.0$ whereas for $B$ it is $\beta_B = 20$, corresponding to relative risks of 7.4 and close to 500 million, respectively. Using an obvious notation, we find that $\Omega^2(A) = 0.25$ whereas $\Omega^2(B) = 0.16$. This very unintuitive result is explained by the fact that for this model there is an upper bound on $\Omega^2$ and this upper bound depends heavily on the distribution of the covariate $Z$. Although it is not realistic to want to entirely eliminate the dependence of the covariable, such a strong dependence, and an upper bound that is very sensitive to this distribution is problematic. For $A$, the covariate is balanced leading to an upper bound of 0.33 whereas for $B$, where one of the covariate values occurs in less than 10% of the cases, the upper bound is slightly greater than 0.16. Some authors (Nagelkerke, 1991) propose a general $R^2$ measure in which we rescale the coefficients to take a maximum value of 1. This is a beginning but is not enough since we are still not really able to claim that a rescaled value 0.30, for instance, corresponds to greater predictive power than a rescaled value 0.25. We obtain greater insight when we consider how "far away" the null model is from that generating the observations and, for this, we need to consider appropriate distance measures when dealing with random variables. This leads to the concept of explained randomness. The ideal situation is where our measure can be given an interpretation in both terms of explained variation and explained randomness.

### 27.1.4 EXPLAINED RANDOMNESS

Whereas explained variation contrasts the variance of different models, the idea of explained randomness is to measure the distance between different distributions. This is more general, although in special cases a measure of explained randomness can reduce to a measure of explained variation. The most well-known example is the multivariate normal model. There are a number of different possible measures of distance between distributions and these give rise to different measures of explained randomness. Those most commonly used (Efron, 1977) correspond to the Fisher information and the Kullback–Leibler information. The $R^2$ coefficient, presented by O'Quigley and Flandre (1994), corresponds to the Fisher information measure although that aspect was not brought out or emphasized in that work. The $R^2$ measure of the next section derives from the Fisher distance, based on $E\{\partial \log f(;\beta)/\partial \beta\}^2$, evaluated at the population value, $\beta = \beta_0$ and the value corresponding to absence of regression effect, $\beta = 0$. Since the measure is based on a measure of information, we consider it a measure of explained randomness. However, it can also be interpreted as a measure of explained variation albeit in terms of $Z$ given $T$ rather than the other way around. We can write the proportional hazards model as

$$f\left(t \mid z;\beta\right) = \lambda_0(t) \exp\left\{\beta z - e^{\beta z} \int_0^t \lambda_0(u)\, du\right\}. \qquad (27.7)$$

The baseline hazard function $\lambda_0(t)$ could be specified to be of a power form or a constant, in which cases the Weibull and exponential models are recovered (Kalbfleisch and Prentice, 1980, Cox and Oakes, 1984). These were the first cases studied by Kent and O'Quigley (1988). Under the model, when $\beta = 0$ there is no association between $T$ and $Z$. Another measure of the strength of association, or the distance between the two models indexed by $\beta = 0$ and $\beta = \beta_0$, can be provided by twice the Kullback–Leibler information gain given via $\Gamma_1(\beta) = 2\{I_1(\beta) - I_1(0)\}$, where

$$I_1(\theta) = \iint_{Z\ T} \log\left\{f\left(t \mid z;\theta\right)\right\} f\left(t \mid z;\beta\right) dt\, dG(z).$$

In the previous expression, the domains of definition of $T$ and $Z$ are denoted by $\mathcal{T}$ and $\mathcal{Z}$, respectively, and $G(z)$ is the marginal distribution function of $Z$. Considered as a function of $\beta$, the asymmetric $I_1(\theta)$ is maximized at $\theta = \beta$, a quantity that directly reflects the strength of association. Compared though to the regression coefficient $\beta$, an information gain measure has the advantage of not depending on scale and a coefficient of explained randomness is defined by $\rho_1^2(\beta) = 1 - \exp\{-\Gamma_1(\beta)\}$. The interpretation of $\rho_1^2(\beta)$, where in practice $\beta_0$ will be replaced by a consistent estimate $\hat{\beta}$, as the proportion of randomness explained by the regression was given by Kent (1983). For normal models and maximum likelihood or least squares estimation, $\rho_1^2(\hat{\beta})$ is the usual coefficient of correlation squared when, instead of working with $f(t \mid z;\beta)\, dt\, dG(z)$, we use the observed empirical distribution of $(T, Z)$. Assuming no censoring, a standard estimate of information gain will be provided by $n^{-1}$ times the usual likelihood ratio statistic. An alternative estimate, having similar statistical properties, is provided by the fitted information (Kent and O'Quigley, 1988) in which $I_1(0)$ and $I_1(\beta)$ are estimated by

$$\hat{I}_1(\theta) = n^{-1}\sum_{i=1}^{n}\int_T \log\{f(t|Z_i;\theta)\} f\left(t|Z_i;\hat{\beta}\right)dt, \qquad (27.8)$$

with $\theta=0$ and $\theta=\hat{\beta}$, a consistent estimate of $\beta$, respectively. Earlier, the marginal distribution of $Z$ has been replaced by its empirical estimate.

In the context of proportional hazards regression, and the requirement to obtain procedures that remain rank invariant to monotonic increasing transformations on time, it is more appropriate to consider the distribution of the variable $Z$ given $T$. We can let the information for $Z$ given $T$ be given by (Xu and O'Quigley, 1999)

$$I_2(\theta) = \int_T\int_Z \log\{g(z|t;\theta)\} g(z|t;\beta)dz\, dF(t), \qquad (27.9)$$

where
   $F(t)$ is the marginal distribution function of $T$
   $g(z|t)$ is the conditional density or conditional probability function of $Z$ given $T$

This alternative information measure has advantages over the earlier definition. Censoring is taken to be independent of the failure time. We define $\Gamma_2(\beta)=2\{I_2(\beta) - I_2(0)\}$ and the explained randomness of $Z$ given $T$ is given by

$$\rho_2^2(\beta) = 1-\exp\{-\Gamma_2(\beta)\}.$$

The measure extends to multiple covariates, where $g(\cdot\,|\,\cdot)$ would be the joint conditional density or joint conditional probability function of $Z$ given $T$. We can estimate the conditional distribution of $Z$ given $T$ by $\{\pi_j(\hat{\beta}, t)\}$ (Xu and O'Quigley 2000a), and the marginal distribution of $T$ by the Kaplan–Meier estimate. Take $W(X_i)$ to be the step of the Kaplan–Meier curve at time $t = X_i$. We then have

$$\Gamma_2(\beta) = 2\int_T\int_Z \log\left\{\frac{g(z|t;\beta)}{g(z|t;0)}\right\} g(z|t;\beta)dz\, dF(t). \qquad (27.10)$$

The information gain, $\Gamma_2(\beta)$ can be consistently estimated by

$$\hat{\Gamma}_2(\hat{\beta}) = 2\sum_{i=1}^{k}W(X_i)\sum_{j=1}^{n}\pi_j(\hat{\beta}, X_i)\log\left\{\frac{\pi_j(\hat{\beta}, X_i)}{\pi_j(0, X_i)}\right\}.$$

When the model generates the observations, we would anticipate $\rho_1^2$ and $\rho_2^2$ to be close to one another as well as the coefficient of explained randomness based on the Fisher information.

## 27.2  EXPLAINED VARIATION/RANDOMNESS BASED ON FISHER INFORMATION

Let us first assume $Z$ of dimension one. In (27.3) the expectation $\varepsilon_\beta(Z|X_i)$ is worked out with respect to an exponentially tilted distribution. The stronger the regression effects the greater the tilting, and the smaller we might expect, on average, the values $r_i^2(\beta)$ to be when compared with the residuals under the null model $\beta=0$. Based on these residuals, a measure of explained randomness based on the Fisher information can be defined (O'Quigley and Flandre, 1994). In the absence of censoring, the quantity $\sum_{i=1}^{n} r_i^2(\hat\beta)/n$ is a residual sum of squares and can be viewed as the average discrepancy between the observed covariate and its expected value under the model, whereas $\sum_{i=1}^{n} r_i^2(0)/n$ is a total sum of squares, and can be viewed as the average discrepancy without a model. Since the semiparametric model leaves inference depending only on the failure time rankings, and being able to predict failure rankings of all the failed subjects is equivalent to being able to predict at each failure time which subject is to fail, it is sensible to measure the discrepancy between the observed covariate at a given failure time and its expected value under the model. Thus we can define $I(b)$ for $b=0,\beta$ by

$$\mathcal{I}(b) = \sum_{i=1}^{n} \delta_i r_i^2(b), \tag{27.11}$$

so that $\mathcal{I}(\hat\beta) = \sum_{i=1}^{n} \delta_i r_i^2(\hat\beta)$, the sum of the squared residuals whereas $\mathcal{I}(0) = \sum_{i=1}^{n} \delta_i r_i^2(0)$ is the sum of the squared "null" residuals, or the total sum of squares (made more precise as follows). We then define

$$R^2(\beta) = 1 - \frac{\mathcal{I}(\beta)}{\mathcal{I}(0)}. \tag{27.12}$$

This corresponds to the definition given by O'Quigley and Flandre (1994). For a normal model, considering the residuals in the previous formula to be the usual normal residuals, then this definition coincides exactly with the usual coefficient of correlation, also interpretable as a percentage of explained variation. Generalizing that definition is then very natural. For the multivariate case, when $Z(t)$ is a $p \times 1$ vector, the dependence of the survival time variable on the covariates is best expressed via the prognostic index (Andersen et al., 1983; Altman and Andersen, 1986):

$$\eta(t) = \beta Z(t).$$

Two individuals with possibly different $Z$ values but the same $\eta$ will have the same survival probabilities. So we can imagine that each subject in the study is now labeled by $\eta$. $R^2$ as a measure of explained variation or, predictive capability, should evaluate how well the model predicts which individual or equivalently, its label, is chosen to fail at each observed failure time. This is equivalent to predicting the failure rankings given the prognostic indices. When $p=1$, $Z$ is equivalent to $\eta$, therefore we can construct the $R^2$ using residuals of the $Z$ values. But for $p>1$, the model does not distinguish between different vector $Z$ values as long as the corresponding $\eta$'s are the same. So instead of residuals of $Z$, we define the multiple coefficient using residuals of $\eta$. Analogous to the univariate definition, we have, once again, $R^2(\beta) = 1 - I(\beta)/I(0)$ where, for the multivariate case,

$$\mathcal{I}(b) = \sum_{i=1}^{n} \delta_i \left\{ \beta r_i(b) \right\}^2 . \tag{27.13}$$

### 27.2.1 POPULATION PARAMETER $\Omega^2$

The population parameter $\Omega^2(\beta)$ of $R^2(\hat{\beta})$ was originally given in O'Quigley and Flandre (1994). However, as discussed in Xu (1996), in order to completely eliminate any asymptotic dependence upon censoring, it is necessary to weight the squared Schoenfeld residuals by the increments of any consistent estimate of the marginal failure time distribution function $F$. The practical impact of this on numerical values would typically be small and, in routine analysis, we might choose to work with the simpler calculation. Our main purpose in giving consideration to this weighting of the residuals is to provide a mathematically tight framework to the large sample theory. Therefore, let $\hat{F}$ be the left-continuous Kaplan–Meier (KM) estimate of $F$, and define $W(t) = \hat{S}(t)/\sum_{1}^{n} Y_i(t)$ where $\hat{S} = 1 - \hat{F}$. Then $W(t)$ is a non-negative predictable stochastic process and, assuming there are no ties, it is straightforward to verify that $W(X_i) = \hat{F}(X_i +) - \hat{F}(X_i)$ at each observed failure time $X_i$, that is, the jump of the KM curve. In practice, ties, if they exist, are split randomly. So, in place of the previous definition of $\mathcal{I}(b)$ for $b=0,\beta$, we use a more general definition in which

$$\mathcal{I}(b) = \sum_{i=1}^{n} \int_0^{\infty} W(t) \left\{ Z_i(t) - \varepsilon_b \left( Z \mid t \right) \right\}^2 dN_i(t) = \sum_{i=1}^{n} \delta_i W(X_i) r_i^2(b). \tag{27.14}$$

We now define

$$R^2(\beta) = 1 - \frac{\sum_{i=1}^{n} \delta_i W(X_i) r_i^2(\beta)}{\sum_{i=1}^{n} \delta_i W(X_i) r_i^2(0)} = 1 - \frac{\mathcal{I}(\beta)}{\mathcal{I}(0)}. \tag{27.15}$$

The definition given by O'Quigley and Flandre (1994) would be the same as previous one if we defined $W(t)$ to be constant and, of course, the two definitions coincide in the absence of censoring. The motivation for the introduction of the weight $W(t)$ is to obtain large sample properties of $R^2$ that are unaffected by an independent censoring mechanism. Viewing $R^2$ as a function of $\beta$ turns out to be useful in theoretical studies. In practice, we are mostly interested in $R^2(\hat{\beta})$, where $\hat{\beta}$ is a consistent estimate of $\beta$ such as the partial likelihood estimate. Let

$$S^{(r)}(\beta,t) = n^{-1}\sum_{i=1}^{n}Y_i(t)e^{\beta Z_i(t)}Z_i(t)^{\otimes r}, \quad s^{(r)}(\beta,t) = ES^{(r)}(\beta,t), \qquad (27.16)$$

for $r=0,1,2$. Here $a^{\otimes 2}=a'a$ and $a\otimes b=ab'$ for vectors $a$ and $b$. Notice that $\varepsilon_\beta(Z|t)=S^{(1)}(\beta, t)/S^{(0)}(\beta, t)$. Let

$$J(\beta,b) = \int w(t)\beta\left\{\frac{s^{(2)}(\beta,t)}{s^{(0)}(\beta,t)} - 2\frac{s^{(1)}(\beta,t)\otimes s^{(1)}(b,t)}{s^{(0)}(\beta,t)s^{(0)}(b,t)} + \frac{s^{(1)}(b,t)^{\otimes 2}}{s^{(0)}(b,t)^2}\right\}\beta s^{(0)}(\beta,t)\lambda_0(t)\,dt,$$

$$(27.17)$$

where $w(t)=S(t)/s^{(0)}(0,t)$. Then

$$\Omega^2(\beta) = 1 - \frac{J(\beta,\beta)}{J(\beta,0)}. \qquad (27.18)$$

Notice that although (27.18) is not immediately defined for $\beta=0$, the limits exist and are equal to zero as $\beta\to 0$. So we can define $R^2(0)=\Omega^2(0)=0$.

It has been shown (Xu, 1996) that $\Omega^2(\beta)$ is unaffected by an independent censorship mechanism, that is, when $C$ is independent of $T$ and $Z$, and in this case it can be written (O'Quigley and Flandre, 1994) as

$$\Omega^2(\beta) = 1 - \frac{\int E_\beta\left\{\left[Z(t) - E_\beta\left(Z(t)|t\right)\right]^2 | t\right\}dF(t)}{\int E_\beta\left\{\left[Z(t) - E_0\left(Z(t)|t\right)\right]^2 | t\right\}dF(t)}. \qquad (27.19)$$

If, in addition, $Z$ is time-invariant, we will see that $\Omega^2(\beta)$ has the interpretation of the proportion of explained variation (Section 27.3.2). O'Quigley and Flandre showed that, having standardized for the mean and the variance, $\Omega^2(\beta)$ depends only relatively weakly on different covariate distributions, and values of $\Omega^2(\beta)$ appear to give a good reflection of strength of association as measured by $\beta$ and tend to 1 for high but plausible values of $\beta$ (see also Table 27.1). Their numerical results support the conjecture that $\Omega^2$ increases with the strength of effect, thereby agreeing with the third stipulation of Kendall (1975, p. 4) for a measure of rank correlation. The conjecture was proven to be true in Xu (1996); see also Section 27.3.1. The first two stipulations were that perfect agreement or disagreement should reflect itself in a coefficient of absolute value 1; the third stipulation that for other cases the coefficient should have absolute value less than 1, and in some acceptable sense increasing values of the coefficient should correspond to increasing agreement between the ranks. Here we have a squared coefficient, and Kendall's stipulations are considered

**TABLE 27.1**

**$\Omega^2$ as Explained Variation**

| Covariate[a] | c | c | d | c | c | c | d |
|---|---|---|---|---|---|---|---|
| $\beta$ | 0 | 0.7 | 0.7 | 1.4 | 2.8 | 4.2 | 4.2 |
| $R^2(\beta)$ | 0.0002 | 0.0990 | 0.0979 | 0.2844 | 0.5887 | 0.7577 | 0.8728 |
| $\text{Var}\{E(Z\mid T)\}/\text{Var}(Z)$ | 0.0018 | 0.0998 | 0.0985 | 0.2848 | 0.5889 | 0.7578 | 0.8728 |

[a] Covariate distribution: *d*—binary, *c*—uniform. Data are simulated under the same mechanism as in Section 27.4.

in a broader sense because we are not restricted to the ranks of the covariates in the semiparametric context.

## 27.3 PROPERTIES AND INTERPRETATION

In this section, we show that the measure defined earlier has the desired properties and the interpretation as a measure of explained variation. We omit all the proofs here. They can be found in Xu (1996).

### 27.3.1 PROPERTIES OF $R^2$ AND $\Omega^2$

The $R^2$ defined earlier can be shown to have the following properties:

1. $R^2(0) = 0$.
2. $R^2(\hat{\beta}) \leq 1$.
3. $R^2(\hat{\beta})$ is invariant under linear transformations of $Z$ and monotonically increasing transformations of $T$.
4. $R^2(\hat{\beta})$ consistently estimates $\Omega^2(\beta)$. In particular, $\mathcal{I}(\hat{\beta})$ and $\mathcal{I}(0)$ consistently estimate $J(\beta,\beta)$ and $J(\beta,0)$, respectively.
5. $R^2(\hat{\beta})$ is asymptotically normal.

Note that in finite samples $R^2$, unlike $\Omega^2$, cannot be guaranteed to be non-negative. A negative value for $R^2$ would correspond to the unusual case in which the best fitting model, in a least squares sense, provides a poorer fit than the null model. Our experience is that $R^2(\hat{\beta})$ will only be slightly negative in finite samples if $\hat{\beta}$ is very close to zero.

Similarly, we have the following properties for $\Omega^2$:

1. $\Omega^2(0) = 0$.
2. $0 <= \Omega^2(\beta) <= 1$.
3. $\Omega^2(\beta)$ is invariant under linear transformations of $Z$ and monotonically increasing transformations of $T$.
4. For a scalar $\beta$, $\Omega^2(\beta)$ as a function of $\beta$, increases with $|\beta|$; and as $|\beta| \to \infty$, $\Omega^2(\beta) \to 1$.

From the last property, one can show that $\Omega^2$ increases with the predictability of survival rankings, that is, $P(T_i > T_j)$ for given $Z_i$ and $Z_j$ (assuming without loss of generality that $\beta > 0$). This corresponds to Kendall's third stipulation, in the context of semiparametric Cox regression.

### 27.3.2 INTERPRETATION

In order to be completely assured before using $R^2$ in practice, it is important to know that $R^2$ is consistent for $\Omega^2$, that $\Omega^2(0) = R^2(0) = 0$, $\Omega^2(\infty) = 1$, that $\Omega^2$ increases as strength of effect increases, and that $\Omega^2$ is unaffected by an independent censoring mechanism. This enables us to state that an $\Omega^2$ of 0.4 translates greater predictability than an $\Omega^2$ of 0.3. We do, however, need one more thing. We would like to be able to say precisely just what a value such as 0.4 corresponds to. That is the purpose of this subsection.

#### 27.3.2.1 Sum of Squares Decomposition

In definition (27.15) of $R^2(\beta)$, $\sum_{i=1}^{n} \delta_i W(X_i) \{\beta r_i(\beta)\}^2$ can be considered as a residual sum of squares analogous to the linear regression case, while $\sum_{i=1}^{n} \delta_i W(X_i) \{\beta r_i(0)\}^2$ is the total sum of squares. So define

$$SS_{tot} = \sum_{i=1}^{n} \delta_i W(X_i) \{\hat{\beta} r_i(0)\}^2,$$

$$SS_{res} = \sum_{i=1}^{n} \delta_i W(X_i) \{\hat{\beta} r_i(\hat{\beta})\}^2,$$

$$SS_{reg} = \sum_{i=1}^{n} \delta_i W(X_i) \{\hat{\beta} E_{\hat{\beta}}(Z \mid X_i) - \hat{\beta} E_0(Z \mid X_i)\}^2.$$

It can be shown that an asymptotic decomposition holds of the total sum of squares into the residual sum of squares and the regression sum of squares, that is,

$$SS_{tot} \overset{asymp.}{=} SS_{res} + SS_{reg}, \tag{27.20}$$

the difference between the two sides of the equation converging to zero in probability as $n \to \infty$. So $R^2$ is asymptotically equivalent to the ratio of the regression sum of squares to the total sum of squares.

#### 27.3.2.2 Explained Variation

For time-invariant covariates and independent censoring, the coefficient $\Omega^2(\beta)$ has a simple interpretation in terms of explained variation, that is,

$$\Omega^2(\beta) \approx 1 - \frac{E\{\mathrm{Var}(Z \mid T)\}}{\mathrm{Var}(Z)} = \frac{\mathrm{Var}\{E(Z \mid T)\}}{\mathrm{Var}(Z)}. \tag{27.21}$$

Here we again omit the technical argument leading to the previous approximation, but rather show the simulation results of Table 27.1. Indeed there is nothing to stop us defining explained variation as in the right hand side of (27.21), since the marginal distribution of $Z$ and $T$ can be estimated by the empirical and the KM estimator, while the conditional distribution of $Z$ given $T = t$ by the $\{\pi_i(\hat{\beta}, t)\}_i$. However, we can see no advantage to this and recommend that all calculations be done via the Schoenfeld residuals, evaluated at $\beta = \hat{\beta}$ and $\beta = 0$.

## 27.4  EXTENSIONS

### 27.4.1  PARTIAL COEFFICIENTS

The partial coefficient can be defined via a ratio of multiple coefficients of different orders. Specifically, and in an obvious change of notation just for the purposes of this subsection, let $R^2(Z_1, \ldots, Z_p)$ and $R^2(Z_1, \ldots, Z_q)$ $(q < p)$ denote the multiple coefficients with covariates $Z_1$ to $Z_p$ and covariates $Z_1$ to $Z_q$, respectively. Note that $R^2(Z_1, \ldots, Z_p)$ is calculated using $\hat{\beta}_1, \ldots, \hat{\beta}_p$ estimated when $Z_1, \ldots, Z_p$ are included in the model, and $R^2(Z_1, \ldots, Z_q)$ using $\hat{\beta}_{10}, \ldots, \hat{\beta}_{q0}$ estimated when only $Z_1, \ldots, Z_q$ are included. Define the partial coefficient $R^2(Z_{q+1}, \ldots, Z_p | Z_1, \ldots, Z_q)$, the correlation after having accounted for the effects of $Z_1$ to $Z_q$ by

$$1 - R^2(Z_1, \ldots, Z_p) = \left[1 - R^2(Z_1, \ldots, Z_q)\right]\left[1 - R^2\left(Z_{q+1}, \ldots, Z_p | Z_1, \ldots, Z_q\right)\right].$$

(27.22)

The previous coefficient, motivated by an analogous expression for the multivariate normal model, makes intuitive sense in that the value of the partial coefficient increases as the difference between the multiple coefficients increases, and takes the value zero should this difference be zero. Partial $\Omega^2$ can be defined in a similar way.

We can also derive definition (27.22) directly. Following the discussion of multiple coefficients, we can use the prognostic indices obtained under the model with $Z_1, \ldots, Z_p$ and that with $Z_1, \ldots, Z_q$. This would be equivalent to defining $1 - R^2(Z_{q+1}, \ldots, Z_p | Z_1, \ldots, Z_q)$ as $\mathcal{I}(Z_1, \ldots, Z_p)/\mathcal{I}(Z_1, \ldots, Z_q)$, the ratio of the numerators of $1 - R^2(Z_1, \ldots, Z_p)$ and $1 - R^2(Z_1, \ldots, Z_q)$. However, since the two numerators are on different scales, being inner products of vectors of different dimensions, their numerical value require standardization. One natural way to standardize is to divide these numerators by the denominators of $1 - R^2(Z_1, \ldots, Z_p)$ and $1 - R^2(Z_1, \ldots, Z_q)$, respectively. This gives definition (27.22).

Partial coefficients in O'Quigley and Flandre (1994) were defined using a single component of the covariate vector instead of the prognostic index. Although our limited data experience did not show any important discrepancies between that definition and (27.22), there seems to be some arbitrariness as to which component of the vector to use. Furthermore the prognostic index should reflect the best prediction a given model can achieve in the sense we described before. Our recommendation is to use (27.22) as the partial coefficient.

### 27.4.2 STRATIFIED MODEL

The partial coefficients of the previous section enable us to assess the impact of one or more covariates while adjusting for the effects of others. This is carried out in the context of the assumed model. It may sometimes be preferable to make weaker assumptions than the full model and adjust for the effects of other multi-level covariates by stratification. Indeed, it can be interesting and informative to compare adjusted $R^2$ measures, the adjustments having been made either via the model or via stratification. For the stratified model, the definitions of Section 27.2 follow through readily. To be precise, we define a stratum specific residual for stratum $s$ $(s = 1, \ldots, S)$, where, in the following, a subscript is in place of $i$ means the $i$th subject in stratum $s$. Thus we have

$$r_i(b; s) = Z_{is}(X_{is}) - \varepsilon_b(Z \mid X_{is}), \qquad (27.23)$$

where $\varepsilon_b(Z|X_{is})$ is averaged within stratum $s$ over the risk set at time $X_{is}$, and we write

$$\mathcal{I}(b) = \sum_i \sum_s \int_0^\infty W(t) \{ Z_{is}(t) - \varepsilon_b(Z \mid t) \}^2 \, dN_{is}(t) = \sum_i \sum_s \delta_{is} W(X_{is}) r_i^2(b, s).$$

$$(27.24)$$

From this we can define

$$R^2(\beta) = 1 - \frac{\sum_i \sum_s \delta_{is} W(X_{is}) r_i^2(\beta, s)}{\sum_i \sum_s \delta_{is} W(X_{is}) r_i^2(0, s)} = 1 - \frac{\mathcal{I}(\beta)}{\mathcal{I}(0)}. \qquad (27.25)$$

Note that we do not use a stratum specific $W(t)$ and, as before, we work with an assumption of a common underlying marginal survival distribution. The validity of this hinges upon an independent, rather than a conditionally independent, censoring mechanism. Under a conditionally independent censoring mechanism, a weighted Kaplan–Meier estimate (Murray and Tsiatis, 1996) of the marginal survival distribution may be used instead.

### 27.4.3 OTHER RELATIVE RISK MODELS

It is straightforward to generalize the $R^2$ measure to other relative risk models, with the relative risk of forms such as $1 + \beta z$ or $\exp\{\beta(t)z\}$. Denote $r(t;z)$ a general form of the relative risk. Assume that the regression parameters involved have been estimated, and define $\pi_i(t) = Y_i(t) \hat{r}(t; Z_i) / \sum_{j=1}^n Y_j(t) \hat{r}(t; Z_j)$. Then we can similarly define $\varepsilon_\beta(Z|t)$ and form the residuals, thereby defining an $R^2$ measure similar to (27.15). In addition, it can be shown that under an independent censorship, the conditional distribution of $Z(t)$ given $T = t$ is consistently estimated by $\{\pi_i(t)\}_i$ (Xu and O'Quigley 2000b), so properties such as being unaffected by an independent censorship are maintained.

It is particularly interesting to study the use of such an $R^2$ measure under the time-varying regression effects model, where the relative risk is $\exp\{\beta(t)z\}$. Different approaches have been proposed to estimate $\beta(t)$ (Sleeper and Harrington, 1990; Zucker and Karr, 1990; Murphy and Sen, 1991; Gray, 1992; Hastie and Tibshirani, 1993; Verweij and Van Houwelingen, 1995; Sargent, 1997; Gustafson, 1998; Xu and Adak, 2001). In this case, we can use $R^2$ to compare the predictability of different covariates as we do under the proportional hazards model; we can also use it to guide the choice of the amount of smoothness, or the "effective degrees of freedom" as it is called by the some of the aforementioned authors, in estimating $\beta(t)$. As a brief illustration, suppose that we estimate $\beta(t)$ as a step function, and that we are to choose between two different partitions of the time axis, perhaps one finer than the other. Denote the two estimates obtained under these two partitions by $\hat{\beta}_1(t)$ and $\hat{\beta}_2(t)$, the latter corresponding to the finer partition. We can measure the extra amount of variation explained by fitting $\hat{\beta}_2(t)$ versus fitting $\hat{\beta}_1(t)$, by

$$R_{ex}^2 = 1 - \frac{\mathcal{I}(\hat{\beta}_2(\cdot))}{\mathcal{I}(\hat{\beta}_1(\cdot))}. \tag{27.26}$$

This can be thought of as a partial coefficient, if we look at the "dimension" of $\beta(t)$ through time. The use of $R_{ex}^2$ in estimating $\beta(t)$ was adopted in Xu and Adak (2001).

## 27.5  ILLUSTRATION

A Cox model analysis of breast cancer data was carried out, initially based on the inclusion of single prognostic factors and, subsequently, based on a multivariate analysis. These results are summarized in Table 27.2. All variables are highly significant. The predictive power though is quite different. Stage and tumor size, as one might expect, have reasonably high predictability. Histology grade also has predictive power, although this covariate has been shown to have a nonproportional regression

TABLE 27.2

Breast Cancer—Univariate Analysis

| Covariate | $\hat{\beta}$ | p-Value | $R^2$ |
|-----------|------|---------|-------|
| Age | −0.24 | <0.01 | 0.005 |
| Hist | 0.37 | <0.01 | 0.12 |
| Stage | 0.53 | <0.01 | 0.20 |
| Prog | −0.73 | <0.01 | 0.07 |
| Size | 0.02 | <0.01 | 0.18 |

**TABLE 27.3**

**Breast Cancer: Multivariate Analysis**

| Covariates | $R^2$ | Partial $R^2$ |
|---|---|---|
| Age | 0.01 | |
| Age and hist | 0.12 | 0.12 |
| Age, hist, and stage | 0.26 | 0.16 |
| Age, hist, stage, and prog | 0.33 | 0.09 |
| Age, hist, stage, prog, and size | 0.33 | 0.01 |

effect. We investigated a more complex model in which the coefficient for histology was allowed to decay with time. The value of $R^2$ increased from 0.12 to 0.24, the improvement in explained variation reflecting an improvement in fit. This case also underlines the relationship between predictability and goodness-of-fit. On the other hand, age has very weak predictive capability, though significant. This estimated weak effect could be due to (1) a population weak effect or (2) a suboptimal coding of the covariate. We investigated this second possibility via two recoded models. The first, making a strong trend assumption, coded age as 1 (0–33), 2 (34–40), and 3 (41 and above). The second model, making no assumptions about trend, used two binary variables to code the three groups. All three models gave very similar values of $R^2$. In consequence, only the simplest model is retained for subsequent analysis, that is, the age groups 1–3. In addition, we calculated the multiple $R^2$ for a set of nested models. These results are illustrated in Table 27.3. Table 27.3 also contains the values of the partial $R^2$ defined in (27.22), when each additional covariate is added to the existing model. The partial coefficient for tumor size having accounted for the other four variables is 0.01, suggesting that the extra amount of variation in survival explained by the patient's tumor size is quite limited.

The example helps illustrate the usefulness of $R^2$ in practice. The analysis is by no means a thorough one and, typically, deeper study would be useful. For instance, the combinatorial problem of examining all possible subgroups of different sizes raises both statistical and computational challenges. The statistical question, also present in the earlier limited analyses, is that of bias, or inflation, of multiple $R^2$ away from zero, when viewed as an estimate of the corresponding multiple $\Omega^2$. This question is not specific to the survival setting and arises in the standard case of linear regression. Bias reduction techniques, such as bootstrap resampling, would also be helpful for our application. The described $R^2$ measure, based on explained randomness, can be considered a natural analogue to the usual $R^2$ for linear regression. It has the properties desirable for such a measure, as well as concrete interpretations including predictability of survival rankings, sums of squares decomposition, and proportion of explained variation. The measure naturally accommodates time-dependent covariates, and can be easily computed after the proportional hazards regression model has been fitted. All that is required is the squaring and summing of the Schoenfeld residuals, under the null and the fitted models. Extensions to other relative risk models are straightforward. We recommend the measure for routine use.

# REFERENCES

Altman, D.G. and Andersen P.K. (1986) A note on the uncertainty of a survival probability estimated from Cox's regression model. *Biometrika* 73, 722–724.

Andersen, P.K., Christensen, E., Fauerholdt, L., and Schlichting, P. (1983) Measuring prognosis using the proportional hazards model. *Scand. J. Stat.* 10, 49–52.

Cox, D.R. (1972) Regression models and life tables (with discussion). *J. R. Stat. Soc., Ser. B* 34, 187–220.

Cox, D.R. (1975) Partial likelihood. *Biometrika* 62, 269–276.

Cox, D.R. and Oakes, D. (1984) Analysis of Survival Data. Chapman and Hall, London.

Efron, B. (1977) The efficiency of Cox's likelihood function for censored data. *Journal of the American Statistical Association*, 72, 557–565.

Gray, R.J. (1992) Flexible methods for analyzing survival data using splines, with application to breast cancer prognosis. *J. Am. Stat. Assoc.* 87, 942–951.

Gustafson, P. (1998) Flexible Bayesian modelling for survival data. *Lifetime Data Anal.* 4, 281–299.

Hastie, T. and Tibshirani, R. (1993) Varying-coefficient models. *J. R. Stat. Soc., Ser. B* 55, 757–796.

Kalbfleisch, J.D. and Prentice, R.L. (1980) The Statistical Analysis of Failure Time Data. Wiley, New York.

Kendall, M. (1975) *Rank Correlation Methods*. 4th edn., Griffin, London, U.K.

Kent, J.T. (1983) Information gain and a general measure of correlation. *Biometrika* 70(1), 163–174.

Kent, J.T. and O'Quigley, J. (1988) Measure of dependence for censored survival data. *Biometrika* 75, 525–534.

Murphy, S.A. and Sen, P.K. (1991) Time-dependent coefficients in a Cox-type regression model. *Stoch. Process. Appl.* 39, 153–180.

Murray, S. and Tsiatis, A.A. (1996) Nonparametric survival estimation using prognostic longitudinal covariates. *Biometrics* 52, 137–151.

Nagelkerke, N.J.D. (1991) A note on a general definition of the coefficient of determination. *Biometrika* 78, 691–692.

O'Quigley, J. and Flandre, P. (1994) Predictive capability of proportional hazards regression. *Proc. Natl Acad. Sci. U.S.A.* 91, 2310–2314.

Sargent, D.J. (1997) A flexible approach to time-varying coefficients in the Cox regression setting. *Lifetime Data Anal.* 3, 13–25.

Schoenfeld, D.A. (1982) Partial residuals for the proportional hazards regression model. *Biometrika* 69, 239–241.

Sleeper, L.A. and Harrington, D.P. (1990) Regression splines in the Cox model with application to covariate effects in liver disease. *J. Am. Stat. Assoc.* 85, 941–949.

Verweij, J.A. and Van Houwelingen, H.A. (1995) Time-dependent effects of fixed covariates in Cox regression. *Biometrics* 51, 1550–1556.

Xu, R. (1996) Inference for the proportional hazards model. PhD thesis of University of California, San Diego, CA.

Xu, R. and Adak, S. (2001) Survival analysis with time-varying relative risks: A tree-based approach. *Methods Inf. Med.* 40, 141–147.

Xu, R. and O'Quigley, J. (1999) A $R^2$ type of measure of dependence for proportional hazards models. *Nonparam. Stat.* 12, 83–107.

Xu, R., O'Quigley, J. (2000a) Estimating average regression effect under non-proportional hazards. *Biostatistics* 1, 423–439.

Xu, R., O'Quigley, J. (2000b) Proportional hazards estimate of the conditional survival function. *Journal of the Royal Statistical Society, Series B.* 62, 667–680.

Zucker, D.M. and Karr, A.F. (1990) Nonparametric survival analysis with time-dependent covariate effects: A penalized partial likelihood approach. *Ann. Stat.* 18, 329–353.

# 28 Prognostic Groups by Tree-Based Partitioning and Data Refinement Methods

*Michael LeBlanc and John J. Crowley*

## CONTENTS

## 28.1   INTRODUCTION

The proportional hazards (PH) model of Cox (1972) has long been used to identify prognostic groups of patients by using the linear component of the model (prognostic index), or informally through counting up the number of poor prognostic factors corresponding to terms in the fitted model. However, the model does not directly lead to an easily interpretable description of patient prognostic groups. An alternative to using prognostic indices constructed from the PH model is a rule that can be expressed as simple logical combinations of covariate values. For example, an individual with some hypothetical type of cancer may have a poor prognosis if ((age ≥ 60) and (*serum creatinine* ≥ 2)) or (*serum calcium* < 5). This chapter presents two general classes of methodologies for constructing these logical rules for prognosis: (1) tree-based methods which partition the data into multiple prognostic groups and (2) peeling or extreme regression which both lead to sequential refinement the data into patient subsets with either very good or very poor prognosis.

*Tree-based partitioning.* Tree-based methods were formalized and extensively studied by Breiman et al. (1984). Trees have also been of interest in machine learning; one example is the C4.5 algorithm due to Quinlan (1993). Tree-based methods recursively split the data into groups, leading to a fitted model that is piecewise constant function approximation over regions of the covariate space. Each region is represented by a terminal node in a binary decision tree. Tree-based methods have been extended to censored survival data for the goal of finding groups of patients with differing prognosis (Gordon and Olshen 1985, Ciampi et al. 1988, Segal 1988, LeBlanc and Crowley 1992, 1993, Fan et al. 2006). Further extensions and examples for tree-based rules in a wide variety of medical research problems were considered by Zhang and Singer (1999). Some examples of tree-based methods for survival data in clinical studies are given in (Albain et al. 1990, Lerner et al. 2009, Wiener et al. 2010).

*Prognostic peeling.* Trees are useful methods for constructing multiple prognostic groups. However, in some cases the goal is to construct a simple decision rule to describe a single patient subset with either very good or very poor prognosis. For that objective, complementary techniques to tree-based methods have recently been developed. These methods are related to the patient rule induction method (PRIM) proposed by Friedman and Fisher (1999). The basic idea of the PRIM algorithm and extensions is to describe a region in the covariate space corresponding to the most extreme expected outcome. PRIM was developed for uncensored data and works best with very large data sets, but has been extended by LeBlanc et al. (2002) to better address survival data, and to other low signal applications by LeBlanc et al. (2005). The main components of the algorithm are common between the published methods. Initially the entire data set is considered and then a fraction α of the data is removed from either extreme of a variable distribution among all variables. This process, called peeling, is repeated until only small fraction of the data remains. The data corresponding to a rule with sufficiently extreme outcome are removed and the remaining data are peeled again. The end result is a logical rule representing an extreme outcome group.

*Extreme regression.* We also discuss another strategy for constructing a poor or good prognostic group which we call extreme regression (LeBlanc et al. 2006). This method combines the function approximation aspects of trees and can yield prognostic groups where one can control either the level of prognosis in the group or the fraction of patients identified. The method obtains prognostic groups by first constructing a regression function that consists of minimum and maximum (extreme) functions of simple univariate functions of the predictors. Prognostic groups are defined by threshold decisions on the regression function $\eta(x) \geq c$, yielding simple decision rules analogous to trees. However, unlike trees, which work well with both categorical and continuous variables, peeling, and extreme regression are best suited for ordered or continuous predictor variables.

In this chapter we discuss the general methodological aspects of these prognostic modeling strategies. We illustrate the methods with a subset of patients ($n = 2678$) from the large data set collected by the International Myeloma Foundation (IMF) for the goal of constructing a reliable staging system for multiple myeloma (Greipp et al. 2005). Clinical and laboratory data were gathered on previously untreated myeloma patients from 17 institutions, including sites in North America, Europe, and Asia. Patient characteristics were typical for symptomatic myeloma, including age, sex, and clinical as well as laboratory parameters. Given the results in this chapter are only based on a subset of patients for methodologic illustrative purposes, the split points differ from the published IMF results.

## 28.2  NOTATION AND PROGNOSTIC MODELS

We assume that $X$ is the true survival time, $C$ is the random censoring time, and $Z$ is a $p$-vector of covariates. The observed variables are the triple ($T = (X, C)$, $\Delta = I\{X \leq C\}$, $Z$) where $T$ is the time under observation and $\Delta$ is an indicator of failure. Given $Z$ we assume that $X$ and $C$ are independent. The data consist of a sample of independent observations $\{(t_i, \delta_i, z_i): i = 1, 2, \ldots, N\}$ distributed as the vector ($T$, $\Delta$, $Z$). The survival probability at time $t$ is denoted by

$$S(t \mid z) = P\left(X > t \mid z\right).$$

### 28.2.1  FUNCTION APPROXIMATION

Typically, survival data regression models vary smoothly as a function of the covariates. For instance, the PH model specifies the hazard function as

$$\lambda(t \mid z) = \lambda_0(t) \exp\left(\eta(z)\right),$$

where
   $\lambda_0(t)$ is a baseline hazard function
   $\eta(z)$ is the logarithm of the relative risk

The relative risk function is sometimes referred to as the "prognostic index" and is typically a linear function of the covariates $\eta(z) = z'\beta$. More general additive models for the logarithm of the relative risk function are also used for modeling survival data. While additive function expansions are useful for variable interpretation, rules describing patients with differing prognosis, which are typically of the form $\{z: \eta(z) \geq q\}$ or $\{z: \eta(z) \leq q\}$ are difficult to describe because they are a weighted combination of patient characteristics. A tree-based method is also a function approximation method, except that the piecewise constant approximating model is homogeneous over regions of the prediction space. For example, a tree, $T(x)$, assigns the same value for all cases within each region, $x \in T_m \Rightarrow T(x) = \eta_m$. Therefore, tree rules can be described as follows: $\{x: T(x) \geq q\}$ will just be the union of those regions $T_m$ for which $\eta_m \geq q$. It is this easily described as inverse property that makes trees so desirable for constructing prognostic rules for clinical applications. A tree-based model for survival can be represented as

$$S(t \mid z) = \sum_{h=1}^{H} S_h(t) I\{z \in B_h\},$$

where

$B_h$ is a "box"-shaped region in the predictor space, represented by a terminal node, $h$

the function $S_h(t)$ is the survival function corresponding to region $B_h$

$H$ is the number of overlapping regions

Importantly, each terminal node can be described by a logical rule, for instance, $(z_1 < 3) \cap (z_2 \geq 6) \cap (z_5 < 2)$. With the sample sizes typically available for clinical applications, a piecewise constant model can yield quite poor approximations to the conditional survival function, $S(t|z)$, which is likely a smooth function of the underlying covariates. Therefore, methods using smooth models such as linear Cox regression or ensembles of trees such as boosted trees (e.g., Buhlmann and Hohorn 2007) or random survival forests by Ishwaran et al. (2008) likely yield better approximations than piecewise constant tree-based methods. However, the primary motivation for using tree-based models is the potentially easy interpretation of decision rules.

### 28.2.2 EXTREME REGION SUMMARY

An alternative strategy does not attempt to model the entire regression function, but instead describes the survival function in one region, $R$, $S(t|R) = S_R(t) I\{z \in R\}$ corresponding to patients expected to have an extreme good or poor outcome. Unlike tree-based methods there is no attempt at describing the other regions. However, as with trees, $R$ is defined by logic rules. An important attribute is the mass or fraction of the sample within the region, $R$, which can be denoted by

$$\beta(R) = \int_R dP_z,$$

where $dP_z$ represents the probability mass function associated with the covariates.

Estimation of the rules will be reviewed in this chapter. One method called peeling is a nonparametric strategy that does not use an overall regression model.

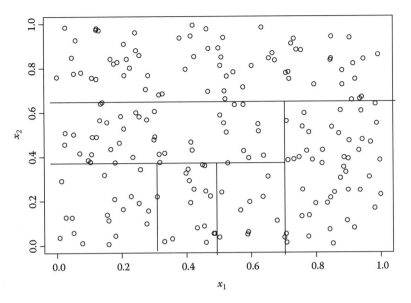

**FIGURE 28.1** Schematic of partitioning of two-dimensional covariate space.

A second method develops a special regression function that allows simple decision rule descriptions of extreme prognostic groups. In summary, tree-based regression constructs regions or boxes $B_h$ by repeatedly partitioning the data, and the extreme region summaries are obtained via sequentially removing small fractions of data along coordinate axes. Figures 28.1 and 28.2 show a schematic of each of the two procedures with two covariates.

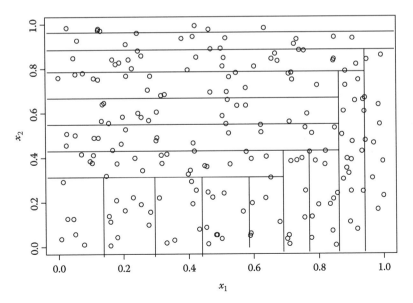

**FIGURE 28.2** Schematic of peeling of two-dimensional covariate space.

$$\max(\min(a_1x_1 + b_1, a_2x_2 + b_2), \min(a_3x_1 + b_3, a_4x_2 + b_4))$$

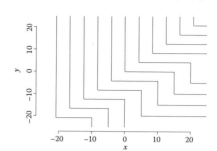

**FIGURE 28.3**  Extreme regression function: sequence of prognostic regions identified from function.

A third method develops regions similar to that presented in Figure 28.2 but it does it by constructing a special "extreme" regression function as displayed in Figure 28.3.

The myeloma data from the IMF presented in this chapter are from 2678 patients with survival outcome and complete covariate data for calcium (CAL), serum β2 microglobulin (B2M), platelets (PLT), serum creatinine (CREAT), serum albumin (ALB), and percent plasma cells in the bone marrow (BMPC).

## 28.3  TREE-BASED PARTITIONING

### 28.3.1  CONSTRUCTING A TREE RULE

A tree-based model is developed by recursively partitioning the data. At the first step, the covariate space is partitioned into two regions and the data are split into two groups. The splitting rule is applied recursively to each of the resulting regions until a large tree has been grown. Splits along a single covariate are used because they are easy to interpret. For an ordered covariate, splits are of the form "$Z_j < c$" or "$Z_j \geq c$," and for a nominal covariate, splits are of the form "$Z_j \in S$" or "$Z_j \notin S$," where $S$ is a nonempty subset of the set of labels for the nominal predictor $Z_j$. Potential splits are evaluated for each of the covariates, and the covariate and the split value resulting in the greatest reduction in impurity are chosen.

The improvement for a split at node $h$ into left and right daughter nodes $l(h)$ and $r(h)$ is

$$G(h) = R(h) - \left[ R\big(l(h)\big) + R\big(r(h)\big) \right],$$

where $R(h)$ is the residual error at node $h$. We assume $G(h) > 0$. For uncensored continuous response problems, $R(h)$ is typically the mean residual sum of squares or mean absolute error. For survival data, it would be reasonable to use deviance corresponding to an assumed survival model. For instance, the exponential model deviance for node $h$ is

$$R(h) = \sum_{i=1}^{N} 2\left[\delta_i \log\left(\frac{\delta_i}{\hat{\lambda}_h \, t_i}\right) - (\delta_i - \hat{\lambda}_h \, t_i)\right],$$

where $\hat{\lambda}_h$ is the maximum likelihood estimate of the hazard rate in node $h$. Often an exponential assumption for survival times is not valid. However, a nonlinear transformation of the survival times may make the distribution of survival times closer to an exponential distribution. LeBlanc and Crowley (1992) investigate a "full-likelihood" method which is equivalent to transforming time by the marginal cumulative hazard function and using the exponential deviance and then using exponential deviance for tree construction.

However, most recursive partitioning schemes for censored survival data use the logrank test statistic of Mantel (1966) for $G(h)$ to measure the separation in survival times between two groups. Simulation studies of the performance of splitting with the logrank and other between-node statistics are given in (LeBlanc and Crowley 1993) and (Crowley et al. 1995).

Figure 28.4 shows the value of the logrank test statistic for groups defined by partitioning on *serum* $\beta_2$ *microglobulin (B2M)*, $(B2M < c)$, and $(B2M \geq c)$ for range of cut points in the IMF data set. The largest logrank test statistic corresponds to a split at $c = 8.89$ and would lead to the first split in a tree-based model to be $(B2M < 8.89)$ versus $(B2M \geq 8.89)$.

## 28.3.2 SPLITTING

If there are weak associations between the survival times and covariates, splitting on a continuous covariate tends to select splits that send almost all the observations

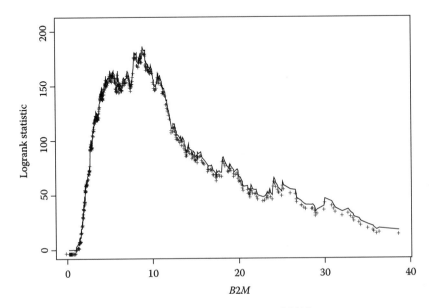

**FIGURE 28.4**   Logrank test statistics at observed values of *B2M*.

to one side of the split. This is called "end-cut" preference by Breiman et al. (1984). When growing survival trees, we restrict both the minimum total number of observations and the minimum number of uncensored observations within any potential node. This restriction is also important for prognostic stratification, since very small groups of patients are usually not of clinical interest.

It is also important that the splitting statistic can be calculated efficiently for all possible split points for continuous covariates. While the logrank test is relatively inexpensive to calculate, the statistic must be calculated many times; hence, we improve computational efficiency by using a simple approximation to the logrank statistic which allows simple updating algorithms to consider all possible splits (Crowley et al. 1995). Updating algorithms can also be constructed for exponential deviance; for instance, refer to the works of LeBlanc and Crowley (1995) and Davis and Anderson (1989).

Figure 28.5 shows a tree grown on the IMF using the logrank test statistic for splitting, with a constraint of a minimum node size of 5% of the sample size. The tree has 15 terminal nodes. The logrank test statistic and permutation $p$-value are presented below each split in the tree. The $p$-value is calculated at each node by permuting the responses over the covariates and recalculating the best split at that node 1000 times and then calculating the proportion of logrank test statistics greater than the observed statistic. At each terminal node, the logarithm of the hazard ratio relative to the leftmost node and the number of cases falling into each terminal node are presented. The logarithm of the hazard ratio is obtained by fitting a Cox

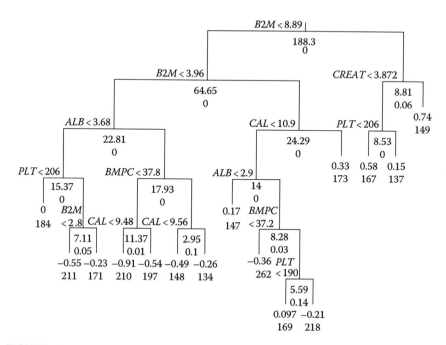

**FIGURE 28.5**  Unpruned survival tree: Below each split are the logrank test statistic and a permutation $p$-value. Below each terminal node is the logarithm of the hazard ratio relative to the leftmost node in the tree and the number of cases in the node.

(1972) model with dummy variables defined by terminal nodes in the tree. The worst prognostic group are patients with very high *B2M* ($B2M \geq 8.89$) and high *CREAT* ($CREAT \geq 3.872$) and corresponds to an estimated logarithm of the hazard ratio relative to the best prognostic group equal to 74. While the minimum node size was set to be quite large (5% of the sample or approximately 134 observations), the logrank test statistics near the bottom of the tree (and permutation *p*-values) indicate there may be several nodes that should be combined to simplify the model.

### 28.3.3 PRUNING AND SELECTING A TREE

Two general methods have been proposed for pruning trees for survival data. The methods which use within-node error or deviance usually adopt the CART pruning algorithm directly.

### 28.3.3.1 Methods Based on within-Node Deviance

In the CART algorithm, the performance of a tree is based on the cost complexity measure

$$R_\alpha(T) = \sum_{h \in \tilde{T}} R(h) + \alpha \, |\tilde{T}|$$

of the binary tree $T$, where $\tilde{T}$ is the set of terminal nodes, $|\tilde{T}|$ is the number terminal nodes, $\alpha$ is a nonnegative parameter, and $R(h)$ is the cost (often deviance) of node $h$.

A subtree (a tree obtained by removing branches) $T_0$ is an optimally pruned subtree for any penalty $\alpha$ of the tree $T$ if

$$R_\alpha(T_0) = \min_{T' \preceq T} R_\alpha(T'),$$

where
  "$\preceq$" means "is a subtree of"
  $T_0$ is the smallest optimally pruned subtree if $T_0 \preceq T''$ for every optimally pruned subtree, $T''$

The cost complexity pruning algorithm obtains the optimally pruned subtree for any $\alpha$. This algorithm finds the sequence of optimally pruned subtrees by repeatedly deleting branches of the tree for which the average reduction in impurity per split in the branch is small.

The deviance will always decrease for larger trees in the nested sequence based on the data used to construct the tree. Therefore, honest estimates of deviance for a new sample are required to select a tree that would have small expected deviance. If a test sample is available, the deviance for the test sample can be calculated for each of the pruned trees in the sequence using the node estimates from the training sample. For instance the deviance at a node would be

$$R(h) = \sum_{i \in N_h} 2 \left[ \delta_i^T \log \left( \frac{\delta_i^T}{\hat{\lambda}_h \, t_i^T} \right) - \left( \delta_i^T - \hat{\lambda}_h \, t_i^T \right) \right],$$

where $\left(t_i^T, \delta_i^T\right)$ are the test sample survival times and status indicators for test sample observations falling into node $h$, $z_i^T \in B_h$, for the tree and node estimate $\hat{\lambda}_h$ calculated from the learning sample.

Given that a test sample is usually not available, the selection of the best tree can be based on resampling-based estimates of prediction error (or expected deviance). The most popular method for tree-based models is the $K$-fold cross-validation estimate of deviance. The training data, $\Lambda$, are divided into $K$ test samples $\Lambda_k$ and training samples $\Lambda_{(k)} = \Lambda - \Lambda_k$, $k = 1, \ldots, K$ of about equal size. Trees are grown with each of the training samples $\Lambda_{(k)}$; each test sample $\Lambda_k$ is used to estimate the deviance using the parameter estimates from the training sample $\Lambda_{(k)}$. The $K$-fold cross-validation estimate of deviance is the sum of the test sample estimates. The tree that minimizes the cross-validation estimate of deviance (or a slightly smaller tree) is selected. While $K$-fold cross-validation is a standard method for selecting tree size, it is subject to considerable variability; this is noted in survival data in simulations given in LeBlanc and Crowley (1993). Therefore, other methods such as those based on bootstrap resampling may be useful alternatives (Efron and Tibshirani 1997). One bootstrap method based on logrank splitting is given in the next section.

### 28.3.3.2  Methods Based on between-Node Separation

LeBlanc and Crowley (1993) developed an optimal pruning algorithm analogous to the cost complexity pruning algorithm of CART for tree performance based on between node separation. Between-node pruning has been extended for the use in multivariate survival data by Fan et al. (2006). They define the split complexity of a tree as

$$G_\alpha(T) = G(T) - \alpha \, |S|,$$

where $G(T)$ is the sum over the standardized splitting statistics $G(h)$ in the tree $T$:

$$G(T) = \sum_{h \in S} G(h),$$

where $S$ represents the internal nodes $T$.

A tree $T_0$ is an optimally pruned subtree of $T$ for complexity parameter $\alpha$ if

$$G_\alpha(T_0) = \max_{T' \preceq T} G_\alpha(T'),$$

and it is the smallest optimally pruned subtree if $T_0 \preceq T'$ for every optimally pruned subtree. The algorithm repeatedly prunes off branches with smallest average logrank test statistics in the branch. An alternative pruning method for trees based on the maximum value of the test statistic within any branch was proposed by Segal (1988).

Since the same data are used to select the split point and variable as used to calculate the test statistic, we use a bias-corrected version of the split complexity described previously:

$$G_\alpha(T) = \sum_{h \in S} G^*(h) - \alpha |S|,$$

where the corrected split statistic is

$$G^*(h) = G(h) - \Delta^*(h),$$

and where the bias is denoted by $\Delta^*(h) = E_{Y^*} G(h; \Lambda^*, \Lambda) - E_{Y^*} G(h; \Lambda^*, \Lambda^*)$. The function $G(h; \Lambda^*, \Lambda)$ denotes the test statistic where the data $\Lambda^*$ were used to determine the split variable and value and the data $\Lambda$ were used to evaluate the statistic. The function $G(h; \Lambda^*, \Lambda^*)$ denotes the statistic where the same data were used to pick the split variable and value, and to calculate the test statistic. The difference $\Delta^*(h)$ is the optimism due to adaptive splitting of the data. We use the bootstrap to obtain an estimate $\widehat{\Delta}^*(h)$, then we select trees which minimize the corrected goodness of split

$$\widetilde{G}_\alpha(T) = \sum_{h \in S} \left( G(h) - \widehat{\Delta}^*(h) \right) - \alpha |S|.$$

$\widetilde{G}_\alpha(T)$ is similar to the bias-corrected version of split complexity used in LeBlanc and Crowley (1993) except here we do the correction locally for each split conditional on splits higher in the tree. We typically choose a complexity parameter $\alpha = 4$. Note that if splits were not selected adaptively, an $\alpha = 4$ would correspond approximately to the .05 significance level for a split and $\alpha = 2$ is in the spirit of Akaike information criterion (AIC) (Akaike 1974). Permutation sampling methods can also be used to add an approximate $p$-value to each split conditional on the tree structure above the split to help the interpretation of individual splits.

Figure 28.6 shows a pruned tree based on the corrected goodness of split using 25 bootstrap samples with $\alpha = 4$. There are 8 terminal nodes.

Usually only a small number of prognostic groups are of interest. Therefore, further recombination of nodes with a similar prognosis from the pruned tree may be required. We select a measure of prognosis (for instance, hazard ratios relative to some node in the tree or median survival for each node) and rank each of the terminal nodes in the pruned tree based on the measure of prognosis selected. After ranking the nodes, there are several options for combining nodes in a pruned tree. One method is to grow another tree on the ranked nodes and only allow the second tree to select three or four nodes; another method is to divide the nodes based on quantiles of the data; and a third method is to evaluate all possible recombinations of nodes into $V$ groups and choose the partition that yields the largest partial likelihood or largest $V$ sample logrank test statistic. The result of recombining to yield the largest partial likelihood for a four group combination of the pruned myeloma tree given in Figure 28.6 is presented in Figure 28.7.

## 28.4   PROGNOSTIC DATA PEELING

Tree-based methods are effective for describing multiple prognostic strata. However, if the goal is find a single poor or good prognostic group with greater

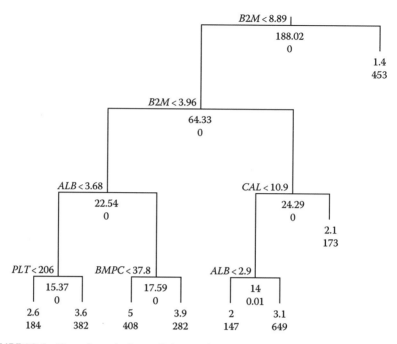

**FIGURE 28.6** Pruned survival tree: Below each split are the logrank test statistic and a permutation $p$-value. Below each terminal node is the median survival (in years) and underneath the number of patients represented by that node.

control of the relative outcome for patients in that group, other strategies may be useful. In developing a clinical trial for a new aggressive therapy, one often must limit the study to only those patients with sufficiently poor prognosis appropriate for the toxicity associated with that therapy. Conversely, if a group of patients can be identified that has very good prognosis, one may want to investigate less toxic therapies for that group. However, the prognostic group must include a sufficient proportion of the patients with that disease to make patient accrual to the clinical trial feasible. Data peeling is a strategy for defining a prognostic group based on several covariates by repeatedly refining rules by removing data along the covariate axes. The method allows one to look at average patient outcome (median survival or $k$-year survival probability) as a function of the fraction of the sample represented by the rule.

## 28.4.1 Region Refinement

Interest focuses on a region, $R$, of the predictor space with extreme patient outcome values. Denote the functional of interest, $Q$, (e.g., mean, median, or 5 year survival probability) for that region by

$$Q(R) = Q_{z \in R}(z).$$

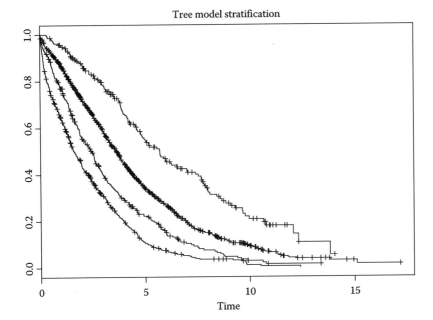

**FIGURE 28.7** Survival for four prognostic groups derived from the pruned survival tree. The top curve corresponds to survival for Node 3, the next curve corresponds to Nodes 2, 4, and 5, the next to Nodes 1 and 6 and the bottom curve to Nodes 7 and 8 (numbered from the left on Figure 28.6).

We assume a PH model with a conditional hazard function defined by

$$\lambda(t;z) = \lambda_0(t)\exp\bigl(\eta(z)\bigr),$$

where

$\lambda_0(t)$ is an unknown baseline hazard function

$\eta(z) = \eta I\{z \in R\}$ with $I\{z \in R\}$ equal to 1 if the covariate value is in $R$ or 0 otherwise

To facilitate description, we focus on a region, $R$, which can be described by a decision rule. For instance, we construct interpretable models based on boxes in the predictor space. If we assume the individual covariates, $z_1, \ldots, z_p$, are ordered, then univariate rules are of the form $D_j = \{z: z_j \geq s_j\}$ or $D_j = \{z: z_j < s_j\}, j = 1, \ldots, p$. Boxes can then be expressed as the intersection of the intervals:

$$B_k = \bigcap_{j=1}^{p} D_j.$$

Quite general regions can be defined using unions of boxes in the predictor space. Such rules are sometimes referred to as rules of disjunctive normal form. A model for two groups can be represented by $\eta(z) = \eta I\{z \in R\}$, where $R = \bigcup_k B_k$ is a union over boxes.

The peeling algorithm constructs rules (boxes) by repeatedly removing small amounts of data along the coordinate axes. Initially the entire data set is considered and then a fraction $\alpha$ of the data is removed along the covariate axis which leaves the largest parameter estimate for the remaining data in the box. The removal of data is continued until some minimum fraction of the observations remain in the box. The fraction of data to be removed at each step is taken to be quite small so that the procedure can recover from bad local decisions. However, a minimum number of observations, $n_{min}$, must be removed at each step to control the variance of the procedure.

Since survival data tend to have low signal, we have found it advantageous to remove data only in one direction for each variable. We refer to this as "directed peeling." The directions for refinement or data removal can be picked based on prior knowledge of the impact of the variables on disease outcome, or based on signs of the coefficients from a fitted linear PH model or a semiparametric method such as local partial likelihood as developed by Gentleman and Crowley (1991).

While $k$-year survival probability or median survival can be used to guide the peeling process, we have found it useful to use the hazard ratio from a Cox model since censoring may make those first quantities inestimable within some regions of the predictor space. The directed peeling algorithm changes the face of a box that maximizes the rate of increase in the estimated hazard ratio parameter associated with a box, $\eta(z) = \eta I\{z \in B\}$. Let

$$d_p = \frac{\hat{\eta}_{B_p} - \hat{\eta}_B}{\hat{\beta}(B) - \hat{\beta}(B_p)}$$

denote the change in the estimated regression parameter, $\hat{\eta}_{B_p}$, from the current value, $\hat{\eta}_B$, for a given proposed new box $B_p$ obtained by changing a box face along one axis. A cut point is changed from $s_p$ to $s_p'$ to modify the box $B_p = B \cap \{z_p < s_{p'}\}$ or $B_p = B \cap \{z_p \geq s_{p'}\}$ depending on the direction of the peeling. Because clinical data often include tied values for some covariates, one cannot remove an exact fraction $\alpha$ of the data at each step. Therefore, we standardize the change in hazard ratio by the difference in support between the current and refined box, $\hat{\beta}(B) - \hat{\beta}(B_p)$.

We note that the peeling process is computationally manageable. An upper bound on the number of steps for a peeling algorithm is $\log(\rho)/\log(1 - \alpha)$ where $\rho$ is the minimum fraction of the data of interest in a risk group. For example, for $\alpha = .1$ and $\rho = .05$ the maximum number of steps is 29. Focusing on the hazard ratio function allows a convenient way to select poor prognosis boxes as a function of the mass of the box. However, the median survival or proportion of sample in the prognostic group are useful summaries and are included as output from our peeling software.

As an example of the directed peeling process, we peel with respect to two variables $B2M$ and $ALB$ to identify a group of myeloma patients with particularly good survival. The first 15 steps of the refinement sequence are given in Table 28.1 for rules of the form

$$B2M \leq c_1 \bigcap ALB > c_2.$$

We call sequence of all the survival estimates the trajectory curve of the procedure.

**TABLE 28.1**

**Sequence of Thresholds for the First 15 Steps of Peeling of the Myeloma Data Set**

| Step | c1 (B2M) | c3 (ALB) | Median Survival |
|------|----------|----------|-----------------|
| 1 | 18.4 | −Inf | 3.17 |
| 2 | 12.4 | −Inf | 3.25 |
| 3 | 9.8 | −Inf | 3.39 |
| 4 | 8.3 | −Inf | 3.42 |
| 5 | 8.3 | 2.5 | 3.53 |
| 6 | 8.3 | 2.8 | 3.55 |
| 7 | 8.3 | 2.9 | 3.62 |
| 8 | 7.4 | 2.9 | 3.70 |
| 9 | 6.6 | 2.9 | 3.73 |
| 10 | 6.0 | 2.9 | 3.78 |
| 11 | 5.5 | 2.9 | 3.82 |
| 12 | 5.2 | 2.9 | 3.85 |
| 13 | 4.8 | 2.9 | 3.85 |
| 14 | 4.6 | 2.9 | 3.92 |
| 15 | 4.6 | 3.1 | 3.95 |

The rules are of the form $B2M \leq c_1 \cap ALB > c_2$

## 28.4.2 VARIABLE SELECTION AND PEELING FRACTION

To limit the amount of data adaptation, we use variable selection to limit the number of variables used in peeling. Options are to select the top $r$ variables based on the most significant univariate partial likelihood score tests or to limit peeling to variables that have been selected by multivariable linear PH modeling. For instance, one can use a forward stepwise model building strategy to select the variables to be used in the subsequent peeling. This simple filtering strategy also constrains the complexity and yields more easily interpreted rules.

Once the variables have been selected, the only tuning parameters that need to be adjusted are the fraction and minimum number of observations to remove at each step of the peeling process and the minimum fraction of the data to be considered in a smallest final group. As a default, we chose to remove 10% ($\alpha = .1$) of the current number of observations available for peeling (minimum 10 observations) at each step and set a smallest final group size to 5% ($\rho = .05$) of the original data set.

Simulations have shown that while selecting a small number of covariates for peeling dramatically reduces estimation bias due to selection (LeBlanc et al. 2002), it is still useful to have less biased estimates for rule selection. Given that one rarely has a test sample available to select the rule, we propose selecting rules using $K$-fold cross-validation. Bootstrap bias correction methods would be an alternative as we described for tree-based methods.

We use $K$-fold cross-validation as previously described for tree-based regression. Peeling is applied to each of the training samples $\Lambda_{(k)}$; each test sample $\Lambda_k$ is used to estimate the quantity of interest, $Q_k$ from the model grown on the training sample $\Lambda_{(k)}$.

For each training sample $\Lambda_{(k)}$, the trajectory curve $Q_k(\cdot)$ is defined as a piecewise constant curve $Q_k(x) = Q_k(\hat{\beta}_{l(k)})$ for $\hat{\beta}_{l(k)} + 1 \leq x < \hat{\beta}_{l(k)}$ where $\hat{\beta}_{l(k)}$ is the support of the $l$th box in the $k$th training sample trajectory. We define $\hat{\beta}_0 = 1$, $Q_k(1)$ as the functional calculated on the entire $k$th test sample and $\hat{\beta}_{L(k)+1} = 0$, where $L(k)$ is the smallest box in the $k$th trajectory.

The cross-validation estimate is the average over the individual curves indexed as a function of the fraction of the sample

$$Q^{cv}(\hat{\beta}_j) = \frac{1}{K} \sum_{k=1}^{K} Q_k(\hat{\beta}_j),$$

where

$\hat{\beta}_j$ is the observed support from the entire training sample for box $B_j$

$Q_k(\cdot)$ is functional of the $k$th test sample applied to the trajectory from the $k$th training sample

It is our experience that $K$-fold cross-validation can yield quite variable results. Therefore, for the peeling method we repeat $K$-fold cross-validation several times and average. The peeling trajectory for the myeloma data set and the 10-fold cross-validated estimates (averaged five times) are presented in Figure 28.8. In this case,

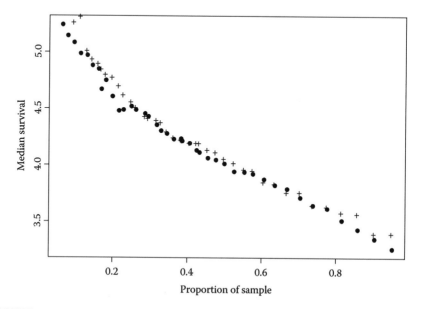

**FIGURE 28.8** First peeling trajectory on the myeloma data focusing on a good prognosis group (• represents training sample estimates and + represents averaged 10-fold cross-validation estimates).

the cross-validation estimates suggest limited selection bias. Here we suppose we are interested in patients with at least 4.5 years of median survival. If we apply the peeling rule and cross-validation, the resulting rule is

$$\text{RULE 1:}\quad B2M \leq 3.5 \bigcap ALB > 3.71,$$

which corresponds to a cross-validated estimate of median survival equal to 4.5 years and represents approximately 20% of the patients.

### 28.4.3 Constructing Multiple Box Rules

We have described the construction of a single box trajectory. The peeling process can be applied again to find additional patients with sufficiently extreme (poor or good) outcome. Therefore, the rules are refined through the addition (union) of other boxes. One removes the data corresponding to the first rule, before the next rule is constructed. At the $M$th iteration the box is constructed by using data not contained in any of the previous boxes:

$$\left\{ (t_i, \delta_i, z_i) \mid z_i \notin \bigcup_{m=1}^{M-1} B_m \right\}.$$

The estimated median survival from the Kaplan-Meier estimator (denoted by $KM_{MED}$) for a box at iteration $M$ is

$$Q_M = KM_{MED} \left\{ t_i, \delta_i \mid z_i \in B_M \cap z_i \notin \bigcup_{m=1}^{M-1} B_m \right\},$$

and the support in the box excluding previous boxes is

$$\beta_M = ave \left\{ I \left\{ z_i \in B_M \cap z_i \notin \bigcup_{m=1}^{M-1} B_m \right\} \right\},$$

where *ave* denotes "average." We applied this strategy to the myeloma data to determine if additional patients could be identified with a median survival of greater than 4.5 years using the 10-fold cross-validation estimates (averaged over five replications). While no additional group of patients could be identified with a survival greater than 4.5 years, the following rule depending on four variables (*B2M, PLT, CREAT,* and *ALB*) describes the next 10% of patients with best overall survival,

$$\text{RULE 2:}\ PLT > 208 \bigcap CREAT \leq 1.43 \bigcap B2M \leq 3.5 \bigcap ALB > 3.0$$

Combined with patients identified with RULE 1, the good prognostic group represents 30% of myeloma patients with estimated median survival of 4.2 years. One can also identify good prognosis patients from the tree-based model. In that case 15% patients were identified with a survival better than 4.5 years, but then adding in the patients with the next best survival leads to a group with 4.4 year median survival consisting of 26% of patients. This somewhat smaller fraction patients compared to peeling is mostly due to the discreteness of the tree-based rules which partition the data in large fractions.

## 28.5 EXTREME REGRESSION PROGNOSTIC MODELS

In the last section we showed that nonparametric data peeling can be an effective method for constructing a single or sequence of groups of patients corresponding to either extreme good or poor prognosis. Here we develop a strategy for finding such groups based on estimation of the entire regression function with a goal of improved performance in moderate sized clinical trials data sets. If one were to use a smooth additive model, even the linear regression model $h(x) = x'\beta$ leads to complex level set rules to describe the cases for which $\{x: x'\beta \geq q\}$. While prognostic rules developed for tree models such as $\{x: T(x) \geq q\}$ will result in decision rules, one potential downside to tree-based models relates to their discreteness. Consider a tree with only a few nodes representing significant fractions of the data. As one changes the threshold $q$ the percentage of sample corresponding to $T(x) \geq q$ often changes in large jumps. Therefore, the goal is to identify a different class of regression functions which is smooth but leads to logical rules if one considers cutpoints $T(x) \geq q$. Such a regression function exists (we call it extreme regression).

Our strategy is to use extreme functions (maximum and minimum) which yield simple interpretations of level sets similar to those from tree-based models. But, similar to linear or additive models, these models are a smooth function of the predictors.

Much like the prognostic peeling method, extreme regression focuses on groups of very good or poor prognosis (rather than a set of prognostic groups like trees), but allows indexing by the size of the prognostic group. Because of the nature of the function approximation method, it tends to give less variable solutions than peeling or trees. Some advantages to using our underlying function approximation approach are that it should work well in situations with a smaller number of cases due to its more parametric form, and it allows construction of a nested sequence of rules as the threshold $q$ varies.

### 28.5.1 EXTREME MODEL FORM

Our proposal is to replace the usual additive main effect and multiplicative interaction regression model with extreme operators of maximum and minimum. An example of such a model is

$$\eta(x) = \max\left(\min(\beta_{01} + \beta_{11}x_1, \beta_{02} + \beta_{12}x_2), \min(\beta_{03} + \beta_{13}x_3, \beta_{04} + \beta_{14}x_4)\right).$$

More generally we can write

$$\eta(x) = \max_j\left(f_1(x), f_2(x), \ldots, f_J(x)\right),$$

where each term $f_j(x) = \min(g_{j,1}(x), \ldots, g_{j,K(j)}(x))$. Each of the component functions, $g_{j,k}(x)$ depends only on a single predictor. Label $k$ denotes the component model of the $j$th "min" term where $j = 1, \ldots, J$ and $k = 1, \ldots, K(j)$ and where $K(j)$ is the number of linear component functions in each "min" term $j$. We use a simple univariate linear predictor

$$g_{j,k}(x) = \beta_{0,k} + \beta_{1,k} x_{l(k)}$$

where $l(k)$ is the label of the predictor in the $k$th term of component model $j$ (formally we should write $l(k,j)$, $\beta_{0,j,k}$, and $\beta_{1,j,k}$, but we suppress the $j$ for presentation). The following development for the linear model could easily be extended to $g_{j,k}(x)$ functions that are more general smooth univariate functions of predictors.

The overall model is a continuous piecewise linear model that locally depends only on a single predictor variable on each partition $R_{j,k}$ defined as $\{x: g_{j,k}(x) = f(x)\}$. We denote the data points which fall into region $R_{j,k}$ as the active set of points associated with function $g_{j,k}(x)$. Adaptive function approximation methods using piecewise linear component functions have been successfully and widely used (e.g., multivariate adaptive regression splines (MARS) Friedman [1991] and Hastie et al. [2009]) and for survival analysis in (e.g., Hazard Regression (Kooperberg et al. 1995) and other adaptive regression splines (LeBlanc and Crowley 1999). However, the extreme function formulation places different constraints on the nature of the piecewise linear model which are useful for describing the inverse of the regression function.

It is easily seen that the description of any $q$-level set $\Omega = \{x: f(x) \geq q\}$ is just

$$\Omega = \left\{ x : \mathrm{OR}_j \left( \left( g_{j,1}(x) \geq q \text{ AND} \cdots \text{AND } g_{j,K(j)}(x) \right) \geq q \right) \right\}.$$

This is referred to as a Boolean expression in disjunctive normal form (a union of intersections of simple terms). It is critical that each component function $g_{j,k(x)}$ is a function of a single predictor for $\Omega$.

### 28.5.2 ESTIMATION

While the algorithm was originally developed for squared error loss, it has been extended to parametric survival models. The estimation problem can be represented as of minimization

$$-L(\beta) = \sum -l\left(T_i, \delta_i \mid f(x_i)\right)$$

where
the $l(\cdot)$ is a log-likelihood function
the model $f(x_i)$ is the particular maximum and minimum form presented earlier

We have implemented the algorithm with exponential likelihood. For estimation, it is helpful to note that the objective function can also be represented as a weighted sum of likelihood observation components of the $M$ linear models

$$-L(\beta) = -\sum h_{(j,k)}(x_{i,l(k)}) l\left(T_i, \delta_i \mid g_{j,k}(x_{i,l(k)})\right),$$

where the weight function is an indicator $h_{(j,k)}(x_{i,l(k)}) = I\{g_{j,k}(x_{i,l(k)}) = f(x_i)\}$. For a fixed partition (or weight function) the ordinary maximum likelihood estimates of the coefficients are straightforward to calculate. In addition, given current parameter estimates one can determine the observations for which $\{x_i\colon g_{j,k}(x_{i,l}(k)) = f(x_i)\}$ to update the partition. An intuitive algorithm can incorporate these two facts as two steps: (1) *estimation* and (2) *partition* (reassignment of observations to groups). This algorithm is similar to the $K$-means algorithm. However, there is no assurance of finding a global optimum. In addition, in our experience during early steps of that algorithm, if many observations are reassigned to other partitions/groups at a single step of the algorithm, the log likelihood may actually decrease from one iteration to the next. This convergence issue can be addressed by introducing a step size $\Delta$ to the updating.

We note that a sufficiently small step size will always lead to an increase in the log likelihood. To see this, for the given partition, we calculate the maximum likelihood solution. Movement toward that solution will increase the likelihood. Continue until an observation is at the edge of two partitions. At that point, the observation can be reassigned to the other partition without any decrease in the likelihood. However, now one can obtain maximum likelihood estimates given the new partition; then movement toward the new least maximum likelihood estimate will again increase the likelihood. For computational reasons such a small step size is typically not practical.

We also constrain the number of observations used to estimate any component function. For instance, if $R_{j,k}$ at any step $m$ identifies fewer than $K_n$ observations, then the $K_n$ observations with the smallest absolute values of $d = g_{j,}k(x) - f(x)$ are used for estimation. Our default is $K_n = \min\{50, \max\{.05n, 25\}\}$.

### 28.5.3 MODEL BUILDING

Model building and variable selection can be implemented using greedy, semigreedy, or stochastic searches. We have implemented a simple stepwise algorithm where the model is expanded at each step by adding one additional linear component. This linear component can be added to an existing "minimum" term or as a new linear component in the outer "maximum" term. We rewrite the model at the $m$th iteration as

$$f^m(x) = \max_{j=1}^{J^m} \left(u_j^m(x)\right),$$

where

$$u_j^m(x) = \min\left(g_{j,1(j)}(x), \ldots, g_{j,K(j,m)}(x)\right).$$

The model size can be chosen using a less biased estimate of the prediction error than the residual error on the training data set such as $k$-fold cross-validation (or resampled averaged $k$-fold cross-validation), a low bias method for selecting complexity.

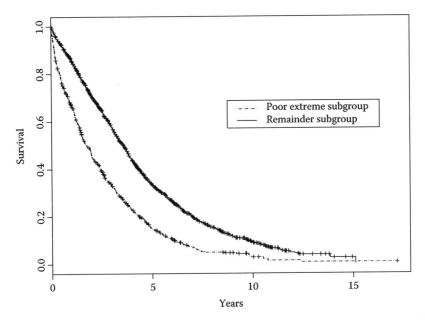

**FIGURE 28.9**   Poor prognostic group identified with extreme regression. Median survival is approximately 1.7 years and represents approximately 25% of patients the remaining patients have a median survival of approximately 3.6 years.

We have used a computationally cheap generalized cross-validation (GCV) estimate with a penalty parameter to acknowledge selection of terms. We use the default penalty of 1.5 per parameter in the model similar in spirit to the default GCV penalty used in the MARS algorithm.

We applied the algorithm to the myeloma data and chose an extreme decision rule with two variables B2M and ALB. The rule describing patients with the worst survival representing 25% of patients is $(ALB < 4.5)$ AND $(B2M \geq 6.7)$. The median survival for this poor prognostic group is 1.7 years versus 3.6 years for the remaining patients. The survival curves are given in Figure 28.9 and the sequence of all rules is shown in Figure 28.10.

## 28.6   DISCUSSION

Both the tree-based and data refinement methods describe prognostic groups using decision rules which we believe are useful for interpretation and for use in clinical settings. The primary objective of tree-based methods with censored survival data is to provide an easy to understand description of multiple prognostic groups of patients. By contrast, the peeling method and extreme regression focus on a single extreme outcome group. For problems where one wants to control either the proportion of patients in a poor/good prognostic group or the prognosis (e.g., median survival or 5 year survival probability), peeling or extreme regression can be a useful complement to tree-based methods, which give more discrete answers.

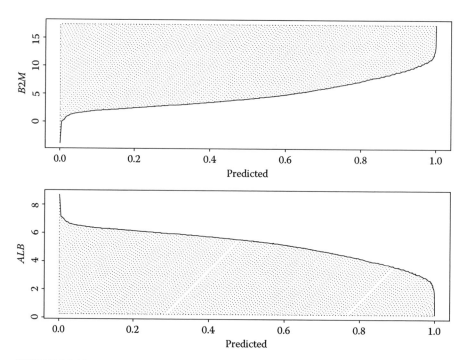

**FIGURE 28.10** Plot of sequence of decision rules as a function of extreme quantiles for myeloma data. Shading indicates the direction of decision rule.

We have chosen to focus on methods for constructing prognostic groups for predictor variables that are ordered. For binary data predictors, for example, including single nucleotide polymorphism (SNP) data then other methods are available for constructing prognostic decision rules. One related method that has been developed for constructing prognostic rules is called logic regression, which is a very general technique for constructing logic or Boolean rules for regression models using binary covariates (Ruczinski et al. 2003). The algorithm uses stochastic searches to avoid getting caught in local optima.

Software implementing tree-based methods based on logrank splitting using SPLUS™ are available from the first author. Other software has been written for tree-based modeling for survival data. The RPART program implements a recursive partitioning based on within-node error which includes exponential model-based survival trees (Therneau and Atkinson 1997). Software implementing peeling and for extreme regression are available from the first author and on CRAN.

## ACKNOWLEDGMENTS

This work was supported by the U.S. NIH through R01-CA90998, R01-HG006124, and P01 CA53996.

# REFERENCES

Akaike H. 1974. A new look at model identification. *IEEE Transactions on Automatic Control*, **19**, 716–723.

Albain K, Crowley J, LeBlanc M, and Livingston R. 1990. Determinants of improved outcome in small cell lung cancer: An analysis of the 2580 patient Southwest Oncology Group data base. *Journal of Clinical Oncology*, **8**, 1563–1574.

Breiman L, Friedman JH, Olshen RA, and Stone CJ. 1984. *Classification and Regression Trees*. Wadsworth, Belmont, CA.

Buhlmann P and Hohorn T. 2007. Boosting algorithms: Regularization, prediction and model fitting (with discussion). *Statistical Science*, **98**, 477–515.

Ciampi A, Hogg S, McKinney S, and Thiffaut J. 1988. RECPAM: A computer program for recursive partition and amalgamation for censored survival data. *Computer Methods and Programs in Biomedicine*, **26**, 239–256.

Cox DR. 1972. Regression models and life-tables (with discussion). *Journal of the Royal Statistical Society, Series B*, **34**, 187–220.

Crowley J, LeBlanc M, Gentleman R, and Salmon S. 1995. Exploratory methods in survival analysis. In *Analysis of Censored Data*, IMS Lecture Notes—Monograph Series 27, H. L. Koul and J. V. Deshpande, Eds., pp. 55–77, Institute of Mathematical Statistics, Hayward, CA.

Davis R and Anderson J. 1989. Exponential survival trees. *Statistics in Medicine*, **8**, 947–962.

Efron B and Tibshirani R. 1997. Improvements on cross-validation: The .632 Bootstrap method. *Journal of the American Statistical Association*, **92**, 548–560.

Fan J, Su XG, Levine R, Nunn M, and LeBlanc M. 2006. Trees for correlated survival data by goodness of split, with applications to tooth prognosis. *Journal of the American Statistical Association*, **101**(475), 959–967.

Friedman JH. 1991. Multivariate adaptive regression splines. *Annals of Statistics*, **19**, 1–67.

Friedman J and Fisher N. 1999. Bump hunting in high dimensional data (with discussion). *Statistics and Computing*, **9**,123–162.

Gentleman R and Crowley J. 1991. Local full likelihood estimation for the proportional hazards model. *Biometrics*, **47**, 1283–1296.

Gordon L and Olshen RA. 1985. Tree-structured survival analysis. *Cancer Treatment Reports*, **69**, 1065–1069.

Greipp P, San Miguel J, Durie B, Avet-Loiseau H, Facon T, Fonseca1 R, Rasmussen E et al. 2005. An International Staging System (ISS) for multiple myeloma (MM). *Journal of Clinical Oncology*, **23**, 3412–3420.

Hastie T, Tibshirani R, and Friedman J. 2009. *Elements of Statistical Learning*, 2nd edn. Springer, New York.

Ishwaran H, Kogalur UB, Blackstone EH, and Lauer MS. 2008. Random survival forests. *Annals of Applied Statistics*, **2**, 841–860.

Kooperberg C, Stone C, and Truong Y. 1995. Hazard regression, *Journal of the American Statistical Association*, **90**, 78–94.

LeBlanc M and Crowley J. 1992. Relative risk regression trees for censored survival data. *Biometrics*, **48**, 411–425.

LeBlanc M and Crowley J. 1993. Survival trees by goodness of split. *Journal of the American Statistical Association*, **88**, 457–467.

LeBlanc M and Crowley J. 1995. Step-function covariate effects in the proportional-hazards model. *The Canadian Journal of Statistics*, **23**, 109–129.

LeBlanc M and Crowley J. 1999. Adaptive regression splines in the Cox model, **55**, 204–215.

LeBlanc M, Jacobson J, and Crowley J. 2002. Partitioning and peeling for constructing patient outcome groups. *Statistical Methods for Medical Research*, **11**, 247–274.

LeBlanc M, Moon J, and Crowley J. 2005. Adaptive risk group refinement. *Biometrics*, **61**, 370–378.

LeBlanc M, Moon J, and Kooperberg C. 2006. Extreme regression. *Biostatistics*, **13**, 106–122.

Lerner S, Tangen C, Sucharew H, Wood D, and Crawford E. 2009. Failure to achieve a complete response to induction BCG therapy is associated with increased risk of disease worsening and death in patients with high risk non-muscle invasive bladder cancer. *Urologic Oncology: Seminars and Original Investigations*, **27**, 155–159.

Mantel N. 1966. Evaluation of survival data and two new rank order statistics arising in its consideration. *Cancer Chemotherapy Reports*, **50**, 163–170.

Quinlan JR. 1993. *C4.5 Programs for Machine Learning*. Morgan Kaufman, San Mateo, CA.

Ruczinski I, Kooperberg C, and LeBlanc M. 2003. Logic regression. *Journal of Graphical and Computational Statistics*, **12**, 475–511.

Segal MR. (1988). Regression trees for censored data. *Biometrics*, **44**, 35–48.

Therneau TM and Atkinson EJ. 1997. An introduction to recursive partitioning using the RPART routines. Technical report, Mayo Foundation (Distributed in PostScript with the RPART package).

Wiener M, Acland K, Shaw H, Soong SJ, Lin HY, Chen DT, Scolyer R, Winstanley J, and Thompson J. 2010. Sentinel node positive melanoma patients: Prediction and prognostic significance of nonsentinel node metastases and development of a survival tree model. *Annals of Surgical Oncology*, **17**, 1068–9265.

Zhang H and Singer B. 1999. *Recursive Partitioning in the Health Sciences*, Springer-Verlag, New York.

# 29 Risk Calculators

*Donna Pauler Ankerst and Yuanyuan Liang*

## CONTENTS

## 29.1 INTRODUCTION

As all roads of modern living, from business, to shopping to making friends, now run through the internet, it is not surprising that simple-to-use online tools are available at the fingertips for addressing almost any medical issue, from the simple question of "how long am I going to live?" (enter gender and date of birth at the U.S. Social Security life expectation calculator (http://www.ssa.gov/oact/population/longevity.html) to "what is my 30 day risk of postoperative surgical site infection after colorectal surgery?" (input some general information about yourself, including whether or not you smoke, pull some information from your medical chart, such as your albumin level, find out some specifics on your surgery, such as the duration in minutes, and enter at the appropriate calculator on http://www.lerner.ccf.org/qhs/risk_calculator/).

Two reasonable questions that are never asked but should be are how did these calculators get built in the first place and can they be blindly trusted? This chapter answers the first question in the context of risk calculators in oncology; the answer to the second is the same as with anything posted on the internet, no. Anyone can post an online calculator on the internet and there is no regulation of the accuracy (for an online tool to make an online tool, click on Make Your Own! at the top of the clinical calculator website http://www.lerner.ccf.org/qhs/risk_calculator/). Trustworthy online risk calculators should be accompanied by scientific peer-reviewed articles, which clearly elucidate the protocol by which they were created. They should have been constructed based on analyses from large representative cohorts and have had generalizability repeatedly confirmed by multiple external validations. After giving a reader-friendly tutorial on how risk calculators are built, this chapter reviews validation metrics and then provides a summary of some of the most currently widely assessed online risk calculators for oncology available on the internet.

## 29.2 BUILDING RISK CALCULATORS

Risk calculators most typically predict the probability of an event, such as having prostate cancer on biopsy, developing infection in a specified period of time, or surviving past 5 years after a treatment, though other types of outcomes can also be found, such as entire survival curves showing the probability of survival past individual times ranging from short- to long-term or velocities of a cancer biomarker. As such, the statistical model underpinning most modern risk models is logistic regression. Therefore this section describes this statistical model; other statistical models, such as Cox's proportional hazards survival model, might be used and the same model selection and validation principles would apply. To make the discussion concrete, the Prostate Cancer Prevention Trial (PCPT) risk calculator for prostate cancer is used continuously throughout as an example.

In 2006, the PCPT risk calculator was posted on the internet (now located at several locations including prostate-cancer-risk-calculator.com) in conjunction with simultaneous publication of its algorithm in the *Journal of the National Cancer Institute* (Thompson et al. 2006). The calculator was developed based on analysis of data from 5519 placebo arm participants who had undergone annual prostate-specific antigen (PSA) and digital rectal examination (DRE) screening as part of the 7 year PCPT. A noteworthy feature of the PCPT was that all participants were requested to undergo prostate biopsy, both during the trial when prompted by a high PSA or abnormal DRE and at the end of the trial regardless of PSA and DRE findings. Hence the PCPT cohort was unique among the existing prostate cancer cohorts in the world in that it was not prone to verification bias, which is the bias that results when only selected members of a population are ascertained for disease status, with selection determined by risk factors.

For predicting prostate cancer outcome, all potential risk factors measured on participants during the trial were identified, including age, family history of prostate cancer in a first degree relative, whether or not a prior prostate biopsy had been performed that was negative for prostate cancer, race, ethnicity, and PSA and DRE outcomes within 1 year prior to the biopsy result used in the analysis. Participants could have multiple biopsies up until either a positive diagnosis or the end-of-study required biopsy; only the last biopsy of each participant was used. The PCPT risk calculator additionally provides estimates of the risk of high-grade prostate cancer, defined as Gleason grade $\geq 7$ disease, but this calculation is not discussed further in this chapter.

### 29.2.1 LOGISTIC REGRESSION

Logistic regression is a method for relating multiple risk factors to a dichotomous outcome. In the context of this chapter, the dichotomous outcome is the presence or absence of prostate cancer on biopsy, and the multiple risk factors include PSA, DRE, family history of prostate cancer, and any other demographic or clinical variables that might be hypothesized to be associated with prostate cancer. Denoting the dichotomous outcome by $Y$, with $Y=1$ indicating prostate cancer and $Y=0$ no prostate cancer, and collecting potential risk factors into a vector $X$, the model for logistic regression relates the log odds of prostate cancer to the risk factors $X$ through

$$\log \frac{P(Y=1|X)}{1-P(Y=1|X)} = \alpha + \beta'X, \qquad (29.1)$$

where

log denotes the natural logarithm (base e)

$\alpha$ is an intercept

$\beta$ is a vector of log odds ratios, one for each risk factor assembled in $X$

To understand why $\beta$ defines log odds ratios, it is helpful to consider the simple scenario of just one dichotomous risk factor, $X=$ DRE result, where $X=1$ if the DRE test is abnormal, suspicious for cancer and 0 otherwise. In this case $\beta$ is a single number. Then, based on the logistic model, the odds of prostate cancer based on DRE is

$$\frac{P(Y=1|X)}{1-P(Y=1|X)} = \exp\{\alpha + \beta X\},$$

where exp denotes the exponential function. This equation implies that for the individual with DRE outcome $X$, the probability of prostate cancer equals $\exp\{\alpha + \beta X\}$ times the probability of no prostate cancer. The odds of prostate cancer for individuals with abnormal DRE ($X=1$) and normal DRE ($X=0$) are given by

$$\frac{P(Y=1|X=1)}{1-P(Y=1|X=1)} = \exp\{\alpha+\beta\}, \quad \frac{P(Y=1|X=0)}{1-P(Y=1|X=0)} = \exp\{\alpha\},$$

respectively. From these expressions, one might expect $\beta$ to be greater than 0 since individuals with an abnormal DRE should have a higher probability, and hence odds, of prostate cancer on biopsy than individuals with a normal DRE. The ratio of odds for individuals with abnormal ($X=1$) to normal ($X=0$) DRE describes the magnitude by which the odds of prostate cancer change for an individual with abnormal compared to normal DRE:

$$\frac{P(Y=1|X=1)/(1-P(Y=1|X=1))}{P(Y=1|X=0)/(1-P(Y=1|X=0))} = \frac{\exp\{\alpha+\beta\}}{\exp\{\alpha\}} = \exp\{\beta\}.$$

Therefore, exp{β} is the odds ratio (OR) for individuals with abnormal compared to normal DRE.

For the case of a single predictor $X$ that is continuous rather than dichotomous, the OR gives the ratio of odds of outcome $Y$ for a unit-increase in $X$ (to see this compute the OR for $X = x + 1$ compared to $X = x$). An OR > 1 implies that an increase in the risk factor increases the odds of prostate cancer, OR < 1 means it decreases the odds and OR = 1 means it has no impact. From the previous relationship, $\beta = \log\{\exp\{\beta\}\}$ is the log odds ratio (log OR), and values of $\beta > 0$, $< 0$, and $= 0$ have the same interpretations as for OR > 1, < 1 and = 1, respectively.

If $X$ were a categorical risk factor with more than two levels, such as race with levels African American, Caucasian, and Other, the logistic model can still be fit by choosing one level as a reference (say Caucasian) and then returning two odds ratios, one for the comparison of each of the remaining levels, African American and Other, to the reference. In many aspects such as this logistic regression operates similarly as for linear regression. In the general case of multiple risk factors (29.1), $\beta = (\beta_1, \beta_2, \ldots, \beta_p)$ is the vector of respective log ORs for each of the multiple risk factors comprising $X = (X_1, X_2, \ldots, X_p)$:

$$\log \frac{P(Y = 1 \mid X)}{1 - P(Y = 1 \mid X)} = \alpha + \beta_1 X_1 + \beta_2 X_2 + \cdots + \beta_p X_p.$$

The interpretation of each parameter $\beta_i$ is the log OR corresponding to a unit increase in the respective risk variable $X_i$, with all other risk variables in the model held constant.

Statistical packages return estimates of log odds ratios (β's), their standard errors, and $p$-values for tests of the null hypotheses that they equal 0 (no effect) versus two-sided alternative hypotheses that they do not equal 0. From these approximate 95% confidence intervals for log ORs can be constructed as (estimated log OR) ± 1.96 × (standard error); to obtain estimates and confidence intervals for the ORs, take the exponent of the estimates and 95% confidence interval bounds, respectively.

### 29.2.2 Model Selection

The developer of a risk prediction tool, particularly one that plans to post on the internet, should want a model that validates well to external populations. Once the calculator is in cyberspace, it is open season for validation by third parties, which is a good thing for ensuring the most accurate tool is available for the intended users. Contrary to what many think, the most-likely-to-validate calculator is not the one that contains all possible risk factors. Models that are over-parameterized, containing statistically insignificant effects or statistically significant effects that bring little to model fit at the expense of a sizable loss to effective sample size, sometimes referred to as degrees of freedom, are not going to validate as well as parsimonious models that optimize the balance between good fit to the development dataset and likelihood to generalize to completely external datasets. For this purpose, a variety of model selection techniques are available in statistical packages, many of which automatically sort through large numbers of models. Some of the most commonly used model selection techniques are based on finding the model with the lowest Akaike's information criterion, AIC $= -2 \times$ maximized log likelihood $+ 2 \times$ number of parameters, or the lowest Bayesian information criterion, BIC $= -2 \times$ maximized log likelihood $+ \log$(sample size) $\times$ number of parameters (Akaike 1974, Schwarz 1978). The first terms of both criteria seek to find the model maximizing goodness-of-fit to the developmental data set, while the second terms penalize for over-parameterization, with the BIC tending to penalize more, and hence selecting smaller models with fewer parameters than the AIC on average. Both criteria were developed in the context of choosing between two models, with one nested in the other, and are only technically applicable for this case. Similarly, extensions to their formulas are required for consistency in handling non-(independent and identically distributed) data, such as that arising from random effects models, or for high-dimensional predictor problems as arising in genomic applications. But this has not prevented these techniques from being used as approximate methods for selecting among vast sets of possible models in a wide array of contexts.

### 29.2.3 INTERNAL VALIDATION

Internal validation can be used as a final selection criterion for choosing between a small number of preselected risk models or for an evaluation of the external validation potential of a model-building procedure. One of the simpler forms is $K$-fold cross-validation, which randomly splits the data into $K$ approximately equally sized sets, $S_k$, $k = 1, \ldots, K$. For each $S_k$, a validation metric $\text{VAL}_{(k)}$, which can be any of the external validation metrics described in Section 29.3, is estimated using the risk model fit on all observations not in $S_k$ and then applied to all observations in $S_k$ as the mock external validation sample. The estimate of validation performance is the sample average of the $K$ internal estimates:

$$\text{VAL} = \frac{1}{K} \sum_{k=1}^{K} \text{VAL}_{(k)}.$$

Standard errors for VAL can be approximated by standard errors estimated from the developmental dataset (Tian et al. 2007).

Alternatively internal validation can be performed using the bootstrap (Efron 1979). For a large number of $K$ iterations, a random sample of the same size as the developmental dataset is drawn with replacement, the risk model is estimated on the random sample and evaluated on the same sample to yield $\text{VAL}_{(k)}$ for $k = 1, \ldots, K$. As for cross-validation, the average VAL is the validation performance estimate. The bootstrap estimate of the standard error of VAL is simply the standard deviation of the $\text{VAL}_{(k)}$ for $k = 1, \ldots, K$ (Efron 1981).

Internal validation approaches do not account for the model uncertainty in arriving at the handful of models under consideration, which contributes to their overoptimistic bias for estimating potential external validation (Copas and Corbett 2002). Instead of application to preselected models, an alternative use of internal validation is for estimating the validation potential for the entire model-building process. For each split or random draw of the developmental dataset, a model is built from scratch on the training set and then evaluated on the test set. The process is more computationally intensive and results in several different models, one for each iteration, but evaluating similarities among the internal models can be useful in identifying risk factors that appear often and hence are most likely to be relevant for external prediction. Many algorithms for supervised and machine-based learning for high-dimensional predictor spaces intrinsically perform some type of internal validation in the model fitting process, thus integrating automatic model selection into the final product, or average over multiply selected models from different internal validation iterations. Some examples include boosting, Bayesian ensembles, bootstrap aggregating (bagging), neural networks, support vector machines, and random forests, all available in the statistical package *R*. While internal validation may provide more safeguards to protect against over-fitting than pure likelihood-based model selection procedures, it is no substitute for external validation on a completely separate dataset to that used to build the model, as described in Section 29.3.

### 29.2.4 PCPT RISK CALCULATOR

As reported in Thompson et al. (2006), the BIC and average cross-validated area underneath the receiver operating characteristic curve (AUC) were used to find the optimal multivariable logistic regression model relating potential risk factors to prostate cancer outcome on biopsy on data from the 5519 PCPT placebo arm participants used to develop the PCPT risk calculator. The AUC is a rank-based measure of how well a risk model discriminates prostate cancer cases from controls and is defined in Section 29.3. Specifically, fourfold cross-validation of VAL = average(AUC) was used, whereby the developmental dataset of 5519 observations was randomly partitioned into four subsets, three of size 1380 and one of size 1379, with randomization stratified to keep the proportion of prostate cancer cases between 20% and 23% in each subset. For logistic regression, randomization stratified by outcome ensures adequate power for each of the training and test sets. Over 50 models, some including two-way interactions, were evaluated by a combination of forward, backward, and stepwise selection and subjective measures. BIC and cross-validated AUC values were tabulated for each of the models. The five models with the lowest BIC values additionally had the highest AUC values. The AUC values fell within one standard error of each other and hence were deemed equivalent according to this metric. The model with the lowest BIC value contained only main effects and no interactions among risk factors. Therefore, this model was selected to form the PCPT risk calculator. This example illustrates the subjectivity that is ultimately exercised in choosing a single model among several that are empirically indistinguishable under a variety of criteria.

The equation for the final selected multivariable logistic model can be accessed on the PCPT risk calculator website and the list of included risk factors and their odds ratio estimates are detailed in Thompson et al. (2006). There are four risk factors included in the model: PSA (OR = 2.34 for logPSA), DRE (OR = 2.47), family history of prostate cancer (OR = 1.31), and history of a prior negative prostate biopsy (OR = 0.64). All were statistically significant with a *p*-value less than .001 except for family history with a *p*-value of .002. As predicted, among the 5519 PCPT placebo arm participants, the risk of prostate cancer increased with increasing PSA, abnormal DRE result, and a positive family history of prostate cancer. More of an initial surprise at the time was the decreased risk among participants with a prior biopsy of the prostate. Upon retrospection, this could be explained as a screening effect.

## 29.3  EXTERNAL VALIDATION

Most risk models underpinning online calculators have been constructed from analysis of data from either a single cohort or a multi-institutional study, and hence may suffer from lack of power due to small sample size of the developmental dataset, or lack of generalizability due to specificity of the cohort. Performance evaluation on a completely distinct population is the only proof of principle for whether or not the calculator has been validated, so only online calculators built on sound published studies and that have been extensively validated using unbiased methods should be trusted. A variety of evaluation methods for risk models have been proposed in the literature, and these can be grouped into those that measure discrimination, calibration, or both. Steyerberg et al. (2010) provide a recent review, detangling the different objectives of the many metrics currently employed to evaluate risk prediction models. To keep the presentation concrete, the PCPT risk calculator for prostate cancer on biopsy will be used throughout as an example. In addition, the presentation will be limited to the foundational components of discrimination and calibration. Composite measures, such as the Brier score and $R^2$ statistics, combine these two concepts into a single measure; newer measures focused on clinical interpretation, such as net benefit, are direct functions of discrimination metrics (Nagelkerke 1991; Vickers and Elkin 2006; Gerds et al. 2008).

The National Cancer Institute dictionary of cancer terms available on the internet defines a marker as a diagnostic indication that disease may develop. In this case, a risk prediction for cancer such as output of the PCPT risk calculator can be viewed itself as an integrative marker, which merges risk factors, such as family history of prostate cancer with other biomarkers, such as PSA and DRE. As seen in (29.1) the weighting of the risk factors is linear on the logit scale. Therefore, all the machinery developed for evaluating continuous markers of disease can be applied to evaluate outputs of risk models with one important exception. Unlike typical markers of disease, which are biological quantities measured in bodily fluids or tissues, risk predictions have been estimated statistically on a developmental dataset, often called the training set. Therefore, evaluation of their accuracy on the same training dataset is inherently biased, a fact that unfortunately still goes unnoticed in many peer-reviewed scientific articles proposing new prediction models. The metrics for evaluating prediction models reviewed in this section should be evaluated on external datasets, often referred to as test sets, to those used to develop the model, in order to obtain an unbiased assessment of performance.

### 29.3.1  DISCRIMINATION

There are two key aspects that characterize the discriminatory ability of a risk prediction for cancer. First, an accurate prediction should be able to "rule in" those who truly have cancer, since missing or delaying a cancer diagnosis can have grave consequences. Second, an accurate prediction should be able to "rule out" persons that do not have cancer, removing potential emotional and financial burdens associated with more invasive testing. Discrimination metrics concern themselves only with how well the risk prediction operates for hard classification: ruling in the cancer cases and ruling out the noncancer cases. They report simply the misclassification error for cancers and noncancers separately, with no judgment given to how close the risk prediction is to the actual risk in the test set, the target of calibration described later. A simple exploratory data analysis tool for investigating how well risk probabilities discriminate between cancer cases and noncancer cases in an external dataset is to plot histograms of the risk predictions for cancer and noncancer cases on the same scale and see the extent to which they overlap. Cancer cases should have notably higher risks than noncancer cases; if there are a substantial fraction of cancer cases with similar estimated risks to the noncancer cases, then discrimination of the risk calculator is poor.

Moving from a risk prediction, which is a probability or percent varying from 0% to 100%, to a recommendation that rules in a patient as a cancer diagnosis or rules out one requires selection of a threshold $c$ such that a risk above $c$ would correspond to ruling in cancer and a risk less than or equal to $c$, ruling out. This is typically not easy to do since no single optimal $c$ will minimize all possible errors and error rates will vary by cohort. At the end, some subjectivity is required. Dilemmas on threshold selection have predominated diagnostic medicine based on continuous markers of disease. For instance, there is an ongoing debate as to whether to lower the 4.0 ng/mL threshold of PSA for referral to prostate biopsy to 2.5 ng/mL. As a first pass, discrimination is evaluated for all possible thresholds $c$ ranging from 0% to 100%.

How successfully the risk prediction rules in cancer cases is termed sensitivity and on the test set is estimated by the percent correct diagnoses among the cancer cases:

$$\text{Sensitivity}(c) = \frac{\text{Number of cancer cases with risk} > c}{\text{Number of cancer cases}},$$

where sensitivity is indexed by $c$ as a reminder that it depends on the user-selected $c$. How successfully the risk prediction rules out noncancer cases is termed specificity and is accordingly estimated by

$$\text{Specificity}(c) = \frac{\text{Number of noncancer cases with risk} \leq c}{\text{Number of noncancer cases}}.$$

Ideally a good risk prediction tool would be one for which a threshold $c$ exists that yields 100% sensitivity and specificity, which, as remarked earlier, is not typically achievable in practice. As seen from the formulas, as the threshold $c$ for a positive diagnosis would increase on any given test set, the sensitivity would decrease to the limit 0% and specificity would increase to the limit 100%. One minus the sensitivity is often referred to as the false-negative rate (FNR) and one minus the specificity, the false-positive rate (FPR).

The receiver operating characteristic (ROC) curve provides a summary of sensitivity and specificity for all choices of $c$ ranging from 0% to 100%; it typically displays sensitivity on the $y$-axis and FPRs on the $x$-axis, with both axes ranging from 0% to 100%. The ROC curve has been widely applied in diagnostic medicine as a standard summary of diagnostic accuracy since its origination from signal detection theory in psychophysics (Swets and Pickett 1982; Hanley 1989; Begg 1991; Zweg and Campbell 1993). There are many appealing features of an ROC curve. First, it provides a way to visualize the notion of diagnostic accuracy in a straightforward way. The higher the ROC curve, the better its capacity for distinguishing cancer from noncancer cases. Second, ROC curves are invariant with respect to measurement scales, for example, risks and the logits of risks (29.1) will yield the same ROC curve. This makes ROC curves particularly useful when comparing tests on completely different measurement scales, for example, for directly comparing risk predictions from a model to the leading biomarker in the model. Finally, as rank-based measures, ROC curves are by definition independent of disease prevalence and hence can be applied to the case-control study situation in addition to prospective studies.

In addition to showing the ROC curve, it is common to present summary points on the curve in a table, such as specificities and sensitivities by selected thresholds of the risk predictions, such as 5%, 10%, and 25%. Alternatively since many applications of diagnostic testing in oncology have maximum allowable FPRs, sensitivities for thresholds obtaining a range of specificities are reported. Finally, it is common to report a summary measure of the ROC curve, as the area under the curve (AUC), which in addition, conveniently holds the intuitive definition as the probability that a randomly chosen cancer case has a higher risk prediction than a randomly chosen noncancer case.

To estimate the ROC curve nonparametrically suppose there are $n_D$ risk predictions from the cancer cases among the test set represented as $\{Y_{Di}: i=1, \ldots, n_D\}$ and $n_H$ risk predictions from the noncancer cases among the test set represented as $\{Y_{Hj}: j=1,\ldots, n_H\}$. Set the collection of thresholds to be $C=\{Y_{Di}: i=1, \ldots, n_D; Y_{Hj}: j=1,\ldots, n_H\}$ and for each $c \in C$, estimate the sensitivity and FPR by

$$\text{Sensitivity}(c) = \frac{\sum_{i=1}^{n_D} I(Y_{Di} > c)}{n_D}$$

$$\text{FPR}(c) = \frac{\sum_{j=1}^{n_H} I(Y_{Hj} > c)}{n_H},$$

where $I(Y_{Di}>c)$ equals 1 if $Y_{Di}>c$ and 0 otherwise and similarly for $I(Y_{Hj}>c)$. To obtain the empirical ROC curve, plot the collection of (sensitivity($c$), FPR($c$)) pairs for all $c \in C$. The AUC is calculated from the empirical ROC curve by averaging sensitivity($c$) across $c$. Alternatively, as the AUC is by definition is $P(Y_D>Y_H)$ where $Y_D$ and $Y_H$ are risk prediction values from randomly selected cases and controls, respectively, it can be calculated by the Mann–Whitney $U$-statistic:

$$A\hat{U}C = \sum_{j=1}^{n_H} \sum_{i=1}^{n_D} \frac{I[Y_{Di} > Y_{Hj}]}{n_D n_H}.$$

Since the Mann–Whitney statistic is a function of the Wilcoxon rank sum statistic, it follows that the nonparametric Wilcoxon test can be used for testing the null hypothesis that the AUC equals 0.5 (meaning the risk predictions do no better than flipping a two-sided coin in distinguishing cancer from noncancer cases) versus the alternative that it exceeds 0.5. These statistics and tests are available in most statistical packages. The standard deviation of the AUC is more complicated to compute, requiring either a $U$-statistic approach (DeLong et al. 1988), or the bootstrap resampling method (Efron and Tibshirani 1993). Other statistical tests, such as tests of the null hypothesis that two risk models have the same AUC on the same dataset versus the alternative that they differ can also be programmed by extending these methods.

A recent validation of the PCPT risk calculator illustrates discrimination concepts. In 2009 the generalizability of the PCPT risk calculator for potential applicability to other populations than for which it was developed was investigated. The PCPT was developed on a relatively healthy population of predominantly Caucasian men. Among the entry requirements were that they be 55 years of age or older, have a normal DRE exam, and a PSA level less than or equal to 3.0 ng/mL. As part of the study they underwent annual screening for 7 years. In contrast, the Early Detection Research Network (EDRN) clinical cohort comprised 645 men who had been referred to multiple urology practices across five states in the northeastern United States and had received a prostate biopsy due to some clinical indication (Eyre et al. 2009). Some of the men in the EDRN cohort were younger than 55 years of age and as Table 1 of Eyre et al. (2009) showed, the cohort differed statistically significantly ($p < .0001$) in distribution of every risk factor compared to the 5519 manned PCPT cohort used to develop the PCPT risk model. PCPT risks were calculated for each member of the EDRN cohort and compared to the actual clinical outcome on biopsy for assessment of discrimination performance of the PCPT risk calculator. The PCPT risk calculator demonstrated statistically significant superior discrimination for detecting prostate cancer cases compared to PSA (AUC = 69.1% compared to 65.5%, respectively, $p$-value = .009), and the ROC curve for the PCPT risk calculator consistently fell at or above that for PSA for all FPRs, with the greatest difference for FPRs less than 25%. For example, the thresholds of the PCPT risk calculator and PSA, which obtained a FPR of 20%, were 48.4% and 6.9 ng/mL, respectively (Table 2 of Eyre et al. 2009). One can view these as two competing tests for referral to further intensive diagnostic testing by prostate biopsy, each with equal specificities: the PCPT risk calculator refers a patient to prostate biopsy if his PCPT risk exceeds approximately 50% and the PSA test if his PSA exceeds 6.9 ng/mL. If these two diagnostic tests had been implemented in the EDRN population to "rule in" patients who should undergo prostate biopsy and "rule out" patients who should not, the PCPT risk calculator would have correctly referred 47.1% of the prostate cancer cases (sensitivity) and the PSA test 35.4% of the prostate cancer cases. Although better than PSA, the PCPT risk calculator would still have missed 50% of the prostate cancer cases. Insisting that 80% of prostate cancer cases get caught for both tests would have meant that the thresholds for referral would have had to be lowered, to 38.0% and 4.0 ng/mL, for the PCPT risk calculator and PSA test, respectively (Table 3, Eyre et al. 2009). But this would have approximately halved the specificity of both tests, to 40.3% for the PCPT risk calculator and 44.1% for PSA. In other words, approximately 60% of the men who did not have prostate cancer would have been referred to a prostate biopsy unnecessarily (FPR), an error rate unacceptable from a public health perspective.

This example illustrates the poor discrimination performance of the currently recommended diagnostic tools for prostate cancer, as well as the difficulty in comparing tests when there is a wide range of possible thresholds. Unfortunately, currently most risk tools across oncology also suffer from poor discrimination performance.

## 29.3.2 CALIBRATION

Calibration concerns itself with how close risk predictions are to the actual risks observed in an external population that is used for validation. For example, the PCPT risk calculator returns a 23% risk of finding prostate cancer on biopsy for a 65 year old Caucasian man with a PSA 2.0 ng/mL, normal DRE, no family history of prostate cancer, and who has never had a prostate biopsy. If the calculator were properly calibrated, then among all such 65 year old Caucasian men with a PSA 2.0 ng/mL, normal DRE, no family history of prostate cancer, and who have never had a prostate biopsy, 23% of them would have prostate cancer on biopsy. In other words, the observed risk would match the predicted risk among homogenous groups defined by the same risk profile. Obtaining a proper external validation set large enough to have enough men in each risk category to make comparisons quickly becomes infeasible as the number of risk factors increases, hence approximations are made by further grouping. To illustrate calibration principles, validation of the PCPT risk calculator on the EDRN cohort comprising 645 men is again used.

Eyre et al. (2009) reported that the average PCPT risk over the EDRN cohort was 45.1%, which is fairly high in keeping with the nature of the cohort as elicited from multiple urology practices. As a first indication of calibration, the average PCPT risk among the cohort should correspond to the actual percent of the cohort that did have prostate cancer on biopsy. This percentage was 43.4%, fairly close to the average PCPT risk.

Table 4 of Eyre et al. (2009) provided further descriptive analyses of the degree to which the PCPT risk calculator calibrated to actual risks for specific subgroups, such as for Caucasians, African Americans, men with a positive family history, and men with PSA less than 4.0 ng/mL. Across all subgroups the average PCPT risk never varied by more than approximately 5 or 6 percentage points from the observed risk but there were some subgroups where PCPT risks were better calibrated to actual risks than others. For example, among the 47 African American participants in the cohort, 51.1% had prostate cancer but the average PCPT risk among these men was only 45.4%. A more systematic method for comparing observed to expected risks is to tabulate observed risks obtained in deciles of expected risks for the individuals of the validation set as done in Table 5 of Eyre et al. (2009). As an example, the minimum PCPT risk observed in the EDRN cohort was 4.1% and 67 of the EDRN participants (10% of 675) had PCPT risks below 30%. Among these 67 participants, 17.9% had prostate cancer on biopsy, a number falling fairly centrally in the interval 4.1%–30%. An approximation to Pearson's chi-square goodness-of-fit test recommended by Lemeshow and Hosmer (1982),

$$\chi^2 = \sum_{i=1}^{k} \frac{(O_i - n_i\pi_i)^2}{n_i\pi_i(1-\pi_i)},$$

was performed by comparing the observed numbers of prostate cancer cases $O_i$ to expected numbers, calculated as the median PCPT risk $\pi_i$ multiplied by the number of observations in each group $n_i$, in each of the $k=10$ decile groups, and assuming a chi-square distribution with $k$ degrees of freedom. This yielded a $p$-value of .10, not rejecting the null hypothesis of a good fit at the .05 level of statistical significance.

A rather intuitive test for what is termed reliability was proposed by Cox (1958) and elaborated upon in Miller et al. (1991). The approach requires logistic regression of the cancer outcomes ($Y_i=0$ no cancer, $Y_i=1$ cancer) on the logit of the predicted risks ($\pi_i$) as covariates for the $i=1, \ldots, N$ individuals in the validation set:

$$\log \frac{P(Y_i = 1)}{1 - P(Y_i = 1)} = \alpha + \beta \log \frac{\pi_i}{1-\pi_i}.$$

A perfect match of predicted to actual risks would occur when $\alpha=0$ and $\beta=1$. Therefore, a test of the composite null hypothesis $H_0$: $\alpha=0$, $\beta=1$ provides an overall reliability test for the predictions. More specifically, the intercept $\alpha$ controls the calibration of the model, which is most clearly seen when $\beta=1$. When $\beta=1$, $\alpha<0$ implies the predicted risks are too high and $\alpha>0$, too low. When $\beta \neq 1$, noting that for $\pi_i=0.5$:

$$\log \frac{P(Y_i = 1)}{1 - P(Y_i = 1)} = \alpha,$$

one can interpret the intercept $\alpha$ as a calibration measure at $\pi_i=0.5$. The slope parameter $\beta$ is referred to as the refinement parameter: $\beta>1$ implies the predicted risks do not vary enough, $0<\beta<1$ they vary too much, and $\beta<0$ they show the wrong direction. Therefore, additional tests of calibration given appropriate refinement, $H_0$: $\alpha=0|\beta=1$, and of refinement given appropriate calibration, $H_0$: $\beta=1|\alpha=0$, can be performed.

In the analysis of Eyre et al. (2009), a logistic regression of observed prostate cancer status on logits of predicted PCPT risks was performed for the 645 men comprising the EDRN validation set. While the exact hypotheses tests reported earlier were not performed, the intercept from the logistic regression was estimated by −0.014 with standard error 0.091 and the slope by 1.291 with standard error 0.159. Separate 95% confidence intervals for these estimates overlapped with 0 and 1, respectively, indicating that PCPT risks were reliable estimates of observed risks in the EDRN population.

## 29.4   EXAMPLES

In this section, examples of some of the currently most widely accessed and validated online calculators dedicated to oncology are given. The list is not exhaustive and the field is rapidly picking up pace, resulting in a continuous stream of new online calculators as they are developed and validated.

### 29.4.1   EARLY PROSTATE CANCER DETECTION

Numerous studies have developed prostate cancer risk calculators based on different cohorts of patients from varying geographical locations and amounts of prior prostate cancer screening, such as by prior prostate biopsy. Shariat and Kattan provided a comprehensive overview of prostate cancer predictive tools published during the period January 1966 to July 2007 (Shariat and Kattan 2009). As alternatives to risk calculators, which hide the calculation in a black box, many of the developed prostate cancer tools are the more old-fashioned yet more transparent nomograms. In its simplest form, a nomogram is a graph, usually containing three parallel scales graduated for relating two risk factors to the risk, so that when a straight line connects the value of the two risk factor scales, the related risk value may be read directly from the third at the point intersected by the line. For more than two risk factors, nomograms can be expanded by assigning points to risk factors, followed by summation of the points to determine the risk category. The advantages of nomograms are that they are model-free, may be used without a computer, and intuitively disclose how each risk factor contributes to the risk. Disadvantages are their lack of accuracy compared to model-based risk calculators. Table 29.1 summarizes a list of online prostate cancer risk calculators developed in Europe, North America, and Asia over the past 3 years. Some risk calculators were developed on clinical cohorts with numerous patients with high PSA or abnormal DRE, which are clinical indicators of preexisting conditions, such as benign hyperplastic dysplasia (Nam et al. 2007; Chun et al. 2009; Cao et al. 2011). In contrast, others were developed on large population-based studies comprising primarily healthy symptom-free men with lower PSA distributions and lower abnormal DRE rates (Thompson et al. 2006, 2007; Ankerst et al. 2008; Liang et al. 2010; Roobol et al. 2010).

As outlined previously, the PCPT risk calculator requires minimal information routinely collected in the clinic (age, race, PSA, DRE, family and prior biopsy history) for predicting the risk of prostate cancer and the risk of high-grade prostate cancer and applies to healthy men with no prior cancer diagnosis and no known clinical symptoms of benign prostatic disease. Other available risk calculators involve more specialized inputs that are not routinely collected, including prostate volume (Nam et al. 2007; Chun et al. 2009; Roobol et al. 2010), the urinary prostate cancer gene 3 (PCA3) (Ankerst et al. 2008; Chun et al. 2009; Cao et al. 2011), and %freePSA (Nam et al. 2007), and were developed for men presenting at clinics with symptoms. These calculators, intended for more specialized clinical populations and with less commonly collected risk factors, are less applicable for the general population of healthy older males that might be targeted for prostate cancer screening.

**TABLE 29.1**

**Review of Currently Available Risk Calculators for Early Prostate Cancer Detection**

| Name | Study Design Sample Size | Source Population Inclusion Criteria | Predictors for Biopsy-Detectable PCA | Notes |
|---|---|---|---|---|
| PCPT risk calculator (Thompson et al. 2006, 2007) | Prospective multicenter RCT from America; $n = 5519$ (1211 PCA; 257 HG PCA) | Healthy screening patients; placebo arm of the PCPT; age ≥ 55 years; biopsied; at least one PSA and DRE measurement within 1 year before biopsy; at least 2 PSA measurements within 3 years before biopsy | PCPT risk factors: age at biopsy, PSA, race, family history, DRE, and prior negative biopsy | Available online at deb.uthscsa.edu/URORiskCalc/Pages/uroriskcalc.jsp; validated in external populations (Parekh et al. 2006, Eyre et al. 2009, Hernandez et al. 2009, Nguyen et al. 2010) |
| PCA3 adjusted PCPT risk calculator (Ankerst et al. 2008) | Prospective multicenter cohort from America; $n = 521$ (182 PCA; 73 HG PCA) | American patients with info on PCA3, PSA, DRE, age (31–87 years), race, negative biopsy history and family history; biopsied | PCPT risk factors and urinary PCA3 | Available online at deb.uthscsa.edu/URORiskCalc/Pages/uroriskcalc.jsp; validated in external populations (Ankerst et al. 2008, Perdona et al. 2011) |
| BMI-adjusted PCPT risk calculator (Liang et al. 2010) | Prospective cohort from SABOR; $n = 3697$ (265 PCA; 81 HG PCA) | Texan screening patients with age, PSA, BMI, DRE, race, family history, and negative biopsy history collected within 2.5 years before diagnosis or last visit | PCPT risk factors and BMI | Screening-detected PCA cohort, not all controls were biopsy-confirmed negative; available online at deb.uthscsa.edu/URORiskCalc/Pages/uroriskcalc.jsp |
| Chun's prostate cancer nomogram (Chun et al. 2009) | Two prospective multicenter studies from Europe and North America; $n = 809$ (316 PCA) | Clinical patients who had been referred for prostatic (re)evaluation due to suspicious DRE/abnormal PSA; with info on age (32–85 years), PSA, DRE, prostate volume, history of previous biopsy, and PCA3 | Age, DRE, PSA, prostate volume, history of previous biopsy, and PCA3 | Not available online; validated in external populations (Aupruch et al. 2010, Perdona et al. 2011); TRUS-derived total prostate volume was calculated via the prolate ellipse formula ($0.52 \times$ length $\times$ width $\times$ height) (Eskew et al. 1997) |

| | | | | |
|---|---|---|---|---|
| ERSPC multistep graphic device: Riskindicator (Kranse et al. 1999, 2008, Roobol et al. 2006, 2010, Steyerberg et al. 2007) | Prospective cohort from Europe; at initial screening 1850 were biopsied (541 PCA; 240 potentially indolent PCA); at repeated screening 1201 were biopsied (225 PCA; 146 potentially indolent PCA) | European men, age 55–74 years, PSA ≥ 3 ng/mL; Step 1–3: Men never screened; Step 4: PCA patients treated with radical prostatectomy; Step 5: Men previously screened; Step 6: Men previously screened and biopsied | Step 3 of the Riskindicator: PSA, prostate volume, DRE and TRUS (i.e., a hypoechoic lesion) | Available online at www.prostate-riskcalculator.com; Step 3 of the Riskindicator was validated in an external population (Roobol et al. 2009) |
| Kattan's nomogram predicting PCA risk following initial biopsy (Nam et al. 2007) | Cross-sectional cohort from Canada; $n=3108$ (1304 PCA; 751 HG PCA) | Canadian men; 2700 clinical patients with abnormal DRE or PSA ≥ 4; 408 volunteers with PSA<4 | Age, race, DRE, PSA, %freePSA, number of biopsy cores, prostate volume, family history, symptom score | Available online at www.lerner.ccf.org/qhs/risk_calculator; PSA between 0.2 and 123 ng/mL; 17%, 12%, and 43% are assigned for unknown %freePSA, number of cores, and prostate volume, respectively |
| Urine-based markers (Cao et al. 2011) | Prospective cohort from China; $n=131$ (86 PCA; 43 HG PCA) | Clinical patients with PSA>4 or abnormal DRE, age (53–82 years) | PCA3, TMPRSS2: ERG, Annexin A3, Sarcosine | Not available online; the first voided urines after DRE were used for marker measurements |

*Abbreviations*: PCPT, Prostate cancer prevention trial; RCT, randomized control trial; PCA, prostate cancer; HG PCA, high-grade prostate cancer (Gleason score ≥ 7); PSA, prostate-specific antigen; DRE, digital rectal examination; PCA3, prostate cancer gene 3; BMI, body mass index; SABOR, San Antonio Center of Biomarkers of Risk for Prostate Cancer; TRUS, Transrectal ultrasound; ERSPC, European Randomized Study of Screening for Prostate Cancer.

The original PCPT risk calculator has been extended to (1) patients receiving finasteride, whereby PSA values are automatically doubled to account for the finasteride effect (Thompson et al. 2007), (2) patients with PCA3 measured, whereby a Bayesian updating algorithm is used to update prior PCPT risks (Ankerst et al. 2008), and (3) patients who know their body mass index (BMI), whereby PSA values of overweight and obese men are inflated to account for the inverse relationship between PSA and BMI (Liang et al. 2010).

Different tools for predicting prostate cancer risk can produce divergent outcomes on the same man (van den Bergh et al. 2008). Even in the absence of tools, a recent large meta-analysis of several of the largest contemporary prostate cancer screening and clinical cohorts revealed significantly different empirical PSA-prostate cancer risk profiles that were only partially explainable by characteristics of the cohort, such as the amount of prior screening (Vickers et al. 2010). In the PCPT, there were few participants with high PSA values exceeding 4.0 ng/mL because of the inclusion criterion $PSA \leq 3$ ng/mL, whereas in the European Randomized Study of Screening for Prostate Cancer (ERSPC) there were fewer participants with lower PSA values due to the biopsy criterion $PSA \geq 3$ ng/mL. Furthermore, both risk calculators have incorporated some variables not shared by the other (Table 29.1). Two recent studies compared diagnostic accuracy of the PCPT and ERSPC online calculators (Cavadas et al. 2010; Oliveira et al. 2011), with both indicating better performance of the ERSPC calculator. However, both studies included patients younger than 55 years (age range = 44–89 and 42–89 years for Oliveira et al. 2011 and Cavadas et al. 2010, respectively), who were outside the validated age range for the PCPT risk calculator; and both studies had significantly higher PSA distributions than that of the PCPT cohort (mean PSA = 12.5 ng/mL for Oliveira et al. 2011; median PSA = 8.12 and 1.5 ng/mL for Cavadas et al. 2010 and the PCPT cohort, respectively). Perdonà et al. (2011) conducted a head-to-head comparison of the PCA3 adjusted PCPT risk calculator (Ankerst et al. 2008) to Chun's nomogram, which also incorporated PCA3 (Chun et al. 2009), using a cohort of 218 Italian men with PSA < 10 ng/mL. They found that the PCA3-adjusted PCPT risk calculator had significantly better discrimination than Chun's nomogram, but Chun's nomogram displayed slightly better calibration in the 10%–40% risk interval. These examples highlight that for selecting the appropriate risk calculator, one must consider the properties of the underlying populations on which the calculator was developed and validated, what risk factors are available, and the notion that one calculator may outperform another on one set of criteria but not on another.

## 29.4.2 Early Breast Cancer Detection

Over the past two decades, a number of statistical models have been developed for predicting the risk of carrying a mutation in a high-risk gene such as the BRCA1 or BRCA2 mutation, and the risk of developing breast cancer with or without such a mutation. Research has been performed to review and compare these models (Amir et al. 2010; Gail and Mai 2010).

The most widely known and commonly used model for breast cancer risk assessment is the Breast Cancer Risk Assessment Tool (BCRAT; Anderson et al. 1992;

Costantino et al. 1999). Also referred to as the Gail Model 2, it is available online at www.cancer.gov/bcrisktool (Table 29.2). The BCRAT estimates a woman's risk of developing invasive breast cancer during the next 5 year period as well as the lifetime risk up to age 90. As a benchmark for comparison, it also computes the 5 year and lifetime risk estimates for a woman of the same age who is at average risk for developing breast cancer. The BCRAT originated from Gail Model 1, which was tailored to Caucasian women with both invasive and in situ cancers as the outcome (Gail et al. 1989) and later extended for applicability to African American women under the names CARE model and Gail Model 2 (Gail et al. 2007, Table 29.2). Both Gail Models 1 and 2 use six established breast cancer risk factors, namely, age, age at menarche, age at first live birth, number of previous breast biopsies, presence of atypical hyperplasia on biopsy, and number of affected first-degree relatives, and only Gail Model 2 accounts for competing risks of mortality. Gail Model 2 has been calibrated in both the general population (Costantino et al. 1999; Rockhill et al. 2001; Chlebowski et al. 2007) and in high-risk clinics (Bondy et al. 1994; Amir et al. 2003). Studies have shown that although the BCRAT is well calibrated, it has limited discriminatory accuracy (Euhus et al. 2002; Amir et al. 2003; Pankratz et al. 2008; Cummings et al. 2009). That is, although a woman's risk may be accurately estimated, one cannot precisely predict which woman will develop breast cancer. In fact, the distribution of risk estimates for women who develop breast cancer overlaps with the distribution for women who do not (Amir et al. 2010). In addition, the BCRAT has not been validated for Hispanic women, Asian women, and other minority populations. Advances in radiographic technology since the publication of Gail Model 1 led to the emergence of mammographic density as a marker for breast cancer. In back-to-back publications in the *Journal of the National Cancer Institute*, Barlow et al. (2006) and Chen et al. (2006) published updates to the BCRAT for incorporating mammographic density into the breast cancer risk calculation, but these have not appeared online to our knowledge.

Breast cancer may also be caused by inherited gene mutations. Hereditary breast cancers account for approximately 5%–10% of all breast cancers (Thull and Vogel 2004). Several genetic risk models are available to estimate the probability of carrying a mutation. The BRCAPRO model computes the likelihood of carrying an autosomal dominant mutation in BRCA1 or BRCA2 (Parmigiani et al. 1998) and online software is available to compute the overall risk of breast cancer using Bayes rule for determining the probability of a mutation given family history (http://www.cyrillicsoftware.com/support/cy3brca.htm). Because none of the nonhereditary risk factors are included in this model, it is likely to underestimate risk in breast-cancer-only families (Amir et al. 2010). The BOADICEA model includes a polygene, which allows for familial correlation that is not captured by mutations in BRCA1 or BRCA2; most recent updates of the model have been described in Antoniou et al. (2008). The model has been validated with respect to the outcome of the germline mutation only (Antoniou et al. 2004) as well as for predicting breast cancer risk (Antoniou et al. 2008). The IBIS model incorporates as risk factors the presence of multiple genes of differing penetrance, including the likelihood of BRCA1 and BRCA2 mutations, while allowing for a lower penetrance of BRCAu (Tyrer et al. 2004). Independent calibration studies are still needed to show that these models yield reliable risk estimates (Gail and Mai 2010).

**TABLE 29.2**

**Review of Selected Models for Predicting Breast Cancer Risk**

| Name | Outcomes Predicted | Dataset Used to Select Risk Factors and Compute Relative Risks | Dataset Used to Compute the Age-Specific Incidence Rates | Risk Factors for Predicting Breast Cancer Risk | Notes |
|------|--------------------|--------------------------------------------------------------|---------------------------------------------------------|------------------------------------------------|-------|
| Gail model 1 (Gail et al. 1989) | Invasive, DCIS, or LCIS breast cancer | Case-control study from BCDDP, $n = 5998$ white women (2852 cases and 3146 controls) | White women from BCDDP, age $\geq 35$ years; under annual mammographic screening, no previous breast cancer and no evidence of breast cancer at the time of their initial screening mammogram ($n = 284,780$) | Age, at menarche, age at first live birth, number of previous breast biopsies, presence of atypical hyperplasia on biopsy, and number of affected first-degree relatives | Validated in the large population-based databases (Bondy et al. 1994, Spiegelman et al. 1994, Costantino et al. 1999); modified later by Costantino et al. (1999) |
| BCRAT (Gail model 2) (Costantino et al. 1999) | Invasive | The same as Gail model 1 | SEER | The same as Gail model 1 | Available online at www.cancer.gov/bcrisktool; calibrated to U.S. SEER; account for competing risks of mortality other than breast cancer; calibrated in general population (Costantino et al. 1999, Rockhill et al. 2001, Chlebowski et al. 2007); and high-risk clinic (Bondy et al. 1994, Amir et al. 2003) |

| CARE model (Gail et al. 2007) | Invasive | Case-control study from CARE study, $n = 3254$ African American women (1607 women with invasive breast cancer and 1647 without) | African American women in 11 SEER registries | Age at menarche, number of previous benign biopsies, and number of affected first-degree relatives | Available online at www.cancer.gov/bcrisktool; calibrated to U.S. SEER; validated with data from Women's Health Initiative (Gail et al. 2007) |

*Abbreviations*: BCDDP, Breast cancer detection demonstration project; DCIS, ductal carcinoma in situ; LCIS, lobular carcinoma in situ; BCRAT, breast cancer risk assessment tool; SEER, surveillance epidemiology and end results; CARE, contraceptive and reproductive experiences.

### 29.4.3 CLINICAL CALCULATORS

Numerous risk calculators for predicting all sorts of diagnostic, prognostic and treatment outcomes for many types of cancers are available online. The website http://www.lerner.ccf.org/qhs/risk_calculator very actively collects, posts and hosts calculators, not just calculators developed at the hosting institution, the Cleveland Clinic Foundation, but from any institution that would like to provide a calculator. The website provides a valuable service since constructing and maintaining an online calculator requires ongoing technical support, and hence will encourage the expansion of translational research through online calculators. Recently, the site has even provided an online tool that allows a user to create their own online tool remotely, further promoting the fast expansion of online tools in oncology. The scientific publication supporting each calculator appears at the bottom of the calculator website page, providing some assurance of quality and a reference for further investigation of the validity of the calculator.

A few concrete examples of the various types of calculators on the website give an idea of the expansive range of predictions provided there. A group of researchers at Baylor College of Medicine developed an online risk calculator for predicting the probability that a man with benign prostatic hyperplasia would experience acute urinary retention or require surgical intervention within 2 years, with or without dutasteride therapy (Kevin et al. 2006). Researchers at the International Bladder Cancer Nomogram Consortium developed a bladder cancer nomogram for predicting recurrence risk after radical cystectomy for bladder cancer (Consortium IBCN 2006). Tools are available to predict the risk of colon cancer recurrence after curative surgery (Weiser et al. 2008) and disease-specific survival after hepatic resection for metastatic colorectal cancer (Kattan et al. 2008). An online nomogram was developed to predict 5 year disease-specific survival after R0 resection for gastric cancer (Kattan et al. 2003). For kidney cancer, there are risk calculators to predict the likelihood of benign, likely indolent, or potentially aggressive pathological findings based only on readily identifiable preoperative factors (Brian et al. 2007; Ganesh et al. 2008), and on postoperative factors (Kattan et al. 2001; Maximiliano et al. 2005; Sorbellini et al. 2006). For oral cancer, a nomogram was developed to predict the likelihood of locoregional recurrence–free survival after treatment for oral cavity squamous cell carcinoma (Gross et al. 2008). For ovarian cancer, a tool is available to predict 5 year disease-specific survival for bulky stage IIIC epithelial ovarian carcinoma (Chi et al. 2008). For pancreatic cancer, a tool is available to predict 12, 24, and 36 month survival after resection for adenocarcinoma of the pancreas (Brennan et al. 2004). For penile cancer, an online tool is available for predicting 5 year survival and lymph-node involvement (Michael et al. 2006; Vincenzo et al. 2006). Continuing efforts are needed to improve and validate these risk calculators so they can play a significant role in reducing the burden of cancer.

## 29.5 HARMS AND BENEFITS

Online risk calculators are a tremendous step forward for translational medicine. One of the biggest advantages they concur is to bring top state-of-the art medicine to doctors all over the world, including those in remote and isolated corners. Between

2007 and 2010, the PCPT risk calculator received 51,000 hits and the helpdesk received numerous emails from physicians in Europe, the United States, Africa, and Australia. Online tools expedite external validation and fast dissemination to the scientific community, which can then more quickly direct research to the right areas, thus continually improving upon the state of the art. Most tools, including the PCPT risk calculator, have their formulas posted on the website for batch validation at local sites. Whereas initially the PCPT statistical team had a hand in all external validations of the PCPT risk calculator, now they first hear about them in scientific peer-reviewed journals. Online tools and formulas foster unbiased comparisons of competing calculators by independent parties, fostering objectivity and creating avenues for research for all members of the oncology community.

But online calculators are not without their potential harms. They should never be used in place of a doctor's opinion nor acted upon without consultation with a health professional. Responsible websites make this clear, most by requiring acceptance of Terms of Use before proceeding to the calculator. It is also incumbent upon responsible sites to provide detailed support on their use as well as a contact, either email or hotline, for questions and concerns.

As with any type of information on the internet, there is no standard regulation and technical errors can occur, so that the information produced cannot be blindly trusted. One early experience with the PCPT risk calculator was an error with European operating systems, which use a comma in place of a decimal. This resulted in very high-risk estimates that were incorrect for European-based users. The error was brought to the attention of the calculator helpdesk from a treating physician, whose patient had requested a check-up from him after calculating his own high risk. One can imagine the huge psychological and then economic burden to this patient, resulting in an unplanned and unnecessary trip to the physician, all because of a computer glitch.

Other experiences from the PCPT risk calculator helpdesk have led to the decision to not report individual risks or confidence intervals exceeding 75%, but rather a generic message that the risk exceeds 75%. There are several reasons for this. The first is concern for the patient who might think they have a fast certain risk of a bad outcome and take an unfavorable action before consulting a physician. A high risk can result from a typo on the input, such as accidentally entering 100 ng/mL instead of 10 ng/mL for PSA into the PCPT risk calculator. While the PCPT risk calculator repeats the input factors along with the estimated risk output, there is no assurance that the user double-checks this information. Also a statistical property of logistic regression risk estimates is that the confidence intervals narrow for probabilities close to the boundaries at 0% and 100%. After an African American patient with several other risk factors for prostate cancer emailed the helpdesk in distress that he had a 100% percent risk of high-grade prostate cancer, with a confidence interval ranging from 100% to 100%, all risk information exceeding 75% was eliminated from the PCPT risk calculator website.

# REFERENCES

Akaike, H. 1974. A new look at the statistical model identification. *IEEE Transactions on Automatic Control* 19(6):716–723.

Amir, E., Evans, D.G., Shenton, A. et al. 2003. Evaluation of breast cancer risk assessment packages in the family history evaluation and screening programme. *Journal of Medical Genetics* 40(11):807–814.

Amir, E., Freedman, O.C., Seruga, B., Evans, D.G. 2010. Assessing women at high risk of breast cancer: A review of risk assessment models. *Journal of the National Cancer Institute* 102(10):680–691.

Anderson, S.J., Ahn, S., Duff, K. 1992. NSABP Breast Cancer Prevention Trial risk assessment program, version 2. NSABP Biostatistical Center Technical Report.

Ankerst, D.P., Groskopf, J., Day, J.R. et al. 2008. Predicting prostate cancer risk through incorporation of prostate cancer gene 3. *Journal of Urology* 180(4):1303–1308.

Antoniou, A.C., Cunningham, A.P., Peto, J. et al. 2008. The BOADICEA model of genetic susceptibility to breast and ovarian cancers: Updates and extensions. *British Journal of Cancer* 98(8):1457–1466.

Antoniou, A.C., Pharoah, P.P.D., Smith, P., Easton, D.F. 2004. The BOADICEA model of genetic susceptibility to breast and ovarian cancer. *British Journal of Cancer* 91(8):1580–1590.

Aupruch, M., Haese, A., Walz, J. et al. 2010. External validation of urinary-based nomograms to individually predict prostate biopsy outcome. *European Urology* 58(5):727–732.

Barlow, W.E., White, E., Ballard-Barbash, R. et al. 2006. Prospective breast cancer risk prediction model for women undergoing screening mammography. *Journal of the National Cancer Institute* 98(17):1204–1214.

Begg, C.B. 1991. Advances in statistical methodology for diagnostic medicine in the 1980's. *Statistics in Medicine* 10:1887–1895.

Bondy, M.L., Lustbader, E.D., Halabi, S., Ross, E., Vogel, V.G. 1994. Validation of a breast cancer risk assessment model in women with a positive family history. *Journal of the National Cancer Institute* 86(8):620–625.

Brennan, M.F, Kattan, M.W., Klimstra, D., Conlon, K. 2004. Prognostic nomogram for patients undergoing resection for adenocarcinoma of the pancreas. *Annals of Surgery* 240(2):293–298.

Brian, R.L., Denise, B., Michael, W.K. et al. 2007. A preoperative prognostic nomogram for solid enhancing renal tumors 7 cm or less amenable to partial nephrectomy. *Journal of Urology* 178(2):429–434.

Cao, D.L., Ye, D.W., Zhang, H.L., Zhu, Y., Wang, Y.X., Yao, X.D. 2011. A multiplex model of combining gene-based, protein-based, and metabolite-based with positive and negative markers in urine for the early diagnosis of prostate cancer. *The Prostate* 71(7):700–710.

Cavadas, V., Osório, L., Sabell, F., Teves, F., Branco, F., Silva-Ramos, M. 2010. Prostate Cancer Prevention Trial and European Randomized Study of screening for prostate cancer risk calculators: A performance comparison in a contemporary screened cohort. *European Urology* 58(4):551–558.

Chen, J., Pee, D., Ayyagari, R. et al. 2006. Projecting absolute invasive breast cancer risk in white women with a model that includes mammographic density. *Journal of the National Cancer Institute* 98(17):1215–1226.

Chi, D.S., Palayekar, M.J., Sonoda, Y. et al. 2008 Nomogram for survival after primary surgery for bulky stage IIIC ovarian carcinoma. *Gynecologic Oncology* 108(1):191–194.

Chlebowski, R.T., Anderson, G.L., Lane, D.S. et al. 2007. Predicting risk of breast cancer in postmenopausal women by hormone receptor status. *Journal of the National Cancer Institute* 99(22):1695–1705.

Chun, F.K., de la Taille, A., van Poppel, H. et al. 2009. Prostate Cancer Gene 3 (PCA3): Development and internal validation of a novel biopsy nomogram. *European Urology* 56(4):659–668.

Consortium IBCN. 2006. Postoperative nomogram predicting risk of recurrence after radical cystectomy for bladder cancer. *Journal of Clinical Oncology* 24(24):3967–3972.

Copas, J.B. and Corbett, P. 2002. Overestimation of the receiver operating characteristic curve for logistic regression. *Biometrika* 89, 315–331.

Costantino, J.P., Gail, M.H., Pee, D. et al. 1999. Validation studies for models projecting the risk of invasive and total breast cancer incidence. *Journal of the National Cancer Institute* 91(18):1541–1548.

Cox, D.R. 1958. Two further applications of a model for binary regression. *Biometrika* 45:562–565.

Cummings, S.R., Tice, J.A., Bauer, S. et al. 2009. Prevention of breast cancer in postmenopausal women: Approaches to estimating and reducing risk. *Journal of the National Cancer Institute* 101(6):384–398.

DeLong, E.R., DeLong, D.M., Clarke-Pearson, D.L. 1988. Comparing the areas under two or more correlated receiver operating characteristic curves: a nonparametric approach. *Biometrics* 44, 837–845.

Efron, B. 1979. Bootstrap methods: another look at the jackknife. *Annals of Statistics* 7:1–26.

Efron, B. 1981. Nonparametric estimates of standard error: The jackknife, the bootstrap, and other methods. *Biometrika* 68: 589–599.

Efron, B. and Tibshirani, R. 1993. *An Introduction to the Bootstrap*. London, U.K.: Chapman & Hall Ltd.

Eskew, L.A., Bare, R.L., Mccullough, D.L., Stamey, T.A. 1997. *Systematic 5 Region Prostate Biopsy is Superior to Sextant Method for Diagnosing Carcinoma of the Prostate*. Commentary. Authors' reply. New York, Elsevier.

Euhus, D.M., Leitch, A.M., Huth, J.F., Peters, G.N. 2002. Limitations of the Gail model in the specialized breast cancer risk assessment clinic. *Breast Journal* 8(1):23–27.

Eyre, S.J., Ankerst, D.P., Wei, J.T. et al. 2009. Validation in a multiple urology practice setting of the Prostate Cancer Prevention Trial calculator for predicting prostate cancer detection. *Journal of Urology* 182(6):2653–2658.

Gail, M.H., Brinton, L.A., Byar, D.P. et al. 1989. Projecting individualized probabilities of developing breast cancer for white females who are being examined annually. *Journal of the National Cancer Institute* 81(24):1879–1886.

Gail, M.H., Costantino, J.P., Pee, D. et al. 2007. Projecting individualized absolute invasive breast cancer risk in African American women. *Journal of the National Cancer Institute* 99(23):1782–1792.

Gail, M.H. and Mai, P.L. 2010. Comparing breast cancer risk assessment models. *Journal of the National Cancer Institute* 102(10):665–668.

Ganesh, V.R., Thompson, R.H., Bradley, C.L., Michael, L.B., Paul, R., Michael, W.K. 2008. Preoperative nomogram predicting 12-year probability of metastatic renal cancer. *Journal of Urology* 179(6):2146–2151.

Gerds, T.A., Cai, T., Schumacher, M. 2008. The performance of risk prediction models. *Biometrical Journal* 50:457–479.

Gross, N.D., Patel, S.G., Carvalho, A.L. et al. 2008. Nomogram for deciding adjuvant treatment after surgery for oral cavity squamous cell carcinoma. *Head Neck* 30(10):1352–1360.

Hanley, J.A. 1989. Receiver operating characteristic (ROC) methodology: The state of the art. *Critical Reviews in Diagnostic Imaging* 29, 307–335.

Hernandez, D.J., Han, M., Humphreys, E.B. et al. 2009. Predicting the outcome of prostate biopsy: Comparison of a novel logistic regression-based model, the prostate cancer risk calculator, and prostate-specific antigen level alone. *British Journal of Urology International* 103(5):609–614.

Kattan, M.W., Gönen, M., Jarnagin, W.R. et al. 2008. A nomogram for predicting disease-specific survival after hepatic resection for metastatic colorectal cancer. *Annals of Surgery* 247(2):282–287.

Kattan, M.W., Karpeh, M.S., Mazumdar, M., Brennan, M.F. 2003. Postoperative nomogram for disease-specific survival after an R0 resection for gastric carcinoma. *Journal of Clinical Oncology* 21(19):3647–3650.

Kattan, M.W., Reuter, V., Motzer, R.J., Katz, J., Russo, P. 2001. A postoperative prognostic nomogram for renal cell carcinoma. *Journal of Urology* 166(1):63–67.

Kevin, M.S., Michael, W.K., Claus, G.R., Timothy, W. 2006. Development of nomogram to predict acute urinary retention or surgical intervention, with or without dutasteride therapy, in men with benign prostatic hyperplasia. *Urology* 67(1):84–88.

Kranse, R., Beemsterboer, P., Rietbergen, J., Habbema, D., Hugosson, J., Schröder, F.H. 1999. Predictors for biopsy outcome in the European Randomized Study of Screening for Prostate Cancer (Rotterdam Region). *The Prostate* 39(4):316–322.

Kranse, R., Roobol, M., Schröder, F.H. 2008. A graphical device to represent the outcomes of a logistic regression analysis *The Prostate* 68(15):1674–1680.

Lemeshow, S., Hosmer, D.W. Jr. 1982. A review of goodness of fit statistics for use in the development of logistic regression models. *American Journal of Epidemiology* 115:92–106.

Liang, Y., Ankerst, D.P., Sanchez, M., Leach, R.J., Thompson, I.M. 2010. Body mass index adjusted prostate-specific antigen and its application for prostate cancer screening. *Urology* 76(5):1268.e1–1268.e 6.

Maximiliano, S., Michael, W.K., Mark E.S. et al. 2005. A postoperative prognostic nomogram predicting recurrence for patients with conventional clear cell renal cell carcinoma. *Journal of Urology* 173(1):48–51.

Michael, W.K., Vincenzo, F., Walter, A. et al. 2006. Nomogram predictive of cancer specific survival in patients undergoing partial or total amputation for squamous cell carcinoma of the penis. *Journal of Urology* 175(6):2103–2108.

Miller M.E., Hui, S.L., Tierney, W.M. 1991. Validation techniques for logistic regression models. *Statistics in Medicine* 10:1213–1226.

Nagelkerke, N.J. 1991. A note on a general definition of the coefficient of determination. *Biometrika* 78:691–692.

Nam, R.K., Toi, A., Klotz, L.H. et al. 2007. Assessing individual risk for prostate cancer. *Journal of Clinical Oncology* 25(24):3582–3588.

Nguyen, C.T., Yu, C., Moussa, A., Kattan, M.W., Jones, J.S. 2010. Performance of Prostate Cancer Prevention Trial Risk Calculator in a contemporary cohort screened for prostate cancer and diagnosed by extended prostate biopsy. *Journal of Urology* 183(2):529–533.

Oliveira, M., Marques, V., Carvalho, A.P., Santos, A. 2011. Head-to-head comparison of two online nomograms for prostate biopsy outcome prediction. *British Journal of Urology International* 107(11):1780–1783.

Pankratz, V.S., Hartmann, L.C., Degnim, A.C. et al. 2008. Assessment of the accuracy of the Gail model in women with atypical hyperplasia. *Journal of Clinical Oncology* 26(33):5374–5379.

Parekh, D.J., Ankerst D.P., Higgins, B.A. et al. 2006. External validation of the Prostate Cancer Prevention Trial Risk Calculator in a screened population *Urology* 68:1153–1155.

Parmigiani, G., Berry, D., Aguilar, O. 1998. Determining carrier probabilities for breast cancer-susceptibility genes BRCA1 and BRCA2. *American Journal of Human Genetics* 62(1):145–158.

Perdonà, S., Cavadas, V., Lorenzo, G.D. et al. 2011. Prostate cancer detection in the grey area of prostate-specific antigen below 10 ng/mL: head-to-head comparison of the updated PCPT calculator and Chun's nomogram, two risk estimators incorporating prostate cancer antigen 3. *European Urology* 59(1):81–87.

Rockhill, B., Spiegelman, D., Byrne, C., Hunter, D.J., Colditz, G.A. 2001. Validation of the Gail et al. model of breast cancer risk prediction and implications for chemoprevention. *Journal of the National Cancer Institute* 93(5):358–366.

Roobol, M.J., Kranse, R., Maattanen, L., Schröder, F.H. 2009. External validation of the risk indicator. *European Urology Supplements* 8(4):192.

Roobol, M.J., Schröder, F.H., Kranse, R. 2006. A comparison of first and repeat (four years later) prostate cancer screening in a randomized cohort of a symptomatic men aged 55–75 years using a biopsy indication of 3.0 ng/mL (results of ERSPC, Rotterdam). *The Prostate* 66(6):604–612.

Roobol, M.J., Steyerberg, E.W., Kranse, R. et al. 2010. A risk-based strategy improves prostate-specific antigen-driven detection of prostate cancer. *European Urology* 57(1):79–85.

Schwarz, G. 1978. Estimating the dimension of a model. *Annals of Statistics* 6(2):461–464.

Shariat, S.F. and Kattan, M.W. 2009. Nomograms for prostate cancer. In *Prostate Cancer Screening*, eds. D.P. Ankerst, C. Tangen, and I.M. Thompson, pp. 117–180. New York: Humana Press.

Sorbellini, M., Kattan, M.W., Snyder, M.E., Hakimi, A.A., Sarasohn, D.M., Russo, P. 2006. Prognostic nomogram for renal insufficiency after radical or partial nephrectomy. *Journal of Urology* 176(2):472–476; discussion 476.

Spiegelman, D., Colditz, G.A., Hunter, D., Hertzmark, E. 1994. Validation of the Gail et al. model for predicting individual breast cancer risk. *Journal of the National Cancer Institute* 86(8):600–607.

Steyerberg, E.W., Roobol, M.J., Kattan, M.W., Kwast, T.H., Koning, H., Schröder, F.H. 2007. Prediction of indolent prostate cancer: Validation and updating of a prognostic nomogram. *Journal of Urology* 177(1):107–112.

Steyerberg, E.W., Vickers, A.J., Cook, N.R. et al. 2010. Assessing the performance of prediction models: A framework for traditional and novel measures. *Epidemiology* 21(1):128–138.

Swets, J.A. and Pickett, R.M. 1982. *Evaluation of Diagnostic Systems: Methods from Signal Detection Theory.* New York: Academic Press.

Thompson, I.M., Ankerst, D.P., Chi, C. et al. 2006. Assessing prostate cancer risk: Results from the Prostate Cancer Prevention Trial. *Journal of the National Cancer Institute* 98(8):529–534.

Thompson, I.M., Ankerst, D.P., Chi, C. et al. 2007. Prediction of prostate cancer for patients receiving finasteride: Results from the Prostate Cancer Prevention Trial. *Journal of Clinical Oncology* 25(21):3076–3081.

Thull, D.L. and Vogel, V.G. 2004. Recognition and management of hereditary breast cancer syndromes. *Oncologist* 9(1):13–24.

Tian, L., Cai, T., Goetghebeur E., Wei, L.J. 2007. Model evaluation based on the distribution of estimated absolute prediction error. *Biometrika* 94:297–311.

Tyrer, J., Duffy, S.W., Cuzick, J. 2004. A breast cancer prediction model incorporating familial and personal risk factors. *Statistics in Medicine* 23(7):1111–1130.

van den Bergh, R.C., Roobol, M.J., Wolters, T., van Leeuwen, P.J., Schroder, F.H. 2008. The Prostate Cancer Prevention Trial and European Randomized Study of Screening for Prostate Cancer risk calculators indicating a positive prostate biopsy: A comparison. *British Journal of Urology International* 102(9):1068–1073.

Vickers, A.J., Cronin, A.M., Roobol, M.J. et al. 2010. The relationship between prostate-specific antigen and prostate cancer risk: The Prostate Biopsy Collaborative Group. *Clinical Cancer Research* 16(17):4374–4381.

Vickers, A.J. and Elkin, E.B. 2006. Decision curve analysis: A novel method for evaluating prediction models. *Medical Decision Making* 26:565–574.

Vincenzo, F., Filiberto, Z., Walter, A. et al. 2006. Nomogram predictive of pathological inguinal lymph node involvement in patients with squamous cell carcinoma of the penis. *Journal of Urology* 175(5):1700–1705.

Weiser M.R., Landmann, R.G., Kattan, M.W. et al. 2008. Individualized prediction of colon cancer recurrence using a nomogram. *Journal of Clinical Oncology* 26(3):380–385.

Zweg, M.H. and Campbell, G. 1993. Receiver-operating characteristic (ROC) plots: A fundamental evaluation tool in clinical medicine. *Clinical Chemistry* 3d9:561–577.

# 30 Developing a Score Based upon Gene Expression Profiling and Validation

*Pingping Qu, John D. Shaughnessy Jr.,*
*Bart Barlogie, and John J. Crowley*

## CONTENTS

## 30.1 INTRODUCTION

DNA microarray technology provides methodology for simultaneously measuring tens of thousands of gene expression levels within cellular samples. Gene expression level profiles so produced provide great insight into the initiation, progression, and treatment of many types of cancer. In the last decade, gene expression profiling (GEP) has indeed become one of the most widely used and powerful tools in cancer research, with applications including subtype discovery [1–5], gene identification, and outcome prediction [6–12].

Due to the high-dimensional features of microarray data, where the number of predictor variables can be tens to hundreds of times greater than the number of samples, traditional multivariate statistical methods may work poorly or prove unsuitable for direct application. Consequently, there has been a proliferation of new statistical methods designed specifically for handling high-dimensional data. A common approach is to select genes by their marginal association with the clinical outcome followed by selecting a predetermined number of top genes, or a subset of genes meeting a prespecified threshold of *p*-value or false discovery rate [13,14]. However, oftentimes, the number of individual genes selected in this manner still exceeds the sample size, or is too large to obtain reliable estimates in subsequent multivariate regression analysis. In such cases, a linear combination of the selected genes would reduce the feature dimension to 1 and be useful for prediction purposes. Such dimension reduction techniques are conceptually related to principal component analysis (PCA) and partial least squares, among others. On the other hand, by limiting the linear combination to only significant gene expression levels, we may facilitate interpretation over PCA. Such a linear combination of top selected genes can be a sensible summary score as the genes selected may come from the same pathway, or share similar functions in the cell (co-expression and co-regulation).

In the statistical literature, class prediction methods based on linear combinations of predictor variables include Fisher's linear discriminant analysis [15], diagonal linear discriminant analysis (DLDA) [16], and Tukey's compound covariate predictor (CCP) [17], among others [18]. In this chapter, we briefly review several such linear approaches and propose another powerful linear approach for class prediction using microarray gene expression profiles. We focus here on the 2-class prediction problems that are frequently encountered in practice, for example, distinguishing two cancer subtypes or treatment responders from nonresponders. We then extend this approach to handle prognostic prediction problems with survival outcome where we are interested in identifying a high-risk group that has very poor prognosis. We also discuss a cross-validation procedure for selecting model parameters. Finally, we illustrate the methods under discussion with two multiple myeloma (MM) GEP data sets.

## 30.2 MULTIPLE MYELOMA DATA SETS

MM is a malignancy of terminally differentiated plasma cells in the bone marrow. The data sets in this chapter come from newly diagnosed MM patients enrolled on Total Therapy 2 (TT2) and Total Therapy 3 (TT3) protocols at the Myeloma Institute of Research and Therapy of the University of Arkansas for Medical Sciences (MIRT/UAMS). These protocols are the foundations of three clinical trials sponsored by the National Institute of Health, where TT3 comprises two consecutive trials, TT3a and TT3b, with essentially similar treatment.

At diagnosis, GEP utilizing the Affymetrix U133Plus2 microarrays (www. affymetrix.com) was performed on purified plasma cells prior to therapy initiation. The GEP data were then derived and normalized using the Affymetrix Microarray Suite GCOS1.1 software, and log2 transformed before subsequent analysis. Clinical data available at diagnosis included treatments, serum LDH, albumin, creatinine,

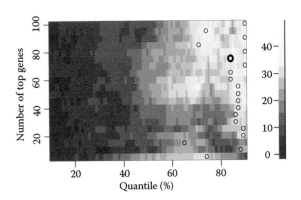

**FIGURE 30.4** A heatmap of log rank statistics comparing survival distributions of the high- and low-risk groups predicted by cross validation (based on training set of data set 2) when using the top 5, 10, ..., 100 genes (represented in rows) to calculate scores and dichotomize from the 10th through 90th percentile with increments of 1 (represented in columns). The color bar on the right shows the colors representing the log rank statistics ranging from 0.3 to 47.55, that is, lighter colors correspond to higher log rank statistics. Each black circle in the heatmap indicates the percentile to achieve maximum log rank statistic for the corresponding gene score, and the single circle highlighted in bold indicates where the maximum log rank statistic was achieved among all.

hemoglobin, and cytogenetic abnormalities (CA), and at follow-up, treatment response and survival time.

## 30.2.1 DATA SET 1

In the first study, we considered a class prediction problem using GEP data. In MM, the adverse consequences of CA at diagnosis have been well established and link to a more aggressive clinical behavior. Although the prognosis of MM patients has been best captured by a GEP-defined 70-gene model [19], metaphase CAs have remained an independent adverse effect. The objective here was to examine whether gene expression profiles within tumor plasma cells can identify MM-associated CA. We will use 350 TT2 cases and 441 TT3 cases as the training and test sets, respectively, for whom both GEP and CA data were available. The proportions of patients with chromosome abnormalities in the two data sets were 32% and 37%, respectively.

## 30.2.2 DATA SET 2

In the second study, the goal was to build a prognostic model using baseline GEP data to predict patient survival. As briefly mentioned in Data Set 1, the GEP 70-gene model [19] has successfully identified high-risk groups of MM patients, though it was originally developed using baseline TT2 GEP data and validated on TT3. Our studies have shown that TT3, utilizing a different drug therapy than TT2, achieved better clinical outcome. We hypothesized that the prognostic genes for TT3 would be quite different from those for TT2, and so our objective was to build a prognostic model using TT3a as the training set ($n = 275$) and TT3b as the test set ($n = 166$). This study utilized GEP data at diagnosis and the duration of progression-free survival (PFS).

## 30.3 GENE SCORING APPROACHES FOR CLASS PREDICTION

Consider a class predication problem. Assume we are given $n$ training pairs,

$$L = \{(x_1, y_1), ..., (x_n, y_n)\},$$

which are independent and identically distributed (iid) realizations of a random vector $(x, y)$ whose distribution is unknown. The feature vector $x_j = (x_{1j}, ..., x_{pj}) \in R^p$ is the gene expression profile for the $j$th sample where $j = 1, ..., n$ and $y_j = \{0, 1\}$ coding for a binary response describing two classes such as cancer versus normal, or responders versus nonresponders to a treatment. Here we assume the gene expression profiles have been properly preprocessed, normalized, and log2 transformed. To predict the outcome $y_j$'s, we begin by ordering the genes by their univariate association with the outcome $y$ using a $t$-test or a Wilcoxon rank sum test, followed by selecting a predetermined number of top genes or a subset of genes meeting a significance criterion (e.g., false discovery rate $<.05$). Classifiers can then be built based on linear combinations of the significant gene expressions of dimension $G$ (usually $G \ll p$).

### 30.3.1 DISCRIMINANT ANALYSIS AND VARIANTS

By performing a linear combination, such as $z = \sum_{i=1}^{G} w_i x_i$ with $w = (w_1, w_2, \ldots, w_G)'$ representing weights, the $G$-dimensional expression profile $x = (x_1, x_2, \ldots, x_G)'$ can be transformed to a scalar or score $z$. In Fisher's linear discriminant analysis [15], the score can be expressed as

$$z = (\bar{x}_{(1)} - \bar{x}_{(0)})' S^{-1} x, \qquad (30.1)$$

where

$\bar{x}_{(k)}$ is the mean expression profile for class $k$ (=1 or 0)

$S$ is the pooled within-class covariance matrix of the gene expression levels

After each gene expression profile is converted to a score, one can calculate the mean score of each class $\bar{z}_{(k)} = (\bar{x}_{(1)} - \bar{x}_{(0)})' S^{-1} \bar{x}_{(k)}$, where $k = 1$ or 0, as well as the midpoint value $c = (\bar{z}_{(1)} + \bar{z}_{(0)})/2$. The weights $(\bar{x}_{(1)} - \bar{x}_{(0)}) S^{-1}$ in (30.1) are designed to maximize the absolute difference between $\bar{z}_{(0)}$ and $\bar{z}_{(1)}$. To predict the class of a new sample with expression profile $x_{new} = (x_{1, new}, \ldots, x_{G, new})'$, first calculate the score, $z_{new} = (\bar{x}_{(1)} - \bar{x}_{(0)})'$ $S^{-1} x_{new}$, and then examine its proximity to the mean scores of class 1 and class 0. If it is closer to the mean score of class 1, the new sample will be assigned to class 1, otherwise class 0. This classification rule is also equivalent to assigning the new sample to class 1 if $z_{new} \geq c$ and class 0, otherwise.

Fisher's linear discriminant analysis is a classical nonparametric prediction method. However, it requires estimating a large number of unknown quantities. For microarray data, the number of significant genes $G$ can easily exceed the sample size, making estimating $S$ impossible. For example, if $G = 10$, the number of unknown variances and covariances to be estimated for $S$ is 55, which would require the sample size to be several times larger than 55 to obtain stable estimates of $S$. This sample size requirement is often unrealistic in practical microarray studies.

DLDA is a good alternative where correlations between genes are taken to be 0; therefore the only unknown parameters to be estimated are the class means and variance of each gene. In DLDA, the score is calculated as

$$z = \sum_{i=1}^{G} \frac{\bar{x}_{i(1)} - \bar{x}_{i(0)}}{s_i^2} x_i, \qquad (30.2)$$

where

$s_i^2$ is the pooled within-class variance estimate for gene $i$

$\bar{x}_{i(k)}$ is the mean expression level for gene $i$ in class $k$ (=0 or 1)

The rest of the classification method is the same as Fisher's linear discriminant analysis. That is, after each gene expression profile in the training set is transformed to a score according to (30.2), one can calculate the mean scores corresponding to class 1 and class 0. A new sample is assigned to class 1 if its score is closer to the mean score of that class, otherwise class 0.

Although the assumption of zero correlations among genes is untrue biologically, DLDA has shown to be a useful approach for making predictions on microarray data. With three microarray data sets, Dudoit et al. [16] compared several classification methods including Fisher's linear discriminant analysis, DLDA, nearest neighbor classifiers, and classification trees. They found that DLDA and nearest neighbor performed as well as the more advanced methods, such as classification trees, while Fisher's linear discriminant analysis performed the worst.

A variant of DLDA is Tukey's CCP [15] where the weights are the two sample $t$-statistics of the corresponding genes. The score is calculated as

$$z = \sum_{i=1}^{G} \frac{\bar{x}_{i(1)} - \bar{x}_{i(0)}}{s_i \sqrt{1/n_1 + 1/n_0}} x_i, \tag{30.3}$$

where $n_k$ is the sample size for class $k$ (=0 or 1), and the rest of the classification method is the same as Fisher's linear discriminant analysis or DLDA.

Another scoring approach closely related to DLDA is Golub's weighted voting scheme [2] where the weight for gene $i$ is

$$w_i = \frac{\bar{x}_{i(1)} - \bar{x}_{i(0)}}{s_{i(1)} + s_{i(0)}}, \tag{30.4}$$

where $s_{i(k)}$ is the standard deviation for class $k$ (=0 or 1) with respect to gene $i$. An equal number of most up- and down-regulated genes according to $w_i$ in (30.4) are taken to form the score $z = \sum_{i=1}^{G} w_i x_i$ where $G$ is an even number. The rest of their classification method is the same as Fisher's linear discriminant analysis or DLDA.

## 30.3.2    RATIO-BASED SCORING APPROACH

Shaughnessy et al. [19] employed a simpler scoring approach for predicting survival that can also be applied to class prediction problems. The score is calculated as the mean difference in expression levels of the most up- and down-regulated genes

$$z = \frac{1}{|R^+|} \sum_{i \in R^+} x_i - \frac{1}{|R^-|} \sum_{i \in R^-} x_i, \tag{30.5}$$

where $R^+$ and $R^-$ denote the gene sets of most up- and down-regulated genes with respect to class 1. Since the expression levels $x_i$ are log2-based, this is equivalent to calculating a ratio of the geometric mean of up- and down-regulated gene expression on the original scale, followed by taking logarithm of base 2. Two major differences exist between this score and the scores for discriminant analysis and variants: (1) its weights depend on the numbers of up- and down-regulated genes rather than the $t$-statistic or the like, and (2) its value does not change as the expression profile on the original scale is multiplied by a constant. This second feature is attractive when expression profiles from the same biological sample processed at two laboratories are not exactly the same but roughly proportional to each other—the ratio-based approach has a better chance of producing the same scores than the other approaches. It combines expression levels from the most up- and down-regulated genes in a simple and intuitive manner. Higher scores favor $y=1$ and lower scores favor $y=0$; thus, it is logical to assign samples with higher scores to class 1 and lower scores to class 0. To define a cut point $c$ for class predictions, one can use the midpoint of class mean scores such that a new sample is assigned to class 1 if its score is greater than $c$, otherwise 0. Our experience has shown that sometimes a more powerful approach is to use an optimal cut point on the basis of maximum likelihood. We refer to the former and latter ratio-based approaches by GMR.m and GMR.p (where m in GMR.m stands for midpoint and p in GMR.p stands for $p$ value), respectively.

### 30.3.3 PREDICTION ACCURACY ASSESSMENT

Common measures to evaluate the accuracy of a prediction model include proportion of misclassified samples, sensitivity, and specificity. Accurate estimation of predictive accuracy is particularly important in class prediction with microarray data. As in most microarray studies, the majority of genes are not differentially expressed and do not contribute to prediction. Overfitting can be a problem where a prediction model fits to noise that is specific to a training set, resulting in perfect fitting on the training set but validation failure on independent data sets.

Ideally, estimation of predictive accuracy should be conducted on a large independent test set. However, in practice, such data sets may not exist, neither may it be feasible to split all available data into large training and test sets. In this case, resampling techniques such as cross validation and the bootstrap are useful methods for evaluating the performance of a predictive model (e.g., see Efron and Tibshirani [20]). A key concept is to avoid building and evaluating a classifier based on the same data set, leading to so called resubstitution error estimate, which is downwardly biased. In cross validation, for example, every sample is predicted using other samples in the same data set, and the final error estimate is a nearly unbiased estimate for the true error. The bootstrap can be thought of as a smoothed version of cross validation. See Molinaro et al. [21] for a comparison of resampling-based methods for error estimation, and Boulesteix et al. [22] for a review of these methods.

### 30.3.4 ILLUSTRATION USING DATA SET 1

We first ranked genes by the two-sample $t$-statistic on the training set ($n=350$) and selected the 200 most significant genes to best discriminate between samples with and without chromosome abnormalities. Among the 200 genes, 150 were up-regulated and 50 were down-regulated with respect to chromosome abnormalities (with false discovery rate $< .001$). Using the top 4, 8, ..., 200 genes we built classifiers using DLDA, CCP, and the two ratio-based scoring methods GMR.m and GMR.p. For Golub's method (Golub), we reordered the genes by Golub's weights (30.4) and selected the top 4, 8, ..., 200 genes by Golub's criterion to compute the scores. Fisher's linear discriminant analysis was not implemented due to its large sample size requirement. To compare the performance of DLDA, CCP, Golub, and the ratio-based methods, we estimated their misclassification errors by 10-fold cross validation on the training set, followed by independent validation on the test set ($n = 441$).

To reduce variation in the error estimates due to choice of data partition, we repeated 10-fold cross validation 10 times and took the averaged error estimate as the final estimate. This method, denoted by CV10, was examined and recommended by Braga-Neto and Dougherty [23]. The final estimated error rates are shown in Figure 30.1 using the top 4, 8, ... and 200 genes for each method based on the training set. All of the methods behaved similarly in that the error estimate curves begin to drop and flatten as more than approximately 20 genes were used to form the scores. The maximum likelihood ratio-based approach GMR.p gave the lowest error estimates regardless of the number of genes used, while the midpoint ratio-based approach gave the highest error estimates when fewer than approximately 100 genes were used and performed closely to the other nonratio-based approaches when more than 100 genes were used. Figure 30.2 presents the box plots of all of the error estimates from top 4, 8, ... and 200 genes for each

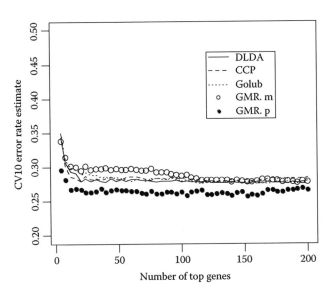

**FIGURE 30.1** (Based on training set of data set 1) Misclassification error rate estimates obtained by using CV10 and the top 4, 8, ..., and 200 genes on the training set with DLDA, CCP, Golub's weighted vote method (Golub), and ratio-based approaches, where GMR.m and GMR.p refer to the midpoint and maximum likelihood methods for determining cut points, respectively.

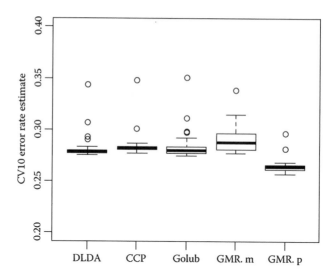

**FIGURE 30.2** (Based on training set of data set 1) Box plots of all CV10 error rate estimates using the top 4, 8, ..., and 200 genes with DLDA, CCP, Golub's weighted vote method (Golub), and ratio-based approaches, where GMR.m and GMR.p refer to the midpoint and maximum likelihood methods for determining cut points, respectively.

method. Table 30.1 summarizes the average error estimates over the top 20, 24, ..., 200 genes, excluding those from the top 4, 8, 12, and16 genes due to their relatively higher estimates, with the GMR.p approach having the lowest error estimate (~26.3%). When validating the classifiers on the independent test set ($n = 441$), we found that both of the ratio-based methods as well as the CCP method had lower error estimates than the DLDA and Golub methods (Table 30.2), and that the GMR.m approach gave even lower error rates than the GMR.p approach when more than 50 genes were used (Figure 30.3).

**TABLE 30.1**

**Based on Training Set of Data Set 1**

|                     | DLDA  | CCP   | Golub | GMR.m | GMR.p |
|---------------------|-------|-------|-------|-------|-------|
| Error rate estimate | 0.278 | 0.282 | 0.280 | 0.287 | 0.263 |

Average error rate estimates obtained using the top 20, 24, ..., 200 genes by CV10 on the training set with diagonal linear discriminant analysis (DLDA), compound covariate predictor (CCP), Golub's weighted vote method (Golub), and ratio-based approaches GMR.m and GMR.p, where GMR.m and GMR.p refer to the midpoint and maximum likelihood methods for determining cut points, respectively.

**TABLE 30.2**
**Based on Test Set of Data Set 1**

|                     | DLDA  | CCP   | Golub | GMR.m | GMR.p |
| ------------------- | ----- | ----- | ----- | ----- | ----- |
| Error rate estimate | 0.309 | 0.301 | 0.341 | 0.291 | 0.301 |

Average error rate estimates obtained using the top 20, 24, ..., 200 training genes to make predictions on the test set with diagonal linear discriminant analysis (DLDA), compound covariate predictor (CCP), Golub's weighted vote method (Golub), and ratio-based approaches GMR.m and GMR.p, where GMR.m and GMR.p refer to the midpoint and maximum likelihood methods for determining cut points, respectively.

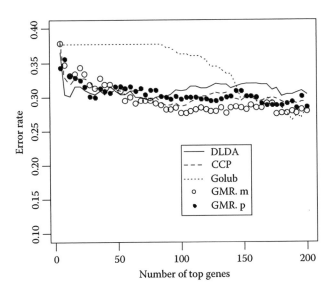

**FIGURE 30.3**    (Based on test set of data set 1) Error rates obtained from the test set when using the top 4, 8, ..., 200 genes derived from the training set, with DLDA, CCP, Golub's weighted vote method (Golub), and ratio-based approaches, where GMR.m and GMR.p refer to the midpoint and maximum likelihood methods for determining cut points, respectively.

## 30.4    EXTENSIONS TO PROGNOSTIC PREDICTION

In recent years, microarray data have also been linked to survival in clinical trials and long-term observational studies [24–29]. The objective in these cases is to select a small subset of genes, out of tens of thousands, and build a prognostic model to predict patient survival. Cox proportional hazards model [30] can be used to order and select genes that are significantly associated with survival in a univariate fashion. Given that, for example, a total of $G$ genes have been identified as significant, one can construct a

**TABLE 30.3**
**Tenfold Cross Validation for Selecting Gene Complexity and Optimal Threshold**

Divide the training set randomly into 10 parts of approximately equal size. Given $(m,q)$, where $m$ and $q$ are in reasonable ranges, repeat the following steps:

1. Use nine parts of the data to order genes and calculate the ratio-based gene score based on the top $m$ genes as well as the $q$th percentile of this score, which we denote by $w$.

2. Predict the risk group label in the remaining part by calculating the gene scores using the $m$ genes identified in step 1 and dichotomizing at $w$, so that those with scores larger than $w$ are assigned to the high-risk group (=1), otherwise low-risk group (=0).

3. Repeat step 1–2 10 times. Every sample in the training set will now be assigned a label of 0 for low risk or 1 for high risk. Compute the log rank statistic between group 0 and 1 and denote it by logrank $(m,q)$.

Select $(m^*,q^*)$ such that $(m^*, q^*) = \arg\min_{(m,q)} \left( \mathrm{logrank}(m,q) \right)$ .

prognostic index or score in analogy to compound covariate or the ratio-based score described in Section 30.3. Such a score can then be used to classify patients into high- and low-risk groups, for example, patients with scores greater than the median are assigned to the high-risk group, otherwise low-risk group, as we saw earlier.

However, in some cases, it is desirable to identify a high-risk group with very poor prognosis. Using median score as a threshold may not be optimal for that purpose. Here we consider a 10-fold cross-validation approach that simultaneously selects the number of genes for calculating a score along with an optimal threshold to dichotomize the score. The details of this procedure are presented in Table 30.3. We illustrate it by using data set 2 as described in Section 30.2.

### 30.4.1  ILLUSTRATION USING DATA SET 2

We began by ordering genes with univariate Cox regression analysis. Out of 54,675 Affymetrix U133Plus2 probes, 304 were significantly associated with PFS with $p$-value <.0001. To select an optimal subset of these probes, we carried out 10-fold cross validation following the procedure described in Table 30.3 to select the best combination of genes for calculating a ratio-based score, and a threshold for dichotomizing that score. We considered the top 5, 10...and 100 genes and examined the 10th through 90th percentile with increments of 1. For every combination, all of the training samples were predicted to belong to either the high- or low-risk group by using some other samples on the training set. Figure 30.4 shows the log rank statistics comparing all of the predicted high- and low-risk groups after cross validation; the best prognostic score used 75 genes to compute a score and dichotomized at the 84th percentile. The Kaplan–Meier survival curves [31] of the high- and low-risk cross-validated groups were presented (Figure 30.5) according to the best score. After cross validation, a final score was calculated based on the entire training set with the top 75 genes dichotomized at the 84th percentile equaling −0.27.

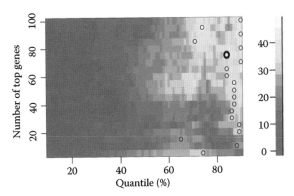

**FIGURE 30.4 (See color insert.)**    A heatmap of log rank statistics comparing survival distributions of the high- and low-risk groups predicted by cross validation (based on training set of data set 2) when using the top 5, 10, …, 100 genes (represented in rows) to calculate scores and dichotomize from the 10th through 90th percentile with increments of 1 (represented in columns). The color bar on the right shows the colors representing the log rank statistics ranging from 0.3 to 47.55, that is, lighter colors correspond to higher log rank statistics. Each black circle in the heatmap indicates the percentile to achieve maximum log rank statistic for the corresponding gene score, and the single circle highlighted in bold indicates where the maximum log rank statistic was achieved among all.

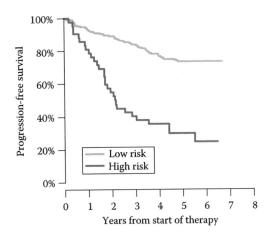

**FIGURE 30.5**    Kaplan–Meier estimates of PFS distributions for the high- and low-risk groups defined by the optimal 75-gene-84th-percentile score from cross validation on the training set of data set 2.

To assess the predictive ability of this score, we validated it on the independent test set ($n = 166$). For each sample in the test set, we computed its ratio-based score based on the 75 genes and dichotomized it at $-0.27$ so that patients with higher scores were classified as high risk, otherwise low risk. Figure 30.6 shows the Kaplan–Meier curves of the predicted risk groups in the test set. Approximately 22% (36 out of 166)

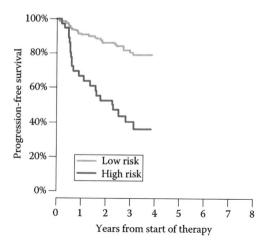

**FIGURE 30.6** Kaplan–Meier estimates of PFS distributions for the high- and low-risk groups, predicted on the test set of data set 2, using the optimal 75-gene-84th-percentile score derived from the training set of data set 2.

of the patients were classified as high risk with 53% survival probability at 2 years after treatment, as opposed to the remaining low-risk patients with 86%. The survival differences between the two risk groups were highly significant by the log rank test [32] with $p$ value $< .0001$.

## 30.5   CONCLUDING REMARKS

In this chapter, we discussed some linear approaches to compute a gene score for class and prognostic predictions using microarray GEP data. We focused on a ratio-based scoring approach and illustrated it with two myeloma data sets. Using data set 1, we compared two ratio-based methods with several other classifiers, including DLDA, CCP, and Golub's method, finding that the ratio-based methods were comparable to the other methods in terms of error rate estimates by cross validation. More data sets would have to be used in order to evaluate their performance thoroughly. Using data set 2, we demonstrated how to employ a cross-validation approach for simultaneously identifying an optimal subset of genes and an associated threshold to classify patients into good and bad prognosis groups. In both examples, we tested the methods on independent data sets, as validation is an important step when using microarray data to build classifiers. With the number of genes tens to hundreds of times greater than the number of samples, overfitting can be a serious problem with microarray-based classifiers. The clinical usefulness of a microarray-based classifier can only be established after tests on independent data sets.

There are many factors involved in the establishment of a clinically useful classifier. Both training and test sets should be based on sufficiently homogeneous groups of patients [33]. An optimal situation occurs when training and test sets come from a single large clinical trial, as patients in such trials are recruited with strict criterion and therefore have a good chance of being homogeneous. However, validation can fail if the distribution of a test set is very different from that of the training set. The more similar training and test sets are, the more accurate validation will be. Sometimes when a test set is significantly different from the training set, one may need to seek an understanding of the differences and seek resolution. For example, perhaps the genes are predictive but a new cutoff needs to be redefined to accommodate the changes in new data, or perhaps certain confounding variables exist and need to be adjusted for, and so on. For more discussion on validation considerations see Boulesteix et al. [22].

## ACKNOWLEDGMENTS

This work was supported in part by grant #CA055819 from the National Cancer Institute. The authors thank Dr. Mike LeBlanc, Full Member at Fred Hutchinson Cancer Research Center, Seattle, Washington USA, for some very helpful discussions. The authors also thank the M.J. Murdock Charitable Trust for providing support for a genomics server at Cancer Research And Biostatistics (CRAB), Seattle, where the statistical analysis for this research was conducted.

## REFERENCES

1. Eisen MB, Spellman PT, Brown PO, Botstein D. Cluster analysis and display of genome-wide expression patterns. *Proc. Natl Acad. Sci.* 1998, 95:14863–14868.
2. Golub T, Slonim D, Tamayo P, Huard C, Gaasenbeek M, Mesirov J, Coller H et al. Molecular classification of cancer: Class discovery and class prediction by gene expression monitoring. *Science* 1999, 286:531–537.
3. Alizadeh AA, Eisen MB, Davis RE, Ma C, Lossos IS, Rosenwald A, Boldrick JC et al. Distinct types of diffuse large B-cell lymphoma identified by gene expression profiling. *Nature* 2000, 403:503–511.
4. Bittner M, Meltzer P, Chen Y, Jiang Y, Seftor E, Hendrix M, Radmacher M et al. Molecular classification of cutaneous malignant melanoma by gene expression profiling. *Nature* 2000, 406:536–540.
5. Zhan FH, Huang YS, Colla S, Stewart JP, Hanamura I, Gupta S, Epstein J et al. The molecular classification of multiple myeloma. *Blood* 2006, 108(6):2020–2028.
6. Tusher VG, Tibshirani R, Chu G. Significance analysis of microarrays applied to the ionizing radiation response. *Proc. Natl Acad. Sci.* 2001, 98:5116–5121.
7. Hedenfalk I, Duggan D, Chen Y, Radmacher M, Bittner M, Simon R, Meltzer P et al. Gene- expression profiles in hereditary breast cancer. *N. Engl. J. Med.* 2001, 344:539–548.
8. Tibshirani R, Hastie T, Narasimhan B, Chu G. Diagnosis of multiple cancer types by shrunken centroids of gene expression. *Proc. Natl Acad. Sci.* 2002, 99:6567–6572.
9. Smyth G. Linear models and empirical Bayes methods for assessing differential expression in microarray experiments. *Stat. Appl. Genet. Mol. Biol.* 2004, 3:3.
10. Jansen M, Foekens JA, van Staveren IL, Dirkzwager-Kiel MM, Ritstier K, Look MP, Meijer-van Gelder ME et al. Molecular classification of Tamoxifen-resistant breast carcinomas by gene expression profiling. *J. Clin. Oncol.* 2005, 23:732–740.
11. Chanrion M, Negre V, Fontaine, H, Salvetat N, Bibeau F, Grogan GM, Mauriac L et al. A gene expression signature that can predict the recurrence of Tamoxifen-treated primary breast cancer. *Clin. Cancer Res.* 2008, 14:1744.

12. Rosenfeld N, Aharonov R, Meiri E, Rosenwald S, Spector Y, Zepeniuk M, Benjamin H et al. MicroRNAs accurately identify cancer tissue origin. *Nat. Biotechnol.* 2008, 26:462–469.

13. Benjamini Y, Hochberg Y. Controlling the false discovery rate: A practical and powerful approach to multiple testing. *J. R. Stat. Soc. Ser. B* 1995, 57:289–300.

14. Storey JD. A direct approach to false discovery rates. *J. R. Stat. Soc. Ser. B* 2002, 64:479–498.

15. Fisher RA. The use of multiple measurements in taxonomic problems. *Ann. Eugenics* 1936, 7:179–188.

16. Dudoit S, Fridlyand J, Speed TP. Comparison of discrimination methods for the classification of tumors using gene expression data. *J. Am. Stat. Assoc.* 2002, 97:77–87.

17. Tukey JW. Tightening the clinical trial. *Control. Clin. Trials* 1993, 14:266–285.

18. Simon R, Korn E, McShane L, Radmacher M, Wright G, Zhao YD. *Design and Analysis of DNA Microarray Investigations.* Springer, Berlin, Germany, 2003.

19. Shaughnessy Jr. J, Zhan F, Burington BE, Huang Y, Colla S, Hanamura I, Stewart JP et al. A validated gene expression signature of high risk multiple myeloma is defined by deregulated expression of genes mapping to chromosome 1. *Blood* 2007, 109:2276–2284.

20. Efron B, Tibshirani R. Improvements on cross-validation: The .632+ bootstrap method. *J. Am. Stat. Assoc.* 1997, 92:548–560.

21. Molinaro AM, Simon R, Pfeiffer RM. Prediction error estimation: A comparison of resampling methods. *Bioinformatics* 2005, 21:3301–3307.

22. Boulesteix AL, Strobl C, Augustin T, Daumer M. Evaluating microarray-based classifiers: An overview. *Cancer Inf.* 2008, 6:77–97.

23. Braga-Neto U, Dougherty ER. Is cross-validation valid for small-sample microarray classification? *Bioinformatics* 2004, 20:374–380.

24. Rosenwald A, Wright G, Chan WC, Connors JM, Campo E, Fisher RI, Gascoyne RD et al. The use of molecular profiling to predict survival after chemotherapy for diffuse large-B-cell lymphoma. *N. Engl. J. Med.* 2002, 346:1937–1947.

25. van't Veer LJ, Dai H, van de Vijver MJ, He YD, Hart AAM, Mao M, Peterse HL et al. Gene expression profiling predicts clinical outcome of breast cancer. *Nature* 2002, 415:530–536.

26. Bair E, Tibshirani R. Semi-supervised methods to predict patient survival from gene expression data. *PLoS Biol.* 2004, 2:511–522.

27. Pauler DK, Hardin J, Faulkner JR, LeBlanc M, Crowley JJ. Survival analysis with gene expression arrays. Advances in survival analysis. In *Handbook of Statistics*, Vol. 23. Amsterdam, the Netherlands: Elsevier, 2004, pp. 675–688.

28. Finak G, Bertos N, Pepin F, Sadekova S, Souleimanova M, Zhao H, Chen H et al. Stromal gene expression predicts clinical outcome in breast cancer. *Nat. Med.* 2008, 14:518–527.

29. Shedden K, Taylor JMG, Enkemann SA, Tsao MS, Yeatman TJ, Gerald WL, Eschrich S et al. Gene expression–based survival prediction in lung adenocarcinoma: A multi-site, blinded validation study. *Nat. Med.* 2008, 14:822–827.

30. Cox DR. Regression models and life tables. *J. R. Stat. Soc. Ser. B*, 1972, 34:187–220.

31. Kaplan EL, Meier P. Nonparametric estimation from incomplete observations. *J. Am. Stat. Assoc.* 1958, 53:457–481.

32. Mantel N. Evaluation of survival data and two new rank order statistics arising in its consideration. *Cancer Chemother. Rep.* 1966, 50:163–170.

33. Simon R. Development and validation of therapeutically relevant multi-gene biomarker classifiers. *J. Natl Cancer Inst.* 2006, 97:866–867.

# 31 Analysis of DNA Microarrays

*Shigeyuki Matsui and Hisashi Noma*

## CONTENTS

## 31.1 INTRODUCTION

Cancer is a highly complex disease caused by altered DNA. Some of these alterations may be inherited from parent by offspring and some somatic resulting from mutational and epigenetic events (Ponder 2001). The genomics of cancer cells are studied in order to characterize the disease at the molecular level, identify new therapeutic targets, and develop new molecular diagnostics for optimizing individualized treatment. The advent of high-throughput DNA microarrays, which allow the simultaneous measurements of the level of expression for tens of thousands of genes present in a collection of cells, has greatly stimulated these studies.

From previous clinical studies with microarrays, we can identify three types of objectives: class discovery, gene identification, and prediction. Class discovery refers to discovering novel subclasses of cancer based on tumor gene expression profiling (Alizadeh et al. 2000; Bittner et al. 2000; Perou et al. 2000). For example,

Alizadeh et al. (2000) identified two previously unrecognized subgroups of diffuse large B-cell lymphoma by hierarchical clustering of patients based on gene expression profiling, and interestingly, these subgroups had different outcomes after chemotherapy. Gene identification refers to selecting genes that are differentially expressed across predefined classes (Hedenfalk et al. 2001; Sotiriou et al. 2003; Setlur et al. 2008). Hedenfalk et al. (2001) identified different groups of genes expressed by breast tumors with BRCA1 mutations and those with BRCA2 mutations. Prediction corresponds to developing expression-based prediction systems for diagnostic classification (Golub et al. 1999; Setlur et al. 2008; Den Boer et al. 2009), prognostic prediction (Rosenwald et al. 2002; van't Veer et al. 2002; Shaughnessy et al. 2007), and treatment selection (Ayers et al. 2004; Takata et al. 2005). Golub et al. (1999) developed predictors for classification of acute leukemia arising from lymphoid and myeloid precursors. Shaughnessy et al. (2007) developed a gene expression model for predicting high-risk multiple myeloma. Ayers et al. (2004) developed a predictor of complete pathologic response to neoadjuvant chemotherapy for breast cancer.

In this chapter, we shall focus on statistical issues in the analysis of microarray data from cancer clinical studies. After providing a summary of initial processing of microarray data in Section 31.2, we outline statistical methods for class discovery, gene identification, and prediction in Sections 31.3 through 31.5, respectively. Concluding remarks appear in Section 31.6.

## 31.2 INITIAL DATA PROCESSING

Microarrays measure the abundance of messenger RNA (mRNA) transcripts present in a cell or set of cells. In many microarray experiments, the mRNA extracted from a set of cells is reverse-transcribed into fluorescently labeled complementary DNA (cDNA). When the labeled cDNA is placed on a solid surface on which specific DNA probes composed of nucleotide sequences are immobilized, it will tend to form hydrogen bonds with or *hybridize* to the probes with sufficient sequence complementarity. The amount of cDNA bound to each probe is quantified by detecting the intensity of fluorescence of each probe on the array using a fluorescent scanner. The quantified intensity is considered a measure of the abundance of mRNA transcripts or gene expression level for each probe on the array. For an introductory overview of biological and technical aspects of microarray assays, see Nguyen et al. (2002).

For spotted cDNA arrays, cDNA molecules from a sample of interest and a reference sample are labeled with two different fluorescent dyes, most commonly cyanine molecules Cy 3 (green) and Cy 5 (red). After co-hybridization of two pools of cDNA, a measure of abundance of the corresponding probe transcripts in the sample of interest relative to the reference sample is obtained. More specifically, after image analysis that summarizes the foreground and background intensity measurements in each of the two channels for each probe, a log ratio of the background-corrected, foreground intensities in the two channels is calculated for each probe (Yang et al. 2001). The raw data of the relative intensity are processed to remove systematic variation due to various technical reasons, including differential incorporation and emission properties of the recording device, print-tip variation and wear, and uneven hybridization of the cDNA (Kerr and Churchill 2001a; Dudoit et al. 2002b), to ensure that the location and spread of intensity levels across dyes and arrays are comparable. This process is called *normalization*. A number of normalization methods have been proposed, including global normalization and locally weighted scatterplot smoother (Bilban et al. 2002; Yang et al. 2002; Park et al. 2003).

Affymetrix GeneChip arrays use a photolithograph approach to synthesize oligo-nucleotide probes directly on the silicon surface of the array. A GeneChip array contains several oligonucleotide probes to measure the abundance of a target sequence, the perfect match (PM) probes and an equal number of internal controls, the miss match (MM) probes. The set of a PM–MM probe pair for a target sequence is called a *probe set*. A single fluorescently labeled sample is hybridized to the array and scanned to obtain an absolute measure of the fluorescence intensity for each probe. In order to obtain a summary measure of intensity per probe set, various methods have been developed. As the Affymetrix default, the MAS5.0 (Affymetrix 2002) quantifies this intensity from increased binding to PM over MM probes to adjust for the effect of non-specific binding under the assumption of MM measuring the expected background on PM probes. It calculates a robust mean of background corrected, log transformed intensities using Tukey's biweight estimation. However, there is considerable debate over the assumption that MM probes detect only non-specific hybridization, and several authors have proposed model-based methods using PM-only measurements to estimate a common mean background for all probes through information sharing across probes on an array (Huber et al. 2002; Irizarry et al. 2003; Wu et al. 2004). The robust multiarray average (RMA) (Irizarry et al. 2003) is a popular one for such methods. To make the intensity measures across arrays comparable, many normalization methods have been proposed. The simplest kind of normalization is to scale the arrays so that each array has the same mean or median probe intensity, as performed in MAS5.0. Quantile normalization is an expansion of these global methods and makes the empirical distribution of intensities constant across arrays after normalization (Bolstad et al. 2003). All these methods assume that the variation across arrays is affected by only technical factors, not true biological effects. An alternative approach if this assumption is not appropriate is to consider normalization based on a set of probes, such as housekeeping genes or some least variant genes, which is expected to be uniformly expressed for the samples under study (Li and Wong 2001; Calza et al. 2008). The initial data processing methods for oligonucleotide arrays are reviewed by several authors (Irizarry et al. 2006; Wu 2009).

Normalized log-ratios from two-color spotted cDNA arrays or normalized log signals from oligonucleotide arrays are considered the gene expression levels that will be subject to further statistical analysis for class discovery, gene identification, or prediction.

## 31.3  CLASS DISCOVERY

This section discusses unsupervised clustering and dimension reduction techniques for exploring a group of samples with similar gene expression profiles or a group of co-regulated genes in the same pathway to discover gene function.

### 31.3.1 CLUSTERING

The goal of clustering is to group together objects (genes or samples) in such a way that expression patterns within a group are more alike than patterns across groups. Two main types of clustering algorithms can be distinguished: *hierarchical clustering* and *partitioning clustering* (Gordon 1999).

Hierarchical clustering works by producing a series of successively nested clusters, organizing a tree structure or dendrogram, for a prespecified matrix of pairwise dissimilarity or distance between objects (such as one minus the correlation coefficient between two objects), and distance between clusters that is specified by a linkage method (such as average, complete, or single linkage) (Eisen et al. 1998). Agglomerative clustering operates by iteratively joining closest objects and groups of objects, whereas divisive clustering operates by iteratively dividing up groups of objects into subgroups. Agglomerative hierarchical clustering is the most widely applied clustering algorithm for class discovery, mainly because of its simple implementation. However, a major limitation of hierarchical clustering derives from its sequential nature, which may result in a high risk of clustering on noise. For example, agglomerative clustering cannot recover from bad merges that occur at earlier stages and the error is magnified at later stages that handle larger clusters. This problem is exacerbated in microarray data where there are a large number of noisy variables.

Partitioning clustering algorithms produce a single collection of non-nested disjoint clusters for a prespecified number of clusters and initial partitioning. The $k$-means clustering (MacQueen 1967), $k$-medoids clustering (Kaufman and Rousseeuw 1990), and self-organizing maps (SOM) (Tamayo et al. 1999) are such algorithms that have been applied to microarray data. For a given number of clusters $k$ and initial cluster centers, $k$-means clustering partitions the objects so that the sum of squared distances of each object to its closest cluster center is minimized. The $k$-medoids clustering uses medoids instead of centroids for the centers of clusters, which is more robust to outliers than $k$-means. SOM is a neural network procedure that can be viewed as a constrained version of $k$-means clustering that forces the cluster centers to lie in a discrete two-dimensional space to aid interpretation. An advantage of partitioning clustering is that, through utilizing the prior information on the number of clusters, they reduce the risk of clustering on noise, a weakness of hierarchical clustering, although one does not typically know the number of clusters and the prior information can be incorrect. Partitioning clustering is less computationally demanding than hierarchical clustering, which is particularly advantageous for clustering thousands of genes. An important practical issue is how to choose the initial partitioning, which can largely impact the final result. It is generally recommended that a partitioning procedure is repeatedly run for different sets of initial cluster centers and the partition that minimizes the within-cluster sum of square is chosen for a given number of clusters.

Unlike the clustering algorithms described earlier, model-based clustering assumes some underlying probabilistic model for microarray data, which provides a rigorous statistical framework for the clustering problem. Finite mixture models are commonly assumed, where each cluster is represented by a probability distribution (typically, Gaussian) component and the data are viewed as a realization of a mixture distribution of the components (Yeung et al. 2001a; Fraley and Raftery 2002; McLachlan et al. 2002; Pan et al. 2002; Pan 2006).

In clustering microarray data, some dimension reduction is warranted to reduce the impact of noise genes on the clustering result and to aid interpretation. One common, but heuristic approach is filtering out genes with low intensity or minimal variation across samples prior to clustering. Another approach is to apply dimension reduction techniques, such as principal component analysis (PCA) (see Section 31.3.2), before clustering (Ghosh and Chinnaiyan 2002). A different approach is to assign objects different weights in hierarchical clustering, so that the algorism preferentially clusters on subsets of the attribute objects (Friedman and Meulman 2004). In the model-based clustering, the problem can be formulated as a variable selection problem within the Bayesian approach (Liu et al. 2003; Tadesse et al. 2005) and penalized likelihood approach (Pan and Shen 2007). For gene clustering, a component representing a set of noise genes can be introduced in model-based clustering (Fraley and Raftery 2002). See Thalamuthu et al. (2006) for a comparison study of some gene clustering methods for microarray data.

When the gene function related to a particular phenotype is of interest, it is common to explore clustering of genes selected from a gene identification analysis described in Section 31.4 for the phenotype. However, clustering of samples using a set of genes correlated with a phonotype will usually result in clusters associated with the phenotype. This supervised clustering of samples has been erroneously used as evidence on the clinical relevance of the identified clusters (Dupuy and Simon 2007).

Biclustering or two-way clustering, simultaneously, cluster genes and samples with the goal of identifying groups of genes involved in multiple biological activities in subsets of samples. A simple two-way clustering could be found by reordering the genes and samples after independently clustering them, such as available in the Eisen software (Eisen et al. 1998). More complex methods include coupled clustering (Getz et al. 2000), block clustering (Alon et al. 1999), the plaid model (Lazzeroni and Owen 2002), and Bayesian biclustering (Sheng et al. 2003). See Madeira and Oliveira (2004) for a review of biclustering algorithms.

Objective assessment of the validity of clustering is particularly important in clustering high-dimensional data. A number of estimation methods for determining the number of clusters have been proposed in statistical literature (Milligan and Cooper 1985), although it is even more difficult for clustering high-dimensional data (Yeung et al. 2001b; Thalamuthu et al. 2006). In model-based clustering with underlying mixture models, the number of clusters (components) can be selected on the basis of model selection criteria such as the Bayesian information criterion (BIC) and the integrated classification likelihood (ICL) criterion (McLachlan et al. 2004). Dudoit and Fridlyand (2002) proposed a prediction-based resampling method to estimate the number of clusters. Other prediction-based resampling methods include a jackknife-type method (Yeung et al. 2001b) and a stability-based validation (Lange et al. 2004). Another aspect of cluster validation is the assessment of stability or reproducibility of individual clusters. In data perturbation methods, artificial random noise is added to the observed data, the data are re-clustered, and the difference with the original clustering results is evaluated (Kerr and Churchill 2001b;

McShane et al. 2002). A review of cluster validation methods for genomic data is given by Handl et al. (2005).

## 31.3.2 Alternative Dimension Reduction Techniques

PCA, sometimes referred to as singular value decomposition, and multidimensional scaling (MDS) are prototype dimension reduction techniques that have been widely used in microarray studies (Alter et al. 2000; Bittner et al. 2000; Yeung and Ruzzo 2001; Ghosh and Chinnaiyan 2002). However, a drawback to PCA is that summary variables, which are the orthogonal linear combinations of a potentially large numbers of genes showing the greatest variability across samples, do not necessarily have a clear biological interpretation. In addition, the use of first few principal components in clustering may destroy the clustering structure of the original data (Yeung and Ruzzo 2001), and there is generally no guarantee that the data will cluster along the dimensions identified by these techniques when there are a large number of noisy variables.

## 31.4  GENE IDENTIFICATION

Screening for differentially expressed genes among different clinical subtypes or prognostic classes is often a primary aim in microarray experiments in clinical oncology. Typically separate statistical tests are made for each gene for comparing expression levels between two phenotypic classes. To be specific, for gene $j$ from a pool of $m$ genes, we perform a two-sample $t$-test with a type I error rate $\alpha$. For the two-sample $t$-statistic $Y_j$, the null hypothesis on gene $j$ is rejected if $|Y_j| \geq C_\alpha$, the corresponding threshold for $\alpha$. Suppose that, of the $m$ tests, $m_0$ are true null and the rest $m_1$ are non-null. The outcomes of the $m$ tests are summarized in Table 31.1. However, examination of many hypotheses greatly increases the number of false positives.

### 31.4.1  Multiple Testing

One of the multiple testing approaches applied in earlier microarray experiments is to control the probability of at least one false positive in multiple testing, that is, the *family-wise error rate* (FWER). (Westfall and Young 1993). The Bonferroni procedure is the simplest approach. More efficient procedures can be developed by using multivariate permutation methods to take correlation between genes into account

**TABLE 31.1**

**Outcomes of Multiple Testing**

| True Hypothesis | Reject $H_0$ | Accept $H_0$ | Total |
|---|---|---|---|
| $H_0$ is true | $R_0(C_\alpha)$ | $m_0 - R_0(C_\alpha)$ | $m_0$ |
| $H_1$ is true | $R_1(C_\alpha)$ | $m_1 - R_1(C_\alpha)$ | $m_1$ |
| Total | $R(C_\alpha)$ | $m - R(C_\alpha)$ | $m$ |

(Westfall and Young 1993; Dudoit et al. 2003). However, the criterion of controlling the FWER is typically very conservative for testing a large number of hypotheses.

Another criterion is based on the *false discovery rate* (FDR) (Benjamini and Hochberg 1995), defined as the expected proportion of false positives among the genes declared significant or the expected value of *false discovery proportion*, $FDR = E\{FDP\}$, where $FDP = R_0(C_x)/R(C_x)$, using the notation in Table 31.1. When $R(C_x) = 0$, the FDP is defined to be 0, since no null hypothesis is rejected. The FDR offers a less stringent multiple testing criterion than the FWER, thus more acceptable for microarray gene screening. Benjamini and Hochberg (1995) proposed a procedure to control FDR to be less than or equal to the prespecified level, $\gamma$ say, by finding a data-dependent thresholding rule. In this procedure, for the ordered $p$-values of the $m$ tests, $p_{(1)} \le p_{(2)} \ldots \le p_{(m)}$, the quantities $r_{(j)} = p_{(j)}/(j/m)$ and $q_{(j)} = \min_{h \ge j} \{r_{(h)}\}$ are calculated ($j = 1, \ldots, m$), and then the $j$th null hypothesis is rejected if $q_{(j)} \le \gamma$. It can be shown that $FDR \le \gamma m_0/m$ for positively correlated tests as well, indicating the procedure is conservative (Benjamini and Yekutieli 2001). An alternative approach is to first fix the thresholding rule and then estimate the FDR (Storey 2002). This approach of estimating the FDR is more flexible in practice because it is often difficult to specify the level of FDR before exploratory gene screening analysis. In this approach, multivariate permutation methods, which take into account the correlation between genes, can be used for estimating the FDR, as in the popular significance analysis of microarrays (SAM) method (Tusher et al. 2001). The permutation methods are to obtain an average of the number of false positive for a given threshold $C_x$ from a large number of datasets with permutations of the class labels under the complete null hypothesis with $m_0 = m$, thus yielding a conservative estimate of the FDR. For controlling or estimating the FDR more accurately, assessment of the proportion of the null genes, $\pi = m_0/m$, is warranted. For example, in the Benjamini and Hochberg's procedure, we could use $\gamma^* = \gamma/\pi$ instead of $\gamma$, if $\pi$ is known. A simple conservative estimate of $\pi$ is obtained by considering that null statistics are much more abundant than alternatives at large $p$-values close to one (Storey 2002). Many other methods for estimating $\pi$ and the FDR have also been proposed (Langaas et al. 2005; Pounds 2006).

Control of the FDR can provide a false sense of security, because the discrepancy between the FDR and the actual FDP can be substantial when the correlation across genes increases (Korn et al. 2004). Several authors therefore considered controlling actual FDP (Korn et al. 2004, 2007; Genovese and Wasserman 2006).

The efficacy of multiple testing can be improved by modifying the test statistics. One possibility is to borrow the strength across genes to obtain more reliable variance estimates (see Section 31.4.2) (Baldi and Long 2001; Efron et al. 2001; Tusher et al. 2001; Lönnstedt and Speed 2002; Wright and Simon 2003; Smyth 2004). Another possibility is to use an optimal test that maximizes the expected number of true positives for a given expected number of false positives (Storey 2007). The test can also be modified for detecting particular differential patterns, for example, differentially expressed genes in a subset of cancer samples (Tomlins et al. 2005; Tibshirani and Hastie 2007; Hu 2008; Lian 2008) and multiple association patterns for multiple clinical phenotypes (Matsui et al. 2007).

The genes selected from the gene identification analysis are usually annotated for biological interpretation using software packages and genomic websites, such as Gene Ontology (www.geneontology.org) and KEGG pathways (http://www.genome.jp/kegg/pathway.html). However, this approach using the gene sets that pass through a stringent FDR criterion is not necessarily effective for elucidating biological mechanism. A popular alternative approach is to evaluate association of pre-defined biologically meaningful gene sets with the phenotype, which can improve the power in multiple testing through reduction of the number of hypothesis tested, as well as aid biological interpretation. Many such gene set enrichment methods that provide a score for summary statistics on differential expression for each gene set have been proposed (Nam and Kim 2008; Dinu et al. 2009; Irizarry et al. 2009).

### 31.4.2 MODEL-BASED APPROACH

The model-based approach utilizes information sharing across genes by assuming exchangeability across comparable genes and some structure on gene expression data. One commonly assumed structure is a mixture model with two components; one of which represents the "null" genes with no differential expression and the other represents the "non-null" genes with differential expression. This is a mixture prior in the Bayesian framework. The mixture structure is commonly assumed for the parameter of interest (e.g., the difference in gene expression between two classes) in the model of gene expression levels (Lönnstedt and Speed 2002; Newton et al. 2004; Smyth 2004; Do et al. 2005; Gottardo et al. 2006; Lo and Gottardo 2007) or for gene-specific summary statistics of the parameter of interest, such as test statistics used in multiple testing (Efron et al. 2001; McLachlan et al. 2006; Efron 2009; Noma et al. 2010; Matsui and Noma 2011a,b). Another structure is a hierarchical model that incorporates gene-specific effects, in conjunction with the mixture prior (Lönnstedt and Speed 2002; Newton et al. 2004; Smyth 2004; Do et al. 2005; Gottardo et al. 2006; Lo and Gottardo 2007; Efron 2009; Noma et al. 2010; Matsui and Noma 2011a,b) or an unstructured prior (Baldi and Long 2001; Lewin et al. 2006). The hierarchical structure provides a basis for developing efficient methods for gene ranking (Noma et al. 2010) and estimation of the gene-specific effects (Efron 2009; Matsui and Noma 2011a), as well as estimation of the FDR.

The hierarchical mixture models for gene-specific summary statistics (Efron 2009; Noma et al. 2010; Matsui and Noma 2011a,b) need less modeling assumption (without modeling the other nuisance parameters); hence, it is more robust. One example of this type of hierarchical mixture modeling for two-class comparison (Matsui and Noma 2011b) is to model the two sample $t$-statistic, $Y_j = \left(\hat{\mu}_j^{(1)} - \hat{\mu}_j^{(2)}\right)/\hat{\sigma}_j$, aside from the sample size constant $\tau_n^2 = n/(n_1 n_2)$, where $\hat{\mu}_j^{(1)}$ and $\hat{\mu}_j^{(2)}$ are the mean expression levels for classes 1 and 2, respectively, and $\hat{\sigma}_j$ is the usual pooled estimate of standard deviation for gene $j$ ($j = 1, \ldots, m$). We assume a hierarchical mixture model for the distribution of $Y_j$,

$$f(y_j) = \pi f_0(y_j) + (1 - \pi) f_1(y_j), \tag{31.1}$$

where the component for the null genes, $f_0$, is a normal distribution, $N(0, \tau_n^2)$, and the component for the non-null genes, $f_1$, is specified as

$$Y_j \mid \delta_j \sim N(\delta_j, \tau_n^2) \quad \text{and} \quad \delta_j \sim g_1.$$

The $Y_j$ follows the normal distribution with gene-specific mean $\delta_j$ and constant variance of random variation $\tau_n^2$ in the first level, and $\delta_j$ follows the distribution $g_1$ in the second level. The form of $g_1$ is unspecified. In an empirical Bayes framework, we estimate $\pi$ and $g_1$ via an EM algorithm from the data, where the non-parametric estimates of the prior distribution $g_1$ are supported by fixed discrete mass points like the non-parametric estimation method by Shen and Louis (1999). An application of this method to a leukemia dataset is provided in Section 31.4.4.

### 31.4.3 SAMPLE SIZE ESTIMATION

While it is important to eliminate as many nuisance genes from further consideration as possible, it is also important to remove as few relevant genes from consideration prematurely. As the statistical power of the gene identification analysis is generally determined by the number of biological replicates, rather than technical replicates (Simon et al. 2002), determination of the number of biological samples is important. Many methods for sample size estimation have been developed for controlling FDR (Dobbin and Simon 2005; Pawitan et al. 2005; Tsai et al. 2005; Shao and Tseng 2007; Tong and Zhao 2008; Matsui and Noma 2011b) or actual FDP (Oura et al. 2009) or for gene ranking (Pepe et al. 2003; Matsui et al. 2008b). In practical application of these methods, accurate assessment of the strength of "signal" contained in the data, represented by the parameters, such as the proportion of null genes, $\pi$, and the effect size distribution for non-null genes (e.g., $g_1$ in the hierarchical mixture model (31.1)), is crucial because these parameters can largely impact the sample size estimates. An illustration based on the hierarchical mixture model (31.1) is provided in Section 31.4.4.

### 31.4.4 ILLUSTRATION

Kirschner-Schwabe et al. (2006) reported a microarray experiment for childhood acute lymphoblastic leukemia (ALL) that examined underlying biological determinants of early relapse after treatment, which is known to be a prognostic factor related with poor survival. Gene expression analysis using Affymetrix HG-U133A microarrays (Affymetrix, Santa Clara, CA) was performed for 42 patients from the trial, ALL-REZ BFM 2002, of the Berlin-Frankfurt-Münster study group (The data are available from the NCBI GEO database; Accession code: GSE4698). We compared 14 very early relapsed patients with 28 late relapsed patients based on the expression data from $m = 22{,}283$ probe sets (Kirschner-Schwabe et al. 2006).

We fit the hierarchical mixture model (31.1) (Matsui and Noma 2011b) to the distribution of the two-sample $t$-statistic, $Y$, and performed the EM algorithm for parameter estimation. The estimate of $\pi$ was 0.68, and Figure 31.1a shows the estimate of the effect size distribution, $g_1$. As shown in Figure 31.1b, the estimate of the marginal distribution, $f$, fit well to the empirical distribution (histogram) of $Y$. The FDR for a given threshold $C_\alpha$ on $|Y_j|$ is estimated as

$$F\hat{D}R(c_\alpha) = \frac{\hat{\pi}\{F_0(-c_\alpha)+1-F_0(c_\alpha)\}}{\hat{F}(-c_\alpha)+1-\hat{F}(c_\alpha)},$$

where
$F_0$ is the cumulative distribution of $f_0$
$\hat{F} = \hat{\pi}F_0 + (1-\hat{\pi})\hat{F}_1$

For FDR of 5%, 289 genes were significant. In the estimation method based on the hierarchical mixture model (31.1), we can estimate the overall power, $\Psi(C_x)$,

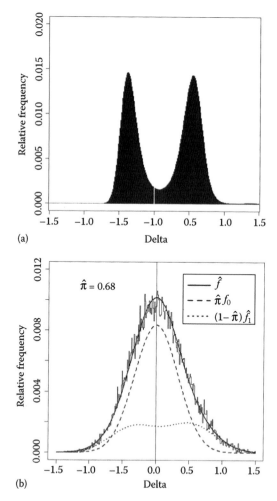

(a)

(b)

**FIGURE 31.1** The estimate of $g_1$ (a) and the estimates of the marginal distribution $f$ and the two components, $\pi f_0$ and $(1-\pi)f_1$, (b) for the ALL dataset.

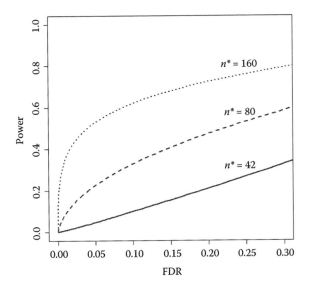

**FIGURE 31.2**  The curve that plots the overall power versus FDR for various values of threshold $C_\alpha$. In addition to the power curve for $n=42$, the original sample size of the ALL dataset, the predicted curves when $n*=80$ and 160 are also given.

which is the average power for all the non-null genes for a given threshold $C_x$, as $\hat{\Psi}(C_x) = \hat{F}_1(-C_x) + 1 - \hat{F}_1(C_x)$. Figure 31.2 shows a curve that plots $\hat{\Psi}(C_x)$ versus $F\hat{D}R(C_x)$ for various values of $C_x$, which allows simultaneous monitoring of true positives and false positives in gene screening. We can also conduct sample size estimation of future microarray experiments. In designing a new, similar or full-scale microarray experiment with sample size $n*$, we can estimate the power curve based on the estimation results with the sample size term, $\tau_{n*}$, instead of $\tau_n$, in the standard deviation in $f_0$ and $f_1$. Figure 31.2 also shows how the larger sample sizes, for example, $n*=80$ or 160, improve the overall power.

## 31.5  PREDICTION

Another clinical application of DNA microarrays is the development of expression-based prediction systems that predict diagnosis classes or outcomes after treatment. A supervised approach is generally more powerful than an unsupervised approach. There are three important components in supervised prediction: selection of relevant genes for prediction, development of prediction models, and assessment of predictive accuracy. Because the number of gene features is much larger than the number of samples, special consideration is needed to avoid overfitting.

### 31.5.1  SELECTION OF GENES

The simplest, but most common approach is a univariate filtering based on marginal association between each gene expression and the response variable as outlined in Section 31.4. Although more complex, computationally demanding multivariate methods were also developed (Saeys et al. 2007), recent studies found that the performance of univariate filtering methods was comparable to that of multivariate methods for microarray datasets with small sample sizes (Lai et al. 2006; Lecocke and Hess 2007).

### 31.5.2 DEVELOPMENT OF PREDICTION MODELS

A variety of class prediction analyses have been applied to microarray data, including linear discriminant analysis (LDA), support vector machines (SVMs), nearest-neighbors, aggregating classifiers (Dudoit and Fridlyand 2003; Simon et al. 2004).

Suppose one has a new sample with the vector of gene expression $x^* = (x_1^*, \ldots, x_G^*)'$ for $G$ selected genes and wishes to assign the sample to one of 2 classes, 1 and 2. The LDA method calculates

$$l(x^*) = (\bar{x}_1 - \bar{x}_2)' S^{-1} x^*, \tag{31.2}$$

where

$\bar{x}_r = (\bar{x}_{r,1}, \ldots, \bar{x}_{r,G})'$ is the mean expression profile for the training set samples with class $r$ for $r = 1, 2$

$S$ is an estimate of the pooled within-class covariance matrix of the expression levels of the genes

The new sample is predicted to be of the class which has the closer average of the linear combination in the training set to $l(x^*)$. A simpler form of LDA is a diagonal linear discriminant analysis (DLDA), in which the diagonal matrix of $S$ is used instead of $S$, resulting in the linear combination,

$$l_D(x^*) = \sum_{g=1}^{G} u_g x_g^*, \tag{31.3}$$

where $u_g = (\bar{x}_{1,g} - \bar{x}_{2,g})/s_g^2$ for $g = 1, \ldots, G$. The DLDA is one approach to overcome the singularity problem of the sample covariance matrix $S$ when $G$ is large relative to the number of samples. By ignoring correlations among genes, the DLDA reduces the number of parameters to be estimated. Some authors proposed variants of the DLDA, such as the compound covariates predictors (CCP) with the standardized $t$-statistic for $u_g$ (Simon et al. 2004) and empirical Bayes predictors with a shrinkage estimate (such as posterior mean), $\hat{\delta}_g/s_g$, obtained from the hierarchical modeling in Section 31.4.2 for $u_g$ (Efron 2009; Matsui and Noma 2011a). The nearest shrunken centroid predictor is another shrinkage-based method, but the amount of shrinkage is determined based on the cross-validated prediction error (Tibshirani et al. 2003; Guo et al. 2007).

SVMs are popular machine learning algorithms for classification. Linear kernel SVMs construct a hyperplane for the decision surface as is done in LDA, but the hyperplane is determined such that the margin of separation between the classes is maximized with a penalty for the number of misclassification, where the margin represents distance from the hyperplane to the closest correctly classified samples.

The $k$-nearest-neighbors ($k$-NN) approach is a simple non-parametric method that finds the $k$-nearest neighbors in the training set closest to the gene expressions on a new sample and then decides the classification of this sample by majority vote. The value of $k$ is prespecified or chosen so that the cross-validated predictive error is minimized.

Aggregating predictors are an approach to improve the predictive capability, in which slightly perturbed predictors from the training set are produced by resampling and then aggregated to produce a composite predictor by voting. Bootstrap aggregating or *bagging* (Breiman 1996) and *boosting* (Freund and Schapire 1997) are methods for generating perturbed versions of the training set. The AdaBoost, the most well-known boosting algorithm, sequentially fits weak predictors via a forward-stagewise additive modeling, with optimization of an exponential loss function (e.g., Hastie et al. 2009).

Several comparison studies for class prediction methods reported that simple methods such as DLDA and $k$-NN performed well in terms of predictive accuracy compared with more complex methods such as aggregated classification trees for microarray datasets with small to moderate sample sizes (Ben-Dor et al. 2000; Dudoit et al. 2002a; Shi et al. 2010).

For predicting continuous survival outcomes, various methods to avoid overfitting have been considered in the framework of regression analysis such as Cox proportional hazards regression, including compound covariates (Simon et al. 2004; Matsui 2006), application of dimension reduction techniques such as clustering (Hastie et al. 2001; Matsui et al. 2008a), PCA (Bair and Tibshirani 2004), partial least squares (Li and Gui 2004), and regularized regressions (van Houwelingen et al. 2006; Park and Hastie 2007).

### 31.5.3 Assessment of Predictive Accuracy

Unbiased estimation of the predictive accuracy is particularly important when performing prediction analysis in high dimensions. For class prediction problems, the proportion of correct classification (PCC), sensitivity, and specificity are common measures of predictive accuracy. Measures of accuracy for predicting survival outcomes include separation of survival curves and time-dependent ROC curves (Heagerty et al. 2000). For further discussion about assessment of accuracy in survival risk prediction using microarray data, see, for example, Simon et al. (2011).

For evaluation of internal validity, resampling techniques such as cross-validation and bootstrap are useful, particularly when the sample size is small (Molinaro et al. 2005; Jiang and Simon 2007). When using these techniques, it is critical that all aspects of model building including gene selection are re-performed for each round in resampling (Ambroise and McLachlan 2002; Simon et al. 2003). When selection of genes and prediction models are optimized based on cross-validated predictive accuracy, the optimization process should be included in the cross-validation proce-dure or an independent validation set is needed to have an unbiased estimate of the predictive accuracy (Dudoit and Fridlyand 2003; Varma and Simon 2006).

For a two-class comparison, another approach is to estimate the PCC directly under some probability model without using resampling techniques (Efron 2009; Matsui and Noma 2011a). Under the assumption that genes have a Gaussian distribu-tion within each class with a common within-class covariance between two classes, the PCC in the DLDA can be estimated by $P\hat{C}C = \Phi\left(\hat{\delta}'\hat{\delta}/2\sqrt{\hat{\delta}'\hat{\Omega}\hat{\delta}}\right)$, where $\Phi$ is the cumulative distribution of the standard normal distribution and $\hat{\Omega}$ is an estimate of the common correlation matrix, and $\hat{\delta} = (\hat{\delta}_1, \ldots, \hat{\delta}_G)'$ is a vector of shrinkage estimates (posterior means) of the standardized mean difference between classes derived from a hierarchical model such as (31.1) in Section 31.4.2 for the set of $G$ genes selected using the entire samples. The shrinkage estimates incorporate the selection bias by (non-randomly) selecting the top $G$ genes and the possibility that some of the selected genes are true null (Matsui and Noma 2011a).

When the model building process is complex and not easily specified in an algo-rithmic manner, an independent validation set would be needed (Simon et al. 2004). Some authors discussed determination of sample sizes for the training and validation sets (Dobbin and Simon 2007).

It is also important to establish that the predictive accuracy is statistically higher than that expected when there is no relation between expression profile and the response variable. A permutation procedure is proposed to assess the statisti-cal significance of cross-validated predictive accuracy (Radmacher et al. 2002). Confidence intervals for cross-validated predictive accuracy can be calculated via a bootstrap resampling scheme (Jiang et al. 2008). Confidence intervals of the PCC under the Gaussian model with common within-class covariance can be obtained by a parametric bootstrap method under the estimated hierarchical model (Laird and Louis 1987).

### 31.5.4 ILLUSTRATION

We performed a two-class prediction on early relapse using gene expression data from the 42 ALL patients presented in Section 31.4.4. We adopted the four predic-tors, LDA, DLDA, 3-NN based on Euclidean distance, and linear SVM. We selected the 50 genes with the largest absolute $t$-statistics (univariate filtering) for the three predictors, DLDA, 3-NN, and SVM. The estimated predictive accuracy was gener-ally insensitive to the number of selected genes (data not shown). For the LDA, we limited the number of top genes to be 10 to avoid the singularity problem. We esti-mated the PCC by a leave-one-out cross validation (LOOCV). In LOOCV, for each training set with one sample left out, we selected the specified number of genes from scratch to obtain an unbiased estimate. The estimated PCC for LDA, DLDA, 3-NN, and SVM were 71.4%, 83.3%, 78.6%, and 78.6%, respectively. The LDA performed the worst, while the performance of the other predictors was comparable. For DLDA, the 95% confidence interval of PCC using a bootstrap resampling method with bias reduction proposed by Jiang et al. (2008) was 73.8%–97.6%. We also estimated the

PCC of the DLDA without using LOOCV under the Gaussian model with common within-class covariance. We used posterior means obtained by fitting the hierarchical mixture model (31.1) in Section 31.4.2 for $\hat{\delta}$ for the top 50 genes selected for all 42 samples. The estimated PCC by this method was 76.6%, which was somewhat smaller than the cross-validated estimate for the DLDA, 83.3%. The 95% confidence interval by a parametric bootstrap method was 72.3%–81.8%, which was much narrower than that by Jiang et al. (2008).

## 31.6 CONCLUDING REMARKS

In this chapter, we have outlined statistical methods for the analysis of microarray gene expression data in clinical oncology. Many methods can be implemented using free packages. For example, the Bioconductor (http://www.bioconductor.org/), which is a free, open source and open development software project for the analysis and comprehension of genomic data, provides hundreds of packages for analysis of microarray gene expression data. The BRB-ArrayTools (http://linus.nci.nih.gov/BRB-ArrayTools.html) is an integrated package for the visualization and statistical analysis of microarray gene expression data. R-codes for implementing the estimation methods using the hierarchical mixture model described in Sections 31.4.2, 31.4.4, and 31.5.4 are available upon request from the authors.

The rapid development of high-throughput technologies, which has reduced the cost of microarrays, and infrastructure development for genomic analysis, including embedding of tissue collection in large clinical studies or randomized trials, have allowed the conduction of cancer genomic studies with several hundred of samples. The tendency toward large-scale genomic clinical studies would enhance the potential of statistical analysis of microarray gene expression data, including more powerful detection of cancer heterogeneity and development of expression-based predictive markers for a particular treatment in randomized trials, possibly with some adaptive design (Freidlin et al. 2010). This tendency also emphasizes the importance of designing more efficient genomic studies with multiple phases, involving gene screening, prediction modeling, and validation. The opportunity for serious statistical engagement still increases in this important field for elucidating the mechanisms of oncogenesis and for developing optimized medicine for individual patients.

## REFERENCES

Affymetrix. 2002. *Statistical Algorithms Description Document*. Santa Clara, CA: Affymetrix.

Alizadeh, A. A., Eisen, M. B., Davis, R. E. et al. 2000. Distinct types of diffuse large B-cell lymphoma identified by gene expression profiling. *Nature* 403: 503–511.

Alon, U. N., Barkai, D. A., Notterman, K. et al. 1999. Broad patterns of gene expression revealed by clustering analysis of tumor and normal colon tissues probed by oligonucleotide arrays. *Proc Natl Acad Sci USA* 96: 6745–6750.

Alter, O., Brown, P. O., and Botstein, D. 2000. Singular value decomposition for genome-wide expression data processing and modeling. *Proc Natl Acad Sci USA* 97: 10101–10106.

Ambroise, C. and McLachlan, G. J. 2002. Selection bias in gene extraction on the basis of microarray gene-expression data. *Proc Natl Acad Sci USA* 99: 6562–6566.

Ayers, M., Symmans, W. F., Stec, J. et al. 2004. Gene expression profiles predict complete pathologic response to neoadjuvant paclitaxel and fluorouracil, doxorubicin, and cyclophosphamide chemotherapy in breast cancer. *J Clin Oncol* 22: 2284–2293.

Bair, E. and Tibshirani, R. 2004. Semi-supervised methods to predict patient survival from gene expression data. *PLoS Biol* 2: 511–522.

Baldi, P. and Long, A. D. 2001. A Bayesian framework for the analysis of microarray expression data: Regularized t-test and statistical inferences of gene changes. *Bioinformatics* 17: 509–519.

Ben-Dor, A., Bruhn, L., Friedman, N., Nachman, I., Schummer, M., and Yakhini, Z. 2000. Tissue classification with gene expression profiles. *J Comput Biol* 7: 559–583.

Benjamini, Y. and Hochberg, Y. 1995. Controlling the false discovery rate: A practical and powerful approach to multiple testing. *J R Stat Soc B* 57: 289–300.

Benjamini, Y. and Yekutieli, D. 2001. The control of the false discovery rate under dependency. *Ann Stat* 29: 1165–1188.

Bilban, M., Buehler, L. K., Head, S., Desoye, G., and Quaranta, V. 2002. Normalizing DNA microarray data. *Curr Issues Mol Biol* 4: 57–64.

Bittner, M., Meltzer, P., Chen, Y. et al. 2000. Molecular classification of cutaneous malignant melanoma by gene expression profiling. *Nature* 406: 536–540.

Bolstad, B. M., Irizarry, R. A., Astrand, M., and Speed, T. P. 2003. A comparison of normalization methods for high density oligonucleotide array data based on variance and bias. *Bioinformatics* 19: 185–193.

Breiman, L. 1996. Bagging predictors. *Mach Learn* 24: 123–140.

Calza, S., Valentini, D., and Pawitan, Y. 2008. Normalization of oligonucleotide arrays based on the least-variant set of genes. *BMC Bioinform* 9: 140.

Den Boer, M. L., van Slegtenhorst, M., De Menezes, R. X. et al. 2009. A subtype of childhood acute lymphoblastic leukaemia with poor treatment outcome: A genome-wide classification study. *Lancet Oncol* 10: 125–134.

Dinu, I., Potter, J. D., Mueller, T. et al. 2009. Gene-set analysis and reduction. *Brief Bioinform* 10: 24–34.

Do, K. A., Müller, P., and Tang, F. 2005. A Bayesian mixture model for differential gene expression. *Appl Stat* 54: 627–644.

Dobbin, K. and Simon, R. 2005. Sample size determination in microarray experiments for class comparison and prognostic classification. *Biostatistics* 6: 27–38.

Dobbin, K. and Simon, R. 2007. Sample size planning for developing classifiers using high dimensional data. *Biostatistics* 8: 101–117.

Dudoit, S. and Fridlyand, J. 2002. A prediction-based resampling method for estimating the number of clusters in a dataset. *Genome Biol* 3: 1–36.

Dudoit, S. and Fridlyand, J. 2003. Classification in microarray experiments. In *Statistical Analysis of Gene Expression Microarray Data*, T. P. Speed (ed.), pp. 93–158. Boca Raton, FL: Chapman & Hall/CRC.

Dudoit, S., Fridlyand, J., and Speed, T. P. 2002a. Comparison of discrimination methods for the classification of tumors using gene expression data. *J Am Stat Assoc* 97: 77–87.

Dudoit, S., PopperShaffer, J., and Boldrick, J. C. 2003. Multiple hypothesis testing in microarray experiments. *Stat Sci* 18: 71–103.

Dudoit, S., Yang, Y. H., Speed, T. P., Callow, M. J. 2002b. Statistical methods for identifying differentially expressed genes in replicated cDNA microarray experiments. *Stat Sin* 12: 111–139.

Dupuy, A. and Simon, R. M. 2007. Critical review of published microarray studies for cancer outcome and guidelines on statistical analysis and reporting. *J Natl Cancer Inst* 99: 147–157.

Efron, B. 2009. Empirical Bayes estimates for large-scale prediction problems. *J Am Stat Assoc* 104: 1015–1028.

Efron, B., Tibshirani, R., Storey, J. D., and Tusher, V. 2001. Empirical Bayes analysis of a microarray experiment. *J Am Stat Assoc* 96: 1151–1160.

Eisen, M. B., Spellman, P. T., Brown, P. O., and Botstein, D. 1998. Cluster analysis and display of genome-wide expression patterns. *Proc Natl Acad Sci USA* 95: 14863–14868.

Fraley, C. and Raftery, A. E. 2002. Model-based clustering, discriminant analysis, and density estimation. *J Am Stat Assoc* 458: 611–631.

Freidlin, B., Jiang, W., and Simon, R. 2010. The cross-validated adaptive signature design. *Clin Cancer Res* 16: 691–698.

Freund, Y. and Schapire, R. 1997. A decision-theoretic generalization of on-line learning and an application to boosting. *J Comput Syst Sci* 5: 119–139.

Friedman, J. H. and Meulman, J. J. 2004. Clustering objects on subsets of attributes (with discussion). *J R Stat Soc B* 66: 815–849.

Genovese, C. R. and Wasserman, L. 2006. Exceedance control of the false discovery proportion. *J Am Stat Assoc* 101: 1408–1417.

Getz, G. E., Levine, E., and Domany, E. 2000. Coupled two-way clustering analysis of gene microarray data. *Proc Natl Acad Sci USA* 97: 12079–12084.

Ghosh, D. and Chinnaiyan, A. M. 2002. Mixture modelling of gene expression data from microarray experiments. *Bioinformatics* 18: 275–286.

Golub, T. R., Slonim, D. K., Tamayo, P. et al. 1999. Molecular classification of cancer: Class discovery and class prediction by gene expression monitoring. *Science* 286: 531–536.

Gordon, A. D. 1999. *Classification*. New York: Chapman & Hall/CRC.

Gottardo, R., Raftery, A. E., Yeung, K. Y., and Bumgarner, R. E. 2006. Bayesian robust inference for differential gene expression in cDNA microarrays with multiple samples. *Biometrics* 62: 10–18.

Guo, Y., Hastie, T., and Tibshirani, R. 2007. Regularized linear discriminant analysis and its application in microarrays. *Biostatistics* 8: 86–100.

Handl, J., Knowles, J., and Kell, D. B. 2005. Computational cluster validation in post-genomic data analysis. *Bioinformatics* 21: 3201–3212.

Hastie, T., Tibshirani, R., Botstein, D., and Brown, P. 2001. Supervised harvesting of expression trees. *Genome Biol* 2: 1–12.

Hastie, T., Tibshirani, R., and Friedman, J. 2009. *The Elements of Statistical Learning: Data Mining, Inference and Prediction*, 2nd edn. New York: Springer.

Heagerty, P. J., Lumley, T., and Pepe, M. S. 2000. Time-dependent ROC curves for censored survival data and a diagnostic marker. *Biometrics* 56: 337–344.

Hedenfalk, I., Duggan, D., Chen, Y. et al. 2001. Gene-expression profiles in hereditary breast cancer. *N Engl J Med* 344: 539–548.

van Houwelingen, H. C., Bruinsma, T., Hart, A. A., van't Veer, L. J., and Wessels, L. F. 2006. Cross-validated Cox regression on microarray gene expression data. *Stat Med* 25: 3201–3216.

Hu, J. 2008. Cancer outlier detection based on likelihood ratio test. *Bioinformatics* 24: 2193–2199.

Huber, W., von Heydebreck, A., Sültmann, H., Poustka, A., and Vingron, M. 2002. Variance stabilization applied to microarray data calibration and to the quantification of differential expression. *Bioinformatics* 18: S96–S104.

Irizarry, R. A., Hobbs, B., Collin, F. et al. 2003. Exploration, normalization, and summaries of high density oligonucleotide array probe level data. *Biostatistics* 4: 249–264.

Irizarry, R. A., Wang, C., Zhou, Y., and Speed, T. P. 2009. Gene set enrichment analysis made simple. *Stat Methods Med Res* 18: 565–575.

Irizarry, R. A., Wu, Z., and Jaffee, H. A. 2006. Comparison of Affymetrix GeneChip expression measures. *Bioinformatics* 22: 789–794.

Jiang, W. and Simon, R. 2007. A comparison of bootstrap methods and an adjusted bootstrap approach for estimating the prediction error in microarray classification. *Stat Med* 26: 5320–5334.

Jiang, W., Varma, S., and Simon, R. 2008. Calculating confidence intervals for prediction error in microarray classification using resampling. *Stat Appl Genet Mol Biol* 7: Article 8.

Kaufman, L. and Rousseeuw, P. 1990. *Finding Groups in Data: An Introduction to Cluster Analysis*. New York: John Wiley & Sons.

Kerr, M. K. and Churchill, G. A. 2001a. Experimental design for gene expression microarrays. *Biostatistics* 2: 183–201.

Kerr, M. K. and Churchill, G. A. 2001b. Bootstrapping cluster analysis: Assessing the reliability of conclusions from microarray experiments. *Proc Natl Acad Sci USA* 98: 8961–8965.

Kirschner-Schwabe, R., Lottaz, C., Tödling, J. et al. 2006. Expression of late cell cycle genes and an increased proliferative capacity characterize very early relapse of childhood acute lymphoblastic leukemia. *Clin Cancer Res* 12: 4553–4561.

Korn, E. L., Li, M. C., McShane, L. M., and Simon, R. 2007. An investigation of two multivariate permutation methods for controlling the false discovery proportion. *Stat Med* 26: 4428–4440.

Korn, E. L., Troendle, J. F., McShane, L. M., and Simon, R. 2004. Controlling the number of false discoveries: Application to high-dimensional genomic data. *J Stat Plan Inference* 124: 379–398.

Lai, C., Reinders, M. J., van't Veer, L. J., and Wessels, L. F. 2006. A comparison of univariate and multivariate gene selection techniques for classification of cancer datasets. *BMC Bioinform* 7: 235.

Laird, N. M. and Louis, T. A. 1987. Empirical Bayes confidence intervals based on bootstrap samples. *J Am Stat Assoc* 82: 739–750.

Langaas, M., Lindqvist, B. H., and Ferkingstad, E. 2005. Estimating the proportion of true null hypotheses, with application to DNA microarray data. *J R Stat Soc B* 67: 555–572.

Lange, T., Roth, V., Braun, M. L., and Buhmann, J. M. 2004. Stability-based validation of clustering solutions. *Neural Comput* 16: 1299–1323.

Lazzeroni, L. and Owen, A. 2002. Plaid models for gene expression data. *Stat Sin* 12: 61–86.

Lecocke, M. and Hess, K. 2007. An empirical study of univariate and genetic algorithm-based feature selection in binary classification with microarray data. *Cancer Inform* 2: 313–327.

Lewin, A., Richardson, S., Marshall, C., Glazier, A., and Aitman, T. 2006. Bayesian modelling of differential gene expression. *Biometrics* 62: 1–9.

Li, H. and Gui, J. 2004. Partial Cox regression analysis for high-dimensional microarray gene expression data. *Bioinformatics* 20: i208–i215.

Li, C. and Wong, W. H. 2001. Model-based analysis of oligonucleotide arrays: Model validation, design issues and standard error application. *Genome Biol* 2: 1–11.

Lian, H. 2008. MOST: Detecting cancer differential gene expression. *Biostatistics* 9: 411–418.

Liu, J. S., Zhang, J. L., Palumbo, M. J., and Lawrence, C. E. 2003. Bayesian clustering with variable and transformation selection (with discussion). *Bayesian Anal* 7: 249–275.

Lo, K. and Gottardo, R. 2007. Flexible empirical Bayes models for differential gene expression. *Bioinformatics* 23: 328–335.

Lönnstedt, I. and Speed, T. 2002. Replicated microarray data. *Stat Sin* 12: 31–46.

MacQueen, J. 1967. Some methods for classification and analysis of multivariate observations. In *Proceedings of the Fifth Berkeley Symposium on Mathematical Statistics and Probability*, Vol. 1, Berkeley, CA, pp. 281–297.

Madeira, S. C. and Oliveira, A. L. 2004. Biclustering algorithms for biological data analysis: A survey. *IEEE/ACM Trans Comput Biol Bioinform* 1: 24–45.

Matsui, S. 2006. Predicting survival outcomes using subsets of significant genes in prognostic marker studies with microarrays. *BMC Bioinform* 7: 156.

Matsui, S., Ito, M., Nishiyama, H. et al. 2007. Genomic characterization of multiple clinical phenotypes of cancer using multivariate linear regression models. *Bioinformatics* 23: 732–738.

Matsui, S. and Noma, H. 2011a. Estimation and selection in high-dimensional genomic studies for developing molecular diagnostics. *Biostatistics* 12: 223–233.

Matsui, S. and Noma, H. 2011b. Estimating effect sizes of differentially expressed genes for power and sample size assessments in microarray experiments. *Biometrics* (In press).

Matsui, S., Yamanaka, T., Barlogie, B., Shaughnessy, J. D., and Crowley, J. 2008a. Clustering of significant genes in prognostic studies with microarrays: Application to a clinical study for multiple myeloma. *Stat Med* 27: 1106–1120.

Matsui, S., Zeng, S., Yamanaka, T., and Shaughnessy, J. 2008b. Sample size calculations based on ranking and selection in microarray experiments. *Biometrics* 64: 217–226.

McLachlan, G. J., Bean, R. W., and Jones, L. B. T. 2006. A simple implementation of a normal mixture approach to differential gene expression in multiclass microarrays. *Bioinformatics* 22: 1608–1615.

McLachlan, G. J., Bean, R. W., and Peel, D. 2002. A mixture model-based approach to clustering of microarray expression data. *Bioinformatics* 18: 413–422.

McLachlan, G. J., Do, K.-A., and Ambroise, C. 2004. *Analyzing Microarray Gene Expression Data*. Hoboken, NJ: John Wiley & Sons.

McShane, L. M., Radmacher, M. D., Freidlin, B., Yu, R., Li, M., and Simon, R. 2002. Methods for assessing reproducibility of clustering patterns observed in analyses of microarray data. *Bioinformatics* 18: 1462–1469.

Milligan, G. W. and Cooper, M. C. 1985. An examination of procedures for determining the number of clusters in a data set. *Psychometrika* 50: 159–179.

Molinaro, A. M., Simon, R., and Pfeiffer, R. M. 2005. Prediction error estimation: A comparison of resampling methods. *Bioinformatics* 21: 3301–3307.

Nam, D. and Kim, S. Y. 2008. Gene-set approach for expression pattern analysis. *Brief Bioinform* 9: 189–197. Erratum in: *Brief Bioinform* 2008; 9: 450.

Newton, M. A., Noueiry, A., Sarkar, D., and Ahlquist, P. 2004. Detecting differential gene expression with a semiparametric hierarchical mixture method. *Biostatistics* 5: 155–176.

Nguyen, D. V., Arpat, A. B., Wang, N., and Carroll, R. J. 2002. DNA microarray experiments: Biological and technical aspects. *Biometrics* 58: 701–717.

Noma, H., Matsui, S., Omori, T., and Sato, T. 2010. Bayesian ranking and selection methods using hierarchical mixture models in microarray studies. *Biostatistics* 11: 281–289.

Oura, T., Matsui, S., and Kawakami, K. 2009. Sample size calculations for controlling the distribution of false discovery proportion in microarray experiments. *Biostatistics* 10: 694–705.

Pan, W. 2006. Incorporating gene functions as priors in model-based clustering of microarray gene expression data. *Bioinformatics* 22: 795–801.

Pan, W., Lin, J., and Le, C. 2002. Model-based cluster analysis of microarray gene-expression data. *Genome Biol* 3: research 0009.1–0009.8.

Pan, W. and Shen, X. 2007. Penalized model-based clustering with application to variable selection. *J Mach Learn Res* 8: 1145–1164.

Park, M. Y. and Hastie, T. 2007. L1 regularization path algorithm for generalized linear models. *J R Stat Soc B* 69: 659–677.

Park, T., Yi, S. G., Kang, S. H., Lee, S., Lee, Y. S., and Simon, R. 2003. Evaluation of normalization methods for microarray data. *BMC Bioinform* 4: 33.

Pawitan, Y., Michiels, S., Koscielny, S., Gusnanto, A., and Ploner, A. 2005. False discovery rate, sensitivity and sample size for microarray studies. *Bioinformatics* 21: 3017–3024.

Pepe, M. S., Longton, G., Anderson, G. L., and Schummer, M. 2003. Selecting differentially expressed genes from microarray experiments. *Biometrics* 59: 133–142.

Perou, C. M., Sørlie, T., Eisen, M. B. et al. 2000. Molecular portraits of human breast tumours. *Nature* 406: 747–752.

Ponder, B. A. 2001. Cancer genetics. *Nature* 411: 336–341.

Pounds, S. B. 2006. Estimation and control of multiple testing error rates for microarray studies. *Brief Bioinform* 7: 25–36.

Radmacher, M. D., McShane, L. M., and Simon, R. 2002. A paradigm for class prediction using gene expression profiles. *J Comput Biol* 9: 505–511.

Rosenwald, A., Wright, G., Chan, W. C. et al. 2002. The use of molecular profiling to predict survival after chemotherapy for diffuse large-B-cell lymphoma. *N Eng J Med* 346: 1937–1947.

Saeys, Y., Inza, I., and Larrañaga, P. 2007. A review of feature selection techniques in bioinformatics. *Bioinformatics* 23: 2507–2517.

Setlur, S. R., Mertz, K. D., Hoshida, Y. et al. 2008. Estrogen-dependent signaling in a molecularly distinct subclass of aggressive prostate cancer. *J Natl Cancer Inst* 100: 815–825.

Shao, Y. and Tseng, C. H. 2007. Sample size calculation with dependence adjustment for FDR-control in microarray studies. *Stat Med* 26: 4219–4237.

Shaughnessy, J. D. Jr., Zhan, F., Burington, B. E. et al. 2007. A validated gene expression model of high-risk multiple myeloma is defined by deregulated expression of genes mapping to chromosome 1. *Blood* 109: 2276–2284.

Shen, W. and Louis, T. A. 1999. Empirical Bayes estimation via the smoothing by roughening approach. *J Comput Gr Stat* 8: 800–823.

Sheng, Q., Moreau, Y., and Moor, B. 2003. Biclustering microarray data by Gibbs sampling. *Bioinformatics* 19: ii196–ii205.

Shi, L., Campbell, G., Jones, W. D. et al. 2010. The MicroArray Quality Control (MAQC)-II study of common practices for the development and validation of microarray-based predictive models. *Nat Biotechnol* 28: 827–838.

Simon, R. M., Korn, E. L., McShane, L. M., Radmacher, M. D., Wright, G. W., and Zhao, Y. 2004. *Design and Analysis of DNA Microarray Investigations.* New York: Springer.

Simon, R., Radmacher, M. D., and Dobbin, K. 2002. Design of studies using DNA microarrays. *Genet Epidemiol* 23: 21–36.

Simon, R., Radmacher, M. D., Dobbin, K., and McShane, L. M. 2003. Pitfalls in the use of DNA microarray data for diagnostic and prognostic classification. *J Natl Cancer Inst* 95: 14–18.

Simon, R., Subramanian, J., Li, M. C., and Menezes, S. 2011. Using cross-validation to evaluate predictive accuracy of survival risk classifiers based on high-dimensional data. *Brief Bioinform* 12: 203–214.

Smyth, G. K. 2004. Linear models and empirical Bayes methods for assessing differential expression in microarray experiments. *Stat Appl Genet Mol Biol* 3: Article 3.

Sotiriou, C., Neo, S. Y., McShane, L. M. et al. 2003. Breast cancer classification and prognosis based on gene expression profiles from a population-based study. *Proc Natl Acad Sci USA* 100: 10393–10398.

Storey, J. D. 2002. A direct approach to false discovery rates. *J R Stat Soc B* 64: 479–498.

Storey, J. D. 2007. The optimal discovery procedure: A new approach to simultaneous significance testing. *J R Stat Soc B* 69: 347–368.

Tadesse, M. G., Sha, N., and Vannucci, M. 2005. Bayesian variable selection in clustering high-dimensional data. *J Am Stat Assoc* 100: 602–617.

Takata, R., Katagiri, T., Kanehira, M. et al. 2005. Predicting response to methotrexate, vinblastine, doxorubicin, and cisplatin neoadjuvant chemotherapy for bladder cancers through genome-wide gene expression profiling. *Clin Cancer Res* 11: 2625–2636.

Tamayo, P., Slonim, D., Mesirov, J. et al. 1999. Interpreting patterns of gene expression with self-organizing maps: Methods and application to hematopoietic differentiation. *Proc Natl Acad Sci USA* 96: 2907–2912.

Thalamuthu, A., Mukhopadhyay, I., Zheng, X., and Tseng, G. C. 2006. Evaluation and comparison of gene clustering methods in microarray analysis. *Bioinformatics* 22: 2405–2412.

Tibshirani, R. and Hastie, T. 2007. Outlier sums for differential gene expression analysis. *Biostatistics* 8: 2–8.

Tibshirani, R., Hastie, T., Narasimhan, B., and Chu, G. 2003. Class prediction by nearest shrunken centroids, with applications to DNA microarrays. *Stat Sci* 18: 104–117.

Tomlins, S. A., Rhodes, D. R., Perner, S. et al. 2005. Recurrent fusion of TMPRSS2 and ETS transcription factor genes in prostate cancer. *Science* 310: 644–648.

Tong, T. and Zhao, H. 2008. Practical guidelines for assessing power and false discovery rate for a fixed sample size in microarray experiments. *Stat Med* 27: 1960–1972.

Tsai, C. A., Wang, S. J., Chen, D. T., and Chen, J. J. 2005. Sample size for gene expression microarray experiments. *Bioinformatics* 21: 1502–1508.

Tusher, V. G., Tibshirani, R., and Chu, G. 2001. Significance analysis of microarrays applied to ionizing radiation response. *Proc Natl Acad Sci USA* 98: 5116–5121.

Varma, S. and Simon, R. 2006. Bias in error estimation when using cross-validation for model selection. *BMC Bioinform* 7: 91.

van't Veer, L. J., Dai, H., van de Vijver, M. J. et al. 2002. Gene expression profiling predicts clinical outcome of breast cancer. *Nature* 415: 530–536.

Westfall, P. H. and Young, S. S. 1993. *Resampling-Based Multiple Testing*. New York: Wiley.

Wright, G. and Simon, R. 2003. A random variance model for detection of differential gene expression in small microarray experiments. *Bioinformatics* 19: 2448–2455.

Wu, Z. 2009. A review of statistical methods for preprocessing oligonucleotide microarrays. *Stat Methods Med Res* 18: 533–541.

Wu, Z., Irizarry, R. A., Gentleman, R., Martinez-Murillo, F., and Spencer, F. 2004. A model-based background adjustment for oligonucleotide expression arrays. *J Am Stat Assoc* 99: 909–917.

Yang, Y. H., Buckley, M. J., and Speed, T. P. 2001. Analysis of cDNA microarray images. *Brief Bioinform* 2: 341–349.

Yang, Y. H., Dudoit, S., Luu, P. et al. 2002. Normalization for cDNA microarray data: A robust composite method addressing single and multiple slide systematic variation. *Nucleic Acids Res* 30: e15.

Yeung, K. Y., Fraley, C., Mutua, A., Raftery, A. E., and Ruzzo, W. L. 2001a. Model-based clustering and data transformations for gene expression data. *Bioinformatics* 17: 977–987.

Yeung, K. Y., Haynor, D. R., and Ruzzo, W. L. 2001b. Validating clustering for gene expression data. *Bioinformatics* 17: 309–318.

Yeung, K. Y. and Ruzzo, W. L. 2001. Principal component analysis for clustering gene expression data. *Bioinformatics* 17: 763–774.

# 32 Methods for SNP Regression Analysis in Clinical Studies
## Selection, Shrinkage, and Logic

*Michael LeBlanc, Bryan Goldman, and Charles Kooperberg*

## CONTENTS

## 32.1 INTRODUCTION

Investigations of the association of patient outcome with a few candidate single nucleotide polymorphisms (SNPs) or much larger numbers of SNPs have been undertaken in various therapeutic studies in oncology (e.g., Durie et al. 2009, Song et al. 2010). Since the genomic material often consists of germline DNA, not tumor DNA, the primary associations to therapeutic efficacy are typically not expected to be as strong as those seen for tumor gene expression. However, even with non-tumor

DNA, there could potentially be some strong correlations with disease symptoms at diagnosis, measures of drug metabolism and patient adverse events due to treatment.

While primarily outside the therapeutic setting, there have been many high-dimensional SNP studies which can be useful in defining good statistical strategies. For instance, there are an increasing number of validated associations seen from high throughput SNP studies including genome wide association studies (GWAS) (e.g., Hindorff et al. 2009, Peterson et al. 2010, Thomas et al. 2009). Often these are case-control studies and may include subject level meta-analyses on multiple cohorts to arrive at total numbers in the multiple thousands of cases and controls to achieve power to detect at least modest individual SNP associations with outcome. In addition, there has been some development of multi-SNP risk models from GWAS including Miyake et al. (2009), Zheng et al. (2008), Yang et al. (2010).

In most therapeutic clinical trials, the number of patients are typically only several hundreds, even when combining across studies. These sample sizes are modest enough to make it far more challenging to conduct well powered tests of association or risk modeling. Realistically, only large effects will be reliably identified in these moderately sized studies. However, given sufficient signal, SNP association studies are feasible; therefore, this chapter will consider model building strategies to construct prognostic or disease risk models, trading off variance control as well as interpretation. A good statistical strategy for risk modeling with GWAS data was outlined in Kooperberg et al. (2010) but we think it applies more broadly to smaller scale SNP analyses more typical of cancer therapeutic studies. Our proposal for a straight-forward statistical regression modeling approach can be outlined as follows: (1) data cleaning, (2) selection of a smaller number SNPs (if there are initially a large number under consideration), (3) modeling in some parsimonious fashion; shrinkage methods are one possibility or using a method that combines features in some logical fashion (such as logic regression or regression trees) and (4) a strategy to avoid drawing false positive associations or building models that are overly complex.

We note that there are many options for modeling in this context. Our focus is on SNP regression; we do not address alternatives here in terms of haplotype reconstruction, although algorithms have been developed for that purpose (for instance, see SNP-Haplotype Adaptive Regression [SHARE]) (Dai et al. 2009). Other than direct haplotype methods, there are methods to reduce dimensionality by using regularization to combine SNPs within gene as a component of the modeling procedure (Chen et al. 2010).

We illustrate the methods with a SNP data set from a clinical trial of multiple myeloma patients from the University of Arkansas generated as part of the Bank on a Cure project.

## 32.2 SIMPLE GENOTYPE DATA

Humans have two copies of each autosomal chromosome. The total length is about three billion base pairs. The most common variation between humans are variations in a single locus, known as SNPs. SNPs are typically coded as 0,1, or 2, the number of minor (variant) alleles at a particular locus. These data can be re-coded as a variable for the dominant effect by labeling 1 if $SNP = \{1,2\}$ or 0 otherwise and for the recessive effect as a 1 if $SNP = \{2\}$ or 0 otherwise. Often, given such a large number of SNPs, and hope for mostly cumulative association with subject outcome, the additive code $\{0,1,2\}$ is used in many statistical testing and regression strategies. This coding is often the most powerful in detecting SNP disease associations.

Data quality is, of course, a fundamental issue in any analysis. However, in this chapter we will not address steps to assess the quality of the genotyping calls. These issues are platform dependent and checking quality would likely involve investigation of control and replication samples. In addition, in some cases, depending on the platform, it could involve returning to the images of relative intensities to re-evaluate the calls. Other quality control techniques involve inspection of QQ plots of the associations (where there are sufficient numbers of SNPs being investigated) to check for more global departures from the 45° line than what would be expected for the hypothesized scenarios where only a few SNPs are thought to be associated with patient outcome or toxicity.

Additional filtering of samples and SNPs for subsequent analysis also typically involves removal based on a sufficient number of observed called genotypes. For instance, often all samples with a call rate smaller than some value (say 97% for large arrays, but often this is set somewhat lower for smaller scale genotyping technologies) will be removed for consideration for further analysis. In addition SNPs that substantially fail the assumption of Hardy–Weinberg (HW) equilibrium, for instance, with a $p$-value of $10^{-3}$–$10^{-5}$, are not considered. The extremeness of the $p$-value would need to depend on the number of SNPs under consideration. We note that typically the check of HW is done in control samples only; in our clinical trial settings all patients typically have disease. So while checking HW plays a role in data cleaning, it is not clear that HW equilibrium needs to be valid for all SNPs in the therapeutic "all case" setting. Another filtering option used primarily for power considerations, is to remove SNPs with a low minor allele frequency (say .05) prior to any formal model building.

## 32.3   EXAMPLE: MYELOMA SNP ANALYSIS

To demonstrate methods in this chapter, we use data based on patients with previously untreated multiple myeloma enrolled in the TT2 trial at the University of Arkansas between October 1998 and February 2004. Details of patient characteristics plus treatment and clinical outcomes have been reported previously (Durie et al. 2009). The multiple myeloma baseline evaluation included serum and urine protein electrophoresis, quantitative immunoglobulin measurements, total 24 h urine protein excretion and serum beta-2 microglobulin. The outcome was defined as extensive bone disease defined by x-ray criteria.

While the original study had data on 282 patients, we construct a larger simulated data set which we think is a more appropriate size for demonstrating regression modeling methods in this chapter. In addition to the observed data cases, 118 additional cases were drawn as a simple bootstrap sample to augment the real sample to yield a total of 400 real and simulated patients for analysis. Given the data set we used is partially simulated, the results presented in this chapter do not agree with the prior published results for this data set.

## 32.4   ASSESSING ASSOCIATIONS

Continuous, binary, or survival endpoints are potentially of interest in the SNP association studies in the context of cancer clinical trials. Therefore, to keep the discussion general, we present the models in terms of the regression component of each of the outcome models.

### 32.4.1   Univariate Associations

Most SNP association studies involve, at a minimum, a report of single SNP associations, potentially after adjusting for population heterogeneity; the adjustments may be based on reported race, genomic measurements of racial variation, and/or baseline clinical factors in a therapeutic study. As noted earlier, a single SNP has three levels, so common coding for assessment of association can be as linear $X = \{0,1,2\}$, dominant $X = 1$ if SNP is 1 or 2, 0 otherwise recessive $X = 1$ if $SNP = 2$ or 0 otherwise.

Consider a regression setting, where there are $n$ observations on variables including non-genomic $Z_l:l = 1, ..., L$ and genomic $X_k:k = 1, ..., K$. To simplify presentation, assume only a single adjustment variable denoted as $Z$. Then testing individual SNPs can be reduced to assessing score or likelihood test statistics of $\beta_k = 0$ in the regression model for coded SNP $k$

$$\eta(X,Z) = \beta_0 + \gamma Z + \beta_k X_k.$$

Nominal $p$-values can be calculated for all $k = 1, ..., K$ tests of association. If the goal is to identify univariate associations, then strategies to control the error rates for false positives are of primary importance. The simplest way to control the family wise error rate (FWER) is to use a Bonferroni correction. However, it is often preferable with moderate numbers of SNPs (some chosen that may have relatively high correlation with each other—high linkage disequilibrium) to acknowledge the correlation structure. A simple way to incorporate the correlation structure in testings is by permutation sampling and to compare the observed statistics to those observed from a sample from the permutation distribution. Where the model includes adjustment variables, permutation of the score residuals and recalculating the test statistics is a more relevant null distribution. If the primary objective focuses on risk or prognostic modeling based on multiple SNPs, then the selection of a set of SNPs for further modeling does not require such a stringent selection of SNPs. One may select some limited number regardless of their overall significance. For instance, with a 3000 SNP study, one may select the SNPs with the top 1% or 5% of $p$-values to reduce overall variability of the subsequent modeling method. However, as described later, additional strategies for model selection (such as cross-validation) will ultimately be needed.

#### 32.4.1.1   Example: Univariate Statistics

After filtering for low allele frequency and call rate, 1903 out of 3404 genotyped SNPs remained in the myeloma data set. We calculated univariate statistics for each of the SNPs displayed in Figure 32.1, testing the SNP associations with bone disease. While one could assess significance via permutation sampling here,

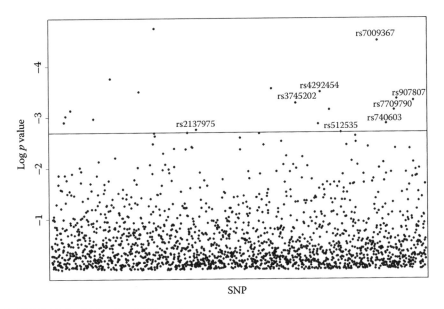

**FIGURE 32.1**   Univariate SNP *p*-values.

Bonferroni-corrected .05 level corresponds to the log10 *p*-value of −4.58 which only includes one SNP. The labels on the plot correspond to the SNPs selected as part of the regularized regression method (least absolute and selection operator [LASSO]) described in a later section. It also demonstrates that it may be useful to include slightly more variables (SNPs) as part of the modeling method, even if they do not achieve significance by multiple comparison adjusted methods.

## 32.5   MULTIVARIATE ASSOCIATIONS

Assume there is interest in combining genetic information across loci. The simplest model is some additive combination of the genotype data. For instance, for binary outcome data or case control studies, a logistic regression model can be used where the probability of disease or toxicity is $P(Y=1|Z, X)=\exp(\eta(X,Z))/(1+\exp(\eta(X,Z)))$ where a linear combination of individual SNPs which is the simplest way to combine information between SNPs adjusting for any baseline factors is

$$\eta(\mathbf{X},\mathbf{Z}) = \beta_0 + \gamma\sum_{l=1}^{L}\gamma_l Z_l + \sum_{k=1}^{K}\beta_k X_k. \tag{32.1}$$

### 32.5.1   PENALIZED REGRESSION

Consider the likelihood-based regression setting. Assume there are *n* independent observations of the genotype and non-genotype data described earlier. Denote the likelihood function as $l(\cdot)$ which would be a binomial likelihood for binary outcomes, partial likelihood for survival endpoints or the typically normal likelihood for continuous outcome data. While step-wise model building is a reasonable strategy for building models (with the Akaike information criteria [AIC] Akaike [1974] or BIC to do the model selection), we believe penalized methods offer the advantage of reduced variability especially in moderate sample size settings. A popular regularization or penalization method is the LASSO (Tibshirani 1996) and its extensions (e.g., Hastie et al. 2009). There has been considerable subsequent work on rapid estimation methods. Suppressing the notation for the adjustment variables, which may or may not be penalized, the LASSO estimate $\tilde{\beta} = (\tilde{\beta}_1, \dots \tilde{\beta}_m)'$ is defined as the maximizer of

$$g(\beta) = \sum_{i=1}^{n} l\left(Y_i, \sum_k \beta_k X_{ik}\right) - \lambda_1 \sum_k |\beta_k|',$$

where $\lambda_1$ is a non-negative penalty parameter. This estimator has the attractive property that as the penalty $\lambda_1$ increases, maximizing $g(\beta)$ with respect to $\beta$ leads to some of the $\beta_k$ set to zero. In addition, the variable selection and regression function estimates tend to have overall less variability than those obtained from forward or backward variable selection methods. Further variance reduction, at the cost of potentially less sparse solution involving more non-zero coefficients, is obtained by using a mixture of $L_1$ and $L_2$ penalty called the "elastic net" proposed by Zou and Hastie (2005). The elastic net can be expressed as an optimization problem with the objective function with both squared and absolute penalty terms

$$g(\beta) = \sum_{i=1}^{n} l\left(Y_i, \sum_k \beta_k X_{ik}\right) - \lambda_1 \sum_k |\beta_k|' - \lambda_2 \sum_k |\beta_k|^2.$$

There is overall shrinking of the linear predictor and setting of some of the coefficients to zero in the model as the penalty parameters $\lambda_1$ and $\lambda_2$ are increased. Flexible software that fits continuous, binary, and survival data is available in $R$ statistical language (GLMNET). In this section, we have described these methods in terms of the original predictors $X_k$; we could generalize to sets of regression splines or even more complex multivariable basis functions, $B_j(X)$, $j = 1, \dots, p$ as described in the next section.

For the case of LASSO, the models are indexed by a single parameter $\lambda_1$ or for the elastic net by two parameters $\lambda_1$ and $\lambda_2$. To objectively choose these tuning parameters, one can either use a separate data set or use a resampling technique such as $K$-fold cross validation. For $K$-fold cross validation, the data are divided in approximately $K$ groups (for instance, $K = 5$ or 10), and fractions $(K-1)/K$ are used to construct the models and index the sequence of models by the tuning parameters, and the log-likelihood is evaluated for each model on the remaining $1/K$ of the data, called the test data. The analysis is repeated for each of the $K$ subsets of the data, and test sample log-likelihoods are averaged over the $K$ subsets. Tuning parameters ($\lambda_1$ and $\lambda_2$ in the case of the elastic net) are chosen that lead to maximum likelihood solutions. It is important that all of the variable selection aspects of the modeling be

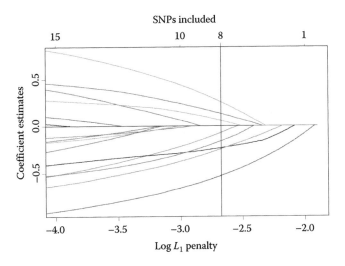

**FIGURE 32.2** $L_1$ penalized regression coefficient paths.

included in the cross-validation loop. For instance, if the initial filter is to use only the top $q$ most significant variables in the penalized regression algorithm, that should be part of the cross-validation loop.

### 32.5.1.1 Example: $L_1$ Penalized Regression Bone Disease Model

We chose to use $L_1$ regression to construct a multi-SNP model of bone disease. Based on prior methodological work we filtered the number of SNPs under consideration prior to using LASSO. For this example we chose only the top 20 SNPs (the top 1% SNPs) with the smallest $p$-values. We left the SNP coding as ordinal {0,1,2}. We applied five fold cross validation over both the variable selection as well as the model building and the final model chosen included eight SNPs. We acknowledge the number of SNPs filtered is another tuning parameter which could also be estimated using cross-validation. The coefficient profile is presented in Figure 32.2. There are eight SNPs remaining in the model; the labels of these SNPs are included in Figure 32.1. Cross-validated log-likelihood is presented in Figure 32.3.

### 32.5.1.2 Example: $L_1$ Penalized Regression Simulation

A concern with the relatively small sample sizes with SNP studies as part of therapeutic cancer studies is that only large effects would be seen. We conducted a small simulation study to investigate this issue. SNP data were generated by resampling from the "observed 400" patient cohort and the disease response was simulated from a single SNP regression model out of the total of 1903 SNPs under consideration. For an odds ratio of 1.75, 91% of the LASSO models (with complexity selected by five fold cross validation) included the true SNP. On average, 5.2 SNPs were selected, indicating at least some tendency for over-fitting. For an odds ratio of 2.0 the probability of selecting the correct SNP increased to 98.6% with a similar level of overfitting. This indicates the potential for identifying moderately strong associations from clinical SNP data.

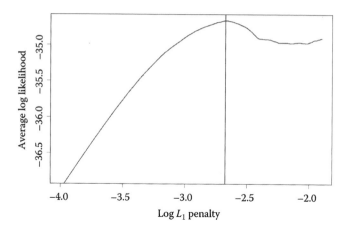

**FIGURE 32.3**   Cross-validated log-likelihood for $L_1$ regression.

## 32.5.2 LOGIC REGRESSION

One way to extend the linear model, described earlier, is to consider more complex SNP combinations. For instance,

$$\eta(\mathbf{X}) = \beta_0 + \sum_h \beta_h B_h(X),$$

where the basis functions $B_h(X)$ could represent nonlinear functions of several of the $X_k$. A specific example of this model is regression trees (Breiman et al. 1984) and extended to survival data, for instance, by Segal (1988) and LeBlanc and Crowley (1993). In that case, the basis functions $B_h(X)$ are products of subset functions of the individual variables, of SNPs. In tree-terminology they would be terminal nodes of a regression tree. Trees are discussed in detail in another chapter and hence are not developed here. Trees have been used in the analysis of SNP data both as single trees (Durie et al. 2009), and as ensembles, such as random forests (Ishwaran et al. 2008).

In this section we describe a method which can be viewed as one that uses alternative interpretable basis functions based on logical or Boolean rules. The method, called "logic regression" is a methodology that is particularly suited for situations where the data are binary or in the case of SNP data "almost binary" and are binary if they are first coded as binary or recessive or dominant codes for each SNP (Ruczinski et al. 2003, Kooperberg and Ruczinski 2005). The resulting model, again suppressing the adjustment variables, can be expressed as basis functions or as Boolean combination of binary predictors $X_j, j = 1, \ldots, p$ such as

$$B_h(X) = \left[ \left( X_1 \text{ OR } X_4^c \right) \text{ AND } X_2 \right],$$

where the $X_j$ are binary coding of the SNP data as either dominant or recessive effects and hence $X_j$ are assumed to be either 0 or 1. $X_j^c$ is the complement function, so $X_j^c = 1 - X_j$. Additional adjustment covariates $Z$ can be included in the model as for the other models described earlier.

Logic regression is usually implemented as a stochastic simulated annealing algorithm which selects those logic terms $B_h(\cdot)$ which maximize the log-likelihood corresponding to the model. Given the potential complexity or adaptivity in fitting each basis function, the number of logic terms $m$ is set to be some small constant (between 1 and 3).

There is a tree-based representation of any logic term, which allows an easy specification for the stochastic optimization algorithm. At each step of the simulated annealing algorithm, one logic tree can be replaced by another logic tree through simple change operations on the tree. These operations are demonstrated in Figure 32.4.

As is true for other simulated annealing algorithms, if the likelihood of the new model is larger than for the current model, then the new model is chosen; if the current model has a smaller likelihood than the new model, then new model is chosen with a probability that is a function of the difference between the current and new model log-likelihood. The probability of choosing the new model is related to the current step number of the algorithm. At early steps of the procedure most of new models are accepted, while after many steps, only improved models are chosen with high probability.

Similar to penalized regression methods, the model complexity (which we have measured as the number of leaves or terms in the logic model) should be selected in such a fashion that acknowledges the significant adaptivity of the logic regression algorithm. Logic regression allows both permutation tests to assess overall association as well as $K$-fold cross validation.

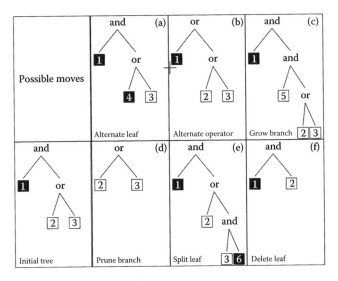

**FIGURE 32.4** Logic regression optimization operations.

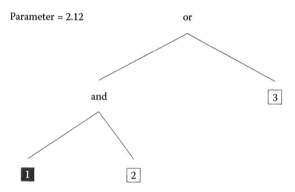

Parameter = 2.12

**FIGURE 32.5** Selected logic regression tree with 3 SNPs (1) rs4292454, (2) rs3745202, and (3) rs7843746.

### 32.5.2.1 Example Revisited: Logic Regression

We return to our example, but now with the goal of constructing a simple logic regression model of Boolean combinations of SNPs. After conducting full cross validation, involving both filtering to the 20 SNPs and application of logic regression, there was no evidence of improvement in prediction over the null model. As expected in the relatively modest sample size setting, the more adaptive and discrete logic regression method suffers somewhat from additional variance, even if the interpretation of a small number of SNPs would be desirable. However, for demonstration purposes we show the three-leaf tree which on the full data set had a deviance of 288 compared to the null model deviance of 321. The model is presented in Figure 32.5. The estimated odds ratio was 2.12 and the logic representation was

$$L = (\text{NOT dominant rs4292454}) \text{ AND } (\text{dominant rs3745202})$$

$$\text{OR } (\text{dominant rs7843746})$$

which represented patients at a higher risk of extensive bone disease.

## 32.6 ASSESSING TREATMENT–GENE INTERACTIONS

In the prior section, we demonstrated logic regression which can be viewed as a procedure which builds models within a special class of interactions. However, there is now an increasing literature for efficiently assessing more simple gene×gene or gene×baseline clinical factor, or gene×treatment interactions. It has been shown that significant gains in power can be obtained in many situations by only considering SNPs with the most significant marginal association prior to testing the interaction. It has been shown that if the test of interaction is independent of the marginal test, then one needs to adjust only for the number of interactions tested rather than the total number of marginal tests conducted (Kooperberg and LeBlanc 2008, Dai et al. 2011). Penalized regression strategies that directly incorporate interactions were considered by Park and Hastie (2008). Several strategies for evaluating and utilizing interactions in genomic studies were described in Kooperberg et al. (2009).

However, potentially the most important class of interactions of interest in therapeutic studies is the interaction of a SNP with the assigned treatment group. A question may arise: Does the impact of treatment (say on toxicity) depend on a gene? A simple case of one treatment and one SNP in a multiplicative model can be represented as

$$\eta(X, Z) = \beta_0 + \gamma Z + \beta_k X_k + \delta Z X_k, \tag{32.2}$$

where
$Z = \{0,1\}$ indicates treatment
$X_k$ represents the specific genetic variable

To assess potential interactions, one can test all $K$ gene by treatment interactions. Another strategy, as noted earlier, is to first test all the gene main effects, and then only test a subset of the interactions corresponding to the top most significant gene main effects. It can be shown that the second stage testing is asymptotically independent of the first stage; so if only $M$ interaction tests are considered at the second stage, then significance only need to be adjusted by the factor of $M$ tests. This can lead to increased power to find interactions in many settings. Of course, if the interaction is "pure" or hidden entirely in the marginal test, then it will be missed at second stage testing (Dai et al. 2011).

If a true interaction is not the primary goal, but rather interest focuses on any gene association that may be modified by baseline clinical factors, then more general weighted tests can be used. For instance, LeBlanc and Kooperberg (2009) constructed adaptively weighted test statistics that can be substantially more powerful than the single tests if interactions are truly present in the data so that within a subset of patients the genetic association is substantially stronger.

## 32.7   DISCUSSION

In this chapter our goal was not to provide an exhaustive review of methods for prognostic or risk modeling with SNP data, but rather to focus on two techniques which have been used and/or developed for SNP data which represent smooth prediction and non-smooth interpretation-based strategies: penalized regression and logic regression. Obviously alternatives to linear penalized models could include regression trees demonstrated in the analysis of clinical SNP data by Durie et al. (2009) or ensembles of trees such as random forests. Other methods have been proposed, including multifactor dimensionality reduction (MDR, Richie et al. 2001) which focuses on low-dimensional combinations of SNPs.

We have not addressed sensible ways to combine SNPs that may be close together; for instance, some sets of SNPs may be thought to correspond to a haplotype block. In that setting, prior to doing some of the modeling proposals we have made in this chapter, one may first want to use a haplotype reconstruction method (e.g., Li et al. 2006). After appropriately acknowledging the haplotype uncertainty, one can use regression methods to predict the outcome. An adaptive technique that does SNP selection and haplotype regression, "SNP and HAplotype REgression" was developed by Dai et al. (2009). An alternative approach is to group using regularized methods on SNPs localized in a region; see, for instance, Chen et al. (2010).

An important issue with the analysis of SNP data in the context of moderate-size clinical studies is an assessment of power to detect meaningful associations. For instance, unlike some large case control studies including meta-analyses used for GWAS studies, our experience is that SNP association studies in therapeutic settings often consist of small numbers of cases. Therefore, statistical methods which control the variability and don't over-fit the data are critically important. In addition, where power to detect reasonable sized effects is limited, combining across clinical studies, where scientifically sensible, may be a useful strategy.

Software for logic regression and GLMNET are currently available at CRAN.

## ACKNOWLEDGMENTS

This work was supported by the U.S. NIH through R01 CA90998, R01 HG006124, and P01 CA53996. The authors thank Dr. Brian Durie and the International Myeloma Foundation and the Bank on a Cure project for use of the data. They acknowledge helpful interactions with Dr. Antje Hoering for information relating to the SNP data.

## REFERENCES

Akaike HA. 1974. New look at model identification. *IEEE Transactions on Automatic Control*, 19:716–723.

Breiman L, Friedman JH, Olshen RA, Stone CJ. 1984. *Classification and Regression Trees*. Wadsworth, Belmont, CA.

Chen LS, Hutter CM, Potter JD, Liu Y, Prentice RL, Peters U, Hsu L. 2010. Insights into colon cancer etiology using a regularized approach to gene set analysis of GWAS data. *American Journal of Human Genetics*, 86:860–871.

Dai JY, Kooperberg C, LeBlanc M, Prentice R. 2011. On two-stage hypothesis testing procedures via asymptotically independent statistics. Submitted to *Biometrika*.

Dai JY, LeBlanc M, Smith NL, Psaty B, Kooperberg C. 2009. SHARE: An adaptive algorithm to select the most informative set of SNPs for candidate genetic association. *Biostatistics*, 10(4):680–693.

Durie BG, Van Ness B, Ramos C, Stephens O, Haznadar M, Hoering A, Haessler J et al. 2009. Genetic polymorphisms of EPHX1, Gsk3beta, TNFSF8 and myeloma cell DKK-1 expression linked to bone disease in myeloma. *Leukemia*, 10:1913–1919.

Hastie T, Tibshirani R, Friedman J. 2009. *Elements of Statistical Learning*, 2nd edn., Springer, New York.

Hindorff LA, Sethupathy P, Junkins HA, Ramos EM, Mehta JP, Collins FS, Manolio TA. 2009. Potential etiologic and functional implications of genome-wide association loci for human diseases and traits. *Proceedings of the National Academy of Sciences USA*, 106:9362–9367.

Ishwaran H, Kogalur UB, Blackstone EH, Lauer MS. 2008. Random survival forests. *Annals of Applied Statistics*, 2:841–860.

Kooperberg C, LeBlanc M. 2008. Increasing the power of identifying gene X gene interactions in genome-wide association studies. *Genetic Epidemiology*, 32:255–263.

Kooperberg C, LeBlanc M, Dai JY, Rajapakse I. 2009. Structures and assumptions: Strategies to harness gene x gene and gene x environment interactions in GWAS. *Statistical Science*, 24(4):472–488.

Kooperberg C, LeBlanc M, Obenchain V. 2010. Risk prediction using genome-wide association studies. *Genetic Epidemiology*, 34(7):643–652.

Kooperberg C, Ruczinski I. 2005. Identifying interacting SNPs using Monte Carlo logic regression. *Genetic Epidemiology*, 28:157–170.

LeBlanc M, Crowley J. 1993. Survival trees by goodness of split. *Journal of the American Statistical Association*, 88:457–467.

LeBlanc M, Kooperberg C. 2009. Adaptively weighted association statistics. *Genetic Epidemiology*, 33(5):442–452.

Li Y, Ding J, Abecasis GR. 2006. Mach 1.0: Rapid haplotype reconstruction and missing genotype inference. *American Journal of Human Genetics*, 79:S2290.

Miyake K, Yang W, Hara K, Yasuda K, Horikawa Y, Osawa H, Furuta H et al. 2009. Construction of a prediction model for type 2 diabetes mellitus in the Japanese population based on 11 genes with strong evidence of the association. *American Journal of Human Genetics*, 54:236–241.

Park MY, Hastie T. 2008. Penalized logistic regression for detecting gene interactions. *Biostatistics*, 9:30–50.

Petersen GM, Amundadottir L, Fuchs CS, Kraft P, Stolzenberg-Solomon RZ, Jacobs KB, Arslan AA et al. 2010. A genome-wide association study identifies pancreatic cancer susceptibility loci on chromosomes 13q22.1, 1q32.1 and 5p15.33., *Nature Genetics*, 42(3):224–228.

Richie MD, Hahn LW, Roodi N, Bailey LR, Dupont WD, Parl FF, Moore JH. 2001. Multifactor-dimensionality reduction reveals high-order interactions among estrogen-metabolism genes in sporadic breast cancer. *American Journal of Human Genetics*, 69:138–147.

Ruczinski I, Kooperberg C, LeBlanc M. 2003. Logic regression. *Journal of Graphical and Computational Statistics*, 12:475–511.

Segal MR. 1988. Regression trees for censored data. *Biometrics*, 44:35–48.

Song Y, Barlow WE, Albain KS, Choi JY, Zhao H, Livingston RB, Davis W et al. 2010. Gene polymorphisms in cyclophosphamide metabolism pathway, treatment-related toxicity, and disease-free survival in SWOG 8897 clinical trial for breast cancer. *Clinical Cancer Research*, 16:6169–6176.

Thomas G, Jacobs KB, Kraft P, Yeager M, Wacholder S, Cox DG, Hankinson SE et al. 2009. A multistage genome-wide association study in breast cancer identifies two new risk alleles at 1p11.2 and 14q24.1 (RAD51L1). *Nature Genetics*, 41(5):579–584.

Tibshirani R. 1996. Regression shrinkage and selection via the lasso. *Journal of the Royal Statistical Society: Series B*, 58:267–288.

Yang et al. 2010. Common SNPs explain a large proportion of the heritability for human height. *Nature Genetics*, 42:565–569.

Zheng SL, Sun J, Wiklund F, Smith S, Stattin P, Li G, Adami HO et al. 2008. Cumulative association of five genetic variants with prostate cancer. *New England Journal of Medicine*, 358:910–919.

Zou H, Hastie T. 2005. Regularization and variable selection via the elastic net. *Journal of the Royal Statistical Society: Series B*, 67:301–320.

# 33 Forensic Bioinformatics

## *Keith A. Baggerly and Kevin R. Coombes*

## CONTENTS

## 33.1  INTRODUCTION

So, what is forensic bioinformatics?

To us, forensic bioinformatics is the art of using raw data and reported results to infer what must have happened to get from one to the other. Ideally, this would never be required, as the reported methods should make this an easy task. Empirically, however, many results from the bioinformatics literature have proved very hard to reproduce, either because some unnoted aspect of the data rendered the conclusions invalid or because steps of the analyses were opaque or undocumented. This lack of transparency is troubling, since our intuition about what "makes sense" fails in high dimensions. We can mention an incorrect gene to an investigator and have him correct us; we can supply an incorrect list of 50 genes and he will be able to construct a seemingly plausible story about why they make sense.

Because of this lack of transparency, we have developed a set of basic tools and checks that we use regularly. Here, we illustrate these in a roughly chronological tour through four case studies. The first two show, in part, why we have learned to approach high-throughput data with a healthy amount of caution, and the latter two show how simple types of errors can have (and have had) very dramatic consequences.

## 33.2  CASE STUDY 1: CAMDA 2002

We have been working with microarray data since about 2000 and have been trying to understand the best ways of processing these data for much of that time. One way we tried to learn what was important was by participating in the Critical Analysis of Microarray Data (CAMDA) competitions in 2001, 2002, and 2003. In these competitions, the organizers assemble and distribute a small number of common datasets for study, and all participants analyze at least one of these. The focus is thus placed on differences between analysis methods, rather than on differences between datasets. Here we focus on the 2002 competition, http://www.camda.duke. edu/camda02/best_presentation/index.html.

In 2002, one of the contest datasets came from a set of mouse studies performed by Pritchard et al. [1] In this study, the authors were trying to characterize the amount of "normal" variation one would see even in the "same" type of samples. Thus, they harvested tissue from three organs (kidney, liver, and testis) from each of 6 C57BL6 male mice, a single inbred line. The arrays were two-channel (red and green), so a pool of material from all 18 organs from all mice was used as a common control. Each individual mouse/organ sample was examined with four arrays: two with the experimental sample in the red channel and the reference in the green channel, and two where the red/green labels were reversed (a dye-swap experiment with replication). Log-ratios from individual arrays were normalized with loess, and the final results were analyzed with F-tests.

Contest data were supplied in both corrected (post-normalization) and uncorrected forms, and the raw array images were also available for reanalysis if desired. In both instances, the data were supplied in three tables, one for each organ, with one row per array spot (5304 rows), four columns (foreground and background spot quantifications in both red and green channels) for each sample, and six additional columns of spot annotation giving the Unigene ID for each cDNA, the clone ID, the corresponding gene name, and the block, column and row numbers giving the physical position of each spot on the arrays. We examined both the corrected and uncorrected data, but did not reexamine the images.

Our first focus was on normalization. Most normalization methods (including the loess approach employed) assume that "most" genes do not change expression very much in the data being examined. However, while this assumption may be reasonable for healthy and diseased versions of the same tissue, it is suspect if the samples are expected to differ drastically, as would be the case with samples from different organs. In the latter case, normalization "adjustments" may actually remove or obscure biology of interest. We chose to normalize the data from each array and channel (red or green) separately, in the hope of recovering differences that might have been hidden.

To test whether our normalization worked, we tried something important: Identifying a question we could ask where we knew a priori what the answer should be. Many differences may seem "plausible," so we find it useful to have gold standard "sanity checks" in place. Here, we used principal component analysis (PCA) to examine the 5304 by 144 matrix of normalized values from the individual array channels. We expected to see four clusters: one for each organ (each with 24 spots), and one for the common reference (with 72 spots). Further, as the reference was derived from a pool of the three organs, we expected the reference cluster to be "in the middle" of the others.

The results of this initial PCA are shown in Figure 33.1. We did not see four clusters. We saw six. While the kidney and liver samples formed distinct clusters as expected, both the testis and the reference samples split into two clusters. Further,

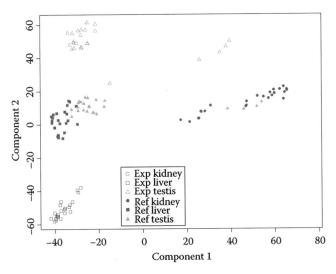

**FIGURE 33.1**    PCA of 144 samples from Project Normal: 24 each from kidney, liver, and testis, and 72 from a common reference assembled as a pool of the individual samples. We expected to see four clusters (one for each organ and one for the reference). We saw six, indicating the presence of either unmodeled structure or errors in the data. (From Stivers, D.N. et al., Organ-specific differences in gene expression and UniGene annotations describing source material, in *Methods of Microarray Data Analysis III*, Johnson K.F. and Lin, S.M. (eds.), pp. 59–72, Kluwer Academic Publishers, Boston, MA, 2003. With permission.)

the "splits" were suggestive: The testis samples split into one group of 20 and another of 4, and the corresponding reference samples also split into 20 and 4 along the same boundaries. The reference samples for the kidney samples were close to the kidney samples, and the reference samples for the liver samples were close to the liver samples. This suggested the presence of a major shift in the data driven by either biology or error.

To understand the problem, we first examined the data for the kidney and liver samples, as these two groups were the most clearly distinct. The answer, as it turned out, lay not with the numbers but with the annotation. For 1932 lines in the two files, the mappings between gene name and spot location were different. This is illustrated for one of the "*villins*" of the piece in Table 33.1. This led us to suspect that one of the two mappings was wrong. It also led us to suspect that the shift had been "introduced" midway through the testis experiments, splitting one group of 20 from the other 4. This "mismapping" hypothesis also suggested some reorderings of the 1932 affected rows that would bring one set of spots (24 kidney and 20 testis) into alignment with the others (4 testis and 20 liver). Some experimentation with these permutations gave a new PCA plot with the four expected clusters.

At the meeting, Colin Pritchard gave an explanation of what had occurred. Since cDNA clones for distinct spots can be "corrupted" over time, their lab regularly did confirmation checks. Midway through the testis experiments, a corrupt entry was identified, and the cell in the Excel file containing the annotation was deleted. *Every other entry in that column then moved up by one row*, effectively scrambling the

---

**TABLE 33.1**

**Annotations for the Gene *villin* from Two Aggregate Quantification Files: One for All Kidney Samples Profiled, the Other for All Liver Samples Profiled**

| Organ | Line # | Unigene ID | Gene Name | Block | Column | Row |
|--------|--------|------------|-----------|-------|--------|-----|
| Kidney | 589 | Mm.4010 | *villin* | 2 | 17 | 5 |
| Liver | 589 | Mm.4010 | *villin* | 4 | 17 | 5 |

The two files give two locations for where *villin* was printed on the arrays: one of the mappings is wrong.

---

mapping for about 40% of the spots. The data were then reordered before export, so the simple nature of the offset was hidden.

There are some key lessons we want to highlight. First, having gold standard or "sanity check" experiments is important. Second, be careful to maintain links between numbers and labels (Excel is dangerous in this regard). Third, do large survey plots of the data early in the analysis, so that major shifts can be identified before too many detailed analyses are performed. We prefer PCA to hierarchical clustering for this purpose, and we like using different colors to mark subgroups known a priori.

More details of this case study (including how we identified which mapping was "correct") are given in Stivers et al. [2]; see also Coombes et al. [3]. We won that year's competition.

## 33.3 CASE STUDY 2: PROTEOMIC DATA MINING

Also in 2002, Duke University hosted a Proteomics Data Mining competition organized along the same lines as CAMDA. (We referred to it internally as "CAPDA.") Two datasets of mass spectrometry traces derived from serum samples were supplied for this competition. In the first dataset, 20 ordered spectra ("fractions"; each spectrum had 60,831 values) from each of 41 patients were supplied, and the goal was to identify biologically relevant subgroups. In the second dataset, 20 fractions per patient were again supplied, but here 24 patients were identified as having cancer and the other 17 were identified as healthy controls, and the goal was to identify specific "peaks" in the spectra that best differentiated the two subgroups. Data were available either as full spectra or as lists of peaks identified by the manufacturer's software.

As readers probably suspect, and as a Perl script confirmed, the two datasets were actually one and the same. Once we knew this, we decided to pursue the peak identification task, as we already "knew" what the subgroups should be and we did not trust ourselves to behave "blindly."

The mass spectra here are traces of intensity (number of hits) at a detector as a function of time; peaks in the spectra correspond to distinct peptides, and on a well-calibrated instrument the mass to charge (m/z) ratio of the peptide can be inferred from the time of detection. Mass spectra data are often reported in text files with two columns: one column for the inferred m/z values (the x-axis), and another for the observed intensity (the y-axis). Sequential observations are, however, often equally spaced in time, so there can be two natural x-axes here: time and m/z.

When we entered this contest, we were not that familiar with mass spectrometry data, so one of the first things we did was take some time and simply plot the data in several different ways. In particular, we plotted early parts of the spectra (with lots of peaks), and late parts of the spectra (with few peaks) from several patients. We superimposed spectra from the same fraction for different patients to see if the problem was "easy." Here, simply looking at the data identified various oddities. As an illustration, the late parts of four spectra, plotted against time index, not m/z, are shown in Figure 33.2.

Several differences not due to biology are immediately apparent. First, there are different baseline intensity levels, which may reflect detector gain settings. Second, the central spectrum has "wiggles" that are quite regular on this scale. This is perfectly sinusoidal noise, and represents an electronic artifact (e.g., feedback from a loose AC power cord). In this case, we wound up estimating and subtracting background separately for each spectrum, and using a Fourier transform to identify and remove the sinusoidal noise from affected spectra (about half). The preprocessed peak data from the manufacturer performed neither of these steps, so the automatically generated peaks included systematic distortions.

The key lessons we want to highlight here involve the importance of simple exploratory data analysis and preprocessing. As it happens, we were the only

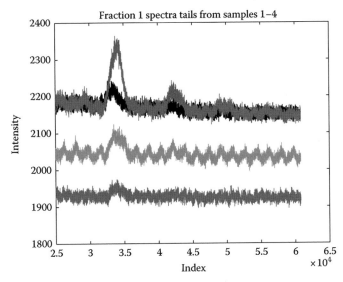

**FIGURE 33.2**   Tail ends of spectra from the first fraction for each of four patients, plotted as a function of time index, not m/z. Several differences not due to biology are immediately apparent. First, there are different baseline intensity levels, which may reflect detector gain settings. Second, the central spectrum has "wiggles" that are quite regular on this scale. This is perfectly sinusoidal noise, and represents an electronic artifact. (From Baggerly, K.A. et al., *Proteomics*, 3(9), 1667, 2003. With permission.)

entrants to identify and remove the sinusoidal noise, and some other types of noise not described in detail here (including a 4K computer buffer "flushing" every 4096th value). The vast majority of our time was spent cleaning and preprocessing the data, with the actual statistical comparison to identify the best peaks coming late in the process. This is typical in our experience.

More details of this case study (including how we actually identified and tested peaks for differential expression) are given in Baggerly et al. [4]; other papers in the same issue of *Proteomics* contain results of other analyses presented at the meeting. We won the competition.

## 33.4   CASE STUDY 3: PROTEOMICS AND EXPERIMENTAL DESIGN

In 2002, Emmanuel Petricoin of the FDA and Lance Liotta of the NCI published a paper in *The Lancet* claiming that patterns of peak expression in mass spectrometry traces derived from serum samples could provide highly sensitive and specific diagnostic tests for ovarian cancer [5]. Such a test could be of great clinical utility, as the lethality of ovarian cancer derives largely from the fact that it typically goes undiagnosed until after it has invaded the abdominal cavity and potentially metastasized, rendering complete surgical resection infeasible, and the fact that our other noninvasive diagnostic tests do not have high enough specificity for general screening.

These results were sufficiently high profile that the NCI announced a Clinical Proteomics initiative, and companies were formed to take these assays to the clinic. In addition, several groups at MD Anderson began parallel work studying their own tumor types of interest, and they asked us for help with implementing the approach. This led us to look at the raw data more closely.

In their *Lancet* paper, Petricoin et al. [5] looked at spectra from 216 serum samples: 100 from women with ovarian cancer, including some cases of early stage disease, 100 from healthy women, and 16 from women with "benign disease" (e.g., ovarian cysts). All of the spectra had 20,514 observations, and covered the same m/z range (roughly up to masses (strictly, m/z values) of 20 kDa). Starting with the previous spectra, they randomly chose 50 cancer spectra and 50 control spectra to train their classifier, and then predicted the status of the samples not used in training the model. They correctly identified all 50 cancer cases, and 47/50 healthy cases (the other three were called cancer). They noted that the 16 benign disease samples were not classified as "cancer," but they were not classified as "control" either—they were sufficiently distinct that they were easily recognizable as "other." This last aspect was part of the allure, as there are actually many proteins that may be high in patients with advanced cancer and low in healthy controls, but the vast majority of these are indicative of systemic distress, and are not specific to ovarian cancer. By classifying the benign disease samples as other, this algorithm implied higher specificity.

Over time, since the results were deemed to be of high clinical relevance, they also generated two more sets of spectra, for a total of three (data set 1 [DS1], the 216 Lancet spectra, DS2, and DS3). The spectra in DS1 were all generated using a particular type of "surface-enhanced" plate for use with mass spectrometers, where the type of coating (here "H4") should make the ionization (and thus detection) of some subsets of peptides easier. After publication, Ciphergen, the company that produced the surface-enhanced chips, suggested that chips with a different type of coating ("WCX2" chips) might give clearer signals. Consequently, all 216 of the DS1 samples were rerun using WCX2 chips, producing the spectra in DS2. Later, to check the approach again, the investigators came back with 162 new cancer samples and 91 new control samples (no new benign disease samples), and ran these 253 samples on WCX2 chips to produce DS3. In each case, the investigators applied their algorithm and were able to find "patterns" separating cancers from controls, but the constituent peaks in these patterns changed from DS1 to DS2 to DS3.

We acquired all three datasets to explore how these spectra could be used. In exploring DS1, we were able to separate the benign samples from the controls and cancers with ease, but we were unable to separate the cancers and controls. Further exploration suggested that data posted to the web had been subjected to processing after the initial analysis, and that this processing destroyed the separation effect of the initial "pattern," calling its robustness into question. In exploring DS2, we noted the same problem of post-analysis processing destroying the pattern, but in these spectra (derived from the same samples used for DS1), we were no longer able to clearly separate the benign disease samples. In order to understand this discrepancy, we tried examining heatmap summaries of both DS1 and DS2 at the same time. These are shown in Figure 33.3.

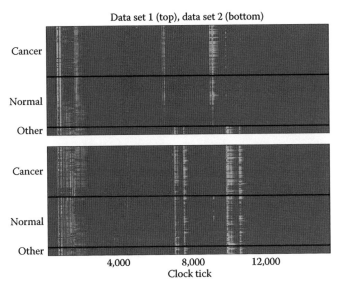

FIGURE 33.3 Heatmaps of spectra from 216 samples run on H4 chips (DS1, top), and later on WCX2 chips (DS2, bottom). In DS1, the "benign disease" or "other" samples are starkly different from both the cancers and controls, as evidenced by the locations of the most intense peaks (vertical bands). In DS2, no such difference is seen. Looking across datasets, however, shows the benign disease samples from DS1 align extremely well with all of the spectra in DS2, leading us to conclude that the experimental conditions changed *before* the benign samples in DS1 were run. (From Baggerly, K.A. et al., *Bioinformatics*, 20(5), 777, 2004. With permission.)

In DS1, the "benign disease" or "other" samples are starkly different from both the cancers and controls, as evidenced by the locations of the most intense peaks (vertical bands). In DS2, no such difference is seen. Looking across datasets, however, shows the benign disease samples from DS1 align extremely well with all of the spectra in DS2, leading us to conclude that the experimental conditions changed *before* the benign samples in DS1 were run. In short, while the benign samples are indeed different in DS1, this difference (and the implied assay specificity) is driven by experimental artifact, not by biology of interest.

The difference we saw in DS1 also made us worry about whether the run order of the other (cancer and control) samples had been randomized, since differences over time could easily be mistaken for the biological changes the investigators expected to see. DS3 was not subjected to the post-analysis processing that broke the "patterns," but with that dataset we were able to separate cancers from controls using peaks in the electronic noise regions of the spectra. The only explanation for this separation was an artifact of poor experimental design (running all of the controls before all of the cancers), not biology.

In this case the apparent clinical importance of the initial results had broad implications. In 2004, the company Correlogic began advertising the "OvaCheck" assay for diagnosing ovarian cancer based on the results discussed earlier, announcing it at the January meeting of the Society of Gynecologic Oncologists. Our objections and others were made available online at the end of January, and the story was covered by the New York Times on February 3. In mid-February, the FDA sent letters to both Correlogic and its collaborators (LabCorp and Quest Diagnostics) requesting consultation before any further advertisement of the assay. In June 2004, the FDA ruled that OvaCheck was a medical "device" in the sense that the outcome of its use would potentially guide medical interventions of high risk. As a device, the algorithm was subject to FDA review and regulation, and OvaCheck was never cleared to be marketed. The FDA has since indicated that other "omic" signatures or "in vitro diagnostic multivariate index assays" (IVDMIAs) are also medical devices [6].

In 2005, this incident was cited by members of the NCI's scientific advisory board when they voted against pursuing an $89 million initiative to discover new diagnostic protein signatures. Rather, they later voted for another initiative focused on better understanding the capabilities of the mass spectrometry approach, with the latter specifically *not* trying to produce diagnostic signatures in the short term and including funding specifically targeting experimental design issues.

The key lessons we want to highlight here involve the importance of basic experimental design and (again) of exploratory data analysis. The two can often be productively combined by plotting clinical variates of interest as a function of assay run date when the latter is available. A surprisingly large number of high-throughput biological studies are subject to complete confounding. This is a major problem since sizable batch effects have been observed with almost every type of high-throughput assay now in use (see Leek et al. [7]). In this light, we note that run date information for Affymetrix experiments is often included in the CEL file headers, where it can be accessed with the read.celfile.header function in the affyio package.

More details of this case study (including other artifacts and an argument in one of the commentaries that the investigators *explicitly chose* to run all samples of one group before all of the other [8]) are given in Baggerly et al. [9] and Baggerly et al. [10]; Hu et al. [11] provide other examples of poor experimental design affecting proteomic studies. The data and code underlying our analyses of these data are available at http://bioinformatics.mdanderson.org/Supplements/ReproducibilitySELDITOF/.

## 33.5 CASE STUDY 4: MICROARRAYS AND REPRODUCIBLE RESEARCH

In November 2006, Potti et al. published a paper in *Nature Medicine* claiming to show how microarray signatures of drug sensitivity could be constructed from cell line profiles and used to predict patient response [12]. In theory, this would allow doctors to personalize therapy by selecting the drugs to which a given patient's tumor would be most sensitive. *Discover* magazine designated this paper one of the top 100 breakthroughs of 2006. The group shortly extended their method to deal with other drugs widely used in treating lung cancer (Hsu et al. [13], dealing with cisplatin and pemetrexed) and with predicting response to combination chemotherapy (Bonnefoi et al. [14]).

Again, there was excitement about using the approach at MD Anderson, and again, we were asked to examine the raw data to figure out how the approach worked. Our first finding was that the analysis was extremely hard to reproduce, even after exchanging emails with the investigators, because various small processing steps were not described in precise detail. In working past that, we found that some of the processing steps included errors contaminating the results: Genes were mislabeled due to an off-by-one indexing error. Some genes identified as "important" were not produced by their software. Worst, "sensitive" and "resistant" labels were apparently reversed for some drugs; if the base method worked, this would result in withholding treatment from those most likely to benefit from it. We concluded that the method didn't actually work at all; it only appeared to work due to poor bookkeeping. We published a short note to that effect in *Nature Medicine* (Coombes et al. [15]), and commented on the need to include code sufficient to allow for complete reproducibility of the analysis. This 750-word note was accompanied by roughly 130 pages of supplementary code and documentation.

We identified further problems in 2007, 2008, and 2009; see, for example, Baggerly et al. [16]. In June 2009, we learned that clinical trials using this approach to guide therapy had been started at Duke University back in 2007, and were still underway. We wrote out our objections and submitted a report to the *Annals of Applied Statistics* at the start of September 2009; the paper [17] was accepted and posted online 2 weeks later. The NCI agreed the issues raised were of serious concern, and forwarded the paper to Duke's Institutional Review Board (IRB). Duke suspended trial accruals in October 2009 and arranged for an external review.

In November 2009, while the investigation was underway, the Duke investigators posted new data to the web. In particular, they posted the array data that had been used to "validate" the performance of the predictive signatures introduced by Hsu et al. [13] for cisplatin and pemetrexed, which were two of the drugs they'd been using in clinical trials for 2 years by that point. We downloaded these data in order to see whether we could also verify the performance.

The cisplatin and pemetrexed validation data involved array profiles from 59 women with ovarian cancer who had been treated with the drugs in question. Hsu et al. [13] had previously indicated that these profiles were drawn from a larger dataset available from the Gene Expression Omnibus (GEO), GSE3149, but they had not named which of the 153 samples in the larger dataset were used. In their November 2009 posting, the 59 array profiles were specifically named. In order to check data provenance, we looked for high pairwise correlations between the profiles posted by the investigators and those given in GSE3149. The results are shown in Figure 33.4.

We reordered the GSE3149 samples so that if all of the sample labels matched, there should be 59 squares (matched profiles) falling on the diagonal line shown. No squares fall on this line. There were no matches at all for the first 16 posted samples. We found matches for the remaining 43, but *none* of the sample names were correct. Using the names posted would in many cases reverse the true response status of the underlying sample. A disconnect between the numbers and the sample names rendered the predictions invalid. We then examined the behavior of the first 16 samples (where we found no matches) in more detail, by plotting the RMA-summarized intensities of the first 100 probesets for each of the 59 arrays. In looking across samples, the identities of the brightest and darkest probesets will generally remain

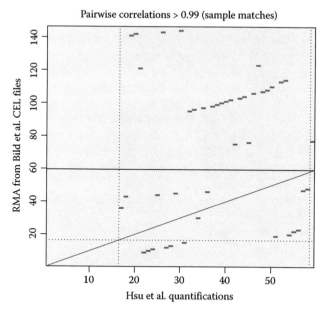

**FIGURE 33.4** Locations of high (0.999+) pairwise correlations between the 59 samples posted by Duke investigators in November 2009 (x-axis) and the 153 samples in GSE3149 (y-axis). We reordered the GSE3149 samples so that if all of the sample labels matched, there should be 59 squares (matched profiles) falling on the diagonal line shown. No squares fall on this line. There were no matches at all for the first 16 posted samples. We found matches for the remaining 43, but *none* of the sample names were correct. Using the names posted would in many cases reverse the true response status of the underlying sample.

fairly stable, because of the differential binding affinities of the various probes for cRNA. Indeed, this is seen for the last 43 samples, which roughly parallel the patterns seen in the rest of GSE3149. For the first 16, however, the pattern is quite different, but consistent across the set. These 16 samples do not match any of the GSE3149 samples because the mapping between the numbers and the gene names has been corrupted, so we do not know what goes where.

In short, all of the validation data were wrong, for two drugs they'd been using in clinical trials for 2 years. We reported this to Duke and to the NCI in mid-November, and the data were stripped from the web within the week.

In January 2010, Duke announced that the findings of their external reviewers were positive, and that they were restarting the clinical trials. We objected, but to no avail. The trials then proceeded until mid-July, at which point the *Cancer Letter* revealed that one of the investigators (Anil Potti) had repeatedly "puffed up" his CV, including claims to have been a Rhodes scholar. A group of prominent bioinformaticians and biostatisticians wrote to Harold Varmus, the newly appointed head of the NCI, requesting that the trials be resuspended, and they were. In October, after another review of the data, the senior author (Joseph Nevins) called to retract the Hsu et al. [13] paper, citing problems identical to those noted earlier: 43/59 validation samples were mislabeled, and they could not match the other 16. In November, the trials were terminated. In January 2011, a *Nature* news feature revealed that the Duke administrators overseeing the initial investigation, in collaboration with the acting head of Duke's institutional review board, had chosen to withhold our report from the external reviewers. All three of the foundational papers cited previously [12–14] have since been retracted, and others are being reviewed.

This case has now led to an Institute of Medicine review of the use of "omics" based signatures in clinical trials, with a focus on what data should be made available and when.

This case is easily the most complex, but one of the key lessons we want to highlight here is that it should not have been—it was hard because poor documentation allowed errors to go unnoticed until after things had proceeded to clinical trials. We advocate more complete availability of data and code (see Baggerly et al. [18] and Baggerly and Coombes [19]) in part because the complexity of high-throughput data is such that inadvertent simple errors are very hard to find without it. This boils down to a simple question: When you report results, are your analyses documented well enough for somebody else to reproduce them? The other lesson we wish to emphasize is the importance of checking data provenance—are the labels correct? As analyses become more complex, involving multiple datasets across the web, being able to track this type of accuracy becomes ever more important. We try to do most of our analyses using data frames in R, which keeps track of row and column labels for us. But, when we encounter cases where disconnects are part of one of the analysis steps, we include explicit spot checks before and after to make sure a sample of the values transform as we expect them to and keep their proper names.

More details of this case study are given in the references cited earlier (Baggerly and Coombes [17] is the most extensive), and are also available at http://bioinformatics.mdanderson.org/Supplements/ReproRsch-All/ and its child links. The full report we sent in November 2009, together with all of the data and code needed to recreate it, is available at http://bioinformatics.mdanderson.org/Supplements/ReproRsch-All/Modified.

## 33.6 GENERAL LESSONS

The tools we have introduced here are, for the most part, simple ones—gold standard tests, PCA, exploratory data analysis, plotting by run date, checking provenance. In this sense, they are parallel to the errors themselves, since, in our experience, *the most common mistakes people make are simple ones*, for example, getting labels transposed, disconnecting labels from data, and confounding the design. No malice of any type is required; the first two mistakes in particular are easy to make in Excel. If the analyses are clear, simple errors are often easy to find and fix. If the analyses are opaque, then the simple errors may go unnoticed, and simple mistakes are still important.

Another general lesson that we have learned is that clarity and reproducibility are vitally important in high-throughput biology. In keeping with this observation, we instituted the requirement in our department that all analysis reports are written in Sweave [20], a literate programming language that combines R and LaTeX in a way that lets others run your reports and get the same numbers you did. (While we like Sweave, we note that other tools such as GenePattern [21] and Galaxy [22] are available; reproducibility is the goal, and Sweave is a tool for reaching it.) To enhance clarity, we have also imposed a regular structure on our reports, the most important of which is that our reports begin with a short (one or two page) "executive summary" organized in the "Introduction, Data and Methods, Results, Conclusions" style of presentation most familiar to our collaborators. Examples of such reports are available at http://bioinformatics.mdanderson.org/Supplements/ReproRsch-All/.

Getting used to checking simple things and making things reproducible requires some initial effort, but we see this effort both as necessary for the field to progress and well worth it from the point of view of enhancing our own productivity.

## REFERENCES

1. Pritchard CC, Hsu L, Delrow J, Nelson PS. Project normal: Defining normal variance in mouse gene expression. *Proc Natl Acad Sci USA* 2001; 98:13266–13271.
2. Stivers DN, Wang J, Rosner GL, Coombes KR. Organ-specific differences in gene expression and UniGene annotations describing source material. In *Methods of Microarray Data Analysis III*, Johnson KF, Lin SM (eds.), 2003, pp. 59–72. Kluwer Academic Publishers, Boston, MA.
3. Coombes KR, Wang J, Abruzzo LV. Monitoring the quality of microarray experiments. In *Methods of Microarray Data Analysis III*, Johnson KF, Lin SM (eds.), 2003, pp. 25–40. Kluwer Academic Publishers, Boston, MA.
4. Baggerly KA, Morris JS, Wang J, Gold D, Xiao LC, Coombes KR. A comprehensive approach to the analysis of matrix-assisted laser desorption/ionization-time of flight proteomics spectra from serum samples. *Proteomics* 2003; 3(9):1667–1672.
5. Petricoin EF, Ardekani AM, Hitt BA, Levine PJ, Fusaro VA, Steinberg SM, Mills GB et al. Use of proteomic patterns in serum to identify ovarian cancer. *Lancet* 2002; 359(9306):572–577.

6. FDA. Draft guidance for industry, clinical laboratories, and FDA staff: In vitro diagnostic multivariate index assays. 2007, http://www.fda.gov/MedicalDevices/DeviceRegulationandGuidance/GuidanceDocuments/ucm079148.htm

7. Leek JT, Scharpf RB, Bravo HC, Simcha D, Langmead B, Johnson WE, Geman D, Baggerly K, Irizarry RA. Tackling the widespread and critical impact of batch effects in high-throughput data. *Nat Rev Genet* 2010; 11(10):733–739.

8. Liotta LA, Lowenthal M, Mehta A, Conrads TP, Veenstra TD, Fishman DA, Petricoin EF, 3rd. Importance of communication between producers and consumers of publicly available experimental data. *J Natl Cancer Inst* 2005; 97(4):310–314.

9. Baggerly KA, Morris JS, Coombes KR. Reproducibility of SELDI-TOF protein patterns in serum: Comparing datasets from different experiments. *Bioinformatics* 2004; 20(5):777–785.

10. Baggerly KA, Morris JS, Edmonson SR, Coombes KR. Signal in noise: Evaluating reported reproducibility of serum proteomic tests for ovarian cancer. *J Natl Cancer Inst* 2005; 97(4):307–309; commentaries: 310–314, 315–319.

11. Hu J, Coombes KR, Morris JS, Baggerly KA. The importance of experimental design in proteomic mass spectrometry experiments: Some cautionary tales. *Brief Funct Genomic Proteomic* 2005; 3(4):322–331.

12. Potti A, Dressman HK, Bild A, Riedel RF, Chan G, Sayer R, Cragun J et al. Genomic signatures to guide the use of chemotherapeutics. *Nat Med* 2006; 12:1294–1300. Retracted January 7, 2011.

13. Hsu DS, Balakumaran BS, Acharya CR, Vlahovic V, Walters KS, Garman K et al. Pharmacogenomic strategies provide a rational approach to the treatment of cisplatin-resistant patients with advanced cancer. *J Clin Oncol* 2007; 25:4350–4357. Retracted November 16, 2010.

14. Bonnefoi H, Potti A, Delorenzi M, Mauriac L, Campone M, Tubiana-Hulin M, Petit T et al. Validation of gene signatures that predict the response of breast cancer to neoadjuvant chemotherapy: A substudy of the EORTC 10994/BIG 00-01 clinical trial. *Lancet Oncol* 2007; 8:1071–1078. Retracted January 29, 2011.

15. Coombes KR, Wang J, Baggerly KA. Microarrays: Retracing steps. *Nat Med* 2007; 13(11):1276–1277; author reply: 1277–1278.

16. Baggerly KA, Coombes KR, Neeley ES. Run batch effects potentially compromise the usefulness of genomic signatures for ovarian cancer. *J Clin Oncol* 2008; 26(7):1186–1187; author reply: 1187–1188.

17. Baggerly KA, Coombes KR. Deriving chemosensitivity from cell lines: Forensic bioinformatics and reproducible research in high-throughput biology. *Ann Appl Stat* 2009; 3(4):1309–1334.

18. Baggerly K. Disclose all data in publications. *Nature* 2010; 467(7314):401.

19. Baggerly KA, Coombes KR. What information should be required to support clinical "omics" publications? *Clin Chem* 2011; 57(5):688–690.

20. Leisch F. Dynamic generation of statistical reports using literate data analysis. In *Compstat 2002—Proceedings in Computational Statistics*, Hardle W, Ronz B (eds.), 2002, pp. 575–580. Physika Verlag, Heidelberg, Germany.

21. Mesirov JP. Accessible reproducible research. *Science* 2010; 327:415–416.

22. Goecks J, Nekrutenko A, Taylor J, Galaxy team. Galaxy: A comprehensive approach for supporting accessible, reproducible, and transparent computational research in the life sciences. *Genome Biol* 2010; 11:R86.

# Index